FUNDAMENTAL CONCEPTS AND SKILLS FOR THE

PATIENT CARE TECHNICIAN

D1245798

ELSEVIER

FUNDAMENTAL CONCEPTS AND SKILLS FOR THE

PATIENT CARE TECHNICIAN

KIMBERLY TOWNSEND LITTLE, PhD, RN, CNE

Chair
MSN Programs
School of Nursing
Liberty University
Lynchburg, Virginia

Consulting Editor
RUSSELL C. MCGUIRE, PhD, RN

Professor
Program Director/Department Chair
Undergraduate and Graduate Campus-based Nursing Programs
South University, Montgomery
Montgomery, Alabama
Formerly Vice President and Dean, Allied Health Programs
Patient Care Technician Program Director
Education Corporation of America

ELSEVIER

ELSEVIER

3251 Riverport Lane
St. Louis, Missouri 63043

Senior Content Strategist: Nancy O'Brien
Senior Content Development Specialist: Maria Broeker
Publishing Services Manager: Julie Eddy
Senior Project Manager: Richard Barber
Design Direction: Paula Catalano

Printed in Canada

Last digit is the print number: 9   8   7   6   5   4   3   2   1

Working together
to grow libraries in
developing countries

www.elsevier.com • www.bookaid.org

I would like to dedicate this first edition to my friends and family, who have offered me their unconditional love and support throughout this journey. To my three daughters who have sacrificed spending time with me, thank you for being my biggest fans and for encouraging me to keep writing when I was ready for a break. To my family, colleagues, students, and peers, thank you for the many texts, notes of encouragement, and prompts to keep me going. Every one of them was just what I needed and received just when I needed to receive it.

To everyone reading this book, I would like to encourage you to follow your dreams and goals. You are given each day as a gift, and you have a choice to spend it as you like. Make the choice to do something to better yourself, to grow yourself professionally. Learn something new every single day. As my father has always told me, there are few things in life which cannot be taken away from you. Your education is one of those. So, I encourage you to reach far and reach wide. Accept a challenge that seems too big or too hard to meet, for you never know your true capabilities until you reach as far as you possibly can. Don't be the person who limits yourself; instead, believe in yourself!

ACKNOWLEDGMENTS

This textbook was created utilizing significant content from Cooper, Gosnell: *Foundations of Nursing*, ed. 8 and *Adult Health Nursing*, ed. 8; Proctor, Adams: *Kinn's the Medical Assistant: An Applied Learning Approach*, ed. 12; Warekois, Robinson: *Phlebotomy: Worktext and Procedures Manual*, ed. 4. The borrowed content includes but is not limited to text, boxes, and illustrations. Limited content was also borrowed from Potter, Perry, Stockert, Hall: *Fundamentals of Nursing*, ed. 8 and Perry, Potter, Ostendorf: *Clinical Nursing Skills and Techniques*, ed. 8.

I am thankful for those who have helped make this first edition possible. Russell McGuire's expertise is greatly appreciated and valued. I am grateful for Nancy O'Brien, Katie Gutierrez, and Maria Broeker, who have all offered their continual support in seeing this first edition come to fruition. Their gentle guidance and encouragement made this process a pleasant one. I will be forever grateful for Dr. Linda Silvestri, who first believed in me enough to recommend me to Elsevier as a potential author. Traversing the PhD with her did not happen because of chance, for everything happens for a reason, and, ultimately, I have had this experience because she saw a strength in me I didn't know existed at the time. Finally, many thanks to Elsevier for believing in this endeavor enough to support it.

PREFACE

The first edition of this book has been written to serve the developing patient care technician with a comprehensive resource in an effort to prepare them for the role. The role of the patient care technician has evolved over the years to include the skills of the nursing assistant, as well as phlebotomy, electrocardiogram, and oxygen therapy. The development of this newer role allows healthcare institutions to employ the patient care technician in fast-paced environments such as the Emergency Care Department. This broader scope of skills allows the patient care technician to work in a variety of environments.

Each chapter stands alone; however, you will note there is, at times, some overlap. For example, a patient is at risk of falls at many different times during your care. You may note that certain content, such as falls, may be reinforced in multiple areas as a way to impress upon you the importance of insuring the patient is kept from injury or harm. It's important to note that not all procedures included in this text may be applicable to, or allowed to be, completed in your particular state of employment. It's important you research how your state governs the role of the patient care technician.

Each chapter in this text contains chapter objectives, key terms, and chapter review questions. Additionally, a focus has been placed on Delegation, Documentation, and Illness/Injury Prevention. Specific detail has been provided regarding delegation guidelines for the patient care technician. These distinctive features are noted in separate boxes within each chapter.

Procedures typically performed by the patient care technician are included within the chapters that contain the content relating to those procedures. Step-by-step detailed instructions are given, which may be used for skills checklists, as well as a way to prepare the patient care technician for the performance component of the PCT certification exam.

A case scenario is included at the end of each chapter as a way to allow students to apply what they have learned to a clinically relevant topic. These may be used as an individual exercise or in a classroom setting as a group discussion.

FEATURES

HELPING YOU MASTER THE CONTENT

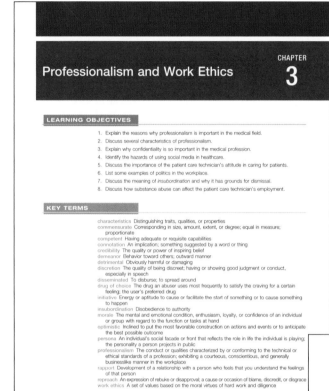

Emphasizing essential terms and concepts to reinforce what you are learning.
Learning Objectives, Key Terms, and Review Questions in each chapter.

Presenting reality-based situations encountered by the patient care technician to encourage you to practice and apply critical thinking.
Each chapter includes a Case Scenario.

---

380   SECTION V   Patient Care and Comfort

CHAPTER SUMMARY

Water is the primary fluid in the body and is necessary for life. One can live longer without adequate food than they can without water. As a PCT, it is important to ensure that each patient has an adequate supply of fresh water.

Sometimes patients do not eat well; this can be when they are ill, in a strange environment, or just do not have an appetite. Encourage patients to eat what is on their plate, but do not become frustrated or pushy with them. Oftentimes, patients are lonely and just want someone to sit with them while they eat. If time allows, provide an opportunity to sit with patients while they eat. Patients who have limited vision may need additional assistance with eating. Those with chronic pain or inflammation in their hands may have difficulty in opening their cartons and condiments on their tray. Assist them as needed. Some patients may use assistive devices to allow them to feed themselves easier. Promote independence as much as possible.

Some patients require IV therapy. As the PCT, you may be asked to discontinue the IV line, either when the patient no longer requires IV fluids or when they are being discharged. Be sure to verify the order for discontinuation of an IV site before performing the procedure.

Accurate record keeping is vital when managing fluid balance in a patient. It is important to be as specific as possible when determining how much a patient drank or ate at each meal, as well as during other times when it is requested by the nurse or ordered by the physician. Keep good notes, and document as soon as possible.

Case Scenario

You have been asked by the nurse to discontinue the IV sites of four patients who will be discharged that day. The nurse has given you the patients' names and room numbers. You gather your supplies and proceed to the first patient's room. When you explain the procedure to the patient, the patient replies, "But the doctor just left my room, and he said he's decided to keep me another day. You go ahead though; I've been wanting to get that thing out of my arm for days." What should you do at this point? Should you proceed with discontinuing the IV site because the nurse told you to do so? Should you move on to the next three patients and then come back to this patient when you are done? Explain your answer and give the reason for your decision.

REVIEW QUESTIONS

1. Normal daily water intake and output (I&O) is approximately how many milliliters?
   a. 1500
   b. 2500
   c. 3500
   d. 6500

2. How many milliliters of urine per hour must the kidneys secrete in order to eliminate waste products from the body?
   a. 30
   b. 60
   c. 20
   d. 100

3. Which of the following statements best describes the risk of fluid and electrolyte imbalances in the older adult?
   a. Most older adults can maintain fluid and electrolyte balance just as well as younger adults.
   b. Older adults have unlimited reserves to maintain fluid balance when abnormal losses occur.

   c. Body water increases with age, which puts the older adult at risk for fluid volume excess.
   d. Physiologic changes in the skin and mucous membranes decrease their reliability as indicators of dehydration.

4. Which of the following is the most important in preventing the introduction of microorganisms to the patient when an IV infusion is discontinued?
   a. Hand hygiene
   b. Checking the identification of the patient
   c. Ensuring the six rights of medication administration
   d. Carefully checking the order for discontinuation

5. When collecting information on a patient's intake, IV fluids should not be included.
   a. True
   b. False

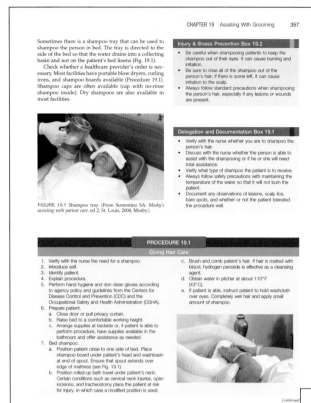

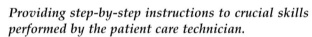

Fostering a safe and effective approach to care.
Delegation and Documentation and *Injury and Illness Prevention* boxes present practical tips that reinforce the importance of providing safe care in a professional and ethical manner.

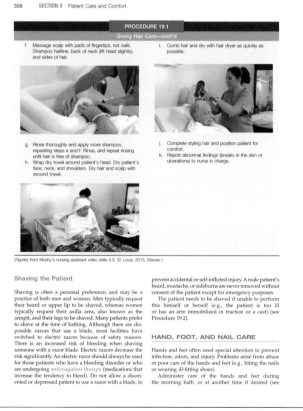

Providing step-by-step instructions to crucial skills performed by the patient care technician.
Procedures are presented in a clear easy-to-understand format. Critical steps are visually reinforced with color illustrations and photographs.

Providing a complete solution to support your endeavor to become an efficient and effective patient care technician.
Workbook for Fundamental Concepts and Skills for the Patient Care Technician includes a variety of activities to reinforce what you will learn in the textbook. In addition, procedure checklists and a practice exam encourage you to master techniques and concepts critical to becoming a patient care technician.
Interactive review questions and video clips in the Student Evolve Learning Resources test your knowledge and visually demonstrate critical procedure steps.

CONTENTS

PROCEDURES LIST

Introduction to Healthcare

Today's Healthcare

LEARNING OBJECTIVES

1. Identify trends in today's healthcare system.
2. Discuss implications of healthcare reform for delivery of patient care.
3. Identify the components of the healthcare system.
4. Describe the complex factors involved in the delivery of patient care.
5. Identify the participants in the healthcare system.

KEY TERMS

Affordable Care Act The landmark health reform legislation passed by the 111th Congress and generally referred to as Obamacare.

certified nursing assistant Someone who helps patients with healthcare needs under the direction of a nurse.

health To be without illness or to be free from disease.

healthcare system A network of agencies, facilities, and providers involved with healthcare in a specified geographic area.

health disparity A greater difference that has been discovered between one group compared with another group, meaning that one group is suffering more than another group.

Health Insurance Portability and Accountability Act (HIPAA) Enacted in 1996 as a way to protect everyone's privacy.

health promotion Strategies that aim at keeping a person healthy from the beginning.

holistic healthcare A system of comprehensive or total patient care that considers the physical, emotional, social, economic, and spiritual needs of a person.

illness A disease or sickness that affects the body and/or mind.

injury prevention Strategies that focus on prevention of injuries.

nurse A licensed person trained to care for the sick.

ombudsman Someone who is appointed to represent a person to ensure that the rights of the patient are being maintained.

Omnibus Budget Reconciliation Act (OBRA) Standards for long-term care facilities and nursing homes or assisted living facilities to ensure that residents would be able to achieve and maintain their highest level of well-being possible.

patient A person receiving medical treatment.

patient care technician A health technician working under the supervision of a registered nurse, physician, or other health professional to provide basic patient care.

physician A person who provides and practices medicine.

wellness The state of being in good physical and mental health.

HEALTH

To be healthy is known to be without illness or to be without disease. Our nation strives to achieve a state of health for all members of society. One way it does this is through the development of the Healthy People goals and objectives, which are reviewed and published every 10 years (www.healthypeople.gov). The objectives focus on areas in the United States that need to improve health outcomes. The areas emphasized will either improve the health of others or focus on improving the quality of life when one is experiencing an illness. In addition, a focus placed upon health disparities and how to remove those disparities is discussed. A health disparity is known as a greater difference that has been discovered between one group compared with another group, meaning that one group is suffering more than another group. This may include race or ethnicity, sex, sexual identity, age, disability, socioeconomic status, and geographic location, or where they live (www.healthypeople.gov). The overall or main goal of the Healthy People 2020 goals and objectives is to achieve health in the person and community.

Over the years, healthcare providers have evolved into a team of individuals who work together to provide good outcomes for the person in need. In the 1900s, the healthcare team was made up of a doctor, who is now known as a physician, and a nurse. Additional members of the team may include a licensed practical or vocational nurse (LPN/LVN), a patient care technician (PCT), a certified nursing assistant (CNA), and a medical office assistant (MOA). This will be discussed further later on in the chapter.

Health Promotion

The method for delivery of care many years ago focused on curing the sick, whereas now more focus is placed on keeping people healthy to begin with in hopes of preventing them from getting sick. This is known as health promotion. An example of a health promotion strategy is the recommendation of exercising at least 30 minutes a day as a way to prevent being significantly overweight, also known as obesity.

Injury Prevention

Instead of focusing on treating the injuries that occur from accidents, the healthcare team focuses on preventing injuries. This is known as injury prevention and is an area addressed in Healthy People 2020. An example of an injury prevention strategy is the use of seatbelts when in a car and wearing helmets when riding a bicycle or all-terrain vehicle. Money spent teaching one how to prevent injuries from occurring in the first place is money saved. Research has shown that with injury prevention education such as helmet use, the number of head traumas experienced from these types of accidents has decreased (http://www.nhtsa.gov/people/injury/pedbimot/motorcycle/safebike/reducing.html).

Looking Ahead to Today

Much has changed over the years regarding healthcare. This section will discuss some of those changes, particularly healthcare coverage, and changes in the healthcare team.

MEDICALLY UNDERSERVED

Increasing rates of homelessness, undocumented workers, and poverty, combined with the enormous rise in healthcare costs, have led to an increased number of individuals in the United States who are unable to afford healthcare. Although unemployment has been a contributing factor, in 2015 the unemployment rate was actually down at 5.1%, from 7% in 2013 (http://www.bls.gov/news.release/pdf/empsit.pdf). Jobs in healthcare are on the rise, whereas jobs in areas such as mining are on the decline. There are still a significant number of immigrants from other countries who come to the United States to live. The Department of Homeland Security estimated in 2013 that approximately 13.1 million illegal immigrants live in the United States. These immigrants are often afraid to seek healthcare because of fear of being sent back to their native country; therefore they are often considered to be medically underserved, causing their illnesses to worsen, often requiring more care and increased expenses to get them back to wellness and health.

AFFORDABLE CARE ACT

In an effort to address those who were unable to afford healthcare, the Affordable Care Act was signed by President Barack Obama on March 23, 2010. It was not until January 1, 2014, though, that the changes to healthcare plans went into effect. The overall goal of the Affordable Care Act was to provide healthcare coverage to those who would otherwise not be able to afford and access healthcare insurance. The main points of the Affordable Care Act include the following:

- Opens Health Benefit Exchange sales of coverage (members could select their choice of coverage)
- Prohibits denial of coverage to adults with preexisting conditions
- Requires large employers to provide coverage to those who work at least 30 hours per week

- Expansion of eligibility for the Medi-Cal program (California's Medicaid program)
- Tax credits for small businesses that provide coverage
- Tax credits for individuals and families with income up to $94,200 (for a family of four) who buy their insurance through the Health Benefit Exchange (http://affordablehealthca.com/timeline-obamacare/)

Limited access to healthcare is another concern that hinders individuals with mental health disorders and those who live in rural areas. Initiatives to provide increased services in rural and community-based clinics offer assistance to these populations. The healthcare team's engagement in health promotion activities to both prevent and manage illness and chronic conditions is one such solution.

Nursing Shortage

The United States continues to face a nursing shortage. With the enactment of the Affordable Care Act, which provides more people with healthcare options, an increase in members of the healthcare team is also required. The nation is expected to need an increase of more than 1.2 million nurses by 2020 (www.aacn.nche.edu). Despite strategies to reduce the shortfall of nurses, the supply is not expected to meet the growing demand. The nursing workforce is aging; the average age of nurses is 50 years (www.nursingworld.org). In the coming decade, many nurses who are currently working are expected to retire.

Nursing, once considered a prime career choice for women, now faces competition as women look at other promising career options (American Association of Colleges of Nursing, 2012). Schools of nursing are also facing a shortage of qualified educators, which further hinders growth of the profession. The cyclic nature of the nursing shortage is forcing healthcare organizations to look for more efficient and safe ways to provide care.

DEVELOPMENT OF THE PATIENT CARE TECHNICIAN

The need for qualified healthcare workers to assist the nurse in the healthcare setting has led to the addition of the PCT to the healthcare team. The role of a PCT has developed over the years as a nurse's assistant who is able to provide higher-level care to patients, such as phlebotomy, electrocardiogram (ECG), and venipuncture. The skills performed by the PCT are delegated by a nurse and are typically performed in a hospital or outpatient setting. (See more about PCTs in Chapter 2.)

Healthcare Delivery Systems

PCTs practice within the healthcare delivery system as a member of the healthcare team. To achieve their greatest potential, PCTs must be aware of the complexity of this system and the vital role that they play in its functioning. It is important that PCTs recognize that they are valued members of the healthcare team; members of this team must work together in order to be effective, in an effort to produce better outcomes for the patient.

HEALTHCARE SYSTEM DEFINED

The healthcare system consists of a network of agencies, facilities, and providers involved with healthcare in a specified geographic area. Many categories of healthcare professionals operate within this system, including the PCT. This healthcare environment includes the patient, the patient's family, the community in which the system operates, technology, governmental and regulatory agencies, the medical profession, third-party participants (e.g., insurance companies), and many other forces that affect the patient's care. The major goal of the system is to achieve optimal levels of healthcare for a defined population. This goal can be achieved by providing safe and appropriate healthcare services. The PCT is an integral member of the team of healthcare professionals who provide these services within the scope of practice. Some states regulate what the PCT can do, as defined by the state's nurse practice act.

Wellness-Illness Continuum

The range of a person's total health is described along the *wellness-illness continuum.* One's position on this continuum is ever-changing and is influenced by the individual's physical condition, mental condition, and social well-being. At one end of the spectrum is wellness (a dynamic state of health in which an individual progresses toward a higher level of functioning, achieving an optimal balance between internal and external environment). Wellness represents the highest level of optimal health. Illness, at the opposite end of the spectrum, represents a diminished or impaired state of health (Fig. 1.1).

A balance of all aspects of life is the key to maintaining one's health. Factors that affect the level of wellness

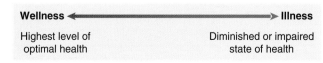

FIGURE 1.1 Healthcare continuum. (From Cooper K, Gosnell K: *Foundations of nursing,* ed. 7, St. Louis, 2015, Mosby.)

include age, gender, family relationships, emotional stressors, ethnic and cultural influences, and economic status. Consideration of the interrelationships among these variables is of paramount importance when the nurse is planning and providing care. An all-inclusive approach to healthcare is known as holistic healthcare (a system of comprehensive or total patient care that considers the physical, emotional, social, economic, and spiritual needs of a person).

Maslow's Model of Health and Illness

Several models of the wellness-illness continuum have been developed. These models enable the PCT to understand the patient's individual level of wellness and position on the continuum. The most common model was developed in the 1940s by Abraham Maslow. He believed that an individual's behavior is formed by the individual's attempts to meet essential human needs, which he identified as physiologic, safety and security, love and belongingness, and esteem and self-actualization. Maslow placed these needs into a conceptual hierarchy or pyramid that ranks them according to how basic each one is. A person has to meet needs at the base of the pyramid before advancing to the needs higher on the pyramid. Those needs placed higher on the pyramid are not requirements for life but rather enhance it. Remember that each patient may view or prioritize individual needs according to his or her own value system (Fig. 1.2).

HEALTH PROMOTION AND ILLNESS PREVENTION

As mentioned earlier in this chapter, from the earliest recorded civilizations to the twentieth century, the primary focus of healthcare was on the care of the sick. Today's focus has broadened to include an emphasis on an awareness of the causes of disease and the prevention of its spread through the use of health promotion activities.

In contrast to their origins as dirty, unsanitary, and poorly kept institutions where unsuspecting patients acquired diseases, hospitals have become clean, increasingly safe locations where patients and their families are cared for with limited fears that they will be exposed to additional illness and medical problems. The U.S. Department of Public Health works to help in the identification of disease types and related risk factors. These statistics identify problem areas for researchers and healthcare providers, who then direct their efforts at developing treatment for the illness, isolating its cause, and establishing methods to decrease its spread. The determination of cause-and-effect relationships provides a starting point for the development and implementation of health promotion initiatives. Although strategies to improve health have certainly helped, there are still areas that affect patient outcomes negatively. Sometimes patients get infections from being in the hospital, perhaps from poor hand washing. Sometimes nursing and pharmacy staff make errors when calculating medications, which results in the patient receiving either too little or too much of the ordered medication. This can result in complications or even death.

Today, three levels of health promotion are recognized. Their purpose is to promote health through maintaining wellness, preventing disease-related complications, and reducing the sickness associated with disease states. *Primary prevention* seeks to avoid disease states through wellness activities such as use of seatbelts and helmets, and preemptive screening programs such as mammograms, colonoscopies, and glucose screening are known as secondary prevention strategies. *Secondary prevention* recognizes the presence of disease but seeks to reduce the impact of the condition by encouraging behaviors to promote health. An example of tertiary prevention would be dietary teaching to a patient with diabetes with intention to reduce episodes of hyperglycemia. The activities of management of care for those with serious health problems who seek to improve the quality of life and reduce further loss of function are captured by tertiary prevention.

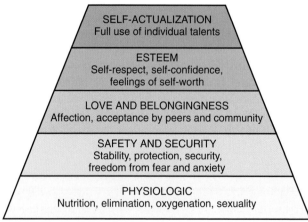

FIGURE 1.2 Maslow's hierarchy of needs. (Data from Maslow A: *Motivation and personality*, ed. 2, New York, 1970, Harper & Row.)

Injury and Illness Prevention Box 1.1

- Influenza (flu) vaccinations are recommended and required by most healthcare facilities for all staff, including the PCT.
- You will come in contact with those who are sick or have a contagious disease. It's important to stay as healthy as possible so that your immune system is not weak.
- Just like in the airplane, where the flight attendant states, "Parents, first place the oxygen mask over your nose and mouth before providing assistance to your children," if you don't first take care of yourself, you won't be able to provide care to others.

Continuity of Care

The patient is the focus of the healthcare system. However, many factors in our healthcare system determine what actually happens in the care of each patient. The number of healthcare providers and healthcare agencies involved in the care and treatment of a single patient is extensive. Increased specialization by healthcare providers and healthcare institutions, reimbursement procedures by third-party payers (e.g., insurance companies), federal regulatory organizations, and state healthcare regulatory agencies all affect the consumer (the patient) and the type and quality of care provided.

One of the greatest challenges for the consumer of medical care (the patient) is navigation of the healthcare delivery system. The consumer faces challenges to maintain autonomy and obtain continuity of care. Patients who are already weakened by the stressors of actual or potential medical conditions can become frightened as they attempt to understand the medical care and related choices available to them. It can be overwhelming to them.

Delivery of Patient Care

The care of patients is a humanistic enterprise. It involves not only treating disease and injury but also preventing disease, restoring optimal wellness through rehabilitation, caring for the chronically ill, and educating patients and families. To identify the individual needs of the patient and to plan a systematic approach to meet those needs, nurses participate in developing an individualized care plan with use of the nursing process. The purpose of the care plan is to meet the expressed needs of the patient. Its development involves the patient and all healthcare providers who, through a coordinated and cooperative effort, work toward meeting the patient's total needs in a holistic caring manner. As a PCT, you will assist with carrying out the nursing care plan by completing the tasks that are delegated to you by the nurse.

Participants in the Healthcare System

There are members of the healthcare team who make up the larger healthcare system. Each member of this team plays an important role in the treatment of the patient.

Professional Healthcare Specialists

The patient is the central focus of activities performed by more than 200 types of healthcare providers identified in the healthcare system in the United States. Many professions require **certification** or licensure of their members. Within many disciplines are subspecialties of individuals who have advanced training and licensure. As a PCT, you may choose to take a certification examination that will give you credentials as a Certified Patient Care Technician.

Currently, the following institutions provide certification examinations for the PCT:

Institution (Web Address)	Title of Certification
National Healthcare Association (www.nhanow.com)	Certified Patient Care Technician/Assistant (CPCT/A)
National Center for Competency Testing (www.ncctinc.com)	Patient Care Technician (NCPCT)
National Certification Career Association (www.nccanow.com)	Certified Patient Care Technician/Assistant (NCCA)

Registered Nurses

The registered nurse (RN) is a direct healthcare provider who is licensed after completion of one of three types of nursing education programs: a 4-year baccalaureate degree program, a 2-year associate degree program, or a 3-year diploma program. RNs practice in a variety of settings inside and outside of the care facility. RN duties and tasks vary according to educational background and the state's nurse practice act. Educational and career opportunities exist for the RN beyond initial licensure. Nurses with master's degrees or doctorates represent a small but growing segment of the profession. These individuals are often termed *advanced practice nurses*. Their roles are expanded and may involve educator, administrator, and prescriber, giving them the authority to write prescriptions.

Licensed Practical/Vocational Nurses

The LPN/LVN practices under the supervision of the RN or the physician. Working together, the LPN/LVN and the RN are the direct patient caregivers in most institutions. The role of the LPN/LVN is based on the scope of practice outlined in each state's nurse practice act.

Nursing Assistant

The nursing assistant practices under the supervision of the LPN or RN. Many states require nursing assistants to be certified (CNA), which means that they have completed coursework and performed a certain number of skills that considers them to be safe and knowledgeable in caring for patients. The PCT is often a CNA who has further training in advanced skills and hence, can perform more than a CNA is typically able to perform, such as phlebotomy and ECG.

Other Caregivers

Other caregivers are also required to be registered or licensed and to have the specialized education and training dictated by their professional organizations. **Holistic care** requires that professionals from different areas come together to provide comprehensive care. When a patient's condition dictates, referral to other care providers may be indicated. For example, social workers are trained to counsel patients who have social, emotional, or environmental problems. Physical therapists use precise methods of massage, exercise, and hydrotherapy to help restore physical function of the body. Dietitians are trained to determine the foods that meet the nutritional requirements of the patient. Respiratory therapists assist the patient by administering oxygen, monitoring and maintaining ventilators, drawing blood for blood gas analysis, and performing other pulmonary function tests.

Technologists, Medical Technicians, and Paraprofessionals

Diagnostic personnel work in the inpatient or outpatient healthcare setting, and may work in patient care areas or in areas such as the laboratory and radiology departments. Their roles involve assisting the medical professional staff in testing for disease states and injury, and in assisting the nurse to carry out the nursing care plan. The term *technologist* refers to those who have a baccalaureate degree, whereas the term *technician* refers to those who have had training and have earned an associate degree or certificate. As a PCT, you may work in the patient care setting located inside a healthcare facility, such as a hospital, or located in an outpatient facility, such as a doctor's office. An unlicensed assistive personnel (UAP) is educated in basic nursing techniques and performs under the supervision of the RN. The PCT is considered to be a UAP, and so is a CNA. The unit secretary prepares and maintains patient records, orders supplies, schedules tests, and performs receptionist duties on the care unit. Some healthcare facilities are cross-training individuals in two or more areas, which means that they may be both a unit secretary and a PCT. This allows the PCT to be more marketable for the healthcare facility, meaning that you are capable of working in multiple areas.

This is only a sample of the healthcare participants in the healthcare system. Each participant has a valuable contribution to make toward ensuring the safety and well-being of the patient.

ECONOMIC FACTORS THAT AFFECT HEALTH AND ILLNESS

Rising Healthcare Costs

Healthcare costs have reached a critical height. A large portion of the country's financial resources are committed to healthcare-related costs. Several factors have been highlighted as playing a role in the increase in costs, including an aging population, increased use of advanced technologies, rising cost of private healthcare insurance, rising cost of medical malpractice insurance, and a struggling economy.

Increasing Number of Aging Americans

As the baby boomer generation nears the age of retirement, their health problems increase; this onset of chronic diseases in a large segment of the population strains the healthcare system. Diseases associated with aging include heart disease, diabetes, and osteoporosis. As the U.S. population ages, an increasing number of older adults need nursing home care, which is costly and has limited coverage under traditional insurance plans.

Advances in Technology

Advances in technology have led to better diagnosis and treatment of illness; however, such progress carries a large price tag. Research and development of technology costs millions of dollars, a price that is passed on to the healthcare consumer in the cost of individual tests or treatments. Technological advances have become a source of concern related to patient privacy as electronic piracy (stealing one's healthcare information) has become increasingly possible. Safeguards for the electronic health records add to the costs for healthcare.

Protecting the Privacy of Patients

The Health Insurance Portability and Accountability Act (HIPAA) was enacted in 1996 as a way to protect everyone's privacy. You may have heard this called HIPAA. The Office for Civil Rights (OCR) enforces the HIPAA Privacy Rule, which protects the privacy of everyone's identifiable health information (http://www.hhs.gov/ocr/office/index.html). Each time a person starts care at a healthcare facility or is admitted to the hospital, the person is provided with the HIPAA regulations, which speak to how his or her privacy will be maintained. These HIPAA guidelines state how your confidential information will be kept private, and it will ask who the patient would like to have access to such information. Additionally, HIPAA guidelines will ask the person to state what forms of information may be shared with anyone, such as laboratory results, diagnoses, and medication information, to name a few. If the person's information is to be shared with anyone, even another physician, the person must give consent to that first. Failure to maintain or keep one's privacy can result in large fines to the healthcare organization. If a person's confidential information is shared in error, the HIPAA Breach Notification Rule requires the facility to notify the patient at minimum. There are other requirements of notification when a breach of confidential information has occurred. (See the U.S. Department of Health and Human Services website for more information: www.hhs.gov)

Delegation and Documentation Box 1.1

- Never ask a coworker for his or her login information, and never give your login information to anyone who asks for it.
- Remember to exit out of the computer you are working at when you walk away so that no one else can enter any information under your name.
- Protect the person's privacy by shielding, or covering, the computer screen so that family members cannot see what you are typing.

Changes in Delivery System

Hospitals throughout the United States are changing delivery systems to make care more cost-effective. Cross-training is a commonly encountered method for modifying the systems used to deliver care.

Cross-training allows employers to maximize the use of available staff. Workers are trained to perform duties that cross traditional role boundaries. Cross-training may involve combining the roles of differing categories of workers or expanding the responsibilities of staff members to cover multiple care units. Two groups of workers frequently cross-trained to expand their roles include unit secretaries and UAPs. This training provides a single worker who is able to perform UAP-related tasks (e.g., ambulating patients and taking vital signs) and receptionist duties (e.g., transcribing orders and ordering unit supplies). Another type of cross-training involves linking patient care units, frequently identified as sister units. Common sister units are maternal childcare, which are for patients delivering babies, and women's health. The staff is trained to work in both areas. Individuals receive training to perform duties that vary according to the needs at a given time. This training can be as narrowly defined as medical training to care for surgical patients or as broadly defined as housekeeping personnel training to give basic morning care to patients. The scope of cross-training is usually defined by the individual institution, and the purpose is to reduce the number or cost of employees without compromising the quality of patient care.

Other trends that affect the economics of healthcare include the development of multisystem healthcare chains or networks that may include several hospitals, clinics, nursing homes, and pharmacies. These systems share expenses and generally achieve an overall reduction in operating expenses. Health maintenance organizations (HMOs) or group healthcare practices provide healthcare to members for a fixed prepaid rate. This service includes medical care, nursing care, diagnostic tests, hospitalization, and various inpatient and outpatient treatments. This service has shown a high quality of low-cost healthcare. This may be of benefit to the PCT in that working for a larger healthcare system or chain could provide the PCT with more opportunity and better healthcare benefits.

Social and Environmental Factors That Affect Health and Illness

Social and environmental factors do not necessarily cause illness, but they do influence the development or progression of an illness. Financial hardship, lifestyle choices, and social pressures all influence an individual's willingness or ability to actively maintain health or prevent illness. In addition, personal behavior choices such as smoking, drug abuse, alcoholism, and obesity affect an individual's health and wellness. The individual's mental state has an influence on patient outcomes. Emotions associated with fear, loss of identity, and loss of control are commonly experienced during illness. An imbalance in body functions can affect one's physical condition and ultimately the position along the wellness-illness continuum. Although there is often a tendency to separate social factors from physical factors, remember that the two areas affect each other reciprocally.

Each patient possesses a unique personality, background, lifestyle, and level of education. Early recognition of the effect of environmental factors on a patient and prompt intervention by family, healthcare providers, or the patients themselves can decrease or keep any negative impact to a minimum.

Health Promotion

Most people in the United States believe that everyone has a right to healthcare, regardless of race, color, creed, or economic status. This healthcare includes the treatment of disease, and health promotion and preventive medicine. In many cases, treatment of illness is less of a concern than its prevention. The acute awareness of preventive medicine has resulted in today's emphasis on education about issues such as smoking, heart disease, drug and alcohol abuse, weight control, and mental health and wellness promotion activities.

During illness or after a change in health status, people often feel that they are not in control of their health, but they do typically trust in the healthcare system. The presumption is that care will be highly satisfactory and lead to a cure. Healthcare providers are expected to provide service in a knowledgeable, safe, and quick manner and to work in a cooperative manner for their benefit. Patients also expect the cost of care to be reasonable and, most importantly, paid by somebody else (an insurance company or the government).

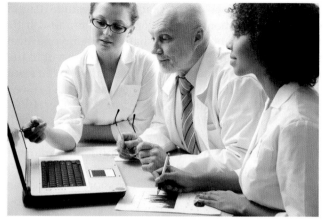

FIGURE 1.3 Collaborating with members of the healthcare team. (Copyright 1999–2012 Thinkstock. All rights reserved.)

Patients' Rights

In 1972, the American Hospital Association (AHA) issued the *Patient's Bill of Rights* in an effort to ensure that the patient's fundamental rights for treatment with dignity and compassion were fulfilled. The document was revised again in the 1990s and was finally replaced in 2003 when the AHA adopted the *Patient Care Partnership*. Under the terms of this document, patients are assured that they can expect high-quality hospital care, a clean and safe environment, involvement in their care and the decision-making process, protection of privacy, help when leaving the hospital, and help with billing concerns (American Hospital Association, 2003). Nursing home patients also have their rights protected. The *Resident's Bill of Rights* is a document that has been developed to provide clarity to the needs and rights of the individual who resides in a long-term care environment (Centers for Medicare and Medicaid Services, 2012). An ombudsman is someone who is appointed to represent a person to ensure that the rights of the person are being maintained. It is someone who is an advocate for another person, or someone who looks out for the person's best interest. Ombudsmen are commonly found in the nursing home setting for the older adult persons who may be unable to ensure that their rights are being protected. The Omnibus Reconciliation Act of 1987 (OBRA) created standards for long-term care facilities and nursing homes or assisted living facilities to ensure that residents would be able to achieve and maintain their highest level of well-being possible.

Healthcare Providers' Rights

The delivery of healthcare has to be a process of mutual exchange between patients and healthcare providers. Patients expect their rights as just outlined to be respected, but healthcare workers have expectations as well. Healthcare professionals expect that patients will do the following to actively participate in their care as much as possible: take an active role in the planning process, have an understanding of the care and the treatment given, ask questions, follow the treatment plan prescribed, act responsibly with respect to their own conditions, and give healthcare workers the same respect to which patients are entitled.

Interdisciplinary Approach to Healthcare

As stated before, the primary goal of the healthcare team is the optimal physical, mental, and social well-being of the patient. This goal is achieved by promoting and restoring health within the wellness-illness continuum. Healthcare personnel, when working to meet the needs of the patient, must work together as a healthcare team. Following this interdisciplinary approach to treatment prevents the fragmentation, or brokenness, of patient care. Just as the plan of care for patients is developed in a holistic manner, so is the actual delivery of healthcare. All healthcare providers must remember that the central focus of all their activity is the patient.

Each member of the team is responsible for coordinating activity with every other member of the team by developing a comprehensive care plan, effectively communicating, and keeping accurate records (Fig. 1.3).

Care Plan

The care plan is a document that outlines the individual needs of the patient and the approach of the healthcare team to meet these needs. It is developed in cooperation with the patient and, in some cases, the patient's family. It further identifies who will assist in treating the patient. The plan of care is a "living document" that is updated as the patient's condition warrants. The goal of the document is to guide and direct the activities surrounding the patient's care, ensure continuity and consistency of care, and eliminate duplication of services. As a PCT, your role is to participate in the care plan by performing tasks that are delegated to you by the RN.

Communication

Good communication is essential for the exchange of information among the members of the healthcare team. Communication is the necessary requirement for meeting the needs of the patient or, if necessary, making appropriate changes to do so. (See Chapter 4 for further discussion of communication with the healthcare team.)

Documentation

Documentation is the permanent record of the patient's progress and treatment while the patient receives care within a healthcare facility. It constitutes the formal and legal record of care received by the patient and the patient's response to that care (Fig. 1.4). The information recorded during the entire course of treatment serves many purposes. It provides a progress record of treatment so that all the involved healthcare members are aware of what treatment the patient is receiving. It also

provides a chronicle of events, which becomes a valued piece of the patient's health history that may be referenced for future healthcare needs. Each piece of information you enter as documentation should always be as clear and accurate as possible.

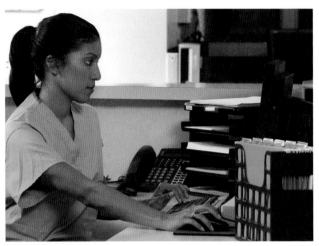

FIGURE 1.4 Documenting patient care at a computer. (Copyright 1999–2012 Thinkstock. All rights reserved.)

CHAPTER SUMMARY

The healthcare team has evolved into a group of people who work together to achieve the best outcome for patients they possibly can. No longer does this team consist of just a doctor and a nurse; each individual member of the healthcare team has a part in the plan of care for the patient, and each member is just as important as the next member. The roles of the healthcare team have expanded over the years to include the use of UAPs, such as the PCT and the CNA. These expanded roles allow for increased productivity without increasing the resources significantly. To be without illness or injury is to be in a state of health, and helping persons achieve that should be each team member's goal. Through health promotion and injury prevention strategies, each member of the healthcare team can work to achieve this for the persons they care for. Barriers, or those things that prevent persons from being able to seek healthcare, are being removed with advances such as the Affordable Care Act. The Healthy People goals and objectives seek to improve our nation's health, which includes removing any barriers that prevent people from being able to seek and actually access the care they need.

Case Scenario

As the PCT, you can have influence on decreasing the number of hospital-acquired infections that occur. The infection rate of your unit has been higher lately than in prior months. Your charge nurse has created a poster showing effective handwashing as a way to decrease infection. You notice one of your co-workers not washing his or her hands after removing the gloves or when he or she enters into the patient's room. How could you handle this situation? Would you address the co-worker, or notify the nurse? Could the handwashing practices of one person make a difference in the overall infection rate of the unit?

REVIEW QUESTIONS

1. To be healthy is to be without disease.
   a. True
   b. False

2. The role that is considered to be a nursing assistant with advanced skills is
   a. Certified nursing assistant
   b. Patient care technician
   c. Licensed practical nurse
   d. Unit secretary

3. Health promotion is known as which of the following?
   a. Attempting to cure an illness without seeking treatment
   b. Strategies that try to prevent illness from occurring
   c. Treatment of a disease with surgery
   d. A promotion or bonus received at work for staying healthy

4. The patient care technician receives tasks delegated by which other member of the healthcare team?
   a. Physician
   b. Pharmacist
   c. Other patient care technician
   d. Unit secretary

5. An ombudsman is known as someone who does what?
   a. Seeks to ensure that resident rights are maintained in the long-term setting
   b. Stands guard outside the resident's door
   c. Is in charge of the finances for the long-term care setting
   d. Does all of the hiring for the long-term facility

6. HIPAA was put into place in an effort to do what?
   a. Assist with payment of a healthcare bill
   b. Provide insurance coverage for healthcare
   c. Protect person's rights to privacy of protected information
   d. Provide an advocate for someone who is unable to care for himself or herself

7. An example of a secondary prevention strategy is which of the following?
   a. Encouraging use of seatbelts
   b. Teaching diabetic patients on good nutrition
   c. Encouraging use of helmets when riding an all-terrain vehicle
   d. Encouraging mammogram screening

8. Which of the following factors has a negative impact on healthcare for the underserved?
   a. Poverty rates increasing
   b. A declining unemployment rate
   c. An increase in access to care
   d. The Affordable Care Act

9. Which is known to be a benefit of the Affordable Care Act?
   a. Members are no longer denied coverage if they have a preexisting condition.
   b. Members are provided insurance coverage at no cost.
   c. Everyone is provided with insurance coverage.
   d. Everyone has the same insurance coverage.

10. When a person can work in multiple areas and in multiple roles, such as a unit secretary who is also trained as a nursing assistant, the person is said to have been cross-trained.
    a. True
    b. False

The Role of the Patient Care Technician

1. Briefly discuss the history of the role of the patient care technician (PCT).
2. Discuss the role of the PCT in the healthcare environment.
3. Comprehend the current employment outlook for the PCT.
4. Identify several considerations to keep in mind, other than financial compensation, when choosing a position as a PCT.
5. Understand the PCT credentialing requirements, the importance of credentialing, and the process of obtaining credentials.
6. Discuss the differences between a certified nursing assistant and a PCT.

benefits A payment or gift made by the healthcare institution, such as healthcare insurance and paid time off

career ladder A stepwise progression from entry level to a more advanced role, and may include more pay, more authority, and more responsibility

certification Confirmation that one has the knowledge and/or skill pertaining to a particular area or subject usually through the successful completion of a certification examination

continuing education units (CEUs) Credits earned for attending sessions that have some educational information relating to a particular topic

cross-training Where one individual is trained to do a variety of skills in a variety of areas

phlebotomy The surgical opening or puncture of a vein in order to withdraw blood or introduce a fluid

simulation The acting out of a scenario or situation on a manikin in an effort to gain confidence and improve skill before participating with a real person

versatile The person can perform multiple tasks in one setting, or in multiple settings

THE PATIENT CARE TECHNICIAN

The role of the patient care technician (PCT) has evolved over the past few years into its own individual role. It is an exciting advancement that has benefited the entire healthcare team through the expansion of skills and level of expertise the PCT can provide to the healthcare team. The PCT is sometimes referred to as a nursing assistant; however, the role encompasses more skills and training than that of a nursing assistant. Skills such as phlebotomy and ECG are often included in the role of the PCT, as well as intravenous therapy and oxygen delivery. The development of this newer role affords healthcare institutions with technicians who are qualified to perform a wider variety of skills and who can function in a variety of patient care environments. The PCT may be employed in an outpatient or inpatient healthcare setting, in an acute-care or long-term care setting, as well as in physician offices.

Although the U.S. Department of Labor has not yet published data on the PCT, it has reported promising growth for both the nursing assistant and the phlebotomist. According to the U.S. Department of Labor's *Occupational Outlook Handbook,* nursing assistant employment will grow 21% from 2012 to 2022, faster than average for all occupations. The employment growth for phlebotomists is expected to grow at a rate of 27%. Much of this growth will be the result of an increase in the number of group practices, clinics, and other facilities that need a high number of support personnel. This makes the PCT who can handle both clinical and administrative duties particularly valuable to the healthcare organization.

A career as a PCT is challenging and offers job satisfaction, opportunities for service, financial reward, and possibilities for advancement. Men and women can be equally successful as PCTs and can become employed in a variety of settings. Individuals considering the PCT role must be dedicated and committed and must have a strong desire to become caregivers. Caregivers are people who have the ability to put the needs of the patient first, and they have a sincere concern for those who are not at their best. A caregiver must feel an obligation to assist the patient in whatever way possible and must have patience with those who, at times, are more difficult. This strong inner desire is one of the most important qualities of the successful professional PCT. Through the development of this "care giving" mentality, many personal rewards will follow, as will a long and beneficial career.

The History of the Patient Care Technician

The first PCT was more than likely working as a nursing assistant who was called on to help when an extra pair of hands was needed. As time passed, and with the incorporation of healthcare reform, the push to do more with less became more apparent. The need to provide specialty training to those working as nursing assistants was never more apparent. Nurses take on heavier patient loads, and the patients are sicker than ever by the time they get to the hospital. Rather than calling three different persons who function in three different roles into the room to perform laboratory specimen collection, an ECG, and phlebotomy procedures such as drawing of admission labs, the patient care technician provides healthcare institutions an individual who possesses more skills to assist the healthcare team. Not only does this save the healthcare institution time and money, but it also decreases the number of staff coming in and out of a patient's room, which may increase patient satisfaction and decrease the risk of infection. Community colleges have begun offering training programs focusing on the PCT and a certification examination.

PCTs are utilized in a variety of patient care settings. One area where utilization of PCTs is growing is with hemodialysis. Hemodialysis is a procedure that removes waste products from the blood, which eases the workload on the kidney. This is a procedure necessary for those who experience end-stage renal disease, also known as ESRD. The PCT has been valuable in this patient population, because the majority of patients receive their hemodialysis from freestanding outpatient dialysis centers, which means that they are not in the physical building of the hospital. In 2014, there were 1,545,200 PCTs in the United States, many of them providing assistance to the nurse in the hemodialysis setting (www.bls.gov). As mentioned before, the change in Medicare and Medicaid reimbursement has led to a large increase in the number of PCTs working in dialysis centers (Vachharajani, 2011).

Another setting where PCTs have been utilized is in the emergency care setting. Many patients need a variety of tests when they come to the emergency room to determine what is wrong with them. In the past, the registered nurse (RN) was the one who performed such diagnostic testing, such as urine pregnancy testing, fingerstick glucose testing, and urinalysis testing with urine dipsticks. With utilization of the PCT in this setting and additional training, the RN is now able to delegate these tasks to the PCT and focus on higher-level care that only the RN can perform. A busy emergency room in the center of Manhattan, New York, added a much-needed diagnostic test to the role of the PCT. There was a need to perform hundreds of HIV screening tests per month. Requiring the RN to perform this test was delaying care the RN could be providing to others. This particular healthcare facility added the HIV testing (rapid oral screening) to the role of the PCT. Once the facility added this to the role of the PCT, the number of completed tests increased dramatically (Egan et al., 2014).

| Table 2.1 | Comparison of the Tasks Completed by the Certified Nursing Assistant and the Patient Care Technician |

Tasks Performed	CNA	PCT
Vital signs	✓	✓
Oral care	✓	✓
Bathing	✓	✓
Bedmaking	✓	✓
Hourly rounding	✓	✓
Phlebotomy (fingersticks, venipuncture)		✓
Urine diagnostic screenings		✓
Electrocardiography		✓

CNA, certified nursing assistant; PCT, patient care technician.

The Difference Between the Certified Nursing Assistant and the Patient Care Technician

The certified nursing assistant (CNA) and PCT have similar roles and responsibilities (Table 2.1). Both care for patients in either inpatient or outpatient settings, and both accept responsibilities delegated by the nurse or physician. The PCT may also be a CNA, or the CNA may work without being a PCT. The main difference between the two roles is that the PCT has a wider variety of skills training, such as the addition of phlebotomy and electrocardiography (ECG). The CNA does not typically perform these skills. Both the CNA and PCT may perform skills such as bathing, dressing, and oral care. Certification is available for both the nursing assistant and the PCT. Some may choose to have both certifications, whereas others may have one or the other.

Training the Patient Care Technician

Historically, training consisted of a 6-week classroom component with an additional 3 to 6 weeks of hands-on training or clinical instruction. This may include the use of simulation as well. Simulation is defined as the acting out of a scenario or situation on a simulation manikin in an effort to gain confidence and improve skill before participating with a real person. Research has shown that human error is less likely to occur with the use of simulating events that may occur in the healthcare setting before the person performs in the healthcare setting. Simulation has been primarily developed and implemented by the U.S. military, where tactics were practiced before going out into the front line of defense.

Today, there are a variety of avenues one can take in order to become trained as a PCT. Many are certificate programs, and most all require that the participant either come into the program as a nursing assistant, or

during the program achieve the certification of nursing assistant. Additional training is provided in phlebotomy and ECG training. Some programs may require certification in both phlebotomy and ECG training as well. Programs typically average 265 hours.

One particular hospital in New York made a decision to upgrade the nursing assistants to PCTs in 2008 (Small et al., 2012). The reason they wanted to do this was so that nurses could focus more of their time and effort on ensuring that patients' medications were delivered on time and adequate teaching was given to the patient and family and not spend time performing tasks that truly a PCT could do. The expansion of the nursing assistant role to the PCT at this hospital meant adding drawing blood (phlebotomy), monitoring blood glucose levels, and performing ECGs to the list of tasks for the PCT. To add these skills to the role of the PCT, adequate training and education must be offered. This particular hospital designed an education program in which the RNs were the ones who taught the information needed to perform these added skills. Ultimately, the RN is responsible and accountable for any care provided by the PCT. The nursing assistant must have additional training, both classroom and hands-on, before they can add on the additional skills of phlebotomy and ECG.

Instructors are important allies of PCT students, and the relationship between instructor and student should be one of mutual respect. Students must realize that instructors have a strong desire to share their knowledge and they want each student to succeed. Individual schools have certain rules and regulations that must be enforced, many of them the result of state or federal regulation or legislation. For example, there is a specific number of clinical hours that must be completed before you can take the certification examination. If you miss clinical and do not have enough clinical hours, you will not be able to take the certification examination. The guidelines students must follow are not designed to hinder their education, but rather to ensure that graduates are competent PCTs. Students should complete assignments accurately, turn them in on time, and take pride in all the work they do for class. They should never miss school days unless absolutely necessary, and they should develop good habits in school so that they become valuable assets to future employers.

Certifications for the Patient Care Technician

The National Healthcareer Association (NHA) offers certification for the PCT. The Certified Patient Care Technician/Assistant (CPCT/A) is a 100-question certification examination consisting of several categories. There are actually 110 questions on the examination; however, 10 of the questions are considered to be pilot or sample questions that are not included in the final score. The categories and the percentage of the 100 questions from each category include the following:

- Patient care (48)
- Safety (10)
- Professional responsibilities (5)
- Infection control (4)
- Phlebotomy (23)
- ECG monitoring (10)

To qualify to take the certification examination for the PCT, the candidate must meet the following:

1. Possess a high school diploma, or General Education Development (GED)
2. Successfully complete a training program or have at least 1 year of supervised work experience in the health field (taken from www.nhanow.com)

National Healthcareer Association

Some schools also offer certification through the NHA. Examinations and credentials available from the NHA include those for Certified Patient Care Technician/ Assistant (CPCT/A), Certified Phlebotomy Technician (CPT), and Certified Electrocardiography Technician (CET). The cost for these certification examinations ranges from about $100 to $150. More information is available on the NHA website at www.nhanow.com.

National Center for Competency Testing

The National Center for Competency Testing (NCCT) is an independent certification agency that has tested more than 240,000 individuals since 1989. The organization offers certification as a medical assistant, billing and coding specialist, medical office assistant, phlebotomy technician, PCT, and ECG technician. To earn an NCCT credential, candidates must meet all eligibility requirements and pass an examination based on the knowledge, skills, and abilities required at job entry. The NCCT's website is www.ncctinc.com.

Taking Certification Examinations

Students should take the examination soon after graduation; the detailed knowledge gained in school is easier to recall the sooner the examination is taken. Although the graduate is not guaranteed higher wages with certification or registration, most employers are willing to pay more for a graduate who has been through formal training and the certification or registration procedure. By registering for certification examinations soon after beginning the PCT training, the student can prepare throughout the classroom experience.

Paying for the Certification Examination

Currently, the cost to take the Patient Care Technician Examination averages between $90 and $149 (http://

www.nhanow.com/certifications/patient-care -technician). Many employers will cover the cost of the examination if there is an agreement to work for the healthcare institution after successful completion of it. Certain certificate programs may include the cost of the certification examination in the overall price of the program. You may be forced to pay for this examination on your own.

Preparing for the PCT Certification Examination

It is important to be adequately prepared before taking the certification examination. There is a test blueprint that outlines the categories and content areas from which the questions are taken (available online at www.nhanow.com/certifications/patient-care -technician). Many programs will offer a review course or session to prepare their students for the certification examination. It is important that before coming to the testing site to take the examination, you have had a good night's rest and have eaten a balanced diet. You may want to consider placing earphones in your ear to block out noise if this may bother you during the test. Currently, the examination is only available in the English language. Translators are not allowed to be present in the testing room with candidates.

Passing the PCT Certification Examination

Examination scores are sent to the candidate approximately 48 hours after taking the examination. If a grade of passing is not achieved, there is a second option to take the examination. If a passing grade is not achieved after the second opportunity, the candidate must wait 30 days before applying to take the examination again. If a passing grade is not achieved on the third attempt, you must wait 12 months before taking the examination again. If a passing grade is not achieved on the fourth attempt, you must wait 12 months between each attempt. Keep in mind that each attempt requires one to pay full price to take the examination. If one does not pass the examination the first time, it is recommended to seek out additional help before testing again.

Continuing Education

Education does not end with the completion of formal training. The amount of medical knowledge generated by research and published in a given year is astounding. The practicing PCT must keep current with the rapid changes in the profession. Most nurses appreciate PCTs who ask questions about unfamiliar conditions and procedures, and they are willing to teach students about the functioning of the body and treatments that benefit the patient. Much can be learned by reading or reviewing the medical literature that arrives in the daily mail or articles that appear in newspapers, magazines, and medically related newsletters.

Continuing education classes are available to enhance the knowledge of the professional PCT. Continuing education units (CEUs) may be required to maintain the PCT's certification. These credits can be obtained through various other agencies and educational institutions. Professional seminars and workshops often offer CEUs. Notices of continuing education classes are sent in bulk to medical facilities and physicians' offices, so staff members should watch for courses that pertain to their particular job duties and take advantage of them. The certified PCT is required to have 10 credits of continuing education before renewing their certification every 2 years (www.nhanow.com).

Some hospitals have chosen to create a career ladder for the PCT as a way to encourage lifelong learning. A career ladder is a stepwise progression from entry level to a more advanced role, and may include more pay and more responsibility. Completion of continuing education classes can be considered one way to advance on the career ladder, depending on the facility where you work. Becoming certified as a PCT can be another step on the ladder.

Delegation and Documentation Box 2.1

- Take charge of your paperwork related to your education. Keep good records and know when your certification is about to expire.
- Plan ahead for recertification; ask your nurse manager if the facility where you work will cover any of the fees associated with certification or recertifying.
- CPR and first aid are required by most, if not all, healthcare institutions. Keep a copy of your identification cards stating that you are CPR and first aid certified. Do not rely on the healthcare institution to keep copies of your records.

The Scope of Practice of a Patient Care Technician

Today's patient care assistant is a versatile professional. This means that the person can perform multiple tasks in one setting or in multiple settings. Individuals with PCT training can accomplish various jobs in the hospital environment, and some are employed by freestanding emergency centers or surgery centers. Opportunities are growing because of the constant change within the medical profession and the surge of cross-training, which means that one individual is trained to do a variety of duties. PCTs work under the direct supervision of a nurse and perform tasks delegated by the nurse.

The duties performed by the PCT do not constitute the practice of medicine. Students should review the definition and requirements of the scope of practice for PCTs in their individual states.

The clinical duties that PCTs perform vary according to the healthcare institution and state. They assist with or perform basic testing procedures and are usually proficient in phlebotomy. PCTs are trained in first aid skills and cardiopulmonary resuscitation. They collect and prepare laboratory specimens, and they know how to follow the regulations established by the U.S. Occupational Safety and Health Administration (OSHA). PCTs also perform ECGs and prepare patients for x-ray evaluations. They assist in minor surgical procedures, prepare sterile trays, and perform autoclave sterilization procedures for instruments. Other clinical duties involve obtaining and recording vital signs.

Duties and restrictions related to PCTs vary from state to state, but in most of the United States, PCTs perform under the nurse and are considered to be unlicensed assistive personnel (UAP).

A Career for Patient Care Technicians

Trained PCTs are equipped with a flexible, adaptable career in which they experience the rewards of helping other people (Fig. 2.1). The skills acquired by the PCT are valuable, and employment is readily available anywhere in the world where medicine is practiced. This career attracts the nontraditional student who may be older than the average postsecondary student by a decade or more. Although many older students feel intimidated by the classroom, they often have excellent experiences in school and reach the top of the class. The job of PCT is more than suitable for the student just exiting high school. Many individuals plan to work as PCTs to earn a viable income while pursuing further academic studies. The experience can be particularly helpful if the PCT desires to further their education in the area of healthcare, such as nursing.

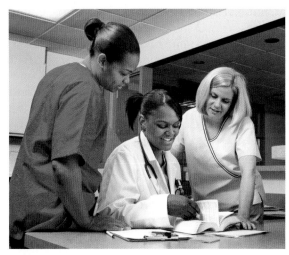

FIGURE 2.1 The role of the patient care technician is a career with benefits and perks, not to mention taking care of those in need. (From Proctor D, Adams A: *Kinn's The Medical Assistant: an applied learning approach*, ed 12, St. Louis, 2014, Saunders.)

The practice of medicine has changed dramatically in the past several decades. Increasing costs have created a trend away from hospital-based treatment and toward the delivery of care in physicians' offices and in outpatient ambulatory clinics. Computerization and technologic advances have created more opportunities for formally trained PCTs, and their responsibilities have similarly increased. Clearly defined educational requirements have been established, and this has resulted in improvement of the quality and accessibility of PCT training. These requirements have also helped create a healthy respect for PCTs, who are considered an integral part of today's allied health field.

Formal training and certification are valuable not only to the PCT but also to the physician-employer. PCTs are compensated in various ways, some by hourly wages and some by salary. The earnings vary from place to place. Overall, PCTs can expect a healthy return on their investment in training, experience, and skills. The *Occupational Outlook Handbook* reports statistics on the average salaries for many different career fields, including PCTs. (This information can be accessed at www.bls.gov/oco. Annual salary updates are also available on the website.) More information on salaries may be obtained by monitoring online job information on sites such as Yahoo! Careers and Monster. PCTs should be aware of what constitutes a realistic entry-level salary for their geographic area.

The medical field offers great benefits to employees. Usually, the larger the organization, the better the benefits. Most employers offer health insurance or managed care plans to their employees. Often a life insurance program is included, and dental insurance can be a valuable benefit if available. Some companies have profit sharing plans, as well as a retirement plan. Some organizations give their employees access to credit unions, and many have discount options at local businesses, such as uniform shops. Other benefits may include uniform stipends or reimbursement, tuition reimbursement, and continuing education allowances.

Remember that you should consider benefits when contemplating a job opportunity. Many PCTs may choose to work for less money if the benefits and the opportunities for advancement are good. Consider driving time, holidays, paid parking, sick days, vacation days, and facilities when choosing a job. Do the co-workers seem to enjoy one another's company and get along? All of these should be weighed carefully before the final decision is made as to which position to accept. Some facilities pay more and offer fewer benefits, whereas others pay less and offer more benefits. It is true that "money is a byproduct of services rendered." Nowhere is this more accurate than in the medical field. When the patients are served well, the PCT becomes more and more valuable to the employer and is compensated accordingly.

Professional Appearance

A well-groomed PCT in appropriate attire has a positive psychological effect on patients. The essentials of a professional appearance are good health, good grooming, and suitable dress.

Good health requires adequate sleep, balanced meals, and enough exercise to keep fit. PCTs can set a good example by living a sensible, healthy lifestyle that includes regular checkups for their own physical condition, both medical and dental.

Injury and Illness Prevention Box 2.1

- Practice safety measures such as wearing a seatbelt when operating a vehicle at all times.
- Stay as healthy as possible. Consider annual well-visits with a physician. Take a multivitamin. Avoid use of alcohol.
- If you work night shift, make arrangements for 6 to 8 hours of sleep during the day, especially if you are returning the next night. This protects you as well as your patients from harm related to your drowsiness.

Good grooming is little more than attention to the details of personal appearance. Personal cleanliness, which includes taking a daily bath or shower, using deodorant, and practicing good oral hygiene, is vital. Perfume and aftershave cologne should not be used or should be applied lightly because patients and co-workers may be allergic to some scents. Makeup should be conservative and applied moderately. Heavy or exaggerated makeup is out of place in the professional office; subtle eye and lip makeup is best. Clear or muted shades of nail polish are best, and long nails are not only inappropriate but also can be dangerous to the patient. Nails must be kept clean and at a very conservative length. The PCT's hair should be shiny, clean, neatly styled, and off the collar.

Medical professionals rarely wear traditional white in today's medical facilities, although it is appropriate if allowed in the policy manual. Fashionable styling makes it possible for the PCT's uniform to be both practical and attractive. Women may choose to wear pantsuits, which are available in white or a variety of colors; a two-piece dress uniform in white or a color; an attractively styled traditional white uniform; or a scrub set. Scrubs have become increasingly popular and much more attractive over the past decade (Fig. 2.2). They now are often made of pretty fabrics in rich colors and patterns, and are much better suited for the healthcare setting than the old green or blue scrubs worn in the surgical suites of hospitals. Healthcare organizations will have policies related to what type of uniform may be worn, and perhaps even what color is to be worn depending on what role you are in and what unit you work on. Some organizations use color of uniforms to

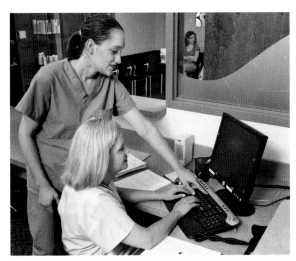

FIGURE 2.2 Scrubs have become the required dress for many healthcare institutions. (From Proctor D, Adams A: *Kinn's The Medical Assistant: an applied learning approach*, ed 12, St. Louis, 2014, Saunders.)

separate the nurses from the UAP, such as the PCT, as well as those working in housekeeping. This helps to cut down on confusion with patients knowing who to ask for help or for pain medication, since most employees wear some type of scrub in the patient care area. It is important to ensure that your scrubs are ironed and wrinkle-free when arriving to work each day. A messy, wrinkled uniform could be a sign of how you will conduct your work for the day.

Men may also wear the newer scrubs or may choose white slacks with a white or colored shirt, jacket, or pullover top. Uniforms should be laundered daily and neatly pressed because PCTs are exposed to ill patients throughout the work period. Shoes should be appropriate for a uniform, spotless, and comfortable. Many attractive styles that resemble running or tennis shoes are available at uniform shops, specially conditioned for the medical professional who is on his or her feet most of the day. White shoes must be kept white by daily cleaning and touchups. Remember that if laced shoes are worn, the laces also need cleaning.

Some psychiatrists and some pediatricians, for example, believe that the clinical appearance of a uniform may affect patients adversely. However, today's uniforms reflect so many styles and patterns that the right one for the particular unit should be readily available. Some of the fabrics depict cartoon characters or drawings that will appeal to children yet still function as a durable uniform.

The garments worn while on duty must be comfortable, allow for easy movement, and still look fresh at the end of a busy day. Whatever uniform style the technician chooses, it should be personally becoming and worn over appropriate undergarments. The lines, colors, and ornamentation of the undergarments should not be seen through the uniform; therefore, it is best to wear undergarments that have a neutral color and not a pattern. Thongs and high-cut underwear should be avoided. When a uniform is worn, jewelry should be limited to an engagement ring, wedding band, and professional pin. No more than two earrings per ear lobe should be worn, and the clothing or hairstyle should always cover tattoos.

Facial and tongue piercings are unacceptable in the medical setting and must be removed during working hours. A name badge will help patients identify each staff person by name.

Make sure that the dress code required in the workplace setting is clearly understood. Adherence to that code is a demonstration of responsibility and willingness to cooperate with workplace rules. Compliance with workplace regulations is a factor in decisions on promotions.

Legal and Ethical Issues

In the course of PCTs' daily work, they must deal with a vast amount of personal and intimate information about the patients who have entrusted their care to the physician and those employed by the practice or healthcare institution. Such information must be held in strict confidence and must never be discussed with or relayed to others, including professional associates, unless the lack of knowledge would hinder the patient's care.

CHAPTER SUMMARY

This chapter has presented the advantages of becoming a trained PCT and some of the many career opportunities available. The skills that must be developed and the general knowledge that must be acquired to perform the duties of a PCT effectively have been presented. However, skills and knowledge alone do not ensure success. Personality traits and professional appearance are also critical. Continuing education is vital to the PCT's career. The individual who chooses this career must be willing to accept the responsibilities inherent in its standards. The importance of obtaining national certification cannot be stressed enough.

Case Scenario

Sandra Ortiz is a single mother who has decided on PCT as a career. She has always been interested in the medical field and wants a job that will allow her flexibility in scheduling time with her 3-year-old son, Roberto. The idea of working in a hospital appeals to her, and she has applied to a school that is close to her apartment and day care provider. She plans to attend day classes and work part-time in the evenings and on weekends.

Sandra is very excited about her new career and has set several goals for her training. First, she hopes to attain perfect attendance and, second, she would like to graduate with honors. She has budgeted her study time and plans to ask her instructors during the first 2 weeks of school for suggestions on how she can better prepare for classes and examinations. Sandra will find the role of PCT to be a rewarding career and respected profession.

- What obstacles might prevent Sandra from attending all her classes, and how can she prepare in advance to overcome them?

- How can Sandra begin to explore the type of patient care unit in which she would enjoy being employed after graduation?
- What goals might Sandra have at the beginning of her training and at the end of training?
- How can Sandra make the most of her time attending school to become a PCT?
- Sandra knows that she needs certain benefits as a single mother. What might she need to look for in a job after she graduates?
- What are some ways Sandra can compare positions and opportunities?
- What types of websites might help Sandra learn about opportunities in her geographic location?

REVIEW QUESTIONS

1. The skills performed by the certified nursing assistant are the same as the skills performed by the patient care technician.
   a. True
   b. False

2. To be able to take the certification examination for the patient care technician, one must have or be which of the following?
   a. Have a high school diploma
   b. Be 21 years of age
   c. Be married
   d. Have 5 years of clinical experience in the healthcare field

3. Who is responsible for paying for the certification examination for the patient care technician?
   a. The future employer
   b. The school where the training is offered
   c. The candidate of the examination
   d. The testing company

4. If ones does not pass the second certification examination for the patient care technician, how soon can the candidate schedule the third examination?
   a. Immediately
   b. 30 days
   c. 12 months
   d. 24 months

5. How many hours of continuing education is required before one can renew the patient care technician certification?
   a. 5
   b. 10
   c. 15
   d. 20

Professionalism and Work Ethics

LEARNING OBJECTIVES

1. Explain the reasons why professionalism is important in the medical field.
2. Discuss several characteristics of professionalism.
3. Explain why confidentiality is so important in the medical profession.
4. Identify the hazards of using social media in healthcare.
5. Discuss the importance of the patient care technician's attitude in caring for patients.
6. List some examples of politics in the workplace.
7. Discuss the meaning of *insubordination* and why it has grounds for dismissal.
8. Discuss how substance abuse can affect the patient care technician's employment.

KEY TERMS

characteristics Distinguishing traits, qualities, or properties

commensurate Corresponding in size, amount, extent, or degree; equal in measure; proportionate

competent Having adequate or requisite capabilities

connotation An implication; something suggested by a word or thing

credibility The quality or power of inspiring belief

demeanor Behavior toward others; outward manner

detrimental Obviously harmful or damaging

discretion The quality of being discreet; having or showing good judgment or conduct, especially in speech

disseminated To disburse; to spread around

drug of choice The drug an abuser uses most frequently to satisfy the craving for a certain feeling; the user's preferred drug

initiative Energy or aptitude to cause or facilitate the start of something or to cause something to happen

insubordination Disobedience to authority

morale The mental and emotional condition, enthusiasm, loyalty, or confidence of an individual or group with regard to the function or tasks at hand

optimistic Inclined to put the most favorable construction on actions and events or to anticipate the best possible outcome

persona An individual's social facade or front that reflects the role in life the individual is playing; the personality a person projects in public

professionalism The conduct or qualities characterized by or conforming to the technical or ethical standards of a profession; exhibiting a courteous, conscientious, and generally businesslike manner in the workplace

rapport Development of a relationship with a person who feels that you understand the feelings of that person

reproach An expression of rebuke or disapproval; a cause or occasion of blame, discredit, or disgrace

work ethics A set of values based on the moral virtues of hard work and diligence

THE MEANING OF PROFESSIONALISM

Professionalism is defined as having a courteous, conscientious, and generally businesslike manner in the workplace. It is characterized by or conforms to the technical or ethical standards of a certain profession. Conducting one's self in a professional manner is essential for being a successful patient care technician (PCT). The attitude of those in the medical profession generally is more conservative than that seen in other career fields. Patients expect professional behavior and base much of their trust and confidence in those who show this type of demeanor in the healthcare setting (Fig. 3.1). There is evidence that patients are less likely to sue those who they like and feel close to. By developing a rapport, the PCT makes the patient feel that their feelings and concerns are valid and true. Patients feel that they matter to the PCT and are the focus of the PCT's attentions and efforts.

Work Ethics

Work ethics are sets of values based on the moral virtues of hard work and diligence, involving a whole range of activities, from individual acts to the philosophy of the entire facility. The PCT should always display initiative and be reliable. A person who has a good work ethic is one who arrives on time, who is rarely absent, whose work output is commensurate with the pay received, and who uses his or her best abilities. The phrase "being early is on-time" is one that is best if practiced. Arriving at the beginning of your shift time does not allow any time to store your belongings before beginning to work. Co-workers become frustrated if another employee consistently arrives late or is absent. This forces the co-workers to take on additional duties and may prevent them from completing their own work. One missing employee can disrupt the entire day because assignments are made based on how many staff are scheduled for the day, and when one is not there, the rest of the staff is shorthanded. All employees should know the attendance policies in their facility as outlined in the policy and procedure manual. Many facilities monitor their employee's absences and tardiness and may implement discipline that includes an option for being terminated, or fired, when there are multiple episodes of calling out sick, arriving late, or not showing up to work.

Most new hires have a probationary period that may last 30 to 90 days. Any absences or tardiness during the probationary period can be grounds to terminate the employee once the probationary period is up or even before that if multiple attendance issues arise. If the PCT has an emergency and must be absent or tardy, he or she should make sure to notify the supervisor according to the healthcare institution's policy. All employees must be on time and in attendance every day they are scheduled.

Work ethics also apply to other situations. If another employee is seen taking drugs from the supply cabinet or money from the cash box, the act should certainly be reported. However, if the guilty employee is also a close friend of the person who witnesses the act, an ethics dilemma arises. A PCT must always act in such a way that his or her actions are above reproach.

Characteristics of Professionalism

Many characteristics make up the professionalism required of PCTs. Students should begin developing these characteristics while in school; these qualities do not appear magically when the student begins working with actual patients. Although we might think that we would always behave appropriately during an externship or in a job setting, the habits developed in school will carry over into these experiences. If the behavior is unacceptable, it will be detrimental to the PCT's professional career. If the PCT wishes to advance and receive wage increases, promotions, and the trust of the employer, the characteristics discussed in the following sections must be a part of his or her persona. Additionally, healthcare facilities sometimes have to make decisions to decrease their staffing personnel. The decision to either keep or let go a PCT could be based on the

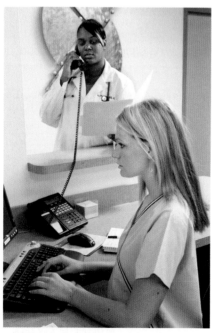

FIGURE 3.1 Maintain professionalism in all that you do. (From Proctor D, Adams A: *Kinn's The Medical Assistant: an applied learning approach*, ed 12, St. Louis, 2014, Saunders.)

professionalism of that person, including his or her attendance record.

Loyalty

Loyalty is faithfulness or allegiance to a cause, ideal, custom, institution, person, or product. Loyalty to an employer means that the employee is appreciative of the opportunity provided by the job and supports the company by giving the best effort possible. Many individuals today are interested only in what the employer can provide for them. However, this is an immature approach to take toward a job. When a person is employed by a company, use of skills is exchanged for different types of compensation. Each benefits the other. Often we forget that experience alone is a great benefit from working. Loyalty to the employer is important, and in return the employee should feel a sense of loyalty from the company.

Courtesy

Show courtesy to the patients and your co-workers in the healthcare setting. Kind words and compassion go far in building trust between the PCT and patient. All visitors and staff are to be shown kindness and consideration. Having a bad day is no excuse for a PCT to inflict anger or irritation onto patients. Always demonstrate a good attitude and offer patients and visitors a sincere smile. Remember that patients are consumers, which means that they are purchasing, or paying, for the healthcare they receive.

Initiative

Lack of initiative is one of the more common complaints from supervisors about employees. Taking initiative means that the PCT looks for opportunities to be of help, assisting others as the workload demands. Instead of waiting to be told to perform a task, the competent PCT looks for tasks that need to be completed. Never remain idle. There is almost always something that can be done in an effort to help someone else out. It is also best to plan ahead, as you don't always know when your patient load will be increased abruptly. Supplies can be inventoried, ordered, or restocked when extra time is available. Cleaning countertops and straightening areas as work is done helps keep the facility tidy. Just because cleaning may not be in the specific job description of a PCT, it does not mean that one should not help keep the area clean. It takes the entire healthcare team to help keep the unit clean.

Flexibility

A PCT must be able to adapt to a wide variety of situations in the healthcare setting. An emergency could occur and the staff must be flexible enough to adjust the assignment to care for all patients. Being flexible also means that staff members are willing to assist one another in the performance of their duties. No one should ever say, "That's not my job." The patients must come first, and every staff member must be willing to lend a hand when needed.

Credibility

Credibility is the perceived competence or character of a person, leading to the belief that the individual can be trusted. Because trust is a vital component of the physician–patient relationship, the credibility of the physician and those who assist should be strong and unquestionable. The information provided to patients must be accurate. Patients expect the physician and healthcare team to instruct and educate them in a manner that enhances their health and provides positive results. A PCT should never discuss personal opinions or communicate negative comments about a particular physician or other healthcare member to the patient. Take care to not instruct the patient on anything that could be seen as teaching. This is the nurse's responsibility. Remember that giving anything that could be construed as medical advice is outside the scope of the duties of the PCT. To avoid facing charges of practicing medicine without a license, a PCT must be sure to suggest only what the physician has authorized.

Delegation and Documentation Box 3.1

- Never state that something has happened unless you are sure it has; hearsay is when you repeat something that was said but you were not witness to it. Avoid taking part in hearsay.
- Communicate clearly any details to the nurse and physician. Avoid using words such as "sort of" and "maybe" as these words can be difficult to determine the meaning.
- Never teach patients how to do something related to their medical care. This is the nurse's responsibility. Once the nurse has taught the patient, you may reinforce the teaching through repeating the same steps the nurse has shown the patient.

Confidentiality

The importance of confidentiality in the healthcare environment cannot be stressed enough. Patients are entitled to privacy where their health is concerned, and they should be confident that healthcare professionals use information only to care for them. Never reveal any information about any patient to anyone without specific permission to do so. Always verify that the person seeking information has the right to see it and that the patient has signed a consent form allowing a third party to view the record. Health Insurance Portability and Accountability Act (HIPAA) guidelines require the patient to sign a release before others can be told any information relating to the health of that patient. Casual conversations in hallways, elevators, and break rooms between staff members can be overheard by a family member or friend of the patient. Confidentiality is often breached in these areas of the healthcare setting. Never assume that no one is around listening to conversations.

The rules regarding confidentiality extend beyond the healthcare setting. At home, PCTs should not discuss with their families and friends the details about patients. Those outside the medical profession do not understand how vital it is to keep information confidential and may pass along private or damaging facts to others. Make it a rule never to discuss a patient with anyone unless information must be shared for the patient's care and treatment.

Social Media

Maintaining a person's confidentiality includes protecting his or her privacy on social media. Social media applications such as Facebook and Twitter have rapidly infused today's society as a whole. As of 2016, there are approximately 1.7 billion users of Facebook, and more than 310 million users of Twitter. It seems very innocent to post a message of encouragement to someone you have cared for while working on the same unit in which he or she was a patient; however, this can be seen as a violation of confidentiality. By posting a message of encouragement, a connection is made to that person's hospital experience. It is best to not make any connections with patients on social media sites in order to maintain the person's right to privacy and confidentiality. There have been staff members who have been fired from the healthcare institution where they were employed because of posting comments on social media sites that refer to the patients under their care. Additionally, the PCT should not make any reference to the workplace climate on social media sites. Workplace climate may include references to the number of patients currently on the unit, number of staff, personnel issues, or cutbacks. These all affect the workplace climate; however, this should not be discussed on social media. If the PCT is concerned about the workplace climate, an appointment should be made to discuss it with his or her manager in a private yet professional manner.

Attitude

Possibly the most important asset a PCT brings to the healthcare institution is a good attitude. A good attitude is characterized by courtesy and kindness to others, refraining from jumping to conclusions, giving the other

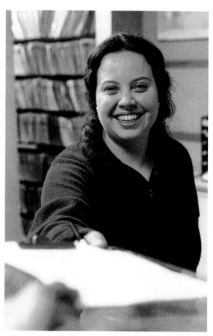

FIGURE 3.2 Having a good attitude goes a long way in developing good patient and staff relationships. (From Proctor D, Adams A: *Kinn's The Medical Assistant: an applied learning approach*, ed 12, St. Louis, 2014, Saunders.)

Delegation and Documentation Box 3.2

- Never, ever post any type of message connecting you to your patient on any form of social media.
- Never take pictures of your patient or patient's body parts using your cell phone or any camera. This includes living or dead material, such as pieces of tissue that were removed from the patient.
- Avoid posting any negative remarks about your shift at work on social media.

person the benefit of the doubt, and being optimistic. This trait alone can influence promotions, terminations, and the entire atmosphere (Fig. 3.2). Individuals are able to control their attitudes with practice. It takes skill to react calmly to people who are very upset rather than to respond in kind, especially if you are being harassed or accused. Speaking in an even tone and perhaps a little softer than normal forces the listener to lower his or her voice to hear. Offer to help resolve the problem and attempt to move to a private room to talk, out of the hearing of other patients. Always have a good attitude with co-workers and be willing to assist them with their duties, especially on hectic days.

Obstructions to Professionalism

At times it is not easy to be a professional. Sometimes patients, co-workers, and supervisors try our patience, and it can be difficult to maintain a professional attitude in these cases. Some of the obstructions to professional behavior are discussed in this section. Never use social media as an outlet to vent frustrations regarding the workplace.

Personal Problems and "Baggage"

Everyone has a life outside the workplace, and sometimes we face challenges and difficult times that are hard to put aside. During working hours, our thoughts should be on the job at hand, especially when we are dealing with patients. However, some situations in our lives may be so critical or distracting that we find ourselves thinking of them constantly. This personal baggage can interfere with our ability to perform job duties properly.

When a situation intrudes on our thoughts at work, it often is best to take the time to talk with a supervisor. It is not always necessary to share the intimate details, but a quick explanation that some difficulties are occurring outside of work helps the supervisor to understand any changes in habit or attitude. Some supervisors are uncaring and are concerned only with satisfactory job performance. The PCT must use some discretion in discussing private affairs with the supervisor.

The professional PCT never transfers personal problems or baggage to anyone at the healthcare institution, especially patients. The workday should be centered on patient care; therefore do not allow personal business to interfere with time that should be spent assisting patients and the physician. The patient must be the prime concern of all the employees in a medical facility.

Rumors and the "Grapevine"

A rumor is considered to be talk or widely disseminated opinions with no discernible source, or a statement that is not known to be true. The definition alone suggests that spreading rumors should be avoided. Most people enjoy working in an environment in which employees cooperate and get along with each other, but rumors can cause problems with employee morale and often are great exaggerations or manipulations of the truth. By promoting the grapevine, rumors are passed along and become more and more outrageous with each retelling. A PCT should refuse to participate in the rumor mill and should attempt to be cordial and friendly to everyone at work (Fig. 3.3). Supervisors regard those who spread or discuss rumors as unprofessional and untrustworthy. Avoid passing along work-related rumors to patients, family, and friends.

Personal Phone Calls and Business

The PCT should not take unnecessary phone calls from friends and family while at work. The healthcare

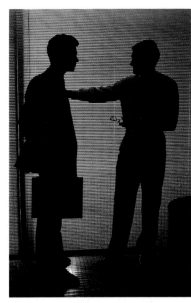

FIGURE 3.3 Gossip and rumors have no place in the healthcare setting. Avoid engaging in this behavior. (From Proctor D, Adams A: *Kinn's The Medical Assistant: an applied learning approach*, ed 12, St. Louis, 2014, Saunders.)

Injury and Illness Prevention Box 3.1

- Protect your mental health by making sure that you have provided for time off during the work week. Working seven straight days in a row is unhealthy for anyone.
- Exercise on your days off and when you have time before or after work. It improves blood flow and is thought to decrease stress.
- Avoid from engaging in negative conversation. There is usually nothing to be gained from it other than stress. Be the one who changes the tone of the conversation to a positive one.

institution's telephone line is a business line and must be used as such, except in emergencies. Using personal cell phones during working hours is not acceptable. Most cellular phones used today are considered to be smart phones, which means that these phones retrieve and push data into the cyber world, rather than just function as a telephone. This provides yet another opportunity to break the patient's privacy and confidentiality. Refrain from using personal cell phones during the shift with the exception of breaks. Never take a personal call or respond to text messages on a cell phone while working with a patient. If a phone must be carried, place it on the vibrate setting and always step into a hall or break area if a call absolutely must be taken. This should happen only in rare cases.

Checking personal e-mail also should be avoided in the workplace. Any type of personal business, such as studying, looking up information on the Internet for personal use, Internet shopping, or checking a personal bank account, should be done at home and not while at work. All of these actions distract the PCT from the job at hand; the focus should be on serving the patients at all times. Employees can and are terminated from their employment for surfing or shopping on the Internet for personal reasons or for checking personal e-mail. Make sure that all personal business is handled outside of business hours.

Workplace Politics

Most people associate workplace politics with some underhanded scheme or plans to move upward in the system in whatever way possible, whether the methods used are ethical or not. The tendency is to give the word politics a negative connotation. Politics can be defined as the art or science of influencing and guiding government or some other organization. The same can be applied to workplace politics. When an individual wishes to move upward in an organization, he or she may use a positive or negative strategy. Many people develop a specific plan regarding how they will advance and in what time they will accomplish their goals. PCTs who want to advance should be productive workers, accept responsibility, be dependable, and always conduct themselves in a professional manner. Using underhanded techniques and instigating trouble is not an effective method of career advancement. Those who use negative workplace politics often find that their methods turn into disasters and they lose the support of co-workers and supervisors, making the work environment tense and anxious. Often, they seek other employment, but if they continue negative politics in their new workplace, they will likely face the same results and find themselves without a job.

Professional Attributes

Teamwork

If managers were asked to name the most important attributes for medical professionals, teamwork would be high on the list (Fig. 3.4). Staff members must work together for the good of the patients. They must be willing to perform duties outside the formal job description if they are needed in other areas of the healthcare institution. Many supervisors frown on employees who state, "That's not in my job description." Any order that is given by a supervisor becomes mandatory, and an individual who refuses to perform an assigned task can have his or her employment terminated for insubordination. A PCT should perform the duty and later discuss with the nurse any valid reasons that the task should have been assigned to someone else. However, if the task is illegal, is unethical, or places the patient or anyone else in danger, it should not be performed.

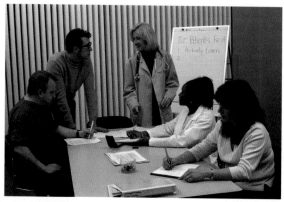

FIGURE 3.4 Teamwork is so important in the healthcare setting. All members must be willing to work together in order to provide the best care possible. (From Proctor D, Adams A: *Kinn's The Medical Assistant: an applied learning approach*, ed 12, St. Louis, 2014, Saunders.)

Although most would enjoy working in an environment where everyone gets along and likes every other employee, this does not always happen. Personal feelings must be set aside at work, and all employees must cooperate with others to get the job done efficiently. If a PCT has an issue with another employee, the first move would be to discuss it privately with the offending employee. If the situation does not improve, perhaps a supervisor should be involved for further discussions.

Time Management

We have often heard the expression "work smart." This means that we are to use our time efficiently and concentrate on the most important duties first. To do this, we must first prioritize our duties and arrange our daily task list to ensure that these duties can be performed. The first way to improve time management is to plan the tasks that need to be done that day. Taking 10 minutes to write down the tasks for the day helps ensure that they are done. Then, stay on schedule throughout the day, unless you are interrupted by emergencies. The key to managing time is prioritizing.

Prioritizing

Prioritizing is simply deciding which tasks are most important and in what order the tasks should be performed. Many people make a "to do" list for the day's activities; however, the secret to success is prioritizing those activities into categories that give order to the tasks.

Most tasks can be prioritized into three general categories: those that *must* be done that day, those that *should* be done that day, and those that *could* be done if time permits. Once a general list of tasks has been established, review the list and further prioritize it, using a code such as *M* for must, *S* for should, and *C* for could (or this might be further simplified by using the letters *A*, *B*, and *C*). Once the tasks have been divided into these categories, they can be further classified in each section. For instance, if category *A* (must be done that day) has six tasks, they can be numbered in the order they should be performed. The same process is completed with the tasks in categories *B* and *C*. As the tasks are completed, they are checked off for that day. Other categories can be added to customize the list. For example, an *H* category can be used for duties to perform at home, *P* could represent phone calls that need to be made, *E* could represent errands to run, and *EM* might represent e-mails to be sent. Customizing the categories makes the list more user-friendly and helps the user to meet his or her individual needs.

Setting Goals

Individuals who succeed in life are planners and goal setters. The first step in becoming a proficient goal setter is to take the time to really think about what is to be accomplished throughout one's lifetime. These goals must be written down and reviewed often. Goals should be set for all areas in a person's life, including personal growth, career, home life, family, spiritual needs, and any others that apply to the individual. The goals should not be unreasonable. They should be measurable and specific, with written steps detailing how they will be reached. Determination and persistence in reaching the goals helps make them happen, along with hard work. The goals should be reviewed often and progress evaluated. Reset goals whenever necessary and celebrate accomplishments.

Knowing the Facility and Its Employees

A much-circulated story tells of a college professor who used to end a critical test with the question, "What is the name of the woman who cleans our wing of the building?" This would perplex most students, but the question makes a good point. A PCT should attempt to get to know the people who work in the healthcare facility and should have a good idea of who handles which duties (Fig. 3.5). When patients have specific problems with which they need help, they can be referred to the person who knows the most about that particular issue. It is wise to express appreciation to others whenever possible. Say "thank you" or "I appreciate your help" often when working with others. This makes co-workers more likely to assist at other times when their help is needed.

Documentation

Charting accurately with legible, neat handwriting can make a difference in the perception of professionalism

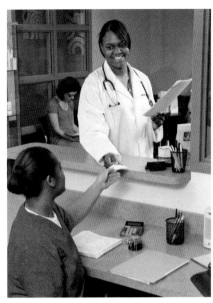

FIGURE 3.5 Attempt to get to know those you work with and the roles that they play. (From Proctor D, Adams A: *Kinn's The Medical Assistant: an applied learning approach*, ed 12, St. Louis, 2014, Saunders.)

in the healthcare setting. Complete, accurate electronic medical record (EMR) entries are critical as well, and a thorough knowledge of the computer program used will enhance the providers' ability to provide competent patient care. Be complete in any narrative regarding patients. Be sure to state facts, not opinions, and never use sarcastic remarks when charting. Use conservative speech, proper wording, and good grammar in all situations in the medical facility.

Note Taking

Keep a small spiral notebook in a pocket with a pen so that if any instructions are given in passing by the nurse, you have a place to jot it down until you have access to the patient's chart. This can help prevent forgetting to do something like discontinuing an intravenous line in addition to many other errors that could be made by relying on memory. Remember to discard any note sheets that contain patient confidential information in a confidential recycling bin or in a shredder.

Hygiene

It is important to maintain a clean, professional look as a PCT. In the healthcare environment, cleanliness is so important in order to make sure that the patients heal and don't get even worse while they are a patient. Hygiene begins at home when preparing to come to work. The PCT should have showered recently and not have a strong body odor. Strong perfumes or body sprays should not be used, as such smells could be offensive to patients. There should not be a smell of cigarette smoke, as this may aggravate the patient's illness further. Hair must be neat and pulled back away from the face so that it does not interfere with the work that has to be done.

The uniform may include hospital-issued scrub tops and pants; if not provided, the PCT may be required to purchase a set of scrub tops and pants. The uniform must be sized appropriately and fit according to the PCT's shape. The hemline of the pants should not drag on the floor. For women, if the top is a V-cut, it is important that it is layered with an undershirt, or that the top does not reveal the chest area. Also, undergarments should be in the color of the PCT's skin tone.

It is important that the uniform be clean and wrinkle-free. A uniform that is stained or wrinkled does not give a professional look. If the uniform has holes or threadbare areas, it probably needs to be replaced.

Some healthcare facilities may have policies in place that require the covering of tattoos and the removal of certain piercings while at work. Be sure to look up the institution's policies regarding the presence of such and follow accordingly.

Interpersonal Skills

Interpersonal skills are so important in working with patients and other health professionals. A PCT should work to perfect his or her communication techniques.

When speaking to patients and providing them with information, remember that most do not have any medical background and do not understand many of the phrases used by the medical community. A PCT must be patient and explain in a courteous manner any aspect of the instructions or details that the patient does not understand. When instructing the patient, the PCT should have a professional attitude of concern and helpfulness. Assure the patient that everyone in the facility is bound by rules of patient confidentiality if the patient seems concerned about revealing information.

A PCT does not share personal information with anyone at the healthcare facility. Refrain from passing along rumors of any type to patients or their families. Be especially careful speaking of any patient when you are in public areas of the healthcare facility, such as the elevator or cafeteria.

Substance Abuse

All employees of medical facilities must avoid drug and alcohol abuse (also called *substance abuse*), which is defined as the repeated and excessive use of a substance, despite its destructive effects, to produce pleasure and escape reality. Substance abuse includes the use of illegal and legal drugs. Many facilities require drug screening before employment, and some perform the screenings randomly during employment. Because drugs and alcohol remain in the body for various lengths of time,

an individual who uses them on a Sunday afternoon may still have residual effects on Monday. This can prevent a PCT from performing at maximum capacity and can cause mistakes that may even be life-threatening to the patient. Also, the drive to and from work can result in an accident because of substance abuse. Fatal or not, substance abuse results in harm to another person, and the user is at risk of lawsuits and legal problems. By abusing drugs even once, the PCT can damage his or her career irreparably.

A person is considered to have a substance abuse problem if at least one of the following four criteria is met:

- Continued use despite social or interpersonal problems
- Repeated use that results in failure to fulfill obligations at work, school, and/or home
- Repeated use that results in physically hazardous situations
- Use that results in legal problems

The PCT should understand the differences between use, dependence, abuse, and addiction. Most people use some type of drug or supplement, many on a daily basis. If a patient takes a blood pressure medication, he or she uses that drug for a specific purpose that provides a health benefit. Physical dependence is not always part of the definition of addiction. Some drugs cause a physical dependence but not an addiction, such as a medication for diabetes. The patient depends on the drug to relieve the symptoms of the disease, but the drug usually is not abused or used in a way that would be considered an addiction. *Abuse* is the use of illegal drugs or the misuse of prescription and over-the-counter drugs.

Anyone who experiences at least three of the following seven criteria in the same 12-month period could be considered an abuser and should seek drug and alcohol counseling:

- Tolerance for the drug
- Withdrawal symptoms
- Difficulty controlling drug use
- Negative consequences from drug use
- Significant time or emotional energy spent seeking drugs
- Neglect of regular activities
- A desire to cut down on the use of a certain drug

Addiction is the compulsive use of a substance despite its negative and sometimes dangerous effects. The abuse of prescription drugs is a growing concern in the United States. Many of these drugs alter brain activity and are highly addictive, and as a result, the user's behavior changes. Opioids, central nervous system depressants, antianxiety drugs, and stimulants are the most common categories of prescription drug abuse. Once users are addicted, their ability to make voluntary decisions changes and a craving leads to a state of constantly seeking the drug of choice. Most healthcare facilities and physicians are opposed to hiring a person with a history of or convictions for substance abuse. Often, personal relationships and careers are destroyed, and this can lead to theft to buy drugs or alcohol.

According to the National Institute on Alcohol Abuse and Alcoholism (NIAAA), alcohol abuse is a disease that has the following four symptoms:

- *Craving*—a strong urge or need to drink
- *Loss of control*—the inability to stop drinking once it has begun
- *Physical dependence*—the occurrence of withdrawal symptoms after drinking (e.g., shakiness, nausea, sweating, and anxiety)
- *Tolerance*—the need to increase the amount of alcohol taken in to get the same effect

The potential to abuse alcohol is partly inherited, and the individual lifestyle may also influence whether a person becomes an alcoholic. This does not mean that a person who is a child of an alcoholic will definitely become an alcoholic, but the risk is greater when alcoholism is prevalent in the family. Treatment for alcoholism works for many people. Some never drink again, but others may go for months or years without drinking and still suffer a relapse; still others are simply unable to stop drinking for any length of time.

Substance abuse has the potential to end a PCT's career and can lead to incarceration, meaning being put in jail. A PCT who is under the influence of controlled substances or alcohol can easily make errors and fail to document correctly and, in addition, cannot care for the patient to his or her optimal ability. Convictions for substance abuse can make finding a job in a healthcare facility almost impossible. Many facilities conduct pre-employment and random drug testing, and the chances of not being caught are extremely slim, especially if a substance is still in the system several days after use. Avoid any behavior that can threaten loss of a career in the medical field and legal action.

CHAPTER SUMMARY

Patients expect and deserve professional behavior from those who work in healthcare facilities. Always show compassion, care, and consideration for a person, whether a patient, visitor, or co-worker. By displaying these traits, the PCT earns the respect of co-workers and becomes indispensable to the physician-employer. Behaving in a professional manner helps gain the patient's trust. Trust is one of the most important factors in preventing cases of medical professional liability. Treating patients with care and not subjecting them to poor attitudes keeps the patient–healthcare professional relationship strong and conducive to the health and recovery of the patient. Professionalism is vital in the medical profession because patients expect and deserve to be treated in a professional way. When the PCT acts in a professional way, he or she creates trust with the patient. Patients notice professional behavior, even when it is not directed at them specifically. They notice how others are treated in the break room and at the nurse's station. Always act in a professional manner while at work. Some of the characteristics of professionalism are loyalty, dependability, courtesy, initiative, flexibility, credibility, confidentiality, and a good attitude.

Confidentiality is crucial in the medical profession because patients depend on medical personnel to keep their health information private. Breach of patient confidentiality is one reason an employee could be terminated immediately and can result in litigation between the patient and the physician-employer.

Workplace politics can be negative or positive. A person who uses others to gain promotion in the company or who takes credit for a team effort may be using workplace politics in a negative way; a person who strategically plans advancement through outstanding performance, dependability, and teamwork uses workplace politics in a positive manner. Knowing when to speak and when to listen helps the PCT play the game of politics well in the healthcare facility.

Substance abuse can lead to arrest and conviction, and it can, and in most cases does, damage a promising career. The PCT may face legal action if he or she is abusing drugs or alcohol. This can lead to the end of a career in the healthcare industry. In extreme cases, patients could die from the PCT's actions while under the influence of controlled substances. Any PCT struggling with a substance abuse problem should seek professional help immediately.

Case Scenario

Karla has recently gone through a divorce and is having a difficult time with being able to pay her bills. She does not have reliable childcare for her young children and her car has been in the shop for several days. She has family who are able to watch her children on the weekends and during the evenings, but her shifts are typically scheduled during the day. How might Karla be proactive in working out a solution so that she can still come to work on time? Should she tell her manager about her situation, or should she try and work it out on her own?

REVIEW QUESTIONS

1. If a patient's family member sends the PCT a picture, it is okay for this picture to be uploaded on social media sites.
   a. True
   b. False

2. At which point can the PCT give test results to the patient's family members?
   a. If the patient says it's okay
   b. If the patient has signed a release indicating which family members are allowed to receive patient information
   c. If the nurse gives you permission to do so
   d. If the family members are present with the patient

3. To say something that is obviously harmful to someone is said to be:
   a. Detrimental
   b. Disseminated
   c. Tolerant
   d. Insubordination

4. Documentation on the patient's record must be which of the following?
   a. Neat and able to be read
   b. Short and sweet
   c. Filled with your opinion of how the patient should be treated
   d. PCTs do not document; therefore no documenting should occur.

5. To be professional, the PCT should act in what way?
   a. Courteous
   b. Lazy
   c. Smart
   d. Sarcastic

Communicating With the Healthcare Team

1. Discuss the concepts of verbal and nonverbal communication.
2. Recognize assertive communication as the most appropriate communication style.
3. Identify various factors that have the potential to affect communication.
4. Discuss potential barriers to communication.
5. Recognize trust as the foundation for all effective interaction.
6. Describe the electronic health record (EHR) and the personal health record (PHR).
7. Determine when the use of situation, background, assessment, and recommendation (SBAR) is beneficial.
8. State important legal aspects of chart ownership, access, confidentiality, and patient care documentation.
9. Describe the basic guidelines for and the mechanics of charting.
10. Discuss issues related to computerization in documentation.

KEY TERMS

aggressive communication Occurs when an individual interacts with another in an overpowering and forceful manner to meet one's own personal needs at the expense of the other

assertive communication Interaction that takes into account the feelings and needs of the patient, yet honors the technician's rights as an individual

assertiveness One's ability to confidently and comfortably express thoughts and feelings while still respecting the legitimate rights of the patient

auditors People appointed to examine patient charts and health records to assess quality of care

chart (healthcare record) A legal record that is used to meet the many demands of the health, accreditation, medical insurance, and legal systems

charting The process of adding information to the chart

closed posture A more formal, distant stance, generally with the arms, and possibly the legs, tightly crossed

communication A reciprocal process in which messages are sent and received between people

computer on wheels Point-of-care computer devices sometimes housed on wheeled carts

connotative meaning When one sometimes receives a message differently from how the sender meant it to be received

denotative meaning The commonly accepted definition of a particular word

documenting Recording the interventions carried out to meet the patient's needs

electronic health record (EHR) The electronic version of a patient's chart; also known as the electronic medical record (EMR)

electronic medical record (EMR) The electronic version of a patient's chart; also known as electronic health record (EHR)

gestures Movements people use to emphasize the idea they are attempting to communicate

informatics The study of information processing

jargon Commonplace "language" or terminology unique to people in a particular work setting, such as a hospital, or to a specific type of work, such as nursing

Kardex (or Rand) A system used by some facilities to consolidate patient orders and care needs in a centralized, concise way

medication administration record (MAR) The report that serves as the legal record of the drugs administered to a patient at a facility by a healthcare professional

narrative charting Recording of patient care in descriptive form

nomenclature Classification system of technical or scientific names and terminology

nonverbal communication Transmitted without the use of words (either oral or written)

nursing care plan Plan that outlines the proposed nursing care based on the nursing assessment and nursing diagnoses to provide continuity of care

one-way communication Communication in which the sender is in control and expects and gets very little response from the receiver

open posture When one takes a relaxed stance with uncrossed arms and legs while facing the other individual

personal health record An extension of the electronic health record (EHR) that allows patients to input their own information into an electronic database

point of care Taking place at the patient rather than away from the patient; typically at the bedside

posture The way that an individual sits, stands, and moves

quality assurance, assessment, and improvement An audit in healthcare that evaluates services provided and the results achieved compared with accepted standards

receiver The person or people to whom the message is conveyed

recording Recording the interventions carried out to meet the patient's needs

SBAR/traditional (block) chart Situation, background, assessment, and recommendation is a method of communication among healthcare workers and is considered to be a part of documentation

sender One who conveys the message in communication

traditional (block) chart A type of chart that contains different categories, such as admission, history & physical, laboratory, or x-ray. This chart may be electronic or may be in paper form

two-way communication Communication that requires that both the sender and the receiver participate in the interaction

unassertive communication A communication style where one does not stand up for what they feel or believe is right

verbal communication Involves the use of spoken or written words or symbols

OVERVIEW OF COMMUNICATION

For communication to occur, both a sender and a receiver of a message are necessary. The sender is the one who conveys the message, whereas the receiver is the person or people to whom the message is conveyed. The individual who receives the message may be the intended receiver and sometimes an unintended receiver. Consider the following scenario:

The night-shift patient care technician (PCT) reports to the day-shift technician outside Ms. B's room: "Ms. B was on her call light all night. She's a real complainer!" Ms. B overhears the exchange.

The day PCT is the intended receiver, or the one with whom the night PCT means to communicate with regarding Ms. B's behavior. Because Ms. B also hears the statement, she becomes an unintended receiver. Consider the possible effect of this message on the relationship between Ms. B and both PCTs. Negative consequences for the relationship between Ms. B and the PCTs is the possible outcome if Ms. B believes that the day technician shares the night technician's view of her.

Both one-way and two-way communication is possible, and the type of communication that actually occurs depends partly on the roles of the individuals in the interaction. One-way communication is highly structured; the sender is in control and expects and gets very little response from the receiver. A speech to a large audience is an example of one-way communication. One-way communication has very little place in the nurse–patient relationship. Two-way communication requires that both the sender and the receiver participate in the interaction. It allows for exchange between the technician and the patient, and its purpose is to meet the needs of both the technician and the patient and to establish a trusting relationship. One should always strive to seek and accept the patient's input and feedback rather than simply talk to the patient.

Communication is one of the most important aspects of care. Some form of communication occurs each time an interaction takes place. Interactions occur between two groups of people, such as the PCT and the patient, or the PCT and a family member, a physician, or a coworker, or any number of other combinations. Remember that the message that is intended is not always the message that is received. One should strive at all times to communicate effectively and minimize miscommunication.

Communication is a reciprocal process in which messages are sent and received between people (Balzer Riley, 2012). Reciprocal means that it goes both ways. Communication takes both verbal and nonverbal forms and conveys a variety of messages (e.g., information, emotions, humor, acceptance, rejection).

Verbal Communication

Verbal communication involves the use of spoken or written words or symbols. Sometimes words have very different meanings, or connotations, for different people. The connotative meaning of a word is subjective and reflects the individual's perception or interpretation. This means that one sometimes receives a message differently from how the sender meant it to be received. It's all in how the receiver takes the message. It can change based on the person receiving it. The PCT should be aware of the potential for miscommunication attributable to this subjective variation and meaning of this type of communication. Take, for example, the word *stable*. If the nurse informs family members that their loved one's condition is stable, they perhaps may understand that, for the moment, the patient's condition is not deteriorating, or getting worse. On the other hand, they may hear a different message, and not the one that was intended: namely, that the patient is doing well and is out of danger.

Denotative meaning refers to the commonly accepted definition of a particular word. For example, the word *telephone* means essentially the same thing to anyone who is familiar with the English language. The key word here is *familiar*. No guarantee exists that both parties know the word, let alone assign the same definition to it. Consider the situation in which the nurse asks the patient when he or she last voided or had a stool. Although these terms and phrasing are familiar to healthcare professionals, the patient may have no idea that the nurse is asking when he or she last urinated or had a bowel movement. This is an example of the nurse using hospital jargon. Jargon is commonplace "language" or terminology unique to people in a particular work setting, such as a hospital, or to a specific type of work, such as nursing. It is as though the nurse and the patient have different dictionaries for what is thought to be a shared language. The PCT must be cautious of the terminology used when communicating with patients.

Nonverbal Communication

Messages transmitted without the use of words (either oral or written) constitute nonverbal communication.

Nonverbal cues include tone and rate of voice, volume of speech, eye contact, physical appearance, and use of touch. Some degree of nonverbal communication usually accompanies verbal communication. It is important to always be aware of any nonverbal cues given when in the presence of patients. Sometimes odors or sights may cause one to want to wrinkle the face or widen the eyes. This may be perceived by patients as being negative, and may cause embarrassment to them.

Voice

The way the voice is delivered can send messages to persons, specifically with tone, volume, and the rate of speech. Characteristics of people's voices vary depending on such things as their emotions, how familiar or comfortable they are with a situation, their confidence level, and geographic and cultural influences. Meaning cannot be accurately interpreted on the basis of tone, rate, and volume alone. For example, a high-pitched, loud voice and rapid speech may indicate that an individual is frightened, but people also speak that way out of excitement or enthusiasm. In fact, some people always tend to use this speech pattern. You cannot always conclude that one is nervous or excited just on the way one speaks. One should consider the voice characteristics in the context of the situation as a whole so that interpretation of the message is accurate. One must be very observant in communication styles and patterns.

Eye Contact

Eye contact is a component of communication that can influence communication and miscommunication. Generally, when one makes eye contact with someone there is a desire to communicate or interact. However, the nature of the interaction and the results of eye contact are not necessarily always positive. Extended eye contact sometimes implies aggression and arouses anxiety. Rolling of the eyes can communicate a sarcastic response and is often viewed as being rude. On the other hand, the person who maintains eye contact for 2 to 6 seconds during interaction helps involve the other person in what is said without being threatening or intimidating. An absence of eye contact communicates many things: shyness, lack of confidence, disinterest, embarrassment, hurt, deference, and respect. Sensitivity to one's own eye contact and that of others helps with perceiving what is actually occurring in an interaction. Culture significantly affects how people interpret eye contact. Americans view eye contact in a positive manner, whereas some cultures, such as persons of Arabic or Native North American descent, view eye contact as impolite, aggressive, or improper (Maier-Lorentz, 2008).

Physical Appearance

The physical appearance of the participants in an interaction has the potential to greatly influence the perceptions they form of each other. Physical appearance includes the attributes of size, color of skin, dress, grooming, posture, and facial expression. Although often these attributes have absolutely nothing to do with any messages the sender intends to convey, they can have a major impact on the receiver's interpretation. Take, for example, the patient with a personal bias against individuals with numerous tattoos or body piercings. The patient may have difficulty in establishing a trusting and therapeutic relationship with a caregiver that has tattoos or piercings.

A professional appearance conveys pride and competence. How one chooses to dress while on duty sends a strong message to the patient. The PCT who chooses to wear wrinkled uniforms or soiled shoes may risk sending the message that the patient is not worth the time it would take for the technician to look professional. This may lead the patient to view the PCT as uncaring or incompetent.

Many healthcare facilities have adopted specific dress codes to convey professionalism in the workplace (see Chapter 3). Scrubs of one design or color are often worn by specific personnel as a means of communicating to the patient the role of that professional. For example, in some facilities, the nurse may wear one color of scrubs, and the unlicensed assistive personnel (UAP) may wear another. Jewelry, piercings, tattoos, and hair may also be addressed in dress codes within healthcare facilities.

Gestures

Gestures are movements people use to emphasize the idea they are attempting to communicate. Gestures also play a useful role in clarifying. A patient is often better able to express where pain is on the body by pointing to a particular area than trying to describe it in words. However, many gestures affect communication negatively. For example, a PCT who frequently looks at a watch while caring for a patient conveys disinterest in what the patient is saying or that the technician has a limited amount of time to spend with the patient. Also, gestures often have very different meanings from individual to individual and from culture to culture. It is essential to be always be aware of gestures the participants use during interactions and to consider the implication of gestures used. Gestures may include hand movements, shrugging of the shoulders, or shaking/nodding of the head.

Posture

The way that an individual sits or stands is called posture. Posture has the potential to convey warmth and acceptance or distance and disinterest. A person is considered to display an open posture when taking a relaxed stance with uncrossed arms and legs while facing the other individual. A slight shift in body position toward an individual, a smile, and direct eye contact are all consistent with open posturing and convey warmth and caring (Balzer Riley, 2012). Closed posture is a more formal, distant stance, generally with the arms, as well as possibly the legs, tightly crossed. A person often interprets closed posture as disinterest, coldness, and even nonacceptance. This may make the patient feel as if the PCT does not want to be there. Standing at the bedside looking down at the patient in the bed places the PCT in a position of authority and control. The patient is likely to experience this as intimidating and condescending. Whenever possible, the PCT should be at the same level as the patient during conversations; this is especially important with pediatric patients. Sitting at the bedside in a relaxed and open posture is one example (Fig. 4.1). Sometimes it is necessary to kneel down in order to be at the same eye level of the patient. It is also necessary with pediatric patients to remove white lab coats, as they can frighten young children. The media has portrayed those in white lab coats to be the ones who deliver the treatment, and in some cases, this can be viewed as causing harm. Although this is in no way accurate, a person may have experience only with seeing television shows that portray this. By removing the white lab coat and assuming an eye-level approach with relaxed posture, the patient may feel more comfortable with the person providing the care.

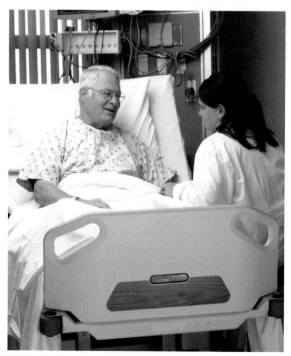

FIGURE 4.1 Open posture. (From Cooper G: *Foundations and adult health nursing*, ed 7, St. Louis, 2015, Mosby.)

Consistency of Verbal and Nonverbal Communication

No definitive studies demonstrate what percentage of communication is verbal or nonverbal; however, most communication experts believe that nonverbal communication makes up the largest percentage of our communication. People choose their verbal communication. Oftentimes, the nonverbal communication comes spontaneously, unless thought about first. Nonverbal communication is very powerful. If nonverbal cues are inconsistent or incongruent with the verbal message, the nonverbal message is most likely the one received. At the very least, this difference between what is seen and what is heard is frequently the cause of misinterpretation and misunderstanding. The following scenario is an example of incongruence between what the PCT is stating and what he or she is demonstrating.

Technician N has been having a very busy morning. While trying to get Ms. D ready to go to surgery, technician N has been interrupted several times by staff members asking for help or advice. Now Mr. R, a patient also assigned to technician N, has put on his call light. As she enters Mr. R's room in an obvious hurry, Mr. R states, "I'm very sorry to bother you, but could you refill my water pitcher?" Technician N grabs the pitcher from the bedside stand and takes it to the sink, while muttering through tight lips, "It's no bother, Mr. R. I'm happy to do it!"

The verbal words spoken by the technician are quite appropriate. However, the nonverbal cues are "speaking" much louder than her words, and Mr. R is sure to pick up on her anger and frustration from her posture, tone of voice, and facial expression. How is it possible for him to really believe that he has not been a bother and that the technician is "happy" to help him?

STYLES OF COMMUNICATION

The manner, or style, in which a message is communicated greatly affects the mood and the overall outcome of an interaction. Every time an interaction occurs between a healthcare provider and a patient, the tone is set for the relationship. The style of communication demonstrated is often what makes the difference between a positive or negative interaction.

Assertive Communication

Assertiveness is one's ability to confidently and comfortably express thoughts and feelings while still respecting the legitimate rights of the patient. An assertive communication style is interaction that takes into account the feelings and needs of the patient, yet honors the technician's rights as an individual (Box 4.1). It

Box 4.1   Assertive Communication

Communicating assertively means the following:
- Being skilled in a variety of communication strategies and able to express your thoughts and feelings in a way that simultaneously protects your rights and those of others
- Having a positive attitude about communicating directly and honestly
- Feeling comfortable and in control of anxiety, tenseness, shyness, or fear
- Feeling confident that you can conduct yourself in a self-respecting way while still respecting others
- Honoring the fact that you and the other person both have rights

Characteristics of an assertive patient care technician are as follows:
- Appears self-confident and composed
- Maintains eye contact
- Uses clear, concise speech
- Speaks firmly and positively
- Speaks genuinely, without sarcasm
- Is unapologetic
- Takes initiative to guide situations
- Gives the same message verbally and nonverbally

From Balzer Riley J: Communication in nursing, ed. 7, St. Louis, 2012, Mosby.

makes interactions more even sided and has positive benefits for all involved (Balzer Riley, 2012).

Aggressive Communication

Aggressive communication occurs when an individual interacts with another in an overpowering and forceful manner to meet one's own personal needs at the expense of the other. Aggressive communication is destructive and nontherapeutic. In the situation just described, technician N responds to Mr. R in an aggressive manner. Neither party benefits from such an interaction. After the fact, technician N most likely feels guilty and disrespectful for having responded to Mr. R in this harsh manner, and Mr. R undoubtedly feels humiliated and unworthy.

Another choice for technician N, although not a favorable one, was to respond unambiguously to Mr. R but in an unassertive communication style. In this style, the technician agrees to do what the patient requests, even though doing so creates additional problems and interrupts her workflow. Use of this style sacrifices one's legitimate personal rights to the needs of the patient, and there is a price to pay: resentment experienced by one or both parties in the scenario.

Imagine that technician N had responded like this to Mr. R's request to have his water pitcher refilled: "Well, I'm really busy right now, but . . . well, I guess I can do it if I hurry. I just don't know how I'm ever going to get my other patient ready for surgery in time. Here, give me your pitcher."

This interaction is much like the previous one, although more out in the open. The problem with this interaction is that no one really benefits from the interaction. Mr. R now has fresh water but probably feels like he has imposed on the staff unduly. Perhaps he even feels angry thinking that his needs are not as important as those of another patient. Technician N now is even further behind than before and is likely to feel resentment toward Mr. R and as guilty or ashamed as before for giving Mr. R the impression he is a "bother."

The most effective way to address the situation is with an assertive communication style. Perhaps the interaction sounds like this: "Mr. R, if you don't mind waiting about 10 minutes, I will be glad to fill your water pitcher with fresh ice and water. If you need it filled before that, I can ask one of the other nursing assistants to fill it for you now."

With assertive communication, the needs of both technician N and Mr. R can be met, with neither of them feeling unworthy, belittled, resentful, or guilty.

ESTABLISHING A THERAPEUTIC RELATIONSHIP

A therapeutic caregiver–patient interaction is one in which the PCT demonstrates caring, sincerity, empathy, and trustworthiness. If the patient senses that the caregiver is not being genuine in conveying these feelings, a therapeutic, trusting relationship does not develop. If one appears hurried or detached from the interaction, a message is sent that the patient is not as important as the other things on the technician's mind, which very likely leaves the patient feeling frustrated and diminished in self-worth.

The PCT must ensure that the *patient* is the focus of each interaction, not the equipment or the task. Upon entering a patient's room, the PCT should look at and address the patient before assessing or adjusting any equipment. In addition, the PCT should be diligent in following through with commitments. If the PCT has promised to assist the patient with a bath in 15 minutes, then this commitment should be carried out. If this is not going to be possible, the PCT should explain this to the patient and establish another mutually agreeable plan for completing the bath. Failure to follow through on commitments undermines the relationship and diminishes trust.

Trust is essential for effective caregiver–patient interaction to occur. Much of the information that the patient shares with the nurse is personal and often highly sensitive. The patient must be able to trust the PCT to treat the information confidentially and share it only with those individuals who need it to provide safe and competent care for the patient. Although confidentiality is

vitally important to maintain, certain limits exist. The PCT is obligated to report a patient's statement of intent to do self-harm or to harm others. This obligation should be made clear to all patients.

Be careful to maintain professional boundaries in caregiver–patient relationships. Sharing of personal information, such as address and phone number, is not advisable. Doing so often leads to situations that the PCT is not prepared to handle.

DOCUMENTATION

The chart (healthcare record) has never been more important in the healthcare system than it is today; it is a legal record that is used to meet the many demands of the health, accreditation, medical insurance, and legal systems. What is recorded on the chart can make the difference in whether or not the healthcare system will get paid, and perhaps how much they will get paid. It also is the record to show that effective care has been given. If vital signs are not documented, then they are considered to have not been taken. If the patient begins to show signs of a complication, the chart is the document that will reflect what led up to this complication. Any incomplete or missing documentation can affect the care the patient receives.

The process of adding information to the chart is called charting, recording, or documenting. Documenting involves recording the interventions carried out to meet the patient's needs. In the charting of interventions, documenting the type of intervention, the time care was given, and the signature and title of the person providing care is essential. Anything written or printed that is a record or proof of activities will, by definition, play a role in this process. Although many details are necessary to remember when documenting in the chart, the process is not difficult but is often time-consuming. Good documentation reflects the character of the person doing the documenting. Documenting something that was not truly done is an issue of one's integrity and is dishonest. Documenting more than was done is also an issue of integrity and shows one is dishonest. Always document exactly what was done and nothing more. Never document something you plan to do until it is done. Documentation is necessary for the evaluation of patient care and for reimbursement, or payment, for the cost of care provided. Whether or not an insurance company or Medicare/Medicaid pays for the patient's care can be dependent on the quality (how accurate) and quantity (how much) of documentation. In the past, all documenting in the patient's health records involved written documentation with an ink pen. Today, a vast majority of facilities use some form of electronic health record (EHR), also sometimes referred to as electronic medical record (EMR). EHRs are used in various settings, including hospitals, long-term care settings, healthcare provider's offices, clinics, and home care agencies.

The PCT must understand how to use medical records effectively and efficiently. This chapter covers the purposes for health records, the common types of records, the basic guidelines and rules for documentation, and legal concerns. The knowledge of these guidelines and the ability to chart completely, accurately, and legibly (when using written records) are requirements for certification and employment of the PCT.

Purposes of Patient Records

There are several reasons for documenting in the patient record. The five basic purposes for accurate and complete patient records are (1) documented communication, (2) permanent record for accountability, (3) legal record of care, (4) teaching, and (5) research and data collection.

The patient's chart provides a concise, accurate, and permanent record of past and current medical and nursing problems, plans for care, care given, and the patient's responses to various treatments. The record facilitates accurate communication and continuity of care among all members of the healthcare team. Continuity of care means that the patient is being cared for without a lapse, or gap. It takes the entire healthcare team to ensure that patient care is continuous.

Recorded information is not as easily lost or altered as the spoken word. Proper charting covers all areas of patient needs and concerns: physical, emotional, psychological, social, and spiritual. If something is said or discussed with patients that may affect their care, it is important that this information is documented. Remember, the patient record is a legal record, and can be used in a court setting if there were ever a liability lawsuit.

This permanent record is sometimes used by various governmental and other agencies to evaluate the institution's patient care, to justify cost reimbursement for care provided, and to establish or review accreditation. Current regulations require chart audits (review of specific chart components for completion and appropriateness) by officially appointed auditors (people appointed to examine patient charts and health records to assess quality of care). Auditors check to see whether all ordered care was charted as given and whether responses to specific care plan items and treatments are noted. Institutions also have specific procedures to provide for quality assurance, assessment, and improvement, which is an audit in healthcare that evaluates services provided and the results achieved compared with accepted standards. Accurate and legible records are the only means institutions have to prove that they are providing care to meet patient needs and established standards. Remember, saying you have done something is not the same as documenting you have done it.

The patient chart or health record is a legal document; when necessary and appropriate, it is used in court proceedings. Although the physician or institution owns the original record, lawyers and courts are able to gain access to it; therefore it is important to chart in a very detailed manner to protect those involved in inpatient care.

Patient health records are also used for teaching. Students in the healthcare professions learn more quickly and easily if examples of good charting are shared. Individuals also learn from their mistakes and the mistakes of others. Be an example to others by choosing to document well, using words that appropriately describe what you see.

ELECTRONIC HEALTH RECORD

In many healthcare settings, the EHR facilitates delivery of patient care and allows for more data analysis to be done so that the care can be coordinated. No longer do physicians have to flip through a paper chart to determine if the patient is getting progressively worse or better, according to their vital signs or their fluid status. EHRs contain information that is identical to that found in traditional records but eliminate repetitive entries and allow more freedom of access to the electronic database. It is much quicker for a physician to click through multiple screens that contain days and days of patient information versus having to search for it within page after page of a paper-based chart. Using an EHR, trends can be identified and color-coded to draw attention to them. For example, if someone's heart rate was 80 yesterday morning, then 95 at 3 PM in the afternoon, and then 100 at 11 PM, that is showing an upward trend. In general, EHRs increase efficiency, consistency, and accuracy and decrease costs. Legibility is an additional benefit of these systems, as the typed word is always neat and without question as to what it is. This is not the same as with the written word. Written words are dependent on someone's handwriting, spelling, and sentence structure. These factors are removed with use of the EHR.

The scope and its use of EHR for documentation in healthcare agencies varies depending on the agency. In addition to documentation of care and interventions, most healthcare agencies have incorporated the EHR into information systems for the management of admissions, billing, and the communication of orders for diet, pharmacy, and diagnostic tests. Use of these information systems allow departments within an institution to interact in a more timely fashion, and it provides a database for research and quality assurance (The Office of the National Coordinator for Health Information Technology [ONC] Office of the Secretary, United States Department of Health and Human Services, 2014).

It also makes it easier for PCTs to serve the patients, perhaps through ordering them something to eat or drink, or entering a lab specimen that needs to be analyzed. In addition, agency-wide computer information systems are more efficient because information entered in the system can be automatically transferred to other areas. In regard to patient care documentation, information systems often include options for generating individualized care plans, automated Kardex forms, and acuity levels and medication administration records (MARs). Although the terms *EMR* and *EHR* are often used interchangeably, a key difference between the EHR and the EMR is that the EHR has the ability to exchange patient data not only within a facility, but also from one facility to another; the EMR typically is set up to exchange patient data within a particular facility (National Alliance for Health Information Technology, 2008).

EHR systems vary in the way they are accessed, depending on the facility. Some systems permit computer input only at the nurse's station; some facilities have bedside systems, also referred to as point-of-care systems; and others use handheld systems that may fit in your pocket. Point-of-care systems are sometimes housed on wheeled carts referred to as a computer on wheels, or COWs (Fig. 4.2). Charting at the bedside saves time and allows current information to be immediately available to all who need it. It is important to always maintain privacy if documenting on a mobile unit, or one that is within view of the patient and family members. Some systems automatically retrieve and record information from electronic devices (e.g., vital signs) and at the same time enter the data in all relevant locations in the record, which cuts down on duplication of effort. In addition, some systems prompt for certain data to be entered, which results in more accurate and complete record keeping.

Electronic charting procedures vary by agency. Data are often recorded in flow-sheet format for easy storage and retrieval. A flow sheet typically has a breakdown of the 24 hours in a day. Activities and vital signs, as well as intake and output, may be included. Some agencies use blank text boxes in which you can type narrative notes in addition to standardized phrases such as "ambulates in hallway," to allow specific and individualized documentation.

Naming conventions, or nomenclature (a classification system of technical or scientific names and terminology), must be considered when choosing computer-based documentation.

The field of medical or nursing informatics (the study of information processing) is constantly evolving, which requires that software programs be updated regularly to stay current with changes in terminology. In addition, considerable time needs to be invested in training personnel, both in charting procedures and the terminology the system uses and in conducting ongoing refresher training. Newly hired personnel need to learn

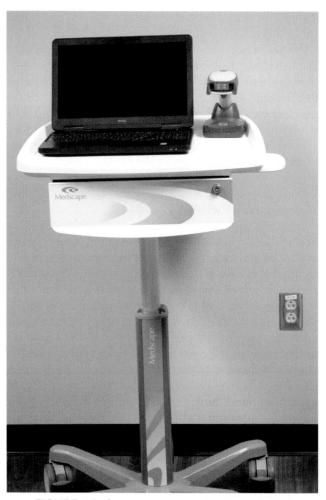

FIGURE 4.2 Computer on wheels. (From Author.)

a new system even if they have already had considerable experience in the field.

In addition to the EHR, a newer concept known as the personal health record (PHR) is an extension of the EHR that allows patients to input their own information into an electronic database. Some outpatient facilities are managing this by allowing the patients to enter their own information by using one of the facility-owned tablets, such as an iPad®. Although the PHR allows for a more complete profile of the patient, issues to consider for the PHR include how the information is going to be stored, who is going to store the information, and what economic costs are involved (Menon, 2012). The PHR may not only contain information submitted by the patient; some systems may allow input of information from other healthcare personnel such as pharmacists, laboratories, and the patient's primary healthcare provider. PHR applications may be managed by various institutions such as private vendors, hospitals, primary care healthcare providers, and insurance companies. These vendors may choose whether or not to charge a fee for storage of this information.

SBAR

SBAR (situation, background, assessment, and recommendation) is a method of communication used among healthcare workers and is considered to be a part of documentation (Kaiser Permanente, 2007). SBAR is considered a safety measure in preventing errors resulting from poor communication during "hand-off" or "handover" interactions, which is the communication that occurs from one shift to the next or when a nurse phones a healthcare provider with information about a patient (Adams, 2012). When a patient is moved from one unit to the other, SBAR is often used to help communicate the patient information to the oncoming healthcare team. SBAR is recognized by The Joint Commission as one method of meeting National Patient Safety Goals (www.jointcommission.org/standards_information/npsgs.aspx).

BASIC GUIDELINES FOR DOCUMENTATION

The quality and accuracy of the documentation is extremely important. Correct choice of words and spelling, grammar, and punctuation, in addition to good penmanship and other writing skills with non–computer-based systems, are critical. The PCT must ensure that information recorded in the chart is clear, concise, complete, and accurate.

The registered nurse (RN) has primary responsibility for each patient's initial admission nursing history, physical assessment, and development of the care plan based on the nursing diagnoses identified. Contributions by all team members during this initial process and during later updating sessions are important.

The forms used to provide documentation of patient care vary based on each healthcare institution's policy. Each facility uses a combination of graphics, care flow sheets, and narrative notes to document observations, care, and responses. The PCT should be sure that his or her notes correlate with the medical orders, Kardex information, and nursing care plan.

Charting Rules

See Box 4.2 for generally accepted documentation rules that provide consistency in documentation between healthcare providers and facilities. These rules also meet the standards expected by the individuals and the agencies that use the charts. Some of the rules apply to handwritten documentation. With a computerized documentation system, generally found with an EHR or EMR, the PCT should follow the guidelines for that particular system.

Box 4.2   Basic Rules for Documentation

- All documents should have the correct patient name, identification number, date of birth, date, and time if appropriate.
- Use only approved abbreviations and medical terms.
- Be timely, specific, accurate, and complete.
- Write legibly (for written documentation).
- Follow rules of grammar and punctuation.
- Fill all spaces; leave no empty lines. Chart consecutively. Go line by line. Do not indent left margin.
- Chart after care is provided, not before.
- Chart as soon and as often as necessary.
- Chart only your own care, observations, and teaching; never chart for anyone else.
- Use direct quotes when appropriate.
- Be objective in charting: only what you hear, see, feel, and smell.
- Describe each item as you see it: for example, "white metal ring with clear stone" (rather than "diamond ring"). Do not speculate, guess, or assume.
- Chart facts; avoid judgmental terms and placing blame.
- Document only what you observe, not opinions. Never use charting to accuse someone else.
- Sign each block of charting or entry as directed by the agency policy.
- When a patient leaves a unit (e.g., to go to x-ray, laboratory, or office), chart the time and the method of transportation on departure and return.
- Chart all ordered care as given or explain the deviation (nothing by mouth [NPO] for laboratory, off unit, refused, etc.).
- Note patient response to treatments and response to analgesics or other special medications.
- If charting in ink, use only hard-pointed, permanent black ink pens; no erasures or correcting fluids are allowed on charts for written patient records.
- If a charting error is made, identify the error according to facility policy and make the correct entry.
- When making a late entry, note it as a late entry and then proceed with your notation: for example, "Late entry _____," or as dictated by the facility policy.
- Follow each institution's policies and procedures for charting.
- Avoid use of generalized empty phrases such as "status unchanged" or "had good day."

Legal Basis of Documentation

Accurate documentation is one of the best defenses in the event of legal claims associated with patient care. To limit liability and the chance of being sued for wrongdoing, the documentation must clearly indicate that individualized care was provided to a patient based on the physician's orders, delegation of the nurse, and following established policy and procedure. The record has to describe exactly what happened to a patient. This is best achieved when the PCT charts immediately after providing care. Although care may have been excellent, in a court of law, if the care was not documented, it would be considered by a jury that the care was not provided. It is the PCT's responsibility to document vital signs, intake and output measurements, and any other delegated tasks by the registered nurse in the medical record.

Inappropriate documentation may lead to malpractice. Some examples of inappropriate documentation include not charting the correct time that events occurred or that an event occurred at all, charting care in advance, and documenting incorrect data. Box 4.2 lists some legal guidelines for documentation that the PCT should keep in mind. Again, some of the rules apply to handwritten documentation. With a computerized documentation system, the PCT should follow the guidelines for that particular system.

Delegation and Documentation Box 4.1

- Never document something that someone else did; always document exactly what you did and nothing more.
- Be as clear and specific as possible in your documentation. Use correct grammar.
- When you are documenting in a patient's room, protect the screen from being visible to visitors in the room as a way to protect the patient's privacy.
- When you are done documenting, always log completely out of the system so that the next person will be unable to view any of your documentation.

Common Medical Abbreviations and Terminology

The PCT must use standard medical abbreviations and terminology to document effectively. The PCT should avoid use of abbreviations or terms that are not standard or approved for use in the documentation system. Use of complete words is always better if one is unsure of the proper abbreviation. Many abbreviations that were once accepted are now considered "abbreviations to avoid" because of the probability of error and misunderstanding with these words or terms. Most facilities have a published list of generally accepted medical abbreviations and the terms approved for use in charting. The PCT should be aware that the use of abbreviations can be confusing if approved abbreviations for a facility are not used (e.g., "BS": breath sounds, or bowel sounds, or blood sugar?). In addition, abbreviations that are used for communication outside of the healthcare facility, such as cell phone texting abbreviations, must never be used in patient records. (See Appendix A for a list of commonly used abbreviations and The Joint Commission's list of abbreviations to avoid.)

METHODS OF RECORDING

The documentation system selected by a healthcare facility optimally reflects the philosophy of the facility and the way care is implemented. Professionally executed charting is legal proof of care given and communicates the patient's status and progress. The nursing process shapes the approach to providing care, and in turn, effective documentation of the care the nurse provides reflects the nursing process. As a PCT, the nursing process is followed through delegation of the nurse.

Traditional Chart

The traditional (block) chart is divided into sections or blocks. Emphasis is placed on specific sections (or sheets for noncomputerized charts) of information. Typical sections are the following: admission information, physician's orders, progress notes, history and physical examination data, nurse's admission information, care plan and nursing notes, graphics, and laboratory and x-ray examination reports. The order, the content, and the number of the sections vary among institutions. The healthcare team uses flow sheets, graphics, and narrative charting (recording of patient care in descriptive form) (Fig. 4.3) to chart observations, care, and responses. Narrative charting is used for both computerized and noncomputerized nurse's notes. Narrative charting includes the data (subjective, objective, or both) about the basic patient need or problem, whether anyone has been contacted or consulted, care and treatments provided (implementation), and the patient's response to treatment (evaluation). This often follows the nursing process, which may be known as the care plan. The nursing process has five categories: assessment, diagnosis, planning, implementation, and evaluation. The descriptive data, such as vital signs, surgical incision, and drain placement, are typically categorized as assessment. The problems, or focus of care, are included under diagnosis. The goals for patient are categorized under planning. The interventions the PCT may be assisting with are part of implementation, and how a patient responds to those interventions comes under evaluation. Information obtained from the nurse's assessment of the patient is organized during the complete head-to-toe assessment.

Record-Keeping Forms and Examples

Each healthcare facility may use a variety of forms to organize the medical record documentation easily and

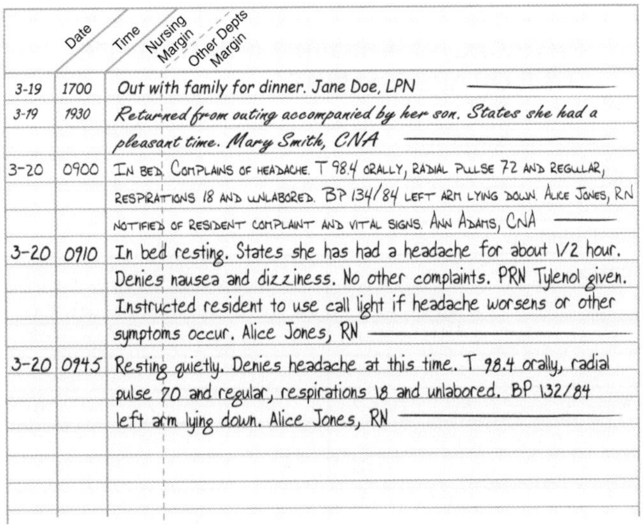

Date	Time	Nursing Margin / Other Depts Margin
3-19	1700	Out with family for dinner. Jane Doe, LPN
3-19	1930	Returned from outing accompanied by her son. States she had a pleasant time. Mary Smith, CNA
3-20	0900	In bed. Complains of headache. T 98.4 orally, radial pulse 72 and regular, respirations 18 and unlabored. BP 134/84 left arm lying down. Alice Jones, RN notified of resident complaint and vital signs. Ann Adams, CNA
3-20	0910	In bed resting. States she has had a headache for about 1/2 hour. Denies nausea and dizziness. No other complaints. PRN Tylenol given. Instructed resident to use call light if headache worsens or other symptoms occur. Alice Jones, RN
3-20	0945	Resting quietly. Denies headache at this time. T 98.4 orally, radial pulse 70 and regular, respirations 18 and unlabored. BP 132/84 left arm lying down. Alice Jones, RN

FIGURE 4.3 Electronic health records. (From Sorrentino SA, Remmert LN: *Mosby's Textbook for Nursing Assistants*, ed 9, St. Louis, 2017, Elsevier.)

quickly, yet comprehensively. Many forms help eliminate the need to duplicate data repeatedly in the nursing notes. The forms present several types of information in a format more accessible than compilation of all progress notes. Most of the forms are self-explanatory as to the type of information required from the nurse (Figs. 4.4).

The nursing Kardex (or Rand) system is a system used by some facilities to consolidate patient orders and care needs in a centralized, concise way. The cumulative care file or Rand is kept at the nursing station for quick reference or is part of the EHR or EMR. Forms vary among institutions based on information required for care. Historically, this was either a flip chart or a Rolodex type of categorized patient information. This information may be categorized according to patient room number or by alphabetizing of the patients' last names (Fig. 4.5).

The nursing care plan (plan that outlines the proposed nursing care based on the nursing assessment and nursing diagnoses to provide continuity of care) is developed to meet the nursing care needs of a patient. Many facilities use standardized care plans for certain conditions or surgeries; however, individualization of the plan of care based on each patient's own needs or circumstances is also important. This kind of plan, developed by nurses for communication among nurses and other members of the healthcare team, is based on nursing assessment and nursing diagnosis. Standardized nursing care plans include the pertinent nursing diagnoses, goals, and plans for care and specific actions for care implementation and evaluation.

Incident Reports

An *incident report* (form used to document any event not consistent with the routine operation of a healthcare unit or the routine care of a patient) (Fig. 4.6) is sometimes necessary to document an unplanned occurrence within a healthcare facility. For example, if a nurse neglects to give a medication or treatment or gives an incorrect dose of a drug, an incident report must be filed. Either of these events has the potential to cause injury. Incident reports are also filled out for any unusual event in a hospital (e.g., injuries to a patient, visitor, or hospital personnel). Many staff members are reluctant to fill out these forms, but this information helps the facility risk manager and unit managers to track occurrences of incidents. One of the benefits of tracking particular incidents is to prevent future problems through education and other corrective measures. If the incident report is completed for a patient, it is typically completed by the nurse. If the incident report is completed because of a personal injury, then the staff member who experienced the personal injury would complete the report.

Injury & Illness Prevention Box 4.1

- Always report any injuries that occur with you or your patients.
- Before you go to your own doctor after a work-related injury, be sure that you have completed an incident report and have contacted the employee health or human resources department of your facility; often they have specific doctors you must see if it is a work-related injury or illness.
- Even if you feel okay after an injury, it is important to complete an incident report.
- Sometimes it is the completion of incident reports that actually prevents future injuries of the same kind.

Text continued on p. 47

PHYSICAL ASSESSMENT (HEAD TO TOE)
TIME OF ASSESSMENT: _____

	NOTES:
1. NEUROLOGIC: Level of consciousness	
Confused	
Oriented x 1. person 2. place 3. time 4. purpose	
PERRLA—Babinski: Positive or Negative	
Hand strength: Strong or Weak	
Leg movement: Strong or Weak	
2. INTEGUMENTARY	
Condition: Moist or Dry	
Temperature:	
Turgor:	
Tenting:	
Incision	
Location:	
Without erythema:	
Exudate:	
Sutures/staples intact	
Sutures/staples not intact	
Open wound:	
Hemovac: Color Amt	
Davol: Color Amt	
Jackson-Pratt: Color Amt	
Penrose: Color Amt	
Wound vac: Color Amt	
Dressing	
Clean & dry:	
Needs change:	
3. CARDIOVASCULAR	
Apical pulse rate:	
Capillary refill <3 sec: Yes or No	
Pedal pulses (1-4+): L & R	
Pedal edema (1-4+): L & R	
Nonpitting edema:	
IV	
Solution:	
Peripheral:	
Central line:	
Rate:	
Site & condition:	
4. RESPIRATORY	
Anteriorly:	
Posteriorly:	
O_2 Saturation level: %	
Crackle:	
Wheezes: Sonorous or Sibilant	
Pleural friction rub:	

FIGURE 4.4 Flowsheets and charts. (From Cooper G: *Foundations and adult health nursing,* ed 7, St. Louis, 2015, Mosby.)

Dyspnea Tachypnea Orthopnea	
O$_2$ Therapy: type:	
Rate: Liters per:	
Incentive spirometer	
Inspiratory capacity: mL	
Chest tube to H$_2$O seal _____ cm	
Chest tube to H$_2$O seal and wall suction _____ mm Hg	
Color and amount _____ mm Hg	
5. GASTROINTESTINAL	
Appetite _____ Type of diet _____	
Dentures: Yes or No	
Oral fluid intake:	
Bowel sounds *4:	
Active Hyper Hypo Absent	
Distention Tympanic Tenderness	
Flatulence	
BM #: Color: Consistency:	
Stoma pink & viable: Yes or No	
N/G	
Amt: mL	
Color of drainage	
Peg tube _____	
Site condition _____ Flush _____ Feeding _____	
Gastrostomy tube _____	
Site condition _____ Flush _____ Feeding _____	
Jejunostomy _____	
Site condition _____ Flush _____ Feeding _____	
6. URINARY	
Output amount: _____ hours of output _____	
Color:	
Odor:	
Catheter	
Type: Foley Ureterostomy	
Suprapubic Nephrostomy	
Urostomy	
CBI credit:	
True urine:	
7. MOBILITY	
Activity level:	
Bed rest. chair. up with assistance. walker.	
crutches. cane	
Up ad lib: Yes or No	
Gait: Unsteady or Steady	
Level of tolerance:	
Traction: Kind: Weight:	

FIGURE 4.4, cont'd

Continued

8. REPRODUCTIVE	
Prostate problems: Yes or No	
Hysterectomy: Yes or No	
Breast—monthly breast self-exam: Yes or No	
Mastectomy:	
____ Rt ____ Left ____ Appearance	
Vaginal drainage: Yes or No	
9. SENSORY	
Hard of hearing: Yes or No	
Hearing aid: Yes or No	
Glasses	
Contacts	

VITALS	VITALS	ADLs
TIME TAKEN: hr	TIME TAKEN: hr	BED BATH-TIME:
Temp:	Temp:	Supplies needed: 1 linen bag
Pulse:	Pulse:	2-3 towels
Respirations:	Respirations:	2-3 washcloths
Blood pressure:	Blood pressure:	4-5 disposable washcloths
How taken:	How taken:	Soap, shampoo, deodorant, comb
Level of pain:	Level of pain:	1 disposable garbage bag
NOTES:	NOTES:	Cotton swabs
		Orange stick/nail file
		Lip conditioner
		Toothbrush, toothettes, toothpaste
		Denture supplies
CHECK:	CHECK:	Other supplies needed by pt:
Water filled & cool	Water filled & cool	
Bed straightened	Bed straightened	
Patient comfortable?	Patient comfortable?	LINEN CHANGE OF BED:
Patient requests:	Patient requests:	1 linen bag (if not doing @ bedtime)
		1 contour sheet
		1 flat sheet
		1 pull sheet
		Pillow case(s) - How many pillows?
		1 blanket
		1 bedspread
		Add'l supplies needed for pt:
___ ALL INFO CHARTED	___ ALL INFO CHARTED	___ ALL INFO CHARTED

FIGURE 4.4, cont'd

Date Activities	Date Elimination	Date Supportive	Date Wounds	Date Hygiene	Date	Diet
7/5 Bed rest 7/6 BRP ___ Dangle ___ Chair ___ w/Chair ___ Crutched ___ Walker ___ Ad. Lib. ___ Turn 7/7 Up with Assistance	7/5 Catheter dc'd 7/6 ___ Commode ___ Adult Diaper ___ Colostomy Old/New ___ Ileostomy Old/New ___ Hematest ___ Save Stools ___ Strain all Urine ___ Urostomy 7/5 Intake/Output ___ Ileo Conduit ___ Enema/Flush PRN ___ CBI	___ Cradle/Footboard ___ Overhead Frame ___ TED Hose ___ Telemetry #___ ___ NG Tube ___ Tracheotomy ___ Traction ___ Oxygen ___ Siderails ___ Restraints ___ Egg Crate 7/5 IV's/Int. lock ___ Isolation ___ PCA Pump ___ Oral Suction ___ K-Pad	___ Packing ___ Hemo drain ___ Drain 7/5 Incision ___ Suction ___ Solcotrans 7/5 T-Tube ___ Chest Tube	7/6 Bed Bath 7/7 Assist ___ Self Bath ___ Shower/Tub ___ Sitz ___ Towel Bath ___ Oral ___ Hair ___ Skin/Decubitus	7/6	Clear liquids

Snacks / Beverages:
- B Hot tea
- D Hot tea
- S Hot tea

Food Allergies: milk

LABORATORY and RADIOLOGY

7/5 Chest x-ray ECG CBC   7/7 Chest x-ray UA/C&S

DATE	TREATMENTS	DISC.
	DAILY WEIGHT SCALE	
7/5	Incentive spirometer q 4 hr while awake.	
7/5	Vital signs q 4 hr.	
7/5	Turn, cough, and deep breath q 2 hr.	
7/5	Reinforce dressings PRN.	
7/6	Chg. abdominal dressings PRN.	
7/6	Record T-tube drainage.	

CONTACT (next of kin)
W.L. Spaur - husband
534-3974
Chaplain/Minister
G Timmons

BLUE DOT:

RECENT/PRESENT SURGERY:
Open Cholecystectomy 7/5/14

ADDITIONAL DIAGNOSIS:
UTI 7/7

| Room: 348A | Age: 59 DOB 11/1/1954 | Name: Serbane, Donna M. | Sex: Fe | S (M) W.D. | Religion Prot | Diagnosis: Cholelithiasis & Cholecystitis | Attending Physician: D. Janeston, MD | Consulting Physician: J.W. Richtey, MD |

FIGURE 4.5 Forms. (From Cooper G: *Foundations and adult health nursing*, ed 7, St. Louis, 2015, Mosby.)

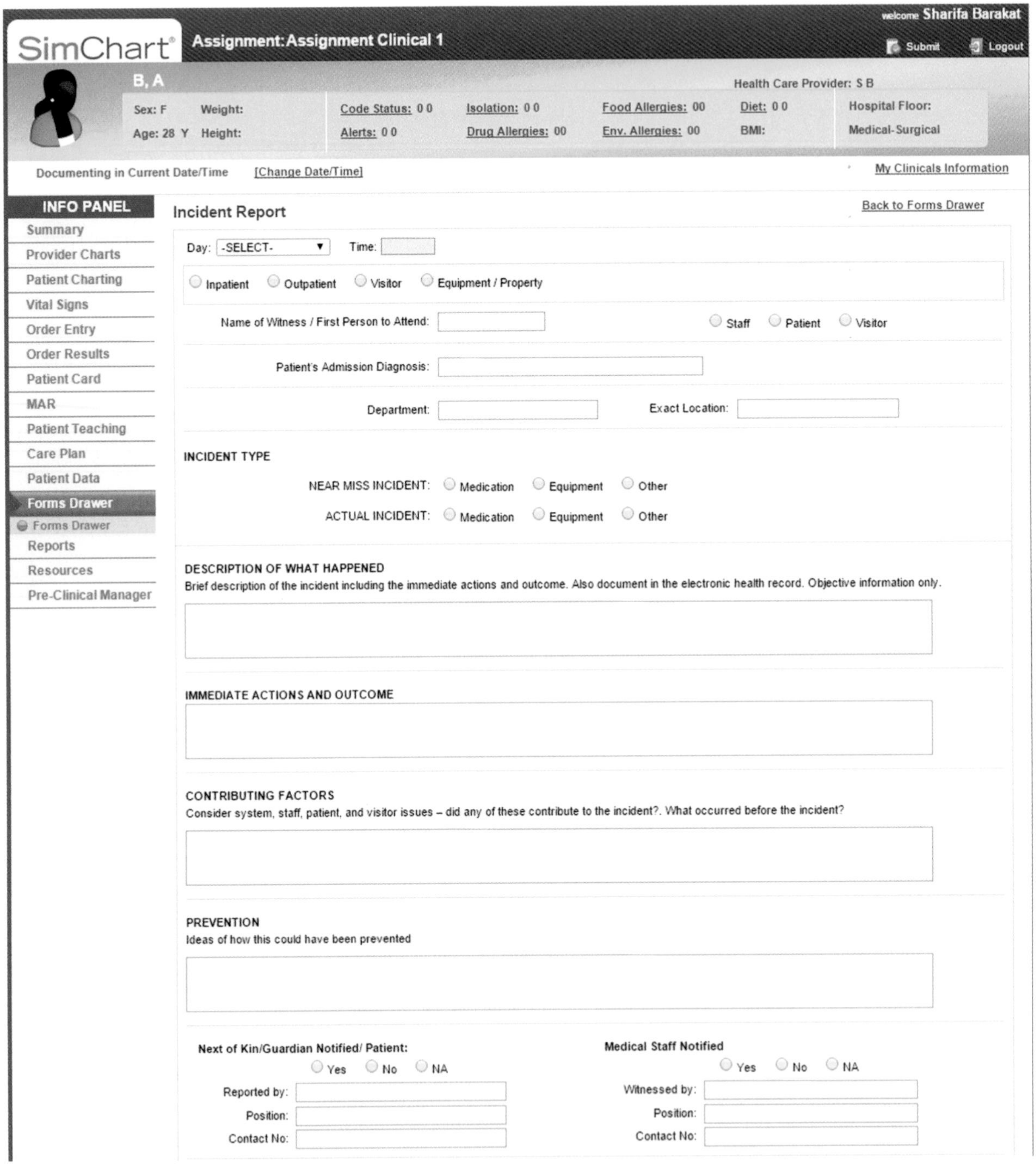

FIGURE 4.6 Electronic incident report. (From SimChart. Copyright 2016 by Elsevier, www.evolve.elsevier.com.)

MEDICAL REPORT
Document patient's assessment and list investigations and treatments. Also document in electronic health record. Objective data only.

Name: [   ]
Designation: [   ]
Day / Time: [-SELECT- ▼] [   ]

STAFF MEMBER RESPONSIBLE FOR AREA AT TIME OF THE INCIDENT
Objective data only.

Has incidence been recorded in the electronic medical record?
○ Yes   ○ No   ○ NA

Name: [   ]
Designation: [   ]
Day / Time: [-SELECT- ▼] [   ]

UNIT MANAGER or DEPARTMENT HEAD:
Document what steps have been taken to prevent reoccurrence

Did the incident occur in another department or is another department responsible?
○ Yes   ○ No   ○ NA

Name: [   ]
Designation: [   ]
Date / Time: [-SELECT- ▼] [   ]

UNIT / DEPARTMENT where incident occurred
(If different from reporting department) Document what steps have been taken to prevent reoccurrence

Name: [   ]
Designation: [   ]
Day / Time: [-SELECT- ▼] [   ]

[Save]   [Print]   [Complete and Submit]   [Cancel]

FIGURE 4.6, cont'd

SPECIAL ISSUES IN DOCUMENTATION

Record Ownership and Access

The original healthcare record or chart is the property of the institution or the healthcare provider. On admission to the healthcare facility, the patient is usually asked to sign a form granting permission to access the record by individuals who have a need to know, such as insurance carriers. Patients may not have immediate access to their full records, depending on the agency policy. Lawyers, with the patient's written permission, are given access to the patient's medical records. Courts have the legal authority to subpoena records for review and use in the case of a lawsuit.

Patients have access rights to their records in most states, but only if they follow the established policy of each facility. A written request for chart access may be required, and institutions can specify a period that allows the physician and the facility to review the record and give a response. Sometimes the institution requires that a staff member or physician be present while the individual looks through the chart to answer questions and to protect the integrity of the record. Patients may also ask for a copy of their medical records. The Office of the National Coordinator for Health Information Technology (ONC), which is part of the Department of Health and Human Services, is continually working on making access to medical records easier and less time-consuming for patients, including electronic access. The department is currently focusing on the issue of personal health records (PHR) (https://www.healthit.gov/).

Confidentiality

Healthcare personnel are mandated to respect the confidentiality of the patient's record. The Patient Care Partnership (information given to patients when admitted to a facility that informs them of their rights and responsibilities) and the law guarantee that medical information is kept private unless the information is needed in providing care or the patient gives permission for others to see it (American Hospital Association, n.d.). The Health Insurance Portability and Accountability Act (HIPAA), an act of Congress passed in 1996, affords certain protections to persons covered by healthcare plans, including continuity of coverage when changing jobs, standards for electronic healthcare transactions, and primary safeguards for the privacy of individually identifiable patient information (see Chapter 1).

Ethics codes of practice also emphasize the PCT's obligation to preserve patient privacy by holding patient information in highest confidentiality. Healthcare personnel may not read a record, or allow others to do so, without a clinical reason, and personnel must hold the information regarding the patient in confidence. Furthermore, trust is necessary for good caregiver–patient relationship, and breaking confidences is a way to lose patient trust. Disregarding policy and procedures and regulations concerning patient confidentiality often leads to job termination, lawsuits, or both (see Chapter 3).

Healthcare students engaged in clinical education are reminded that no information is to leave the clinical site and any documents that have patient-identifying information must be closely guarded at all times within the facility. Any printouts or notes with patient identifiers that have been used by the student must be shredded before leaving the clinical agency. In addition, the student must be vigilant in keeping documents in a safe place when in the clinical agency; documents with patient identifiers should never be left anywhere unattended, such as on bedside tables in the patient's room, at the nurse's station, or on conference room tables. Any information that the student does need for course assignment purposes regarding assigned patients should have no identification information on the documents.

Electronic Documentation Safeguards

Charting using an electronic system is an efficient method of documentation, but the security of the system must be considered when considering legal and ethics issues. Confidentiality, access to information, and inappropriate alterations in patient records are areas of concern. Networks are typically protected by a "firewall" from illegitimate outside access. Some computer systems permit online access from remote sites; however, this further complicates the task of keeping the system secure. To protect the patient's rights and keep the patient's record confidential, anyone who enters data into or views a computerized record has to log on to the system with a secure password. The institution may require the user to change passwords at certain time frames, such as every 90 days, to maintain security. Because the password is assigned only to individual healthcare personnel, any data entered are automatically credited to whoever signed in; thus personnel must never share the password with anyone. The PCT must be sure to log off the system before leaving the terminal to ensure that information about a patient does not remain on the monitor display for others to view. Passwords should never be shared with other staff or written down unless stored in a private, secured space.

It is also necessary to protect computer-generated printouts and prevent the duplication or distribution of information about patients. Most facilities that use computer charting incorporate a system for logging and tracking computer printouts (Box 4.3) and have protocols for shredding the copies that are made. All papers that have protected health information (PHI), such as patient's name, date of birth, and diagnosis should never be taken out of the facility.

Box 4.3   Guidelines for Safe Computer Documentation

- Do not share with another caregiver the password that you use to enter and sign off computer files. (NOTE: A good system requires frequent changes in personal passwords to prevent unauthorized people from accessing and tampering with records. Some facilities use fingerprint scanners instead of passwords.)
- After logging on, never leave the computer terminal unattended without first logging off.
- Follow the correct protocol for correcting errors. To correct an error after storage, follow the facility policy for identifying documentation errors, and then add the correct information and date and initial the entry. If you record information in the wrong chart, follow facility policy for identifying this error.
- Make sure that stored records have backup files, an important safety check. If you inadvertently delete part of the permanent records, type an explanation into the computer file with the date, the time, and your initials, and submit an explanation in writing to your manager.
- Do not leave information about a patient displayed on a monitor where others have the opportunity to see it.
- Follow the agency's confidentiality procedures for documentation.
- Printouts of computerized records also have to be protected. Shredding of printouts and keeping a log that accounts for every copy (whether electronic or printed) of a computerized file that you have generated from the system are ways to keep waste and creation of duplicate records to a minimum and protect the confidentiality of patients.

Use of Fax Machines

Fax machines send written documents over telephone lines to quickly transmit data between healthcare facilities, such as healthcare provider's offices, hospitals, long-term care facilities, and laboratories. HIPAA rules allow for a patient's medical records and information to be faxed. Information can be transmitted from healthcare providers to healthcare facilities and vice versa. For example, laboratory results can be sent via fax, e-mail, or phone to a healthcare provider, or a healthcare provider may fax medical information to another professional for consultation. Various safeguards must be in place to maintain patient confidentiality and privacy. Some facilities require that the sender verify the fax number with the recipient. Similarly, a facility may preprogram frequently faxed numbers into the system to prevent incorrect dialing of the intended number. Although fax machines are still used, they are being used less by facilities that have an EHR system in place.

CHAPTER SUMMARY

Communication is a process that is important to understand. It affects relationships with patients and any member of the healthcare team. A lack of communication can cause a delay in treatment or confusion among those on the healthcare team. It is important to always communicate with patients in a way that they can understand, without using too many medical terms that they do not know. As a PCT, communication with the nurse is important so that the patient can ultimately be taken care of in the best way possible. PCTs carry out written communication through the documentation of care to patients. When each member of the healthcare team communicates in a consistent and clear manner, there is benefit to the patient. It is important to remember that throughout all communications, either regarding patients or personal friends, rights to privacy and confidentiality must be maintained.

Case Scenario

As a PCT, you are responsible for obtaining the vital signs of half the patients on the unit. You have one peer who is obtaining the vital signs for the other half. Your peer grabs a paper towel and a pen and begins rounds. When you question the purpose of the paper towel, the PCT responds stating that it is easier to just write them all down on a paper towel and keep it in his or her pocket than it is to carry a clipboard around. What are your thoughts on this as a documentation practice? Is it safe? Why or why not? Would it be considered acceptable practice?

REVIEW QUESTIONS

1. If a patient care technician uses jargon to describe what the specimen looks like with a patient, the patient should know what that means.
   a. True
   b. False

2. The card system that is used to consolidate patient orders and care needs and is often kept in one central location is known as the
   a. Kardex
   b. Database
   c. SBAR
   d. Personal health record (PHR)

3. Closed posture is generally accepted to mean that one is more accepting, warm, and interested.
   a. True
   b. False

4. If the patient care technician completes a task but forgets to document it in the patient care record, his or her verbal statement saying he or she performed the task will hold up in court if there were a lawsuit.
   a. True
   b. False

5. When a teacher gives a lecture to a large classroom of students, this is known as what type of communication?
   a. Nonverbal communication
   b. Nontherapeutic communication
   c. One-way communication
   d. Two-way communication

The Patient

Understanding the Patient as a Person

LEARNING OBJECTIVES

1. Describe how culture affects the individual.
2. Explain how personal cultural beliefs and practices affect patient relationships.
3. Identify cultural variables that potentially influence health behaviors.
4. Discuss cultural and religious influences as they relate to the older adult.
5. Discuss ethical practices to use when caring for patients.
6. Identify patients with low health literacy.
7. Discuss the use of the interpreter in the care of culturally diverse patients.

KEY TERMS

cultural competence The awareness of one's own cultural beliefs and practices and their relation to those of others, which may be different

culturally competent care Providing care to patients that is individual and specific to their cultural beliefs and practices

culture A set of learned values, beliefs, customs, and practices that are shared by a group and are passed from one generation to another

ethnicity A group of people who share a common social and cultural heritage based on shared traditions, national origin, and physical and biologic characteristics

ethnocentrism A belief that the beliefs and practices of one's particular culture are best

folk health belief system A system that believes health and illness are controlled by supernatural forces; they may be secular or sacred, or a combination of both

health literacy The degree to which people can understand basic health information in order to make their own decisions about treatment options

race A group of people who share biologic physical characteristics

society A nation, community, or broad group of people who establish particular aims, beliefs, or standards of living and conduct

stereotype A generalized expectation about forms of behavior, an individual, or a group

subculture Shares many characteristics with the primary culture but has characteristic patterns of behavior and ideals that distinguish it from the rest of a cultural group

The United States has been described as a "melting pot" of people from many different countries. This description implies that people are so completely blended together that everyone shares the same values, beliefs, health practices, communication styles, and religion. A better example would be to say that the country is like a pot of vegetable soup—many different, but distinct, pieces are combined to form a rich assortment. This assortment makes up our society (a nation, community, or broad group of people who establish particular aims, beliefs, or standards of living and conduct). What's more, the "soup recipe" is no longer what it was; as a result, our societal "flavor" is changing. At the beginning of the 20th century, most immigrants to this country were of European ancestry. Today, according to the 2014 U.S. Census, 37.9% of the population is of African, Asian, Hispanic, American Indian, or some other non-European ancestry (U.S. Census Bureau, www.census.gov).

CULTURE

Culture is a set of learned values, beliefs, customs, and practices that are shared by a group and are passed from one generation to another. Because of the influx of diverse cultures, the United States is rapidly becoming multicultural and multilingual. Many immigrants have come from areas of the world devastated by wars, natural disasters, famine, and poverty. They have had little preparation or time to learn English or American culture before arriving. Many of these immigrant populations have formed subcultures in U.S. society.

Sometimes, separate subcultures exist within a given group. A subculture shares many characteristics with the primary culture but has characteristic patterns of behavior and ideals that distinguish it from the rest of a cultural group. Even among Americans who have lived here for several generations, these subcultures exist. For example, a person who grew up in the mountains of Appalachia has very different cultural practices than a person from New York City. Understanding these practices and acceptance of each person as an individual is the first step in giving holistic care to patients.

Although cultures often differ considerably from one another, they share certain basic characteristics. Box 5.1 identifies four common characteristics of all cultures.

All people within a certain culture do not show the same behaviors. That's because, as people, we are all made differently and are unique. Examples of these differences are as follows:

- Age
- Religion
- Dialect or language spoken
- Gender identity and roles
- Socioeconomic background

Box 5.1	Common Characteristics of Cultures

- Culture is learned, beginning at birth, through language and socialization. Behaviors, values, attitudes, and beliefs are learned within the cultural family system.
- Culture tends to be dynamic and ever changing. Language, traditions, and norms of customs may act as stabilizers for a culture.
- All members of the same cultural group share the patterns that are present in every culture. These include communication, means of economic and physical survival, transportation systems, family systems, social customs and mores, and religious systems. (Morals are accepted traditional customs, moral attitudes, or manners of a particular social group.)
- Culture is an adaptation to specific factors or conditions in a specific location, such as the availability of natural resources. When people are removed from that location, their customs continue even though they are no longer called for in the new setting.

- Geographic location of country of origin or current residence
- Amount and type of interaction between younger and older generations
- Degree to which values in current country are adopted

Cultural influences may be different with each individual. It is best to deliver culturally competent care and avoid stereotyping behaviors. Culture influences each person in various ways. The patient care technician (PCT) is advised to avoid stereotyping members of any cultural group. A stereotype is a generalized expectation about forms of behavior, an individual, or a group. Stereotypes sometimes do and sometimes do not have any relationship to reality.

Cultural Competence and Transcultural Care

Most people look at the world from their own cultural viewpoint. They often believe that the beliefs and practices of their particular culture are best. This belief is called ethnocentrism. The PCT must learn to value the beliefs of others and realize that practices of other cultures can be valuable in healthcare.

When providing care to patients from many different cultures, the PCT is called upon to develop cultural competence, the awareness of one's own cultural beliefs and practices and their relation to those of others, which may be different. One way to identify these beliefs and practices is through a self-assessment, or looking at yourself to determine what your beliefs are toward something or someone. This self-assessment is important. Personal beliefs and practices influence and sometimes put some limits on the ability to care for those from other cultures. Understanding your own personal beliefs allows you to be able to respond to those from different cultures with openness, understanding, and acceptance of cultural differences. The PCT needs to accept that it is not possible to act the same with all patients and still give effective, individualized, holistic care. Rather than ignore the differences, one should include questions about cultural practices during the caregiving process.

Because of the many variations in cultural and sub-cultural practices, culturally appropriate nursing care is a challenge in the 21st century. Understanding these variables and being able to integrate an understanding into all pieces of one's care is known as *transcultural care*. The PCT should strive to achieve a high level of trans-cultural care in day-to-day practices.

It is important to understand that people from different cultures have a variety of practices related to healthcare, treatment methods, and how they respond to illness and death. In many cases, these differences extend to practices related to the lifespan and the ways people of different age groups are cared for. (See Lifespan Considerations: Older Adults Cultural Background section for further information.) In addition, cultural beliefs frequently affect diet and nutrition. Remember to assess areas that are potentially influenced by cultural factors.

Injury & Illness Prevention Box 5.1

- Some herbal and alternative treatments can cause harm to the patient, or can interact with other medications prescribed for the patient. It is important to know any and all treatments the patient is taking. Report any alternative medicines or treatments that are not prescribed by the physician to the nurse.

Lifespan Considerations: Older Adults Cultural Background

- Cultural background has an impact on family dynamics and plays an important role in determining the role and the status of the older person.
- Older adults form a unique cultural group based on shared historical experiences. Often fewer differences are found between two older individuals of diverse cultural backgrounds than between two people of the same culture but from different age groups because of shifts in value systems that occurred over time.
- Some older adults are less tolerant of other cultures as a result of influences or experiences early in their lives, which raises the possibility of misunderstandings and distrust when the caregiver is of a cultural group different from the older person.
- Older people experiencing Alzheimer's disease or other conditions sometimes speak without regard for the cultural sensitivity of others and thus make hurtful comments to caregivers and other people.
- Older adults may value home remedies and cultural practices regarding healthcare and sometimes resist the attempts of caregivers to change even their harmful practices. Practices that are not harmful are left alone out of respect for their wishes.

Learning about cultural differences that exist improves working relationships between members of the healthcare team. In much the same way that this kind of openness helps in caring for patients, it helps in understanding and accepting differences among members of the healthcare team.

RACE AND ETHNICITY

There are various reasons why a person demonstrates a given cultural practice. Perhaps the person is from a foreign country or a region of the United States where that practice is common. Perhaps the person's practice is related to race (a group of people who share biologic physical characteristics) and hereditary factors. Ethnicity refers to a group of people who share a common social and cultural heritage based on shared traditions, national origin, and physical and biologic characteristics. They often share social practices such as language, religion, dress, music, and food. Factors related to culture, race, and ethnicity often overlap, and many people combine a variety of practices related to these. It is important to understand that not everyone in a cultural, racial, or ethnic group has identical practices and that each person should be treated in an individual, holistic manner.

Ethnic and Racial Groups in the United States

The United States is home to people from many cultures. The PCT must not form opinions or make assumptions about a patient's beliefs or practices based on the person's name, skin color, or language.

The census in the United States is taken every 10 years. Changes in the nation's demographic are illustrated in Table 5.1. Significant decreases are noted with the white population accompanied by increases in most other racial groups. The largest increase has occurred in the Hispanic population, which rose from 12.5% to 16.3% of the population between 2000 and 2010. Predictions for the future indicate that this trend will continue

Table 5.1	Changes in Racially Designated and Hispanic Populations, 2000–2010				
	2000		**2010**		
Race	Number	Percent of Total Population	Number	Percent of Total Population	Percent Change
Total population	281,421,906	100.0	308,745,538	100.0	+9.7
White	211,460,626	75.1	223,553,265	72.4	−2.4
Black or African American	34,658,190	12.3	38,929,319	12.6	+12.3
American Indian or Alaska Native	2,475,956	0.9	2,932,248	0.9	+18.4
Asian	10,242,998	3.6	14,674,252	4.8	+43.3
Native Hawaiian and other Pacific Islander	398,835	0.1	540,013	0.2	+35.4
Some other race	15,359,073	5.5	19,107,368	6.2	+24.4
Two or more races	6,826,228	2.4	9,009,073	2.9	+32
Hispanic or Latino (of any race)	35,305,818	12.5	50,477,594	16.3	+3.8

From U.S. Bureau of the Census: Table DP-1: General population and housing characteristics, 2010; and U.S. Bureau of the Census: Profile of general population and housing characteristics, 2010. Available at http://factfinder2.census.gov.

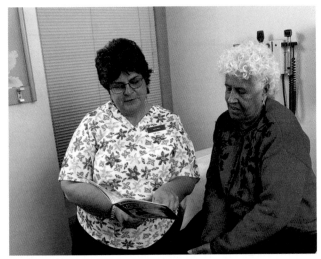

FIGURE 5.1 Manage language barriers with patients who speak a language other than English by providing them written material in their native language, if available. (From Proctor D, Adams A: *Kinn's The Medical Assistant: an applied learning approach*, ed 12, St. Louis, 2014, Saunders.)

and that the minority cultures will, in combination, make up a majority of the U.S. population by the middle of this century (U.S. Census Bureau, Census www .census.gov).

One important aspect of this diversity is the language used to communicate. Many new immigrants from these diverse cultures may not speak English or have a limited comprehension of the language. Often younger members of the family are the ones who help the adults communicate with others outside of the cultural community. Adults frequently bring a young child along as a translator when shopping or seeking healthcare. A professional translator is preferable as opposed to a friend or family member to prevent bias, inaccuracy, or compromises in confidentiality (Fig. 5.1).

COMMUNICATION

The most apparent communication variation is the language spoken. Whether the PCT and the patient can understand each other must be determined. When patients do not understand what is being said, they sometimes say yes or nod the head nonetheless, giving the mistaken impression of agreeing with the PCT. Many people do this to avoid embarrassment or to be polite. You must not assume that the patient or the family understands.

Sometimes, the patient understands some English, or someone else on your unit speaks some of the patient's language. If patients have a poor comprehension of English, they may tire quickly when trying to understand what is being said. Questions and instructions should be kept brief and simple. It is better to come back later and provide more information than to give long explanations. Sometimes, the patient's ability to read written English is better than his or her speaking ability. In such cases, the patient benefits from written explanations accompanied by pictures when possible.

The preferred approach is the use of a professional interpreter. Many healthcare facilities have employees on call to translate when a language barrier exists; however, this is not the preferred method of locating a translator. If there is a problem locating a translator who is available, the healthcare team may have to work with a family member who is able to translate. Note that this is not ideal, in that it affects confidentiality surrounding the patient's care. Use of effective communication techniques is beneficial as the PCT cares for patients from different cultures (Box 5.2).

Even among English-speaking people, different cultural groups assign different meanings to the same words. For example, a person from the United Kingdom may say that he or she is going to take the "lift." An American is not necessarily going to understand that

Box 5.2	Strategies for Communication With Patients From Different Cultures

- Take a little extra time to establish a level of comfort between you and the patient.
- Ask questions in an unhurried and calm manner. Rephrase a question and ask it again if the answer seems inconsistent with other information the patient has provided.
- Observe the cultural differences in communication, and honor those differences. Use eye contact, touch, and seating arrangements that are comfortable for the patient.
- Ask patients about the meaning of health and illness and their understanding of treatments and planned care. Investigate how the illness is likely to affect their life, relationships, and self-concept. Find out what patients consider to be the cause of their illness. Ask how the patient prefers to manage their illness.
- To establish a therapeutic relationship, listen to the patient's perceptions of their needs, and respect the patient's perspectives.
- Listen actively and attentively; try not to anticipate the patient's response.
- Talk to the patient in an unhurried manner that considers social and cultural amenities.
- Give the patient time to answer.
- Use validation techniques to verify that the patient understands. Remember that smiles and head nodding may indicate that the patient is trying to please you, not necessarily that the you are understood.
- Sexual concerns may be difficult for the patient to discuss. Having a patient care technician of the same gender may facilitate communication.
- Use alternative methods of communication, such as a foreign language phrase book, an interpreter, gestures, or pictures, for patients who do not speak English.
- Learn key phrases in languages that are commonly spoken in your community.

From Harkreader H, Hogan MA, Thobaben M: Fundamentals of nursing: caring and clinical judgment, *ed 3, Philadelphia, 2007, Saunders.*

Delegation and Documentation Box 5.1

- Avoid the use of children as interpreters if at all possible. Children often do not have the literacy level high enough to understand what is being told to them, and they may not correctly communicate the information back to the patient because of their age and developmental level.
- When documenting a patient response to a task that was communicated to you through an interpreter, be sure to document something specific like this: "patient tolerated discontinuation of intravenous catheter well with no complaints, according to interpreter," and include the name of the interpreter.

this refers to an elevator ride. Within the United States, the variety of regional accents further complicates the communication picture. People from different areas of the country (e.g., people from the north and the south) sometime struggle to understand each other because of the different accents or regional expressions they use. Some cultural or regional groups speak very rapidly, which adds to the difficulty of understanding.

Other cultural patterns also play a role in communication. In some cultural groups, many family members commonly accompany a person to the healthcare setting. Large groups of family members tend to make communication difficult. They sometimes all try to assist by answering at once. Or perhaps, when in the presence of strangers, a person from another group answers only direct questions and thus appears rude or uncommunicative. Unfortunately, the appearance of rudeness is a common byproduct of a cross-cultural mismatch in communication. Sometimes, a person speaks loudly to make the point known because of the mistaken belief that this helps the receiver of the communication understand better. In fact, it often has the opposite effect of the one desired. Members of some cultures interpret the raised voice as rudeness or aggression and shut out the sound altogether. Never raise your voice just because you think the person will be able to understand you better.

Consider, in contrast, the use of silence. Silence indicates many things to many cultures: a lack of understanding, stubbornness, apprehension, discomfort, agreement, disagreement, respect, or disdain. In some cultures, the presence of silence may result in feelings of discomfort and anxiety. It is not uncommon for people to make attempts to fill periods of silence with conversation. Among Native American, Chinese, and Japanese cultures, silence is sometimes used to allow the listener to consider what the speaker has said before continuing. Members of other cultures, such as Russians, French, and Spanish, tend to become silent to indicate consensus between parties. In Asian cultures, people often use silence as a sign of respect, especially to elders. In contrast, other cultures, such as those of Mexican descent, may use silence when they disagree with a person of authority.

Nonverbal communication is usually expressed through body language. Some groups are more comfortable than others with touching or maintaining eye contact (See Box 5.3). Acceptance of touch may be culturally or regionally related. In parts of the United States, many people consider even casual touching inappropriate. In other regions, casual touch and embracing between acquaintances is the norm. Recent immigrants from England and Germany are even less likely to touch each other in public or allow casual touching by strangers. Spanish, French, Italian, Jewish, and South American individuals are likely to be much more comfortable about touching each other and being touched.

Box 5.3	Cultural Considerations: Culturally Sensitive Communication

- Ask all patients how they like to be addressed. If in doubt, address them formally.
- Determine the patient's preferences for touch. For example, Americans often greet each other with a firm handshake. Many Native Americans, however, see this as a sign of aggression. Touch outside of the marriage is sometimes forbidden in older adults from the Middle East.
- Investigate the patient's preferences for silence. Generally, Eastern cultures value silence, whereas Western cultures are uncomfortable with silence.
- Be aware of the patient's beliefs about eye contact during conversation. Direct eye contact in European American cultures is a sign of honesty and truthfulness. Older Native Americans may avoid eye contact. Asian adults sometimes avoid eye contact with authority figures because this is considered disrespectful, and direct eye contact between the sexes in Middle Eastern cultures is sometimes forbidden except between spouses.

From Potter PA, Perry AG, Stockert P, et al.: Fundamentals of nursing, ed 8, St. Louis, 2012, Mosby, and Meiner SE: Gerontologic nursing, ed 4, St. Louis, 2010, Mosby.

Eye contact also has significant cultural interpretations. Many people in the United States regard maintaining eye contact as an indication of openness, interest in others, attentiveness, and honesty. Lack of eye contact is thus interpreted as a sign of shyness, humility, guilt, embarrassment, rudeness, thoughtlessness, or dishonesty. Other cultures have various other reasons for not maintaining eye contact. Some Asian cultures and American Indians relate eye contact to impoliteness or an invasion of privacy. Certain East Indian cultures avoid eye contact with people of lower or higher socioeconomic classes. Among some Appalachian people, maintaining eye contact indicates hostility or aggressiveness.

Assessing the communication variables of a patient from another culture is important. First, an assessment of cultural factors is performed, and then the caregiver has to respond appropriately. Every effort should be made to communicate with others at their personal level of comfort to establish good rapport. If the patient is from a culture that avoids eye contact, try to look away when talking with the patient. If touch is unacceptable among casual acquaintances, avoid patting the shoulder or touching a hand when talking with the patient.

When the healthcare team violates cultural beliefs and practices, it is likely to interfere with establishing a therapeutic relationship with the patient and the patient's family. Do not expect to completely adjust individual personal cultural practices, but make an effort to understand and accept the differences among practices in various cultures. Do not judge the patient's behavior according to personal practices.

Health Literacy

Health literacy is defined by the U.S. Department of Health and Human Services as the degree to which individuals have the capacity to obtain, process, and understand basic health information needed to make appropriate health decisions and services needed to prevent and treat illness (hrsa.gov). This means that how well the patient can read and understand your instructions will matter as far as whether or not they understand what you are saying. Health literacy can make a difference in whether or not the patient follows your directions. For example, if you explain to patients that they are not able to ambulate in the hall because they have an infusing intravenous line, and they don't know what ambulate or an intravenous line is, they could potentially ignore your instructions and attempt to walk in the halls (Box 5.4).

A portion of the admission assessment completed by the healthcare team should include an assessment of health literacy. No longer is it satisfactory to assume that because someone has a high school diploma, he or she has a high health literacy. Some may be able to understand what is told to them, but may struggle with reading (Fig. 5.2). This can be particularly true with discharge instructions (Fig. 5.3). The nurse may choose to provide alternative methods for teaching the patient their discharge instructions, such as through video, pamphlet, or use of iPad® technology. As the PCT, you may support health literacy by following the recommendations for those with low health literacy.

Box 5.4	Health Literacy

Health Literacy Is More Prevalent Among the Following:	They May Struggle in the Following Areas:
Older adults	Locating health providers and services
Minority populations	Filling out complex health forms
Lower socioeconomic status	Seeking preventative healthcare
Medically underserved	Managing chronic health directions
	Understanding directions on medicine

From Egbert N, Nanna K: Health literacy: challenges and strategies, The online Journal of Issues in Nursing, 14(3), 2009.

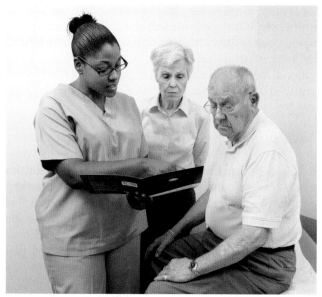

FIGURE 5.2 Demonstrate sensitivity to patients when they may have difficulty understanding the instructions they are given. (From Proctor D, Adams A: *Kinn's The Medical Assistant: an applied learning approach*, ed 12, St. Louis, 2014, Saunders.)

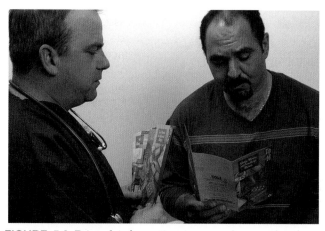

FIGURE 5.3 Printed information is a good example of one way to help patients who have low health literacy. (From Proctor D, Adams A: *Kinn's The Medical Assistant: an applied learning approach*, ed 12, St. Louis, 2014, Saunders.)

Suggestions for Improving Understanding With Those Who Have Low Health Literacy

• Ask the nurse if any of your assigned patients have a low health literacy level.
• Use simple words and short sentences, while avoiding medical and technical terms as much as possible.
• Once the nurse has provided the discharge teaching instructions, be sure that the patient places the written or typed copy in a place where he or she will be able to find them once home.
• If the patient has difficulty filling out required paperwork, ask the nurse for assistance. There are many resources available to help those with lower health literacy with completion of paperwork.

Personal Space

Cultural interpretation of personal space varies and is an important element of assessment. Cultures assign different comfort areas to personal space. Generally, in Western cultures, people in a casual or public setting are most comfortable when they can maintain 3 to 6 feet between them during a conversation (Giger, 2012). Closer contact is reserved for more intimate relationships. Members of some cultures are accustomed to more close contact and sometimes inadvertently invade the space of a person from a Western culture. Occasionally, the need for personal space also manifests itself in a desire to use a certain space. For example, perhaps a resident in a nursing home always wishes to sit in a particular chair or in a specific part of the room. Another resident chooses to sit at the same table for each meal. If someone changes any of these arrangements, either of these residents may become upset.

Body movements are often culturally related. In the United States, certain gestures are generally understood by most longtime citizens. However, some commonly used gestures have the potential to offend someone from another culture. For example, a circle formed with the thumb and forefinger means "A-OK" in the United States. To someone from Brazil, this is an obscene gesture. Traditionally, Italian or Jewish people use more body movements to illustrate or emphasize what they are communicating than do individuals from Asian cultures. As noted previously, touch is used more commonly in some cultures than others (Giger, 2012).

Time

The measurement of time and the rhythms of people's activities and interactions often have different meanings in various cultures. These different meanings have the potential to create some problems in the care of patients from other cultures. Traditional nursing practice emphasizes that medications and treatments are provided on a rigid schedule. The U.S. and many Northern European cultures generally give a high priority to being on time for appointments, and people typically expect everyone to follow this pattern. Japanese American culture also places emphasis on promptness and the adherence to fixed schedules, especially when meeting with a person who is regarded highly. People in many cultures believe that other concerns regarding time are more important. In Eastern cultures, including Chinese, East Indian Hindu, Filipino, and Korean, schedules and time are much more flexible concepts. Some Asians spend a lot of time getting to know someone and view abrupt endings to a conversation as rude. Mexican Americans may be late for an appointment because they focus more on a current activity and are less concerned about a previously planned meeting. According to Giger (2012), this concept, known as "elasticity," implies that future activities are possible to recover but not present ones.

Perception of time or time orientation also varies among cultures. Many people in the United States tend to be future oriented. Present actions are taken based on a future outcome. An example is a person who takes medication to treat hypertension to prevent illness. Among members of other cultures, notably African American or black, Hispanic, and Native American, individuals tend to be more present oriented. Sometimes, like people described previously who prolong a current encounter rather than rushing off to be on time for another one, a present-oriented person chooses to satisfy a current, more urgent need rather than prepare for a less immediate one that is some time away. A Hispanic pregnant woman, for instance, may miss her own healthcare provider's appointments to take care of her family; if her older child needs a ride to school, the mother skips the appointment and drives the child. This type of patient may also view the cost of a medication for hypertension to prevent future problems as an optional expense. Paying the rent or buying food for the family is a current need that takes precedence.

Religious Beliefs and Healthcare

Religious beliefs are frequently entwined with cultural beliefs. Some cultures expect all members to adhere to a particular religion. In these societies, religious and cultural beliefs are difficult to separate. In the United States, wide variations are found in religious practices (Box 5.5). In addition, as people from varying

Text continued on p. 65

| Box 5.5 | Religious Beliefs and Practices That Affect Healthcare in the United States |

American Muslim Mission
Baptism: No baptism is practiced.
Death: The family is contacted before any care of the deceased is performed. Special procedures are observed for washing and shrouding the body.
Dietary habits: In addition to refusing pork, many do not eat foods traditional in black culture such as cornbread and collard greens.
Other practices: Quiet time is necessary to permit prayer. Members are encouraged to use black physicians for healthcare.

Assemblies of God (Pentecostal)
Anointing the sick: Members believe in divine healing through prayer and the laying on of hands. Clergy is notified if the patient or family desires this.
Baptism: Water baptism with complete immersion is practiced when an individual has received Jesus Christ as Savior and Lord based on Acts 2:38.
Death: No special practices are observed.
Dietary habits: Abstinence from alcohol, tobacco, and all illegal drugs is strongly encouraged.
Holy Communion: Notify clergy if the patient desires to receive this sacrament.
Other practices: Faith in God and in the healthcare providers is encouraged. Members pray for divine intervention in health matters. Encourage and allow patients time for prayer. Members sometimes "speak in tongues" during prayer.

Baptist (More Than 27 Different Groups in the United States)
Baptism: Baptists do not practice infant baptism.
Death: No general service is provided, but the clergy does minister through counseling, prayer, and Scripture as requested by the patient or family, and the patient is encouraged to believe in Jesus Christ as Savior and Lord.
Dietary habits: Total abstinence from alcohol is expected.

Holy Communion: Notify clergy if the patient desires to receive this sacrament.
Other practices: The Bible is held to be the word of God, so either allow quiet time for Scripture reading or offer to read to the patient.

Christian Church (Disciples of Christ)
Baptism: These members do not practice infant baptism but do have dedication service. Believers are baptized with immersion.
Death: No special practices are observed.
Holy Communion: Open communion is celebrated each Sunday and is a central part of worship services. Notify the clergy if the patient desires it; sometimes the clergy member suggests it.
Other practices: Church elders and clergy are appropriate to notify to assist with meeting the patient's spiritual needs.

Christian Science
Birth: Physician or nurse-midwife is used during childbirth. No baptism ceremony is practiced.
Death: Autopsy is usually declined unless required by law. Organ donation is unlikely, but is an individual decision.
Dietary habits: Because alcohol and tobacco are considered drugs, they are not used. Coffee and tea are often declined.
Other practices: Members do not normally seek medical care because they approach healthcare in a different, primarily spiritual, framework. They commonly use the services of a surgeon to set a bone but decline drugs and, in general, other medical or surgical procedures. Hypnotism and psychotherapy are also declined. Family planning is left to the family. They seek exemption from vaccinations but obey legal requirements. They report infectious diseases and obey public health quarantines. Nonmedical care facilities are maintained for those needing nursing assistance in the course of a healing. The *Christian Science Journal* lists available Christian

Box 5.5 Religious Beliefs and Practices That Affect Healthcare in the United States—cont'd

Science nurses. When caring for a Christian Science believer, allow and encourage time for prayer and study. Patients often request that a Christian Science practitioner be notified to come.

Church of the Brethren
Anointing the sick: This is practiced for physical healing and spiritual uplift and held in high regard by the church. The clergy is notified if the patient or the family desires.

Baptism: These members do not practice infant baptism but have dedication service.

Death: The clergy is notified for counsel and prayer.

Holy Communion: This is usually received within church, but clergy give it in the hospital when requested.

Church of Jesus Christ of Latter-Day Saints (Mormons)
Anointing the sick: Mormons frequently are anointed and given a blessing before going to the hospital and after admission by laying on of hands.

Baptism: If a child aged above 8 years is very ill, whether baptized or unbaptized, call a member of the church's priesthood.

Birth control and abortion: Abortion is opposed except when the life of the mother is in danger. Only natural means of birth control are recommended. Artificial means are permitted when the health of the woman is at stake (including emotional health).

Death: Mormons prefer burial of the body. Notify a church elder to assist the family. If need be, the elder assists the funeral director in dressing the body in special clothes and gives other help as needed.

Dietary habits: Mormons practice abstinence from the use of tobacco; beverages with caffeine such as cola, coffee, and tea; and alcohol and other substances considered injurious. Mormons eat meat but encourage the intake of fruits, grains, and herbs.

Holy Communion: Hospitalized patients often desire to have a member of the church priesthood administer this sacrament.

Personal care: Cleanliness is very important to Mormons. A sacred undergarment may be worn at all times by Mormons and is removed only in emergency situations.

Other practices: Allow quiet time for prayer and the reading of the sacred writings. The church maintains a welfare system to assist those in need. Families are of great importance, so visiting is important to encourage.

Church of the Nazarene
Baptism: Parents have the choice of baptism or dedication for their infant. Emphasis is on the believer's baptism, which is regarded as a symbol of the New Covenant in Jesus Christ.

Death: Cremation is permitted, and stillborn term infants are buried.

Dietary habits: The use of alcohol and tobacco is forbidden.

Holy Communion: Pastor administers if the patient wishes.

Other practices: The members believe in divine healing but not to the exclusion of medical treatment. Patients sometimes desire quiet time for prayer.

Eastern Orthodox
Anointing the sick: The priest conducts this in the hospital room.

Birth: The infant must be baptized within 40 days after birth. If sprinkling or immersion into water is not possible, baptism is performed by moving the baby in the air in the sign of the cross. Only an ordained priest or a deacon may perform the ritual in this manner.

Birth control and abortion: Birth control and abortion are not permitted.

Dietary habits: Fasting from meat and dairy products is required on Wednesdays and Fridays during Lent and on other holy days. Hospital patients are exempt if fasting is detrimental to health.

Death: Last rites are obligatory and handled by an ordained priest who is notified while the patient is conscious. The Russian Orthodox Church does not encourage autopsy or organ donation. Euthanasia, even for the terminally ill, is discouraged, as is cremation.

Holy Eucharist: The priest is notified if the patient desires this sacrament.

Special days: Christmas is celebrated on January 7, and New Year on January 14. This is important to the care of a patient who is hospitalized on these days.

Episcopal (Anglican)
Anointing the sick: A priest often administers this rite when death is imminent, but it is not considered mandatory.

Baptism: Infant baptism is practiced and is considered urgent if the infant is critically ill. The priest is notified to administer the sacrament. Laypersons are permitted to baptize in an emergency.

Death: No special practices are observed.

Dietary habits: Some patients abstain from meat on Fridays. Others fast before receiving the Eucharist, but fasting is not mandatory.

Holy Communion: Notify the priest if the patient wishes to receive this sacrament.

Other practices: Confession of sins to a priest is optional; if the patient desires this, the clergy should be notified.

Islam
Birth: A baby is bathed immediately after birth, before being given to the mother. The father (or mother if the father is not available) then whispers the call to prayer in the child's ears so that the first sounds heard are about the Muslim faith. Circumcision is culturally recommended before puberty. A baby born prematurely but at least at 130 days of gestation is given the same treatment as any other infant.

Birth control and abortion: Abortion is forbidden, and many conservative Muslims do not encourage the use of contraceptives because they believe that it interferes with God's purpose. Others believe that it is best for a woman to have only as many children as her husband can afford. Contraception is permitted by Islamic law.

Care of women: Because women are not allowed to sign consent forms or make a decision regarding family planning, it is mandatory for the husband to be present.

Continued

Box 5.5   Religious Beliefs and Practices That Affect Healthcare in the United States—cont'd

Women are very modest and frequently wear clothes that cover all of the body. During a medical examination, the woman's modesty must be respected as much as possible. Muslim women prefer female doctors. For 40 days after giving birth and also during menstruation, a woman is exempt from prayer because this is a time of cleansing for her.

Death: Before death, family members ask to be present so that they can read the Koran and pray with the patient. An Imam comes if requested by the patient or family but is not required. Patients face Mecca and confess their sins and beg for forgiveness in the presence of their family. If the family is unavailable, any practicing Muslim is permitted to provide support to the patient. After death, Muslims prefer that the family wash, prepare, and place the body in a position facing Mecca. If necessary, healthcare providers are allowed to perform these procedures as long as they wear gloves. Burial is performed as soon as possible. Cremation is forbidden. Autopsy is also prohibited except for legal reasons, and then no body part is to be removed. Donation of body parts or organs is not allowed because, according to culturally developed law, people do not own their bodies.

Dietary habits: No pork or alcoholic beverages are allowed. All halal (permissible) meat must be blessed and killed in a special way. This is called zabihah (correctly slaughtered). Daytime fasting is practiced during Ramadan.

Personal devotions: At prayer time, washing is required, even by those who are sick. A patient on bed rest sometimes requires assistance with this task before prayer. Provision of privacy is important during prayer.

Religious objects: The Koran is not to be touched by anyone ritually unclean, and nothing is to be placed on top of it. Some Muslims wear taviz, a black string on which words of the Koran are attached. These should not be removed and must remain dry. Certain items of jewelry such as bangles may have religious significance; do not allow them to be removed unnecessarily.

Jehovah's Witness

Baptism: No infant baptism is practiced. Baptism with complete immersion of adults is done as a symbol of dedication to Jehovah because Jesus was baptized.

Birth control and abortion: Use of birth control is a personal decision. Abortion is opposed based on Exodus 21:22–23.

Blood transfusions: Blood transfusions violate God's laws and are therefore not allowed. Patients do respect physicians and accept alternatives to blood transfusions. These include the possible use of nonblood plasma expanders, careful surgical techniques to decrease blood loss, use of autologous transfusions, and autotransfusion through use of a heart-lung machine. Be sure to check unconscious patients for medical-alert cards or bracelets that state that the person does not want a transfusion. Because Jehovah's Witnesses are

prepared to die rather than break God's law, you need to be sensitive to the spiritual as well as the physical needs of the patient.

Death: Autopsy is a private matter to be decided by the persons involved. Burial and cremation are acceptable.

Dietary habits: Use of alcohol and tobacco is discouraged because these harm the physical body.

Organ transplants: Use of organ transplant is a private decision; if used, it is required that the organ be cleansed with a nonblood solution.

Judaism, Observant (Orthodox Judaism and Some Conservative Groups)

Birth: For observant Jews, babies are named by the father. Male children are named 8 days after birth, when ritual circumcision is done. A mohel performs the circumcision. Circumcision is often postponed if the infant is in poor health. Female babies are usually named during the reading of the holy Torah. Patient care technicians need to be sensitive to the wishes of the parents when caring for babies who have not yet been named.

Birth control and abortion: Artificial methods of birth control are not encouraged. Vasectomy is not allowed. Abortion is permitted only to save the mother's life.

Care of women: A woman is considered to be in a ritual state of impurity whenever blood is coming from her uterus, such as during menstrual periods and after the birth of a child. During this time, her husband does not have physical contact with her. When this time is completed, she bathes herself in a pool called a mikvah. Patient care technicians need to be aware of this practice and be sensitive to the husband and wife because the husband does not touch his wife. He cannot assist her in moving in the bed, so the nurse or patient care technician has to do this. An Orthodox Jewish man does not touch any woman other than his wife, daughters, and mother. Home healthcare workers need to be aware of these practices.

Death: Judaism defines death as occurring when respiration and circulation are irreversibly stopped and no movement is apparent. (1) Euthanasia is strictly forbidden by Orthodox Jews, who advocate the strict use of life-support measures. (2) Before death, Jewish faith indicates that visiting of the person by family and friends is a religious duty. The Torah and Psalms are often read, and prayers are recited. A witness needs to be present when a person prays for health so that if death occurs God protects the family and the spirit is committed to God. Extraneous talking and conversation about death are not encouraged unless initiated by the patient or visitors. In Judaism, the belief is that people should have someone with them when the soul leaves the body, so allow family and friends to stay with patients. After death, the body is not to be left alone until burial, usually within 24 hours. (3) When death occurs, the body is to remain untouched for 8 to 30 minutes. Medical personnel are not to touch or wash

Box 5.5   Religious Beliefs and Practices That Affect Healthcare in the United States—cont'd

the body; only an Orthodox person or the Jewish Burial Society is permitted to care for the body. Handling of a corpse on the Sabbath is forbidden to Jewish persons. If need be, the nursing staff is permitted to provide routine care of the body while wearing gloves. Water receptacles in the room have to be emptied, and the family often requests that mirrors be covered to symbolize that a death has occurred. (4) Orthodox Jews and some Conservative Jews do not approve of autopsies. If an autopsy is necessary, all body parts are required to remain with the body. (5) For Orthodox Jews, the body is required to be buried within 24 hours. No flowers are permitted. A fetus is required to be buried. (6) A 7-day mourning period is required by the immediate family. They stay at home except for Sabbath worship. (7) Ensure that organs or other body parts such as amputated limbs are made available for burial for Orthodox Jews because they believe that all of the body must be returned to the earth.

Dietary rules: (1) Kosher dietary laws include the following: no mixing of milk and meat at a meal; no consumption of food or any derivative thereof from animals not slaughtered in accordance with Jewish law; use of separate cooking utensils for meat and milk products; and if for medical reasons a patient requires milk and meat products for a meal, the dairy foods should be served first, followed later by the meat. (2) During Yom Kippur (Day of Atonement), a 24-hour fast is required, but exceptions are made for those who cannot fast because of medical reasons or age. (3) During Passover, no leavened products are eaten. (4) Observant Jewish patients often wish to say prayers over the bread and wine before meals. Time and a quiet environment should be provided for this.

Head covering: Orthodox men wear skullcaps at all times, and women cover their hair after marriage. Some Orthodox women wear wigs as a mark of piety. Conservative Jews cover their heads only during acts of worship and prayer.

Organ transplants: Donor organ transplants generally are not permitted by Orthodox Jews but with rabbinical consent are sometimes allowed.

Prayer: Praying directly to God, including a prayer of confession, is required for Orthodox Jews. Provide quiet time for prayer.

Sabbath: Observed from sunset Friday until sunset Saturday. Orthodox law prohibits riding in a car, smoking, turning lights on and off, handling money, and using television and telephone. Patient care technicians need to be aware of this when caring for observant Jews at home and in the hospital. Medical or surgical treatments should be postponed if possible.

Shaving: The beard is regarded as a mark of piety among observant Jews. For very Orthodox Jews, shaving is never done with a razor, but with scissors or an electric razor, because no blade is to contact the skin.

Lutheran (10 Different Branches [Synods])

Anointing the sick: Patients sometimes request an anointing and blessing from the minister when the prognosis is poor.

Baptism: Lutherans baptize only living infants any time, but usually 6 to 8 weeks after birth. Adults are also baptized, and modes of baptism, as appropriate, include sprinkling, pouring, and immersion.

Death: A service of Commendation of the Dying is performed at the patient's or family's request.

Holy Communion: Notify the clergy if the patient desires this sacrament. Clergy sometimes also inquire about the patient's wishes.

Mennonite (12 Different Groups)

Baptism: No infant baptism is observed, but the child is sometimes dedicated if requested by the parents.

Death: Prayer is important at time of crisis, so contacting a minister is important.

Dietary habits: Abstinence from alcohol is urged for all.

Holy Communion: Communion is served twice a year, with foot washing as part of ceremony.

Other practices: Women sometimes wear head coverings during hospitalization. Anointing with oil is administered in harmony with James 5:14 when requested.

Methodist (More Than 20 Different Groups)

Anointing of sick: If requested, the clergy comes to pray and sprinkle the patient with olive oil.

Baptism: Notify the clergy if the parent desires baptism for a sick infant.

Death: Scripture reading and prayer are important at this time. Donation of one's body or part of the body at death is encouraged.

Holy Communion: Notify the clergy if a patient requests communion before surgery or another health crisis.

Presbyterian (10 Different Groups)

Baptism: Infant baptism is practiced with pouring or sprinkling. Immersion is also practiced at times for adults.

Death: Notify a local pastor or elder for prayer and Scripture reading if desired by the family or patient.

Holy Communion: Communion is given when appropriate and convenient, at the hospitalized patient's request.

Quaker (Friends)

Baptism and Holy Communion: Friends have no creed; therefore a diversity of personal beliefs exists, one of which is that outward sacraments are usually not necessary because there is the ministry of the Spirit inwardly in such areas as baptism and communion. A few Friends baptize with water.

Death: Friends believe that the present life is part of God's kingdom and generally have no rite of passage from this life to the next. Ascertain the patient's personal beliefs and wishes, and then act on the patient's wishes.

Continued

Box 5.5   Religious Beliefs and Practices That Affect Healthcare in the United States—cont'd

Other practices: The name of the Quaker infant is recorded in official record books at the local meeting.

Roman Catholic

Anointing the sick: The priest anoints the forehead, hands, and, if desired, the affected area. The rite is performed on any who are ill and desire it. People receiving the sacrament seek complete healing and strength to endure suffering. Before 1963, this sacrament was given only to people at time of imminent death, so the patient care technician must be sensitive to the meaning this has for the patient. The priest should be called before the patient becomes unconscious, but may also be called in the case of sudden death; the sacrament can also be given shortly after death. The nurse should be the one to document that this sacrament has been administered.

Birth: Because Roman Catholics believe that unbaptized children are cut off from Heaven, infant baptism is mandatory. For newborns with a grave prognosis, stillborns, and all aborted fetuses (unless evidence of tissue necrosis and prolonged death are present), emergency baptism is required. The nurse calls a priest to perform the baptism unless the possibility exists that death will occur before the priest arrives. In that case, anyone is permitted to baptize by pouring warm water on the infant's head and saying, "I baptize you in the name of the Father, of the Son, and of the Holy Spirit." All information about the baptism is recorded on the chart, and the priest and family are notified.

Birth control: Contraception is prohibited except for abstinence or natural family planning methods. Referral to a priest for questions about this is often of great help. Nurses teach the techniques of natural family planning if they are familiar with them; otherwise, the nurse should make referral to the physician or to a support group of the Church that instructs couples in this method of birth control. Sterilization is prohibited unless an overriding medical reason exists.

Death: Each Roman Catholic is to participate in the anointing of the sick and the Eucharist and penance before death. The body is not to be shrouded until after these sacraments are performed. All body parts that retain human quality are required to be appropriately buried or cremated.

Dietary habits: Obligatory fasting is excused during hospitalization. However, if no health restrictions exist, some Catholics still observe the following guidelines: (1) Anyone 14 years of age or older has to abstain from eating meat on Ash Wednesday and all Fridays during Lent. Some older Catholics still abstain from meat on all Fridays of the year. (2) In addition to abstinence from meat, people 21 to 59 years of age are required to limit themselves to one full meal and two light meals on Ash Wednesday and Good Friday. (3) Eastern Rite Catholics are stricter about fasting and fast more frequently than Western Rite Catholics, so the patient care technician should know whether a patient is Eastern or Western.

Holy Eucharist: For patients and healthcare providers who are to receive communion, abstinence from solid food and alcohol is required for 15 minutes (if possible) before reception of the consecrated wafer. Medicine, water, and nonalcoholic drinks are permitted at any time. If a patient is in danger of death, the fasting requirement is waived because the reception of the Eucharist at this time is very important.

Organ donation: Donation and transplantation of organs are acceptable as long as the donor is not harmed and is not deprived of life.

Religious objects: Rosary prayers are said using rosary beads. Medals bearing the images of saints, relics, statues, and scapulars are important objects that are often pinned to a hospital gown or pillow or kept at the bedside. Ensure that extreme care is taken not to lose these objects because they have special meaning to the patient.

Seventh-Day Adventist

Anointing the sick: The clergy are contacted for prayer and anointing with oil.

Baptism: No infant baptism is practiced, but dedication services are.

Death: No special procedures are required.

Dietary habits: Because the body is viewed as the temple of the Holy Spirit, healthy living is essential. Therefore the use of alcohol, tobacco, coffee, and tea and the promiscuous (careless) use of drugs are prohibited. Some are vegetarians, and most avoid pork.

Holy Communion: Although this is not required of hospitalized patients, the clergy is notified if the patient desires.

Special days: The Sabbath is observed on Saturday.

Other practices: Use of hypnotism is opposed by some. People of homosexual or lesbian orientation are ministered to in the hope of "correction" of these practices, which are believed to be wrong. Ensure that a Bible is always available for Scripture reading.

Unification Church

Baptism: No baptism is practiced.

Death: Members believe that after death one's place of destiny depends on his or her spirit's quality of life and goodness while on Earth. In the afterlife, one will have the same aspirations and feelings as before death. Hell is not a concern because it will not be a place as heaven grows in size. People who leave the Unification Church are warned of the possibility that Satan will try to possess them.

Special days: Sunday mornings are used to honor Reverend and Mrs. Moon as the true parents, and members get up at 5 AM, bow before a picture of the Moons three times, and vow to do what is needed to help the Reverend accomplish his mission on Earth.

Other practices: All marriages are required to be solemnized by Reverend Moon to be part of the perfect family and have salvation. The church supplies its faithful members with life's necessities. Members sometimes use occult practices to have spiritual and psychic experiences.

| Box 5.5 | Religious Beliefs and Practices That Affect Healthcare in the United States—cont'd |

Unitarian Universalist Association
Baptism: No baptism is practiced.
Death: Cremation is often preferred rather than burial.
Other practices: Use of birth control is advocated as part of responsible parenting. Strong support for a woman's right to choice regarding abortion is maintained. Unitarian Universalists advocate donation of body parts for research and transplants.

United Church of Christ
Baptism: Members practice infant and adult baptism. Three modes are used as appropriate: pouring, sprinkling, and immersion.
Death: If the patient desires counsel or prayer, notify the clergy.
Holy Communion: Clergy is notified if the patient desires to receive this sacrament.

Modified from Carson VB, Koenig HG: Spiritual dimensions of nursing practice, *revised ed, Philadelphia, 2008, Templeton Press.*

cultures intermarry, religious practices also become more varied.

Data for religious affiliations are not collected by the U.S. Bureau of the Census, making an accurate way to determine the numbers of followers of the various religions in the United States difficult. Despite the inability to quantify the religious preferences in the country, patient care clearly is affected by patients' religious beliefs and practices. The PCT must be aware of and open to the wide range of such beliefs to ensure that care provided is sensitive to the needs of individual patients. For example, Jehovah's Witnesses believe that the Bible prohibits the ingestion of blood, and therefore they are not able to accept blood transfusions. Those who are Jewish will have specific dietary preferences and restrictions that reflect a Kosher diet.

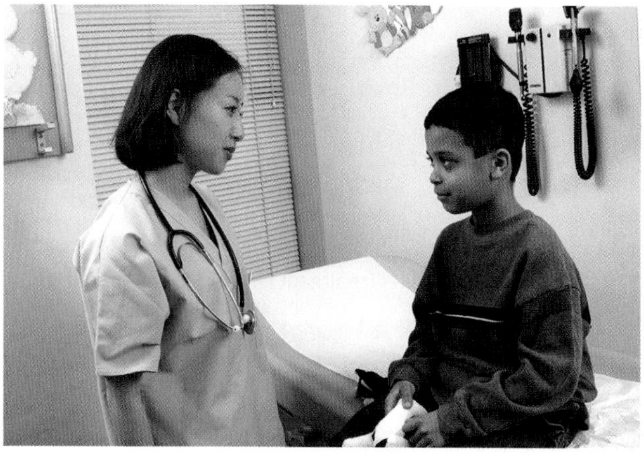

FIGURE 5.4 Consider diversity when providing care to others. The United States has become a very diverse country. (From Proctor D, Adams A: *Kinn's The Medical Assistant: an applied learning approach*, ed 12, St. Louis, 2014, Saunders.)

HEALTH PRACTICES

Today, many healthcare providers still find it difficult to believe that any alternative therapies are as effective as the biomedical methods that they have seen used for many years. In recent years, a variety of alternative health services, such as folk remedies, holistic therapies, and spiritual interventions, have aroused attention and interest in the traditional medical community. Scientific research is being performed in these areas to determine the effectiveness of these methods. Some are now accepted more readily and are sometimes used concurrently with biomedical methods.

Several factors are driving this change in thinking about healthcare. Some of the long-established methods have become less effective, for instance, antibiotics used to treat infections. A number of complementary therapies and folk remedies have been shown to be effective in treatment of certain diseases. Certain herbal therapies have been used as aromatherapy to provide relief. Lavender is an essential oil that has been used to assist with muscular and joint pain, as well as many other digestive and respiratory illnesses. Peppermint oil has been used in the hospital setting to reduce nausea. Folk remedies that have been used for headaches include

soaking your feet in hot water to draw the blood down from your head. Some believe that if you run around the house three times, the headache will go away.

More healthcare providers with varied backgrounds and beliefs about health and illness now practice in the United States. Increasing mobility and use of electronic media have resulted in more sharing of information, which has promoted diversity. Movement of cultural groups to new areas provides exposure of new information and methods of managing health issues (Fig. 5.4). Some healthcare practices among cultures cause no harm but are also ineffective, and others are therapeutic and useful. The concern lies with those that can pose danger to health and wellness. It is important to allow patients to follow practices that are in accordance with their cultural identity and personal beliefs when they are receiving healthcare in the traditional healthcare system, without allowing the effectiveness of either approach to be compromised.

The characteristics of four basic concepts of health beliefs are described in Table 5.2. For many years, Western cultures have almost universally used the biomedical method of treating illness and maintaining health. Folk medicine encompasses many different

Table 5.2	Health Belief Systems

Belief System	Characteristics
Biomedical health belief system	Life is regulated by biomedical and physical processes. Life processes can be manipulated by humans with mechanical interventions. Health is the absence of disease or signs and symptoms of disease. Disease is an alteration of the structure and function of the body. Disease has a specific cause, onset, course, and treatment. It is caused by trauma, pathogens, chemical imbalances, or failure of body parts. Treatment focuses on the use of physical and chemical interventions.
Folk health belief system	This is commonly referred to as "third-world" beliefs and practices. It is often called strange or weird by health professionals who are unfamiliar with folk medicine beliefs. In most instances, these practices do not seem "strange or weird" once healthcare providers become acquainted with them. This system classifies illnesses or diseases as natural or unnatural. According to this belief system, natural events have to do with the world as God made it and as God intended it to be. Thus there is a certain amount of predictability for daily life. Unnatural events imply the exact opposite because they upset the harmony of nature. Thus unnatural events are those events that interrupt the plan intended by God and at their very worst represent the forces of evil and the machinations of the devil. They have no predictability and are beyond the control of ordinary mortals. Treatment is done by carrying out rituals or repentance or giving in to the supernatural force's wishes.
Holistic health belief system	Religious experiences are based on cultural beliefs and may include such things as blessings from spiritual leaders, apparitions of dead relatives, and even miracle cures. Healing powers may also be ascribed to animate or inanimate objects. Religion dictates social, moral, and dietary practices designed to assist an individual in maintaining a health balance and in playing a vital role in illness prevention (e.g., burning of candles, rituals of redemption, and prayer). Baptism may be seen as a ritual of cleansing and dedication and prevention of evil. Anointing the sick may be seen as preparation for death and may also be performed as the hope of a miracle. Circumcision is also viewed as a religious practice. Treatment is designed to restore balance with physical, social, and metaphysical worlds. It may extend beyond treating the person to treating the environment to decrease pollution or prevent hunger, homelessness, and so on.
Alternative or complementary belief system	Today many Americans use one or more nonmedical forms of therapy to treat an illness. Acupuncture, aromatic therapy, meditation, therapeutic touch, and a variety of other techniques prevail as feasible alternative therapies (see Chapter 17). Most of the individuals who use an alternative therapy do so without informing their healthcare provider. Alternative therapies address the whole patient by viewing symptoms as the tip of the iceberg and as the body's means for communicating to the mind that something needs to be changed, removed, or added to one's life. The mind and body are seen as a whole unit.

Data from Giger JM: Transcultural nursing: assessment and intervention, *ed 6, St. Louis, 2012, Mosby.*

traditions in cultures around the world. It often includes native healers who use a variety of methods in treating disorders (Fig. 5.5). At times, this belief system also incorporates religious practices and magic. Within this system, methods are used to manipulate the environment to improve health.

Do not assume that patients born in the United States accept the biomedical view of healthcare. Individuals in many subcultures of the United States practice folk medicine. These people sometimes avoid seeking care from healthcare providers or practice folk medicine while also receiving traditional care.

Biological Variations

Cultural groups are identified in a variety of ways. In some instances, the members share strong biologic characteristics. This is especially true if the cultural group is primarily made up of individuals from a particular race or geographic region. When assessing these individuals, include these characteristics. Some of the

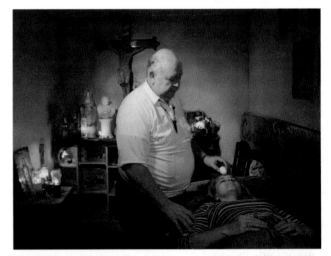

FIGURE 5.5 Within the Mexican American folk medicine system, the *curandero* is the folk healer. (From Harkreader H, Hogan MA: *Fundamentals of nursing: caring and clinical judgment,* ed 3, Philadelphia, 2007, Saunders.)

obvious ones are body structure, skin color, and hair color and texture. For example, you probably expect a cultural group from the Scandinavian region to have many people with blond hair and blue eyes. Asians are likely to have straight, coarse, dark hair. More important to healthcare practice is a family history of diseases that are common within the ethnic group. Some diseases, such as sickle cell anemia, are more frequently found among those of African ancestry. Other diseases, such as diabetes, asthma, or heart disease, tend to be more prevalent among certain cultural groups. Even with consideration of diet, diabetes occurs more frequently among American Indians.

Another important health consideration is the effect of culturally determined dietary practices. Many traditional foods are high in saturated fats, sodium, and sugar. If these foods are eaten frequently, they have the potential to affect patients' health and the health of their family members. In some cases, members of some cultural groups have dietary deficiencies caused by low intake of protein, complex carbohydrates, and fresh fruits and vegetables. Several diverse cultural groups (Chinese, Korean, Mexican, Puerto Rican, and Vietnamese) have beliefs that diseases and foods are classified as either "hot" or "cold." The diet is adjusted according to the perceived balance, and thus diseases are treated with the proper foods. This practice sometimes leads to a failure to meet basic nutritional needs and to dietary problems.

Cultural Practices of Specific Groups

Hispanics make up a large percentage of the population in the United States and account for as much as 50% of the population in some counties (Fig. 5.6). Subcultures also exist within the Hispanic culture, and Hispanics' origins vary as well. According to the 2010 U.S. Census Bureau report, the largest Hispanic populations are found in areas of California, Texas, Illinois, and Arizona. Puerto Ricans are concentrated in New York, Florida, Illinois, and Pennsylvania. About two thirds of all Cubans in the United States live in Florida (U.S. Census Bureau, www.census.gov). Although these groups share some common beliefs, they each have distinct practices. The place of origin is important to determine when caring for an Hispanic patient.

Numerous tribes of Native Americans live throughout various regions of the United States (U.S. Census Bureau, www.census.gov). Care of this population is complicated by the fact that each nation or tribe of American Indians has its own language, religion, and belief system. Practices differ significantly among groups and among members of the same tribe. When the term "American Indian" is used, it is intended to refer to tribes residing within the continental United States.

A complete picture of all cultural practices and beliefs for groups living in the United States is impossible in the context of this chapter. Table 5.3 gives examples of common cultural practices of prevalent minority groups in our culture. Always keep in mind the strong influence culture has on patients, colleagues, and the nurse. An awareness of the community in which the PCT practices is especially important. If the PCT resides in an area that is heavily populated by a culture that is unlike his or her own, it is the PCT's responsibility to learn as much as possible about the people and the culture.

Ethics Principles in Nursing Practice

In healthcare, several common ethics principles are important for consideration when confronted with an ethics question. The first, most fundamental principle is *respect for people.* This principle leads us to view all human life as sacred, with each individual having inherent worth as a person. To the PCT, this principle means that no one person is more important than another; each patient has the same worth and is always entitled to respect. *Autonomy* is another ethics principle; it refers to freedom of personal choice, a right to be independent and make decisions freely. Frequently the patient may ask the nurse for opinions or assistance in making decisions. Neither the nurse nor the PCT has the authority to make decisions for the patient. *Beneficence* means doing good or acting for someone's good; this principle is one of primary importance to healthcare providers. The PCT has an ethical duty to protect life and promote the well-being of all patients. Another ethics principle is *nonmaleficence,* which means to do no harm. It is paramount to act in the patient's best interest and an ethical and legal duty to do nothing that has a harmful effect on the patient. Finally, there is the principle of *justice,* or the concept of what is fair. In the context of nursing, justice means that all patients have the same right to nursing interventions. As the PCT, you assist with carrying out these interventions as delegated to you by the nurse.

It is a great challenge to balance these ethics principles when they seem in conflict. Rarely are options clear or black and white. Decisions often come down to choosing what seems more right and less wrong, more good and less bad.

Values are personal beliefs about the worth of an object, an idea, a custom, or an attitude. Values vary among people and cultures; they develop over time and undergo change in response to changing circumstances and necessity. Each individual adopts a value system that governs what is deemed as right or wrong (or good and bad) and influences behaviors in a given situation.

Values influence everyday decisions. Each person has many values and at times has to choose between

Text continued on p. 73

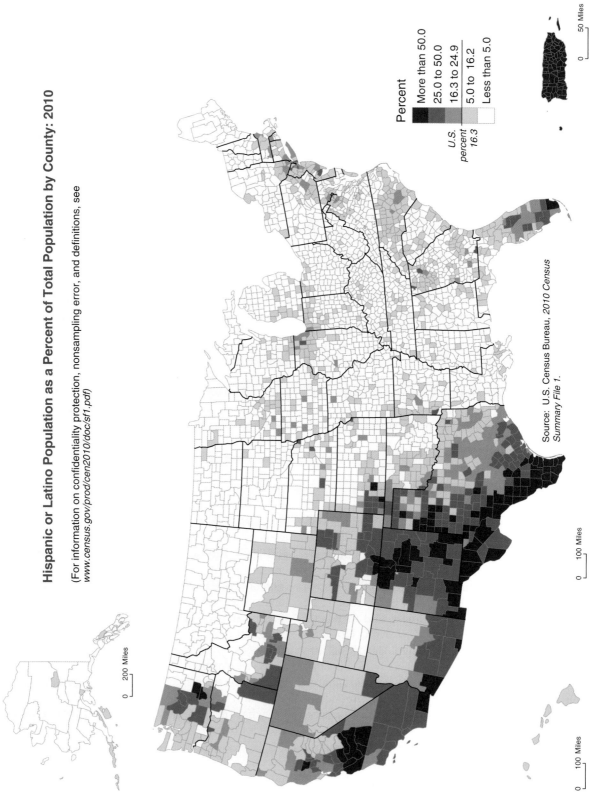

Hispanic or Latino Population as a Percent of Total Population by County: 2010

(For information on confidentiality protection, nonsampling error, and definitions, see *www.census.gov/prod/cen2010/doc/sf1.pdf*)

Percent

More than 50.0
25.0 to 50.0
16.3 to 24.9
5.0 to 16.2
Less than 5.0

U.S.
percent
16.3

Source: U.S. Census Bureau, *2010 Census Summary File 1*.

FIGURE 5.6 Hispanic percentage of the U.S. population according to Census 2010. (From the U.S. Census Bureau.)

Table 5.3 Cultural Beliefs and Practices

Mexican Americans	Blacks (African Americans)	Chinese Americans	Muslim Americans	American Indians
Predominant Health Belief System				
Sometimes accept biomedical, but belief system is often heavily mixed with folk practices.	Highly diverse. Many adhere to biomedical system. Others, particularly from rural areas, more closely follow folk health beliefs. Often the two belief systems are practiced concurrently. Prayer is important.	Holistic belief system is primary influence. Accept biomedical interventions for serious illness, but possibly continue to practice traditional methods to reestablish natural balance.	Holistic. Essential to preserve modesty and privacy. Obligatory to keep body parts covered as much as possible. Use same-sex healthcare providers if at all possible. Always examine a female patient in presence of another female. Patient may wish to have doctor consult with Imam (religious leader) when planning care.	Historically, American Indians have been guided by sacred myths and legends that describe the tribes' evolution from inception to the present time. Supernatural beings portrayed in these stories symbolize the culture, in which religion and healing practices are blended with each other. Values and beliefs intrinsic to culture and religion form the day-to-day living experiences. Traditional American Indian concepts focus on the need for the individual to be in harmony with the surrounding environment and with the family. Health and religion cannot be separated within the American Indian culture.
Language				
Spanish, often mixed with English. Children often are better able to speak English and sometimes translate for adults. Many adults never learn English.	English is understood and used when speaking with those outside of cultural group. Black English dialect is sometimes used when speaking with family and friends. Words commonly used in this dialect are sometimes intermixed with standard English when speaking with those in outside community.	Sometimes continue to speak native language even after many years in United States. It is possible to view this as honoring ancestors and native country. Learning to speak English is often difficult because there is little common basis for pronunciation, written characters, or word order.	Varies with country of origin. New immigrants often need family member or community leader to help with translations.	American Indian language has been shown to be derived from the languages used by the people in northwestern Canada. It is also similar to the language spoken by some people living in Alaska, some on the northern coast of the Pacific Ocean, and some in northern California. The language involves tonal speech in which the pitch is of great importance. Every vowel and consonant is fully sounded, regardless of how many times they are doubled or tripled within a word. Vowels are often interchanged, creating several variations and meanings of a word. Even today, many American Indians still speak the native language and are fluent in English, but some do not speak English and need the assistance of an interpreter.

Continued

Table 5.3 Cultural Beliefs and Practices—cont'd				
	Mexican Americans	Blacks (African Americans)	Chinese Americans	Muslim Americans	American Indians

Communication

Mexican Americans	Blacks (African Americans)	Chinese Americans	Muslim Americans	American Indians
Sustained direct eye contact is considered rude, immodest, or dangerous. Women and children are susceptible to *mal ojo* (evil eye) and so avoid eye contact. Touch is used often. Touch has potential to neutralize mal ojo. Closeness and physical contact are valued in familiar situations. Modesty is highly valued, so it is possible that both men and women will be embarrassed when exposure of body is necessary.	Personal space comfort area tends to be close. Eye contact is sometimes uncomfortable, especially among older generation.	Maintaining eye contact is often considered ill-mannered and disrespectful. Uncomfortable when face-to-face. Prefer to sit side-to-side or at right angles to carry on conversation. Touching is not usual during conversation; it is regarded as disrespectful or impolite. Touch possibly acceptable among same-sex acquaintances, but touching in public between opposite sexes is not acceptable.	Women do not usually shake hands with men. Women prefer to keep head, arms, and legs covered. Allow Imam to visit. Allow privacy to pray. Identify Muslim patients on chart and bracelet. Post signs to alert male staff members to avoid room with female Muslim patient.	Until recently, the Navajo language was unwritten. In World War II, a special branch of the U.S. Marine Corps was developed for Navajos who served as Navajo code talkers. It has been estimated that this highly esteemed group saved millions of lives because the enemy was unable to understand the Navajo language or infiltrate the code. Instead of shaking hands, people of this culture extend a hand and lightly touch the hand of the person they are greeting. Initially these people are silent and reserved, but once they become familiar, warm behavior is usually demonstrated. When introducing themselves by name, they give honor to ancestors by stating the clan and the location of their home area. They avoid eye contact, which is considered a sign of disrespect.

Family Roles

Mexican Americans	Blacks (African Americans)	Chinese Americans	Muslim Americans	American Indians
Families sometimes expect to help care for patient. Male family members are usually consulted before healthcare decisions are made. Only a wife is permitted to give care to husband at home if genitalia are touched.	Women are primary decision makers in family and are frequently head of the household. Extended family plays important role. Even when not related by blood, close ties exist. May refer to these people as "aunt," "uncle," "grandmother," and include them in family decisions.	Loyalty and devotion to family is more important than individual feelings. Taking care of family members brings honor to family. Older children have authority over younger children in family. Decision making is organized in this way, and younger siblings must show respect and deference or it shames the family.	Decision-making unit is the family, not the individual. Husband is consulted in any decisions about family. Imam often included in health-related decisions.	This culture is extremely family oriented, but "family" has a much broader meaning than just father, mother, and children. The biologic family is the center of social organizations and includes all members of the extended family. They are traditionally a matriarchal society. Thus when a couple marries, the husband makes his home with his wife's relatives and his family becomes one of several units that live in a group of adjacent hogans or other type of dwelling. Usually, a male family member who is looked on as having the greatest amount of prestige rises as leader for the extended family and provides necessary direction. However, in settling issues, all sides are listened to and the entire group determines the outcome. To be without relatives is to be really poor.

Birth Rites

Inappropriate for husband to be present during birth. Father not expected to see wife or baby until both are cleaned and dressed. Female family members sometimes request to be present during labor and delivery.	Many folk customs potentially influence birth. Mother often supported through birth process by female family members. Breastfeeding is not readily accepted by new mothers or encouraged by older generations.	Fathers generally are not present in labor and delivery areas. Some mothers prefer acupuncture for birth rather than Western pain-control methods. Traditionally, mother does not see child for 12 to 24 hours.	Men are not present during labor and delivery. Some husbands wish to be present during the birth process. Women seek a female physician. Pregnant women are exempt from fasting during Ramadan, the sacred ninth month during which Muslims fast from food and drink from dawn to dusk.	The tradition of massaging the newborn baby as a bonding experience between the mother and baby is still practiced. Assistance with ceremonies, particularly those associated with birth, is shared and has great importance. After delivery, the umbilical cord is taken from the newborn, dried, and buried near an object or place that symbolizes what the parents want for the child's future. The infant death rate remains disproportionately high for American Indians.

Death Rites

Small children are shielded from the dying and death scene. Families take turns staying around the clock with the dying person. Grief sometimes is expressed with hyperkinetic or seizure type of behavior that serves to release emotions.	Extended family is very supportive during final illness. Family members generally take turns staying with dying person. Some fear touching the body or being present when a person has died.	Often have aversion to death and anything concerning death. Donation of body parts is encouraged. Eldest son is responsible for all arrangements for the deceased. White, yellow, or black clothing is worn as sign of mourning.	Life is unique and precious; any intervention to hasten death is forbidden. Autopsy is acceptable with medical and legal need. It is important to allow family and Imam to follow Islamic practices to prepare body for funeral. Organ donations are permitted.	Assistance with ceremonies, particularly those associated with death, is a shared responsibility and has great importance. People of this culture have a taboo against touching a dead person or any article associated with the deceased individual. Taboos associated with death in a hogan include the need to seal the entry and warn others to stay away; frequently the need to abandon or burn the hogan is observed.

Continued

Table 5.3   Cultural Beliefs and Practices—cont'd

Mexican Americans	Blacks (African Americans)	Chinese Americans	Muslim Americans	American Indians
Dietary Practices				
Lactose intolerance is sometimes present. Rice, corn, and beans are good sources of protein. Meats include beef, pork, poultry, and goat. Diet is high in fat because frying is common method of cooking. Fruits and vegetables that are native are included in diet. Sometimes there is an inadequacy in calcium, iron, vitamin A, folic acid, and vitamin C.	High incidence of lactose intolerance, so intake of milk and milk products is low. Many celebrations and rites revolve around food and feasting on traditional dishes (soul food). Traditional dishes such as collard greens, other leafy and yellow vegetables, legumes, beans, rice, and potatoes are high in nutritive value. Overall, the diet tends to be low in fiber, calcium, and potassium and high in fat. Dietary restrictions sometimes related to religious practices.	Diet is low in fat and sugar. Fat intake is limited because of cooking methods. Fish, pork, and poultry, and nuts, dried beans, and tofu are protein sources. Milk products are avoided because of lactose intolerance. Salt intake sometimes high as a result of eating preserved foods and seasoning with soy sauce. Rice is eaten with almost every meal.	Fasting during daylight hours is practiced during Ramadan. Medical condition often exempts person from fasting. Allow family to provide meals if allowed with treatment. Alcohol and drugs are forbidden. Ensure that no pork products are included in foods.	Lack of food and food storage sometimes contribute to nutritional deficiencies. Lactose intolerance is extremely prevalent, affecting 79% of the American Indian population. One hypothesis suggests that some have a predisposition for diabetes that is seemingly triggered by changes in dietary practices and increasing obesity. Contemporary American Indian diet combines food indigenous to the areas with modern processed foods. Food practices are also influenced by tribal beliefs, practices, geographic area, and local availability of selected food. Foods preferred by many include meat and blue cornmeal. Milk is not a preferred food. The fat intake is primarily of saturated fats, and fiber intake is low. Commodity foods are supplied by the U.S. Department of Agriculture's food distribution program.

Obtained from Cooper K, Gosnell K: Foundations of nursing, ed 7, St. Louis, 2015, Mosby.

competing or conflicting values. Some values are more important than others, and the choices made are based on the priority placed on each particular value. A person's values are learned through experience, observation, and reasoning. Some values are consciously chosen; others are adopted unconsciously. As children, society has a strong influence on behaviors and values retained and learned. Acceptable behavior is rewarded, and unacceptable behavior is punished. The development of an individual value system occurs with maturity and largely reflects culture (see Cultural Considerations box).

CULTURAL CONSIDERATIONS: CULTURE AND ETHICS

People of different cultural backgrounds often define health and illness in different ways. Culture is learned as the individual grows up and is influenced (usually subconsciously) by the surrounding environment. The PCT must be aware of cultural differences and should avoid (1) transferring personal expectations to patients; (2) making generalizations based on personal views; (3) assuming that patients can understand what is being said just because they speak English; and (4) treating each patient the same. To meet the individual's needs, respect for a patient's cultural heritage is vital.

PCTs must reflect on and assess the values held. *Value clarification* is the process of self-evaluation that helps gain insight into personal values. To clarify values, do the following: (1) select the belief or behavior and consciously examine it; (2) decide its value; and (3) incorporate the value into everyday responses and behaviors. These steps exercise freedom of choice and determine which values are of most importance. Patients need to act on their own values, not those of the PCT. Sometimes the patient may be referred to a clergy member or other professional who can help deal with ethics issues. Most healthcare institutions have an ethics committee to help resolve ethics questions that arise and to act as an advising body for issues encountered.

CHAPTER SUMMARY

To achieve cultural competence, the PCT needs an understanding of individual cultural beliefs and practices and an ability to perceive the healthcare setting from the patient's point of view. This understanding helps the PCT to be more open and sensitive to the patient's cultural values. The impact of culture on behaviors, attitudes, and values depends on individual factors and varies among members of a specific cultural group. Beliefs and practices vary among and within cultures.

Try to avoid becoming ethnocentric, as it can interfere with development of cultural competence. It is essential to be open to other cultures and value their beliefs and to recognize that your own cultural beliefs are not necessarily superior to those of others. A preconceived idea that all members of a particular group possess the same attributes is known as stereotyping. Ethnic and racial stereotyping can lead to assumptions about an individual that are often inaccurate. Increased knowledge about cultural groups is imperative as transcultural care continues to be important in healthcare.

Case Scenario

As a PCT, part of your required responsibilities is assisting with preparing the body once the patient has died. A newborn baby has died as a result of sudden infant death syndrome. The parents are Native American, and are refusing to hold the infant or take any of the clothes home that the baby was wearing. You are struggling with this, because you believe that closure can occur if you spend time with your loved one that has just died. How should you handle the parent's request to not see the baby? Should you encourage them, stating this will be their only chance?

REVIEW QUESTIONS

1. A Muslim patient visiting the healthcare provider's office was told that she had to remove her clothes and put on an examination gown. The patient became upset and refused to do so. Why should the PCT allow the patient to remain in her clothes?
   a. The patient is embarrassed.
   b. As a Muslim, the patient must keep as much of her body covered as possible.
   c. The patient is being uncooperative.
   d. The patient cannot disrobe in front of another female.

2. The PCT tells her instructor that she does not understand why a Chinese American family is not grieving for their dying father. What behaviors are being demonstrated by the student PCT?
   a. Subculture orientation
   b. Stereotyping
   c. Ethnocentric
   d. Culturally racist

3. A male PCT is assigned to care for a female Muslim patient. When the nurse enters the room, the patient and her husband become upset. Her husband tells the nurse that the PCT cannot care for his wife. Which statement best describes the patient's spouse's position?
   a. The couple is prejudiced against the PCT's race.
   b. The patient is a Muslim, so only women should be assigned to care for her.
   c. The PCT is not Muslim and therefore cannot care for the patient.
   d. The couple does not speak English.

4. What term describes a person who is aware of her or his own cultural beliefs, the beliefs and practices of other cultures, and has the ability to interact effectively with people from other cultures?
   a. Stereotyping
   b. Ethnocentric
   c. Culturally aware
   d. Culturally competent

5. It is appropriate to use a family member such as a patient's child as an interpreter in the hospital setting.
   a. True
   b. False

Patient Rights, Ethics, and Laws

LEARNING OBJECTIVES

1. Summarize the structure and function of the legal system.
2. Discuss the legal relationship that exists between the patient care technician (PCT) and the patient.
3. Explain the importance of maintaining standards of care.
4. Give examples of legal issues in healthcare.
5. Discuss federal regulations of the Health Insurance Portability and Accountability Act of 1996 (HIPAA) privacy rule and its impact on the healthcare system.
6. Give examples of ways the PCT can avoid being involved in a lawsuit.
7. Explain advance directives.
8. Distinguish between ethical and unethical behavior.
9. Explain the meaning of a code of ethics.
10. Explain the PCT's role in reporting unethical behavior.
11. Give examples of ethical issues common in healthcare.

KEY TERMS

accountability Being responsible for one's own actions

acuity How sick the patients are

beneficence The duty to protect life

deposition When witnesses are required to undergo questioning by the attorneys

doctrine of informed consent Full disclosure of the facts the patient needs to make an intelligent (informed) decision before any invasive treatment or procedure is performed

ethical dilemmas Situations that do not have a clear right or wrong answer

ethics Refers to values that influence a person's behavior and the individual's feelings and beliefs about what is right or wrong

euthanasia The practice of intentionally ending a life in order to relieve pain and suffering

laws Prescribe proper behavior in society; they sanction acceptable behavior and prohibit unacceptable behavior

liability Legal responsibility

liable See liability

malpractice Professional negligence, or not taking care of someone in the manner he or she should be cared for based upon established standards and medical practices

nonmaleficence To do no harm

standards of care Acts whose performance is required, permitted, or prohibited

verdict A decision made in a lawsuit or medical malpractice case

Today's healthcare system is dynamic and complex. It has undergone significant changes over the decades. Healthcare providers are guided by established laws, rules, regulations, and ethical principles. The rising cost of healthcare and growing consumer awareness have had an impact on the practice of nursing and the distribution and use of available healthcare resources. Additional challenges are presented by the rapid advances in technology and communication. Practice opportunities and settings for the patient care technician (PCT) are changing with the focus on managed care, community health, and home healthcare.

The practice of the PCT is guided by a combination of legal principles, established laws, moral standards, and ethical principles. PCTs must understand the legal standards and ethical principles that affect practice. Each state has laws that govern the scope and practice of nursing that are referred to as nurse practice acts. The law sets an obligatory minimum standard in any given situation. Ethical principles, which evolve out of society and culture, frequently impose an even higher duty. These legal standards and ethical principles serve as a support for all members of the healthcare system and help protect the rights of all members of society.

LEGAL ASPECTS OF NURSING

The legal relationship that exists between the nurse and the patient is influenced by the existing laws, rules, and regulations that govern nursing practice. Acting outside the established scope of practice or failing to meet the established standard of care has the potential to result in injury to the patient and give rise to legal liability and the potential loss or sanction of the nursing license. Nurses must be aware of their scope of nursing practice and the standards of care that constitute professional duties. The PCT completes tasks that are assigned by the nurse. It is important that the nurse does not delegate tasks that do not fall within his or her scope of nursing.

Many legal issues are related to healthcare, and healthcare-related litigation that involves nurses and other healthcare workers is common (Fig. 6.1). Today's patients are more educated, are more aware of their rights, and have higher expectations regarding the care they receive. To practice safely, the healthcare team must have a familiarity with common legal issues in healthcare.

Overview of the Legal System

The legal system is a complex set of rules and regulations that have developed in response to the needs of society. Laws prescribe proper behavior in society; they sanction acceptable behavior and prohibit unacceptable behavior. The healthcare team must have a basic

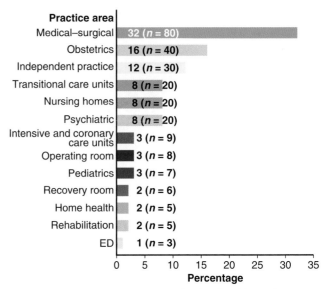

FIGURE 6.1 Practice settings involved in healthcare litigation. (From Croke E: Nurses, negligence and malpractice, *Am J Nurs* 103(9):61, 2003.)

| Box 6.1 | Characteristics of Criminal and Civil Law |

Criminal
- Conduct at issue is offensive to society *in general.*
- Conduct at issue is detrimental to society as a *whole.*
- The law involves *public* offenses (such as robbery, murder, and assault).
- The law's purpose is to *punish* for the crime and deter and *prevent* further crimes.

Civil
- Conduct at issue violates a *person's* rights.
- Conduct at issue is detrimental to that *individual.*
- The law involves an offense that is against an *individual.*
- The law's purpose is to *make the aggrieved person whole again,* to restore the person to where he or she was.

understanding of the legal system, which serves both to mandate and to protect. The law assigns fundamental legal duties and also provides protection for all members of the healthcare system.

The two primary categories of law are criminal and civil (Box 6.1). Matters related to criminal law are those that involve the needs of the public. Cases that concern matters of criminal law are charged by agents that represent either the federal or the state government. Civil cases are between individuals. The charges involved in a civil matter are brought by a person or agency. An important note is that some degree of overlap may exist with the cases. For example, a criminal matter may result in individuals filing a civil lawsuit. The penalties that result from the cases also differ. Criminal cases are resolved with a finding of guilt or innocence. The penalty may involve fines, incarceration, or a combination of the two. Civil matters conclude with a determination of accountability or innocence. Settlements of a monetary nature are assigned based on the type of liability assessed. Civil law and criminal law are established in one of two ways: (1) federal, state, and local governments develop *statutory law*; (2) *common law*, or case law, evolves in response to specific legal questions that come before the court and usually follows *precedent* (previous rulings on an issue).

Negligence

Negligence refers to the failure to act in a manner demonstrating the care and knowledge any prudent individual would. Examples of negligence may include medication errors, patient falls, use of restraints, and equipment injuries (Motacki and Burke, 2011). Nurses and unlicensed assistive personnel (UAP), such as the PCT, may be charged with negligence. Professional-level accountability and judgment are not required elements to establish negligence (see Fig. 6.1). An example of negligence can be found in Box 6.2.

Malpractice

Malpractice refers to professional negligence. PCT responsibilities include both actions taken and those omitted. The concept of malpractice must contain four key elements. Each of the elements must be present for liability to be established.

1. *Duty:* refers to the established relationship between the patient and the nurse.
2. *Breach* of duty: failure to perform the duty in a reasonable, prudent manner.
3. *Harm* has occurred; this does not have to be physical injury.
4. The breach of duty was the *proximate cause* of the harm; the occurrence of harm depended directly on the occurrence of the breach.

If the court finds that malpractice has occurred, the nurse or PCT is subject to legal punishment or restitution as the court determines. The best way to avoid being charged with malpractice is to practice within the rules and regulations, the standards of care, and the employing agency's policies and procedures. The caregiver–patient relationship is also very important; the nurse should strive to maintain a positive relationship. A poor caregiver–patient relationship has been identified as a leading factor in whether a patient seeks legal action. If there is a poor caregiver–patient relationship, the relationship between the PCT and the patient may be strained, or difficult, as well.

Box 6.2 — Busta v Columbus Hospital Corporation (1996)

While he was a postoperative patient at Columbus Hospital in Great Falls, Mr. Busta died from injuries sustained in a fall from his third-floor window; apparently, he had tried to climb down on an improvised rope. At trial, the nurse assigned to care for Mr. Busta testified that, during her last evening visit with him, he had experienced an episode of tachycardia and hypertension. He had also behaved atypically, desiring isolation and refusing all nursing care and his prescribed medication, known to have adverse effects, including confusion, anxiety, and psychosis. The nurse did not report the symptoms and the change in behavior to the physician. She also testified that, when she observed the patient at midnight, he appeared to be sleeping; she did not reassess his vital signs.

Mr. Busta's surgeon testified that, because of the mind-altering adverse effects of the patient's medication, he would have reassessed his patient if he had been notified of the changing signs and symptoms. Expert testimony opined that the nurse was negligent in failing to adequately monitor Mr. Busta on the evening and night before he died and in failing to report the constellation of signs and symptoms to the surgeon, and that the hospital was negligent in failing to maintain a safe environment (evidence presented at trial showed that the hospital had not acted on a directive from The Joint Commission [TJC] to restrict the opening of windows in patients' rooms).

The jury found that the negligence of Columbus Hospital, combined with the patient's contributory negligence, caused the patient's injuries and death; the jury apportioned 70% of the liability to the hospital and 30% to Mr. Busta. The jury found that Mr. Busta and his estate were damaged in the amount of $5000 and his heirs $800,000. On the basis of the jury's apportioned liability, the district court entered a judgment in favor of Mr. Busta's estate in the amount of $3500 and in favor of his heirs $560,000.

(From Croke E: Nurses, negligence and malpractice. Am J Nurs 103[9]:59–60, 2003.)

Overview of the Legal Process

Civil litigation involves the legal exchange between individuals as opposed to legal concerns that involve a criminal matter, which would involve the state or federal government bringing charges. Most legal suits in healthcare involve civil litigation. The process for filing a claim begins when an individual believes that a breach of duty has taken place and resulted in pain, suffering, or injury. At that time, the plaintiff (the complaining party) typically seeks legal representation. In some states, a prelitigation panel may meet to ascertain the validity of the suit being proposed. If this process results in a finding that litigation in this case has a legal basis, the plaintiff writes a statement called a *complaint* and files it in the appropriate court. The complaint names the *defendant* (the person alleged to be liable [legally responsible]) states the facts involved in the case, defines the legal issues the case raises, and outlines the *damages* (compensation that the plaintiff is seeking). The defendant is served a *summons* (a court order that notifies the defendant of the legal action), which constitutes the necessary legal notice, and the defendant usually hires an attorney to represent him or her in the lawsuit. The defendant is asked to provide a response to the charges. This response is either an admission of guilt or a denial of allegations listed in the complaint.

Discovery is the next step in the process. Discovery allows both sides of the case to review documents and interview witnesses. The witnesses may be the defendant being named in the suit or individuals who have facts about the case. Witnesses are required to undergo questioning by the attorneys. This process is referred to as the deposition. Witnesses are under oath. The statements made are recorded. This transcript becomes a part of the evidence.

Other tools also serve the process of discovery. The *interrogatory* is a written question that one party sends to the other party, to which an answer is legally required. A *Request for Production of Documents and Things* is a formal request by the agents filing the charges for all items that are found to be related to the situation, or case, at hand. In a healthcare-related case, these items may include policies and procedures, standards of care, medical records, assignment sheets, personnel files, equipment maintenance records, birth certificates, marriage certificates, medical bills, and other documents pertinent to the issues at hand. A fourth discovery technique is the admission of facts. This tool requests the party to admit or deny certain statements to streamline the factual presentation of the case.

Once the evidence has been presented, the court renders a verdict (a decision) based on the facts of the case, the evidence and testimony presented, the credibility of the witnesses, and the laws that pertain to the issue. Either party has the right, in case of disagreement with the outcome of the lawsuit, to file an *appeal* (request a review of the decision) asking that a higher court review the decision. The outcome of litigation is never certain.

In a criminal trial, the question is whether the defendant (the person accused of the crime) is answerable for a crime against the people (because criminal law concerns crimes against society rather than individuals). At trial, both the people's attorney and the defendant's attorney present their cases. The judge or the jury (if a jury trial) then *deliberates* (considers and decides) the guilt or innocence of the defendant. If the judge or jury reaches a verdict of *not guilty,* the defendant is free to go. If the verdict is *guilty,* the judge passes a *sentence* (penalty) based on the severity of the crime, the defendant's past criminal record, and applicable laws. The defendant who receives a guilty verdict may appeal if there has been an error either (1) in the process in which the conviction was obtained, or (2) by the court during the proceedings. (See Box 6.3 for common legal terminology.)

Legal Relationships

Legal liability for alleged harm may be solely held or shared between multiple parties. The patient or family may choose to pursue charges against the facility, nursing personnel, medical staff, or ancillary departments. Each may be charged separately or in a group. In the past, nurses did not hold legal liability for alleged

Box 6.3	Common Legal Terminology
Abandonment of care	Wrongful termination of providing patient care
Assault	An intentional threat to cause bodily harm to another; does not have to include actual bodily contact
Battery	Unlawful touching of another person without informed consent
Competency	A legal presumption that a person who has reached the age of majority can make decisions for herself or himself unless proved otherwise (if she or he has been legally declared incompetent)
Defamation	Spoken or written statements made maliciously and intentionally that may injure the subject's reputation
Harm	Injury to a person or the person's property that gives rise to a basis for a legal action against the person who caused the damage
Libel	A malicious or untrue writing about another person that is brought to the attention of others
Malpractice	Failure to meet a legal duty, thus causing harm to another
Negligence	The commission (doing) of an act or the omission (not doing) of an act that a reasonably prudent person would have performed in a similar situation, thus causing harm to another person
Slander	Malicious or untrue spoken words about another person that are brought to the attention of others
Tort	A type of civil law that involves wrongs against a person or property; torts include negligence, assault, battery, defamation, fraud, false imprisonment, and invasion of privacy

harm suffered by a patient while receiving medical care, but rather the physician or the hospital did, and sometimes both. As nurses gained recognition for their expertise and gained more autonomy, dissatisfied patients (and their attorneys) began to look at nurses as potential defendants and to seek to hold nurses accountable under the law. As a PCT who works under a nurse, it is important that you follow all procedures and policies related to what tasks can be delegated to you by the nurse. Accountability (being responsible for one's own actions) is a concept that gives rise to a legal duty and thus liability (legal responsibility) in nursing. Indeed, the PCT today is not immune from liability in the healthcare setting. Nurses are facing increased responsibilities in the healthcare arena. The technological advances require more knowledge and competence. Staffing shortages and budgetary constraints may also play a role. High levels of patient acuity (how sick the patients are) and an emphasis on early discharge (how fast they can go home) may result in the need for more comprehensive referrals and improved discharge teaching. Errors in either may result in litigation. Finally, insurance experts believe that some responsibility may rest with the large payout to litigants. The most common areas of litigation against nurses and healthcare workers involve performance failures in the following areas: standards of care, use of equipment, documentation, and patient advocacy (Reising and Allen, 2007).

A landmark case that addressed nursing liability was *Darling v Charleston Community Memorial Hospital* (http://biotech.law.lsu.edu/cases/Medmal/darling.htm). In this case, an 18-year-old man fractured his leg and had a cast applied in the hospital. He was admitted to a room, and the nurses caring for the patient noticed that the toes on his casted leg were edematous and discolored. The patient reported decreased feeling in his toes to the nursing staff. Over the next few days, gangrene developed, and the man's leg had to be amputated. The Illinois Supreme Court heard the case and held that the nurses were liable, along with the physician, because the nursing staff had failed to adhere to the standards of care. This case established a precedent that almost every state has adopted. It is important for the PCT to always stay in communication with the nurse, and communicate to the nurse any signs or symptoms that may not seem right. The PCT plays an important role in keeping the lines of communication open between the nurse and patient. There are times when the PCT may spend more time with the patient during the shift than the nurse is able to. This can prove to enhance, or make better, the care for the patient.

Regulation of Practice

Standards of care define acts whose performance is required, permitted, or prohibited. These standards of care derive from federal and state laws, rules, and regulations and codes that govern other professional agencies and organizations such as the American Nurses Association (ANA) and the Canadian Nurses Association (CNA). These organizations regularly evaluate existing standards and revise them as needed. Standards of care coupled with the *scope of nursing practice* give direction to the practicing nurse. They define the obligations of the nurse, including those activities that are obligation and those that are prohibited. Failure to adhere to these standards gives rise to legal liability. Ignorance of the requirements and limitations does not absolve liability.

Liability for healthcare workers falls into several areas: practice, monitoring, and communication. Box 6.4 shows common breaches of the standards of care. The legal test is the comparison with the hypothetical actions under similar circumstances of a reasonably *prudent* (careful, wise) nurse of similar education and experience. The standards of care follow those laws of the individual state. In reality, application of the standards is not always easy. Nursing shortages in some states have led to a need for individual nurses to take on increased responsibilities and work more hours, and the increased use of UAP, such as the PCT. Personnel cutbacks often leave units short staffed, and nurses feel pressure to take on expanded duties; this raises their risk for liability considerably. In addition, special challenges face entry-level UAPs when they enter the workforce. Orientation programs often fail to adequately cover all the skills needed to be a competent technician. It is the PCT's responsibility to seek additional instruction and supervision when faced with an unfamiliar practice or procedure. The PCT may need to ask the nurse to demonstrate an unfamiliar procedure. Remember that it is not possible for the PCT to meet every single patient's needs.

Delegation and Documentation Box 6.1

- If the nurse asks you to perform a skill that you are unfamiliar with, be sure to seek assistance from the nurse before attempting the skill.
- The registered nurse (RN) should delegate to the PCT. Do not accept delegated tasks from other PCTs. If a PCT asks you to complete a task, first go to your nurse and clarify if you should perform the task.

The laws that formally define and limit the scope of nursing practice are called *nurse practice acts*. All state, provincial, and territorial legislatures in the United States and Canada have adopted nurse practice acts, although the specifics they contain often vary. It is the nurse's responsibility to know the nurse practice act that is in effect for the geographic region. One can write to

Box 6.4   Common Breaches of the Standard of Care

Practice
- Failure to use proper judgment
- Failure to properly assess
- Failure to properly administer medication
- Failure to protect patients from burns
- Failure to properly maintain the airway
- Failure to restock crash cart
- Failure to honor advance directives
- Failure to take an accurate and thorough history
- Failure to provide a safe environment
- Failure to properly administer injections
- Failure to go through hierarchy to get the care needed
- Failure to detect that the patient has an allergy
- Failure to protect the patient from abuse
- Failure to prevent abuse, neglect, or injury by other patients
- Failure to obtain physician orders—practicing outside the scope of nursing practice by writing orders
- Failure to practice safely (by using drugs or alcohol while working)
- Failure to protect and prevent falls

Monitoring
- Failure to properly monitor
- Failure to recognize and report signs and symptoms of patient's deteriorating condition
- Failure to properly use monitoring equipment
- Failure to protect against injuries from monitoring equipment
- Failure to detect or prevent decubitus ulcers
- Failure to monitor and detect polypharmacy effects on patient
- Failure to detect signs and symptoms of a medical condition in a timely and proper fashion
- Failure to detect signs and symptoms of drug toxicity
- Failure to properly use restraints

Communication
- Failure to document in a timely and proper fashion
- Failure to notify physician of laboratory values in a timely and proper fashion
- Failure to report child or elder abuse
- Failure to notify physician of a change in status
- Failure to communicate with other healthcare personnel about advance directives
- Failure to properly give discharge instructions
- Failure to document patient's status or condition in a timely and proper fashion
- Failure to document communications between healthcare providers in a timely and proper fashion
- Failure to document the need for restraints in a timely and proper fashion
- Failure to properly document (precharting)

the board of nursing in a given state or access its website to obtain a free copy of the state's nurse practice act. It is important for PCTs to know and be aware what is contained in their individual state's nurse practice act. It further helps to develop the scope of the PCT.

In addition to the boundaries made by the state's nurse practice act, the employing institution often places limitations on practice. The institution has the right to establish policies and procedures for PCT activities within the confines of the state's nurse practice act. When a question comes before the court regarding whether the standard of care was met in a particular situation, the court uses a variety of resources to answer the question (Box 6.5).

Legal Issues

Many legal issues affect the PCT and influence the level of care delivered to the patient. Both statutory and common law play important roles in defining the rights and responsibilities of the patient and the nursing professionals. The patient has a right to expect the PCT to act in the patient's best interest by providing care that meets and is consistent with the established legal standards and principles.

Box 6.5   Evidence of Nursing Standards

- Practice protocols, contracts, practice agreements, employment agreements, and personnel or employee manuals
- Agency policy and procedure manuals
- State nurse practice acts and regulations
- American Nurses Association Code for Nurses (2001)
- American Nurses Association Standards of Practice (1995)
- Accreditation criteria of The Joint Commission (formerly the Joint Commission on Accreditation of Healthcare Organizations [JCAHO])
- Other accreditation standards depending on the practice setting (e.g., National League for Nursing, National Association of Home Care)
- State and federal licensing laws and regulations that govern healthcare agencies; state, professional, and occupational legislation and regulations
- Nursing specialty standards of care and certification
- Nursing literature, textbooks, and journals
- Education, continuing education, staff development, and orientation
- Experience
- Expert nurse witness, other experts, and peers
- Customs and usual community practices

Patients' Rights

Patients have expectations regarding the healthcare services they receive. In 1972, the American Hospital Association (AHA) developed the Patient's Bill of Rights. Since its inception, the Patient's Bill of Rights has undergone revisions; the modified version of 2003 is called The Patient Care Partnership: Understanding Expectations, Rights, and Responsibilities. The AHA encourages healthcare institutions to adapt the template bill of rights to their particular environments. This involves considering the cultural, religious, linguistic, and educational backgrounds of the population the institution serves. In 1980, the Mental Health Patient's Bill of Rights and the Pregnant Patient's Bill of Rights were adopted into law. The goal of the AHA is to promote the public's understanding of their rights and responsibilities as consumers of healthcare. Failure of the healthcare provider to embrace the outlined rights of the patient can promote breaches in the relationship between the nurse and the patient.

The Joint Commission is an independent accrediting agency responsible for accrediting and certifying more than 19,000 facilities in the United States. The Joint Commission has developed a brochure titled *Know Your Rights,* which is a statement on the rights and responsibilities of patients. The Patient Self-Determination Act (included in the Omnibus Budget Reconciliation Act of 1990, U.S. Code vol. 42, sec. 1395 cc[a][1]) regulates any institution that receives federal funding. The Patient Self-Determination Act requires that institutions maintain written policies and procedures regarding advance directives (including the use of life support if the patient is incapacitated), the right to accept or refuse treatment, and the right to participate fully in healthcare-related decisions.

The Health Insurance Portability and Accountability Act of 1996 (HIPAA), which took effect in 2003, established the duty of the healthcare provider to protect the confidentiality of all health information. Healthcare providers who maintain and transmit healthcare information must provide reasonable and appropriate administrative, technical, and physical safeguards on a patient's health information. The law sets rules and limits on who has permission to look at and receive health information, and assigns penalties for wrongful disclosure of individually identifiable health information. All healthcare providers must be knowledgeable about the HIPAA standards and protect the privacy rights of patients and residents (www.hhs.gov/ocr/hipaa).

Healthcare institutions are obligated to uphold the patient's rights to (1) access to healthcare without any prejudice, (2) treatment with respect and dignity at all times, (3) privacy and confidentiality, (4) personal safety, and (5) complete information about one's own condition and treatment.

Patients' responsibilities to the healthcare institution include (1) providing accurate information about themselves, (2) giving information regarding their known conditions, and (3) participating in decision making regarding treatment and care.

Informed Consent

The Patient Care Partnership establishes the patient's right to make decisions regarding his or her healthcare. The doctrine of informed consent refers to full disclosure of the facts the patient needs to make an intelligent (informed) decision before any invasive treatment or procedure is performed (Fig. 6.2). The patient has the right to accept or reject the proposed care but only after understanding fully what is being proposed—that is, the benefits of the treatment, the risks involved, any alternative treatments, and the consequences of refusing the treatment or procedure. The explanation of the procedure has to be in nontechnical terms and in a language the patient can understand. Failure to secure informed consent may result in civil liability for battery. *Civil battery* (also called technical battery) is the unlawful touching of a person; an intent to harm is not necessary. Consent must be freely given. Coercion negates the spirit of informed consent. Patients who seek treatment sign forms to indicate acceptance of care interventions. Additional consent for treatment may be needed for further invasive actions. Patients may withdraw or limit consent at any time. Consent may be communicated in a variety of ways. Patients may imply consent by their actions. Patients may verbalize their acceptance of treatment interventions. Invasive procedures may require a written consent document to be completed.

Consent must be provided by the appropriate person (Benak and Applegate, 2006). To provide consent, the patient must be at least 18 years of age. Minors under the age of 18 years may consent for treatment in the event they meet certain criteria including the following:

- Marriage
- Court-approved emancipation
- Living apart from parents or guardians for at least 60 days and independent of parental support
- Service in the armed forces

In some situations, a minor may consent for care, including treatment for sexually transmitted infections, drug and alcohol abuse, sexual assault, and family planning.

There must also be competence to consent for care. Competence requires that the patient has sound mind to accept the treatment. In addition, consent cannot be obtained from one who is impaired or under the influence of alcohol or drugs. In the event that the patient is deemed incompetent to provide consent, a legal process exists for the determination of the individual legally

---

AUTHORIZATION FOR AND CONSENT TO OPERATION. ADMINISTRATION OF ANESTHETICS, SPECIAL DIAGNOSTIC OR THERAPEUTIC PROCEDURES AND THE RENDERING OF OTHER MEDICAL SERVICES

Patient ___Jaelyn Cooper___   Date ___January 9, 2014___   Time ___0800___

1. **Operation or Procedure and Alternatives**

   a. I hereby authorize Dr. ___Kelly Gosnell___ and whomever she may designate as her assistants to perform the following procedure and/or alternative procedure necessary to treat my condition: (state nature of procedure(s) to be performed).

   ___Right total hip replacement___

   ___OK for blood transfusion___

   (LIST PROCEDURE(S))

   b. I understand the reason for the procedure is: ___to replace my right hip joint and the head of my right hip bone. OK to receive___

   ___blood transfusion___

   c. For the purpose of advancing medical education and care, I consent to the admittance of observers to the operating room.

   d. It has been explained to me that conditions may arise during this procedure whereby a different procedure or an additional procedure may need to be performed and I authorize my physician and her assistants to do what they feel is needed and necessary.

   e. I understand that no guarantee or assurance has been made as to the results of the procedure and that it may not cure the condition.

   f. I consent to the examination and disposal by hospital authorities of any tissues or body parts that may be removed.

2. **Risks:** This authorization is given with the understanding that any operation or procedure involves some risks and hazards. The more common risks include: infection, bleeding, nerve injury, blood clots, heart attack, allergic reactions, and pneumonia. These risks can be serious and possibly fatal. Specific risks for this procedure and alternative methods of care have been explained to me by my physician.

3. **Anesthesia:** The administration of anesthesia also involves risks, most importantly a rare risk of reaction to medications causing severe injury or death. I consent to the use of such anesthetics as may be considered necessary by the person responsible for these services.

4. **Photography:** I consent to the photographing of operations to be performed, including appropriate portions of my body for medical, scientific, or educational purposes, providing my identity is not revealed by the pictures or by the descriptive texts accompanying them.

5. **Patient's Consent:** I have read and fully understand this consent form, and I understand I should not sign this form if all items, including all my questions, have not been explained or answered to my satisfaction or if I do not understand any of the terms or words contained in this consent form.

   IF YOU HAVE ANY QUESTIONS AS TO THE RISKS OR HAZARDS OF THE PROPOSED SURGERY OR TREATMENT, OR ANY QUESTIONS CONCERNING THE PROPOSED SURGERY OR TREATMENT ASK YOUR SURGEON NOW! **BEFORE SIGNING THIS CONSENT FORM.**

   DO NOT SIGN UNLESS YOU HAVE READ AND THOROUGHLY UNDERSTAND THIS FORM!

6. I certify that I have read and fully understand the above consent after adequate explanations were made to me, and after all blanks were filled in or crossed out before I signed.

   Kim Russell
   (Witness to Signature only)

   Signed   *Jaelyn Cooper*
   (Patient, Parent, or Legal Guardian's Signature)

   Betty Berg RN
   (Second Witness Signature if needed)

   (Doctor Signature)

   (i.e., Telephone Consent)

   AUTHORIZATION AND CONSENT

Valley Regional Medical Center
12 West Industrial Blvd.
Terre Haute, IN 47805
(800) 555-0000

NS-81 (Rev. 2/01)

LABEL

4532

FIGURE 6.2 Sample consent for a special procedure. (From Cooper K, Gosnell K: *Foundations of nursing*, ed 7, St. Louis, 2015, Mosby.)

eligible to provide the consent. In many cases, consent is provided by the spouse. In the absence of the spouse, this role may be passed to another legally identified individual.

It is the duty of the physician or nurse practitioner who is performing the procedure or treatment to provide the needed information to the patient. It is not the duty of the PCT to obtain informed consent. The nurse often has the responsibility to witness the patient signing the consent. In this case, the nurse's responsibility is limited to the actual witnessing of the signature, not provision of information. Neither the nurse nor the PCT discusses with the patient the elements of disclosure that the physician or the nurse practitioner are required to make. Involvement in providing this type of information to the patient potentially places the nurse and PCT in a position of liability. Answers to any unanswered questions that the patient has about the procedure are the responsibility of the healthcare provider who will perform the procedure.

Certain situations may require consent for treatment to be obtained over the telephone. Healthcare facilities have policies that govern telephonic consent. This type of consent is traditionally needed in management of emergency procedures.

Confidentiality

PCTs have a duty to protect information about a patient regardless of how the information is kept. Information should be accessed only on a need-to-know basis. For example, on a patient care unit, only those healthcare personnel directly involved in an individual's care should be able to access that patient's information. Failure to maintain patient confidentiality risks legal liability, and both civil and criminal filings may result. Employers consider violations of confidentiality an offense that justifies termination. The responsibility of maintaining confidentiality is not limited to the work shift. All matters committed to the PCT's keeping are to be held in confidence. Securing the materials that contain confidential information is a responsibility of the PCT. These materials include not only the physical chart forms but the technological resources as well. When accessing computerized patient files, the PCT must ensure that the appropriate log-out information is entered to prevent others from viewing the records. Written notes and chart forms must be stored in restricted areas. Conversations discussing patients and their personal information should be held in private conference rooms. Discussions away from the patient care areas, such as the elevator or cafeteria, are problematic and should be avoided.

Medical Records

Laws govern the collection, maintenance, and disclosure of information in medical records. Each healthcare institution also has policies and procedures regarding patient medical records. Medical records are not public documents, and the information they contain must be kept secure. Any breach in the confidentiality of information kept in a patient's medical record risks legal liability.

In a lawsuit, both parties are permitted to use the patient's medical record to argue facts of the case. Entries made in the chart often show whether the standards of care were met in a given situation. It is essential that the employing institution's policies and procedures regarding the patient's medical record are followed. All entries in the medical record must be permanent, accurate, complete, and legible. Two current trends potentially affect patient confidentiality. Many smaller healthcare organizations are merging to form large corporations in an effort to save resources while continuing to provide services. Also, computer-based healthcare records are becoming common. Together, these two trends have the potential to vastly widen and increase the numbers of people with access to confidential patient information. Those implementing these trends are required to take federal HIPAA privacy standards into consideration and prevent unauthorized release of medical records and patient information.

Invasion of Privacy

The legal concept of invasion of privacy involves a person's right to be left alone and remain anonymous if he or she chooses. Consent for treatment does not mean that the person is giving up his or her right to privacy. Privacy-related concerns may include the physical exposure or disclosure of patient information to others. When providing care, the PCT should protect the patient from unnecessary exposure with the use of drapes and remember to close the door or use available signage to restrict admission to rooms during procedures as needed. Calls and inquiries concerning the patient should be handled with care and in accordance with the healthcare facility's policy and procedures. Providing information such as status of the patient to callers can result in a breach in confidentiality. Calls should be referred to the charge nurse or available family members. PCTs frequently take notes during change of shift report. These notes should be closely monitored during the shift. Report sheets and communication tools should be destroyed at the end of the shift before the PCT leaves the worksite. Use of any patient information (name, photograph, specific facts regarding an illness, and so on) without authorization is a violation of the patient's legal rights. Safeguard the patient's right to privacy at all times.

Reporting Abuse

There are exceptions to the right to privacy. The law stipulates that the healthcare professional is required to report certain information to the appropriate authorities. The report should be given to a supervisor or directly to the police, according to agency policy. When acting in good faith to report mandated information (e.g., certain communicable diseases or gunshot wounds), the healthcare professional is protected from liability.

In an effort to respond to the growing problem of child abuse, the federal Child Abuse Prevention Treatment Act of 1973 made the reporting of child abuse *mandatory.* Healthcare professionals are mandated reporters, meaning that one cannot ignore the presence of abuse. Failure to report suspected cases to the appropriate authorities may result in fines or imprisonment. This means that you can be held responsible for failing to report signs of abuse. Facilities have procedures in place to assist you when making reports. Withholding medical treatment to an infant born with serious life-threatening handicaps is a form of child abuse. Congress enacted the Child Abuse Amendments in 1984 to protect the rights of these handicapped newborns to proper treatment and care. These regulations make any institution that receives federal funds legally responsible to investigate the withholding of medical treatment to an infant. In general, withholding of lifesaving treatment and care is a form of passive euthanasia (letting a person die) and medical neglect. This act carries the risk of professional neglect (medical malpractice) charges.

Spousal and elder abuse may also be a hidden problem within a family. Populations at increased risk include women and older adults (see Lifespan Considerations for Older Adults section). Most states have responded to the issue of spousal and elder abuse by enacting laws to protect victims. Fines, restraining orders that prohibit contact by the abusing person, and even imprisonment are some of the ways often attempted to protect the victims of abuse. Abuse is an underreported crime. Only a portion of abuse cases are ever reported. It is the responsibility of the PCT to know the signs of abuse and the procedures for reporting suspected cases.

LIFESPAN CONSIDERATIONS FOR OLDER ADULTS/ELDER ABUSE

Factors that put older adults at risk for physical, emotional, or financial abuse include the following:

- Declining physical health
- Declining mental ability
- Decreased strength and mobility
- Loss of independence
- Isolation
- Loss of loved ones, friends, and relatives

These factors often make the older adult feel helpless and frightened. Impaired communication, decreased hearing acuity, and anxiety make assessment of an older adult more difficult, but be sure nonetheless to watch for the signs of abuse.

Workplace violence is another form of abuse that occurs at times in the healthcare setting. This form of violence includes verbal abuse, emotional abuse, sexual harassment, physical assault, and threatening behavior. Healthcare institutions are implementing policies and procedures to promote a safe work environment, and education is an important component of the awareness and prevention measures. Strategies to provide adequate supervision, employ security personnel, monitor work areas, and encourage reporting of incidents represent efforts to decrease the incidence of workplace violence.

How to Avoid a Lawsuit

The best defense against a lawsuit is to provide compassionate, competent care. The PCT and patient relationship should be based on trust and respect. Open and honest communication is the key to building a therapeutic relationship and often helps resolve patient dissatisfaction before the patient resorts to legal action. Following the standards of care and the policies and procedures of the facility and adhering to the scope of practice for the PCT reduce the likelihood of lawsuit. Remaining current on practice developments and taking advantage of continuing education opportunities help to ensure competence.

PCTs may find themselves in settings outside of the worksite in which an individual is injured and needs assistance. Concerns may result about the responsibility of the PCT and the decision to offer assistance to a victim. UAPs, such as the PCT or CNA, are not required to offer assistance when they are acting as a "private citizen." If one chooses to offer help, liability may be limited under Good Samaritan laws. These statutes have been developed to provide immunity from liability in certain circumstances. The goal of this protection (except in cases of gross negligence) is to encourage assistance in emergencies that occur outside of a medical facility. State and provincial laws vary, so it is important to know the Good Samaritan laws that apply. A reference with links to individual state positions on Good Samaritan laws can be found at www.heartsafeam.com/pages/faq_good_samaritan.

Proper documentation in the medical record is another important factor in assessment of liability. The medical record is thoroughly examined in the event of a lawsuit, and its use is permitted to demonstrate in court the level of care that was provided to the patient. An important legal presumption to remember is, "Care was not given if it was not charted." Simply stating care was provided does not provide legal protection. Omissions in charting provide a great boost to the team bringing the lawsuit.

ETHICAL ASPECTS OF NURSING

The science of ethical studies the relationships between moral actions and values and how these affect society. The word ethics refers to values that influence a person's behavior and the individual's feelings and beliefs about what is right or wrong. Healthcare ethics involve moral values and principles that affect personal and professional conduct. As previously mentioned, the PCT has the responsibility to practice within the legal and ethical boundaries of practice. Healthcare ethics propose the duties and obligations of PCTs to their patients, other healthcare professionals, the profession itself, and society.

Advance Directives

Advance directives are signed and witnessed documents that provide specific instructions for healthcare treatment in the event that a person is unable to make these decisions personally at the time they are needed.

The two basic types of advance directives are living wills and durable powers of attorney for healthcare. Many patients have instituted one or both.

The Patient Self-Determination Act (PSDA, 1991) requires healthcare institutions to provide written information to patients concerning the patient's rights under state law to make decisions, including the right to refuse treatment and formulate advance directives. It is especially important to understand patients' cultural beliefs and values when explaining advance directives. Regulatory mandates to benefit the public are based on the dominant value in American society of self-determination, which may be in conflict with a patient's cultural heritage.

Under the act, whether the patient has signed an advance directive must be documented in the patient's record. The hospital is also required to ensure that state law is followed. The institution must provide education for the staff and the public concerning living wills and durable powers of attorney. For either type of advance directive to be enforceable, the patient must be legally incompetent or lack capacity to make decisions regarding healthcare treatment. This means that they are mentally unable to make decisions for themselves that are based on sound judgment. The termination of legal competency is made by a judge, and the determination of decisional capacity is usually made by the physician and the family. Therefore the advance directive is implemented within the context of the healthcare team and the healthcare institution. One should be familiar with the institution's policies involving the act.

A living will is a written document that directs treatment in accordance with a patient's wishes in the event of a terminal illness or condition (Fig. 6.3). Living wills are often difficult to interpret and are not clinically specific in unforeseen circumstances. Each state has its own requirements for executing living wills. Generally, the presence of two witnesses is required when the patient signs the document; neither may be a relative or physician. If healthcare workers follow the directions of the living will, they should be safe from liability.

A durable power of attorney for healthcare designates an agent, surrogate, or proxy to make healthcare decisions on the patient's behalf based on the patient's wishes. A proxy is someone who is put in place to make the decisions of the person.

In addition to federal statutes, the ethical doctrine of autonomy ensures the patient the right to refuse medical treatment. This right was upheld in the Bouvia v Superior Court case in 1986. That case allowed the discontinuation of the patient's tube feedings as per the patient's prior request. The courts have also upheld the right of a legally competent patient to refuse medical treatment based on religious beliefs. Jehovah's Witnesses, for example, accept medical treatment but refuse blood transfusions. In the absence of a truly compelling reason otherwise, the right to make such choices is protected. The U.S. Supreme Court stated in the Cruzan v Director, Missouri Department of Health case in 1990 that "we assume that the U.S. Constitution would grant a constitutionally protected competent person the right to refuse lifesaving hydration and nutrition." In cases that involve the patient's right to refuse or withdraw medical treatment, the courts balance the patient's interest with the state's interest in protecting life, preserving medical ethics, preventing suicide, and protecting innocent third parties. Children are generally considered innocent third parties, as they are not old enough to make their own decisions, so someone else has to. Although the courts do not force adults to undergo treatment that is refused for religious reasons, they do grant an order that allows hospitals and physicians to treat children of Christian Scientists or Jehovah's Witnesses who have denied consent for treatment of their minor children.

When patients are legally incompetent and are unable to make healthcare decisions, the court steps in. Balancing the state's interest with that of the patient, the court attempts to deliver a judgment that represents what the patient would have chosen if competent. The Supreme Court held in the Cruzan case that states had the right to require "clear and convincing evidence" of a legally incompetent patient's prior wishes when making determinations to discontinue life-sustaining treatment. In that case, nutrition and hydration were recognized as life-sustaining medical treatment that could be withdrawn.

Every state now requires "clear and convincing" evidence of the patient's choice, but individual states differ as to what standard satisfies the requirement. In the absence of evidence indicating the patient's prior

LIVING WILL DECLARATION OF

If I should lapse into a persistent vegetative state or have an incurable and irreversible condition that, without the administration of life-sustaining treatment, will, in the opinion of my attending physician, cause my death within a relatively short time and I am no longer able to make decisions regarding my medical treatment, I direct my attending physician, pursuant to the Rights of the Terminally Ill Act, to withhold or withdraw life-sustaining treatment that is not necessary for my comfort or to alleviate pain.

Declarant Signature

Signed this_____ day of _____ , 20 _____

Social Security Number: _____ Date of Birth: _____

Address:_____ Signature: _____

City/State:_____

The declarant voluntarily signed this writing in my presence.

Signature of witness: _____ Printed name/Date:_____

Signature of witness: _____ Printed name/Date:_____

-OR-
NOTARY

The declarant voluntarily signed this document in my presence.

STATE OF NEBRASKA   )
) SS.
COUNTY OF_____)   Notary Public

FIGURE 6.3 Example of a living will. (From Cooper K, Gosnell K: *Foundations of nursing,* ed 7, St. Louis, 2015, Mosby.)

choice, most states allow treatment to be stopped based on other factors, including the best interest of the patient balanced with the state's interest (Box 6.6).

Development of Ethical Principles

Ethical dilemmas are situations that do not have a clear right or wrong answer. They are complex, confusing, and often frustrating situations that call for careful rational analysis. First, the problem needs to be identified as an ethical one. This means that the question presented cannot be answered by applying external laws, rules, policies, and procedures. Many situations present a combination of legal and ethical questions. It is important to sort out the questions and seek guidance as needed. The next step is complete assessment of the situation with as much information as possible gathered to aid in the decision-making process. Before a decision is finalized, any ethical principles that might apply to the situation should be considered. Ethical principles are general in nature, but they provide a framework for decision making.

Codes of Ethics

As a member of society and the healthcare community, PCTs use both personal and professional ethical principles to govern professional practice. Professional organizations such as The Joint Commission have developed codes of ethics for the healthcare profession that serve as a way to regulate actions and give guidelines for ethical behavior. By helping healthcare workers become more competent, trustworthy, and accountable, such codes of ethics help safeguard society. The ANA has also developed a code of ethics that specifies the ethical duties required of the nursing professional.

Box 6.6	The Living Will and Durable Power of Attorney

- People who receive extraordinary measures to prolong life are often unconscious or mentally incompetent by the time these measures are put into effect; therefore, only by deciding ahead of time what kind of care you want and communicating these decisions to others can you ensure that you receive the extent of care that you want. This can be done through such documents as a living will and a medical durable power of attorney. If your state has adopted legislation for either or both documents, you should use the legally approved wording.
- Address the living will and send copies of it to your family physician, your attorney, and close family members. It specifies that if the time comes when you can no longer take part in decisions for your own future, this statement will stand as an expression of your wishes and directions while you are still of sound mind.
- You may, for example, direct that if a situation should arise in which there is no reasonable expectation of recovery from extreme physical or mental disability, you be allowed to die and not be kept alive by medications, artificial means, or "heroic measures." You may also, of course, use a living will to request such measures to keep you alive as long as possible. You may request pain-relieving medication, even though it may shorten your life. You may spell out specific provisions with regard to, for example, cardiac resuscitation, mechanical respiration, antibiotics, tube feeding, and permission to offer your organs as transplants to other people.
- Some "living will" legislation applies only to terminally ill patients, not to patients who are incapacitated by illness or injury but may live many years in severe pain, who are in a coma, or who are in some other greatly

disabled state. Thus it is advisable to draw up a durable power of attorney, an instrument that appoints another person (a healthcare surrogate) to make decisions in the event of your incompetence. A number of states have enacted statutes expressly for decisions about healthcare, known as a "medical durable power of attorney." In these states, filling out a form is all that is required; you do not have to consult an attorney.
- Depending on the statute, the agent you appoint (someone you trust and have confidence in) may give, withdraw, or withhold consent to specific medical or surgical measures; hire and fire medical personnel; gain access to your medical records; go to court to carry out your wishes; spend or withhold funds for treatment; and interpret your living will.

Remember
- Both documents must be signed and dated before two witnesses who are not blood relatives and to whom you are not leaving property.
- For the durable power of attorney, you must have your signature notarized. If you choose more than one proxy for decision making on your behalf (a good idea in case your first choice is not available), give an order of priority (1, 2, 3).
- Give a copy to your physician to keep in your medical file, and be sure that the physician agrees with your wishes.
- Give copies to close relatives, friends, or both.
- Tell these people about your intentions now.
- Look over your living will once a year. Redate it and initial the new date to make it clear that your wishes are unchanged.

Reporting Unethical Behavior

PCTs have a duty to report behavior witnessed that does not meet the established standards. Unethical behavior involves failing to perform the duties of a competent caring PCT. When reporting unethical behavior, one should always follow the proper chain of command and explain the facts as clearly as possible. Report any concerns with ethical behavior to the charge nurse. Any documentation of the incident must be objective and accurately state what occurred, when and where it occurred, and any other pertinent facts. Reporting a coworker is never an easy task. Always remember, however, that a PCT's first duty is to the patient's health, safety, and well-being.

Ethical Issues

Ethical issues are difficult for everyone because there is no absolutely right or absolutely wrong answer to the

question the issue presents. Like many other issues in healthcare, ethical issues change as society changes. Some of the current ethical issues in nursing include practitioner-assisted suicide (PAS), the right to refuse treatment, the nurse's right to refuse to provide care, and genetic research.

Practitioner-Assisted Suicide

Healthcare professionals and patient advocacy groups on both sides of the issue are debating the ethics of PAS. Also called physician-assisted suicide, this is a form of active euthanasia in which a healthcare provider takes an active role in ending a patient's life. Two cases, *Vacco v Quill* and *Washington v Glucksberg,* were brought before the U.S. Supreme Court regarding the legality of state bans on assisted suicide. The Supreme Court ruled in 1997 that there is no constitutional right to assisted suicide. This ruling allows each state to decide whether to legalize or ban assisted suicides. The ANA has taken a firm stand on the issue of PAS, holding that PAS is not consistent with the philosophy of nursing. ANA's specific objections to PAS are based on the principle of nonmaleficence, to do no harm, and beneficence, the duty to protect life.

In 1944, the ANA adopted a position statement concerning PAS. The ANA wrote that such an act is in violation of the *Code of Ethics for Nurses* and the ethical tradition of the profession. Nurses have an obligation to provide compassionate end-of-life care that includes providing comfort and pain relief. Proponents of PAS, however, cite the ethical principles of the right to autonomy and the right to self-determination in support of their position. The PCT should be supportive of the nurse's obligation to uphold the position statement of the ANA on PAS.

Right to Refuse Treatment

In the context of healthcare, competent adults have the right to refuse treatment. This right derives from their right to determine what is done, or not done, to them. Medicine's technical capacity to sustain life and postpone death further complicates this complex issue. It is the right of the patient to accept or refuse a treatment, even if the refusal has the potential to or is certain to result in death. To exercise the right to refuse treatment, many patients prepare advance directives. Living wills, one kind of advance directive, become effective when patients are incapacitated and are not able to make their own wishes known; these documents specify which lifesaving treatments are acceptable and which are not. Some patients choose to designate a *healthcare proxy* (assign durable power of attorney) to make decisions regarding medical treatment in the event that the patient becomes unable to make them. The proxy is another person who will speak for the patient and make decisions regarding the patient's care. The proxy is obligated to act on the patient's behalf according to the patient's expressed wishes.

Some states have chosen to enact laws that allow patients to have control in when they end their life, otherwise known as euthanasia. In 1997, the state of Oregon enacted the *Death with Dignity Act*, which allows terminally ill residents to end their lives through the voluntary administration of lethal, or deadly, medications that have been prescribed by a physician. Since origination of this act in the state of Oregon, other states within the United States have followed. In 2008, the state of Washington enacted the *Death with Dignity Act*; in 2013 the state of Vermont enacted the *Patient Choice and Control at the End of Life Act*; and, in 2015, the state of California passed the *End of Life Option Act*, though it is not yet in effect. State laws vary on the legalities of the various forms of advance directives, and PCTs need to know the applicable laws in their state.

Do-Not-Resuscitate Orders

The patient is not usually involved directly at the time a *do-not-resuscitate (DNR) order* is written. Although many people make their wishes regarding DNR status known in an advance directive, at this stage the patient is usually incapacitated with little hope for recovery. The physician, after consultation with the patient's family, writes the DNR order in the medical record. The physician is responsible for following the applicable policies and procedures for writing DNR orders. When a DNR order is written in the chart, the PCT has the duty to follow the order. The nurse should make the PCT aware of any patients who are considered to be a DNR. It is always helpful to make note of this on your assignment sheet. It is difficult to make this determination at times when the patient becomes critical. Knowing ahead of time will save you steps in determining whether or not to begin cardiopulmonary resuscitation (CPR) should the patient require it. In the case of a DNR, the PCT would not begin CPR if the patient suddenly stopped breathing or the heart rate stopped.

Refusal to Treat

Refusal to treat is an issue that arises when a patient's care requires a nurse or other healthcare worker to do something that conflicts with his or her personal moral beliefs. A typical example of this dilemma involves assisting in or caring for a woman having an abortion. There is a legal right to abortion, but this does not establish whether abortion is morally right or wrong. If the PCT has a strong moral or religious belief regarding abortion, these concerns must be communicated with the charge nurse. Do not abandon the patient; instead, ask for another assignment. Remember that the right to disqualify oneself from assisting with an abortion does not extend to the complete ability to avoid caring for the patient after the abortion. Disagreement with care decisions made by patients does not allow the PCT to refuse to care for them.

Patient diagnoses and lifestyles do not allow the PCT the legal right to refuse to care for a person. Examples include an infectious disease, such as HIV, or sexual orientation. The rationale is that the need for standard precautions (infection control measures) applies to every patient, and therefore the PCT is at no greater risk for infection from one patient than from another. The ethical principle of respect for all people without discrimination underlies this issue. The patient has the right to receive care, and the PCT has the responsibility to provide the necessary care as delegated by the nurse.

CHAPTER SUMMARY

There are no easy quick answers to legal or ethical issues. The PCT has the charge of working to effectively manage difficult situations. Today's healthcare system is facing many challenges. The healthcare system will continue to undergo changes in response to the enormous problem of containing healthcare costs while improving quality of care. The PCT profession will experience these changes. The legal system is also undergoing changes. Members of the legal community and the healthcare system have to work together to ensure that the legal and ethical rights of all individuals are considered and protected.

Case Scenario

The following are scenarios with an ethical dilemma. What would you do or say in each one?

1. You see a nursing assistant stealing the patient's ring. She says that she needs money to pay her house note or the bank will foreclose. What should you do?
2. The patient has a do-not-resuscitate order and a living will. He has not designated a healthcare proxy or representative. The patient goes into arrest, and the daughter who has not seen her dad in 10 years yells, "Do something, or I will sue you if he dies!" Whose wishes should you follow?
3. You know that your friend at work is stealing drugs. You have confronted her, but she says that it is not her but for a friend. What should you do?
4. You suspect elder abuse by a family member of one of your relatives. What should you do?
5. You made a mistake, and your charge nurse tells you to just rewrite the notes to protect the unit and the hospital. What should you do?

REVIEW QUESTIONS

1. The PCT knows that one of the best defenses against a lawsuit is for a nurse to
   a. work only in a large hospital or nursing home.
   b. provide for every patient's needs as quickly as possible.
   c. promote a positive relationship with the patient.
   d. carry individual professional liability insurance.

2. The PCT believes that all patients should be treated as individuals. The ethical principle that this belief reflects is
   a. autonomy.
   b. beneficence.
   c. nonmaleficence.
   d. respect for people.

3. The PCT is reviewing the patient's medical record. The nurse notes the presence of an advance directive. The nurse recognizes that the purpose of this documentation is to
   a. help every person exercise the right to die with dignity.
   b. encourage a person to determine how he or she will die.
   c. allow a patient to exercise the right of autonomy.
   d. provide a means to prevent medical maltreatment.

4. The PCT knows that all patients have the right to nursing interventions regardless of their race, religion, or gender. The ethical principle that best describes this concept is
   a. nonmaleficence.
   b. justice.
   c. autonomy.
   d. beneficence.

5. The PCT gets a report, puts his patient assignment notebook in his pocket, and goes on break. His notebook has very specific information about his patients and is missing from his pocket when he returns to the unit. The book is found later on the floor in the cafeteria by a visitor and is returned to the information desk. The PCT
   a. may have breached the Patient Self-Determination Act.
   b. is guilty of criminal misconduct.
   c. could be fired for malpractice.
   d. has violated the Health Insurance Portability and Accountability Act of 1996 (HIPAA).

6. The newly certified PCT is assigned a patient who needs catheterization. The PCT has not performed the procedure before. What would be the best action for the PCT?
   a. Contact the nursing supervisor and explain that the procedure will need to be done by a nurse.
   b. Review the agency procedure for male catheterization in the unit's resource area and ask another experienced nurse to demonstrate the procedure first.
   c. Immediately advise the charge nurse that someone else will need to take on this task.
   d. Promptly notify the staff development office that an instructor needs to do this procedure.

7. Informed consent may be obtained by which of the following persons?
   a. The person's family
   b. The PCT
   c. The nurse
   d. The attending physician

8. The decision to remove someone's legal competency, or ability to make his or her own healthcare decisions, is determined by who?
   a. The person's family
   b. The nurse
   c. The physician
   d. A judge

Body Structure and Function/Growth and Development

CHAPTER 7

LEARNING OBJECTIVES

1. Define the difference between anatomy and physiology.
2. Define the term *anatomical position*.
3. List and define the principal directional terms and sections (planes) used in describing the body and the relationship of body parts to one another.
4. List and discuss in order of increasing complexity the levels of organization of the body.
5. Differentiate among tissues, organs, and systems.
6. Identify and define three major components of the cell.
7. Describe the four types of body tissues.
8. List the 11 major organ systems of the body and briefly describe the major functions of each.
9. Differentiate among the types of family patterns and their functions in society.
10. Describe different types of stresses that commonly affect today's families.
11. Describe the physical characteristics at each stage of the life cycle.
12. List the psychosocial changes at the different stages of development.
13. Describe the normal age-related changes that affect the major body systems.
14. Discuss the effect of the aging process on personality, intelligence, learning, and memory.
15. Discuss Erikson's stages of psychosocial development.
16. Discuss the developmental tasks of the adolescent period.
17. List the developmental tasks for early adulthood.
18. Describe the developmental tasks for middle adulthood.
19. Define aging.

KEY TERMS

active transport Chemical activity that allows the cell to admit larger molecules than would otherwise be possible

adoptive family A family unit with adopted children

ageism A form of discrimination and prejudice against the older adult

anatomy The study, classification, and description of structures and organs of the body

blended (reconstituted) family When adults remarry and bring together children from previous marriages

blood pressure The pressure of blood in the circulatory system

calcium pump Active calcium carriers in the membranes of muscle cells (for example) that allow the cells to force nearly all of the intracellular calcium ions (Ca^{2+}) into special compartments or out of the cell entirely

cell The smallest living unit of structure and function in our body

cephalocaudal Growth and development that proceeds from the head toward the feet

chromosomes Spindle-shaped rods in a cell that carry genetic information in the form of genes

cohabitation Living together without being married

conception (fertilization) The union of a sperm with an ovum (egg)

cytoplasm A sticky, gel-like substance that contains 70% water, as well as nutrients, minerals, enzymes, and other specialized materials

depression A mood disturbance characterized by feelings of sadness, despair, and hopelessness

development A lifelong process that begins at conception, the beginning of pregnancy, and ends with death

diffusion A process in which solid particles in a fluid move from an area of higher concentration to an area of lower concentration, resulting in an even distribution of the particles in the fluid

dorsal Toward the back; see posterior

extended family Consists of the nuclear or traditional family and additional family such as grandparents, grandchildren, aunts, and uncles who live in the same household

filtration The movement of water and particles through a membrane by force from either pressure or gravity

foster family A family formed when the biological parents are unable or unwilling to provide adequate, safe care for their children

grandfamilies Families with children under the age of 18 years who live with or in the custody of grandparents

growth An increase in size and may involve the entire being or parts within

homeostasis The state of achieving a balance or equilibrium within the body

homosexual family A family comprised of a same-sex couple

infant mortality rate The number of childhood deaths that occur before age 1 year

kyphosis An exaggeration of the thoracic curvature

life expectancy The number of years an individual will probably live, based on the average for others with similar characteristics

membrane Permits certain substances to enter and leave while not allowing other substances to cross

mitosis A type of cell division

nuclear family A family unit that consists of parents and their biologic offspring, or children

nucleus The largest organelle within the cell responsible for cell reproduction and control of the other organelles

organ A group of several different kinds of tissues arranged to perform a special function

osmosis The passage of water across a selectively permeable membrane, with the water molecules going from the less concentrated solution to the more concentrated solution

passive transport The movement of small molecules across the membrane of a cell by diffusion

phagocytosis The process that permits a cell to engulf (or surround) any foreign material and to digest it

physiology The processes and functions of the various structures and how they interrelate

pinocytosis The process by which extracellular fluid is taken into the cell

presbycusis A normal progressive, age-associated loss of hearing acuity, speech intelligibility, auditory threshold, and pitch

presbyopia A defect in vision in advancing age that involves loss of accommodation or the recession of the near point caused by loss of elasticity of the crystalline lens and the ensuing change in close vision

proximodistal Growth and development that originates in the center of the body and moves toward the outside

quarks The building blocks of protons and neutrons that comprise the atom

respiratory Relating to respiration, or the act of breathing

school violence Anything that physically or psychologically injures schoolchildren or damages school property

single-parent family The type of family where there is one parent with at least one child

social contract family See cohabitation

sodium-potassium pump The process of actively transporting sodium ions ($Na+$) out of cells and potassium ions ($K+$) into cells

system An organization of varying numbers and kinds of organs arranged to perform complex functions of the body

teratogen A substance, agent, or process that interferes with normal prenatal development, causing the formation of one or more developmental abnormalities in the fetus

tissue An organization of many similar cells that act together to perform a common function

ventral To face forward; the front of the body

widow The remaining spouse when one has died

zygote The developing ovum from the time it is fertilized until, as a blastocyst, it is implanted in the uterus

Caring for a person who is sick or injured requires understanding how the human body normally functions, so patient care technicians must be familiar with basic human anatomy and physiology principles. Anatomy is the study, classification, and description of structures and organs of the body. Physiology explains the processes and functions of the various structures and how they interrelate. The normal, healthy human body is like a finely tuned machine, with each part performing a special function. As with a machine, when the body malfunctions, the repairer must understand how to make the necessary repairs to return the body to homeostasis (normal function), or illness, disease, or death may result.

ANATOMICAL TERMINOLOGY

Study of the human body first requires one to understand the meaning of certain terms that aid in locating specific structures. To understand the following terms, consider the body in a normal anatomical position, that is, standing tall with the face and palms facing forward (Fig. 7.1):

Anterior (or ventral): To face forward; the front of the body. The chest is located anterior to the spine.
Posterior (or dorsal): Toward the back. The kidneys are posterior to the peritoneum.

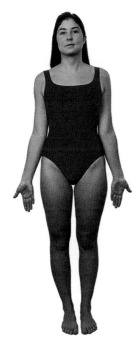

FIGURE 7.1 Anatomical position. The body is in an erect or standing posture with the arms at the sides and palms forward. The head and feet also point forward. The right and left sides of the body are mirror images of each other. (From Frank ED, Long BW, Smith BJ: *Merrill's atlas of radiographic positioning and procedures*, ed 13, St. Louis, 2016, Mosby.)

Cranial: Toward the head. The brain is located in the cranial portion of the body.
Caudal: Toward the distal end of the body. A caudal anesthetic may be given.
Superior: Toward the head, or above. The neck is superior to the shoulders.
Inferior: Lower, toward the feet, or below another. The foot is inferior to the ankle.
Medial: Toward the midline. The sternum (breastbone) is located in the medial portion of the chest.
Lateral: Toward the side. The outer area of the leg, the area located on the side, is called lateral.
Proximal: Nearest the origin of the structure; nearest the trunk. The elbow is proximal to the forearm.
Distal: Farthest from the origin of the structure; farthest from the trunk. The fingers are distal to the palm of the hand.
Superficial: Nearer the surface. The skin of the arm is superficial to the muscles below it.
Deep: Farther away from the body surface. The bone of the upper arm is deep to the muscles that surround and cover it.

Body Planes

To make it easier to study individual organs or the body as a whole, divide the body into three imaginary planes: the sagittal, the coronal (frontal), and the transverse (Fig. 7.2):

1. The sagittal plane runs lengthwise from the front to the back. A sagittal cut gives a right and a left portion of the body. A midsagittal cut gives two equal halves.
2. The coronal (frontal) plane divides the body into a ventral (front) section and a dorsal (back) section.
3. The transverse plane cuts the body horizontal to the sagittal and frontal planes, dividing the body into caudal and cranial portions.

Body Cavities

Although the body appears to be a solid structure, it is not. It is made up of open spaces, or cavities, that contain compact, well-ordered arrangements of internal organs. The body has two major cavities that are subdivided and contain compact, well-ordered arrangements of internal organs. The two major cavities are the ventral and the dorsal body cavities (Fig. 7.3 and Table 7.1).

Ventral Cavity

The ventral cavity consists of the thoracic (or chest) cavity and the abdominopelvic cavity (see Fig. 7.3), which are separated by the diaphragm (a muscle directly beneath the lungs).

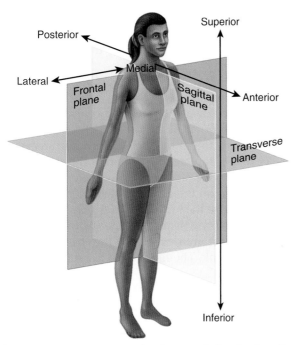

FIGURE 7.2 Directions and planes of the body. (From Harkreader H, Hogan MA, Thobaben M: *Fundamentals of nursing: caring and clinical judgment,* ed 3, St. Louis, 2007, Saunders.)

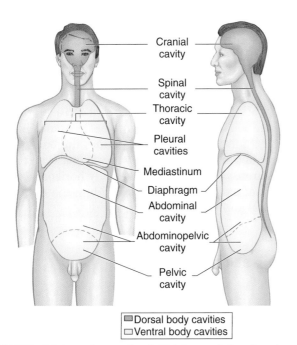

FIGURE 7.3 Location and subdivisions of the dorsal and ventral body cavities as viewed from the front (anterior) and the side (lateral). (From Thibodeau GA, Patton KT: *Structure and function of the body,* ed 14, St. Louis, 2012, Mosby.)

The thoracic cavity contains the heart and the lungs. Its midportion is a subdivision of the thoracic cavity, the mediastinum, which contains the trachea, the heart, and major blood vessels. The subdivisions are the right and left pleural cavities, which contain the lungs.

Table 7.1	Body Cavities
Body Cavity	**Organ(s)**
Ventral Body Cavity	
Thoracic Cavity	
Mediastinum	Trachea, heart, blood vessels
Pleural cavities	Lungs
Abdominopelvic Cavity	
Abdominal cavity	Liver, gallbladder, stomach, spleen, pancreas, small intestine, parts of large intestine
Pelvic cavity	Lower (sigmoid) colon, rectum, urinary bladder, reproductive organs
Dorsal Body Cavity	
Cranial cavity	Brain
Spinal cavity	Spinal cord

The abdominal cavity contains the stomach, the liver, the gallbladder, the spleen, the pancreas, the small intestine, and parts of the large intestine. The pelvic cavity is a subdivision of the abdominal cavity and contains the lower portion of the large intestine (lower sigmoid colon, rectum), the urinary bladder, and the internal structures of the reproductive system. Because the abdominal and pelvic cavities are not separated by any structure, it is referred to as the abdominopelvic cavity (see Table 7.1).

Dorsal Cavity

The **dorsal** cavity is composed of the cranial and spinal body cavities. The cranial body cavity houses the brain, whereas the spinal cavity contains the spinal cord. The dorsal body cavity is smaller than the ventral cavity (see Table 7.1).

ABDOMINAL REGIONS

For convenience in locating abdominal organs, anatomists divide the abdomen into nine imaginary regions. The nine regions are identified from right to left and from top to bottom (Fig. 7.4).

The most superficial (closest to the skin) organs located in each of the nine abdominal regions are shown in Fig. 7.4. The visible organs in each region are as follows: (1) right hypochondriac region, the right lobe of the liver and the gallbladder; (2) epigastric region, parts of the right and left lobes of the liver and a large portion of the stomach; (3) left hypochondriac region, a small portion of the stomach and large intestine; (4) right lumbar region, parts of the large and small intestine; (5) umbilical region, a portion of the transverse colon and loops of the small intestine; (6) left lumbar region, additional loops of the small intestine and a part of the colon; (7) right iliac region, the cecum and parts

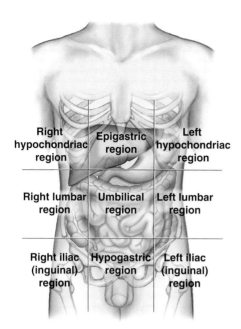

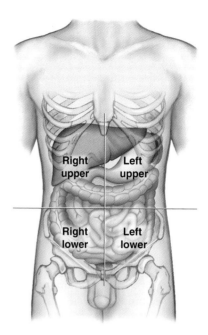

FIGURE 7.4 The nine regions of the abdominopelvic cavity. The most superficial organs are shown. Can you identify the deeper structures in each region? (From Thibodeau GA, Patton KT: *Structure and function of the body,* ed 15, St. Louis, 2016, Mosby.)

FIGURE 7.5 Horizontal and vertical line passing through the umbilicus (navel) divides the abdomen into right and left upper quadrants and right and left lower quadrants. (From Thibodeau GA, Patton KT: *Structure and function of the body,* ed 15, St. Louis, 2016, Mosby.)

of the small intestine; (8) hypogastric region, loops of the small intestine, the urinary bladder, and the appendix; and (9) left iliac region, portions of the colon and the small intestine (Patton, 2013).

ABDOMINOPELVIC QUADRANTS

Health professionals divide the abdomen into four quadrants to describe the site of abdominopelvic pain or to locate an internal pathologic condition such as a tumor or abscess (Fig. 7.5). Horizontal and vertical lines passing through the umbilicus (navel) divide the abdomen into right and left upper quadrants and right and left lower quadrants.

STRUCTURAL LEVELS OF ORGANIZATION

Before studying the structure and function of the human body and its many parts, it is helpful to think about how those parts are organized and how they might fit together into a functioning whole. Fig. 7.6 illustrates the different levels of organization that influence body structure and function. The levels of organization progress from the least complex (chemical level) to the most complex (body as a whole). The structural levels of organization in the body are cells, tissues, organs, and systems.

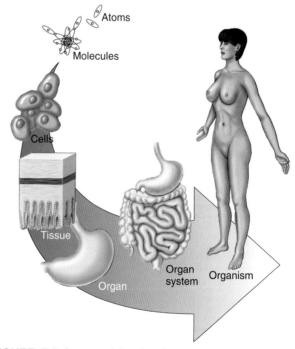

FIGURE 7.6 Structural levels of organization in the body. (From Herlihy B: *The human body in health and illness,* ed 5, St. Louis, 2014, Saunders.)

Although the body is a single structure, it is made up of billions of smaller structures. Atoms and molecules are often referred to as the chemical level of organization (see Fig. 7.6). Atoms are small particles that form the building blocks of matter, once thought to be the smallest complete units of which all matter was made. More recent research has identified the quark. Atoms contain protons, neurons, and electrons; quarks are actually the building blocks of protons and neutrons that comprise the atom (Moskowitz, 2012). When two or more atoms unite through their electron structures, they form a molecule. A molecule can be made of atoms that are alike (e.g., the oxygen molecule is made of two identical atoms), but more often a molecule is made of two or more different atoms (e.g., a molecule of water [H_2O] contains one atom of oxygen [O] and two atoms of hydrogen [H]) (see Fig. 7.6).

The existence of life depends on the proper levels and proportions of many chemical substances in the cytoplasm of cells. The cell is considered the smallest living unit of structure and function in our body. Although cells are considered the simplest units of living matter, they are extremely complex units.

Tissues are even more complex than cells. By definition a tissue is an organization of many similar cells that act together to perform a common function. Cells are held together and surrounded by varying amounts and types of glue-like, nonliving intercellular substances.

Organs are more complex than tissues. An organ is a group of several different kinds of tissues arranged to perform a special function. The stomach and intestines shown in Fig. 7.6 are an example of organization at the organ level.

Systems are the most complex units that make up the body. A system is an organization of varying numbers and kinds of organs arranged to perform complex functions for the body. The organs of the gastrointestinal system, shown in Fig. 7.6, permit digestion of ingested food and excretion of waste products. Major organs of the digestive tract include the mouth, esophagus, stomach, and the small and large intestines.

Cells

Almost 350 years ago Robert Hooke discovered the first cell while examining plant fragments under the microscope. The structures reminded him of the cells in a monastery, so he coined the term *cell* (the fundamental unit of all living tissue) (Fig. 7.7). Many living things are so simple that they consist of just one cell. Conversely, the human body is so complex that it has trillions of cells.

All cells are microscopic but differ greatly in size and shape. Despite their differences, all cells exhibit five unique characteristics of life: growth, metabolism, responsiveness, reproduction, and homeostasis. Homeostasis is achieved when the body's internal environment is relatively constant; this state is naturally maintained by adaptive responses that promote healthy survival.

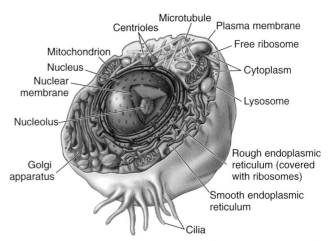

FIGURE 7.7 A typical cell. (From Herlihy B: *The human body in health and illness,* ed 5, St. Louis, 2014, Saunders.)

Structural Parts of Cells

The three main parts of a cell are the plasma membrane, the cytoplasm, and the nucleus (see Fig. 7.7).

Plasma Membrane

The plasma membrane encloses the cytoplasm and forms the outer boundary of the cell. The plasma membrane is an incredibly delicate structure, measuring only about 7 nm (nanometers), or 3/10,000,000 inch thick. Despite its size and delicacy, it has a precise, orderly structure.

Even though it seems fragile, the plasma membrane is strong enough to keep the cell whole and intact. It also performs other life-preserving functions for the cell, serving as a gateway between the fluid inside the cell and the fluid around it. The plasma membrane is selectively permeable. This means that the membrane permits certain substances to enter and leave while not allowing other substances to cross. This membrane separates the cell contents from the dilute saltwater solution called interstitial fluid, or tissue fluid, which surrounds every cell in the body. The plasma membrane also has distinct surface proteins that identify a cell as coming from one particular individual. This fact is the basis of tissue typing, a procedure performed to determine compatibility before an organ transplantation can occur. Carbohydrate chains attached to the surface of cells often help identify cell types.

Cytoplasm

Cytoplasm, found only within cells, is the internal living material of cells. Also known as protoplasm, it is a sticky, gel-like substance that contains 70% water, as well as nutrients, minerals, enzymes, and other specialized materials. Lying between the plasma membrane and the nucleus of the cell, cytoplasm contains

| Table 7.2 | Some Major Cell Structures and Their Functions |

Cell Structure	Function(s)
Plasma membrane	Serves as the cell's boundary; protein and carbohydrate molecules on outer surface of plasma membrane perform various functions (e.g., serve as markers that identify cells of each individual or as receptor molecules for certain hormones)
Endoplasmic reticulum (ER)	Ribosomes attach to rough ER to synthesize proteins; smooth ER synthesizes lipids and certain carbohydrates
Ribosomes	Synthesize proteins; the cell's "protein factories"
Mitochondria	Synthesize adenosine triphosphate (ATP); the cell's "powerhouses"
Lysosomes	Serve as cell's "digestive system"
Golgi apparatus	Synthesizes carbohydrate, combines it with protein, and packages the product as globules of glycoprotein
Centrioles	Function in cell reproduction
Cilia	Short, hairlike extensions on the free surfaces of some cells capable of movement; often have specialized functions such as propelling mucus upward over cells that line the respiratory tract
Flagella	Single projections of cell surfaces, much larger than cilia; an example in humans is the "tail" of a sperm cell; propulsive movement makes it possible for sperm to "swim" or move toward the ovum once they are deposited in the female reproductive tract
Nucleus	Dictates protein synthesis, thereby playing an essential role in other cell activities, namely, active transport, metabolism, growth, and heredity
Nucleoli	Play an essential role in the formation of ribosomes

numerous organelles (tiny functioning structures) that help with the processes of the cell. Because organelles are so small, they were not discovered until the development of the powerful electron microscope. (Table 7.2 lists major cell structures and their functions.)

Nucleus

The nucleus is the largest organelle within the cell. It is responsible for cell reproduction and control of the other organelles. The nucleus is surrounded by the nuclear membrane. It contains nucleoplasm, a refined form of cytoplasm. The nucleus contains two specialized structures: the nucleolus and the chromatin granules. The nucleolus is critical in the formation of protein. The chromatin granules are composed of protein and deoxyribonucleic acid (DNA). DNA contains the genetic code, or blueprint, of the body.

Endoplasmic Reticulum

Throughout the cytoplasm lies a system of membranes, or canals, called the endoplasmic reticulum (ER). ER functions as a miniature circulating system for the cell by carrying substances from one part of the cell to another. There are two types of ER: (1) smooth, which is found in cells that deal with fatty substances, and (2) rough, which is found in cells that manufacture proteins.

Ribosomes

Ribosomes are tiny structures floating free in the cytoplasm or attached to the rough ER. They are called protein factories because they produce enzymes and other proteins.

Mitochondria

The mitochondria are the powerhouses of the cells. They are bean shaped with a folded interior membrane. They take nutrients and convert them to a complex energy form, adenosine triphosphate (ATP), for use by the cell. ATP is described as the "energy currency" of the cells because it supplies the energy for all activities.

Lysosomes

Lysosomes are small saclike structures containing enzymes that digest food compounds and microbes that have invaded the cell.

Golgi Apparatus

The Golgi apparatus is usually located near the nucleus. It is the "packaging plant" of the cell. It packages certain carbohydrate and protein compounds into globules. Then it moves outward through the cell membrane, where it breaks open and releases its contents.

Centrioles

The centrioles are paired, rod-shaped organelles. During cell division (mitosis) they aid in the formation of the spindle, a structure necessary for cell reproduction.

Protein Synthesis

Protein is a vital component of every cell in the body. Protein production relies on nucleic acids in the cell's cytoplasm and nucleus. Two important nucleic acids are (1) deoxyribonucleic acid (DNA), which is located only in the nucleus, and (2) ribonucleic acid (RNA), which is located in both the nucleus and cytoplasm. The DNA encodes a message for protein synthesis as RNA, and sends the RNA to ribosomes in the cytoplasm, where the protein is produced. For this reason DNA is called the chemical blueprint, and RNA is called the chemical messenger.

Cell Division

All cells in the body, except sex cells, reproduce by mitosis, which is a type of somatic (pertaining to non-reproductive cells) cell division in which the original cell divides to form two daughter cells. Each daughter cell has the same characteristics (including both the nucleus and cytoplasm) as the original cell. Each daughter cell contains the same number of chromosomes as the parent cell. Each chromosome in the daughter cells contains the complete genetic information of the original chromosome because of duplication of the DNA molecule during interphase (Fig. 7.8).

The chromosomes (spindle-shaped rods) in the cell's nucleus carry the genes that are responsible for the organism's traits, including such hereditary factors as hair and eye color. These chromosomes are composed of DNA. Each body cell in humans contains 46 chromosomes, which exist in pairs. At the time of fertilization, one member of each pair is received from the father and one is received from the mother to form a total of 23 pairs of chromosomes. These paired chromosomes, except for the pair that determines sex, are alike in size and appearance and carry genes for the same traits.

During mitosis the cell goes through four phases: prophase, metaphase, anaphase, and telophase:

Prophase: In the nucleus the chromosomes form two strands called chromatids. In the cytoplasm the centrioles form a network of spindle fibers.

Metaphase: The nuclear membrane and nucleolus disappear, and the chromosomes are aligned across the center of the cell. The centrioles are at the opposite ends of the cell, and spindle fibers are attached to each chromatid.

Anaphase: The chromosomes are pulled to the opposite ends of the cell, and cell division begins.

Telophase: During this final phase of cell division, the two nuclei appear and the chromosomes disperse. At the end of the phase, two new daughter cells appear.

Movement of Materials Across Cell Membranes

For a cell to survive, it must receive nutrients and oxygen and secrete its waste products. A number of processes allow for mass movement of substances into and out of the cells. These transport processes are classified under two general headings: passive transport and active transport.

The difference between active and passive transport is based on whether energy is required. Active transport involves chemical activity that allows the cell to admit larger molecules than would otherwise be possible. Active processes require the cell to expend energy. Passive transport processes, on the other hand, do not require energy expenditure. The cell obtains energy for active transport from an important chemical substance called ATP. ATP is produced in the cell from nutrients and releases energy so that the cell can work.

Active Transport Processes

Active transport is an extremely important process. It allows cells to move certain ions or other water-soluble particles to specific areas. Certain enzymes play a role in active transport, providing a chemical "pump" that helps move substances through the cell membrane. For

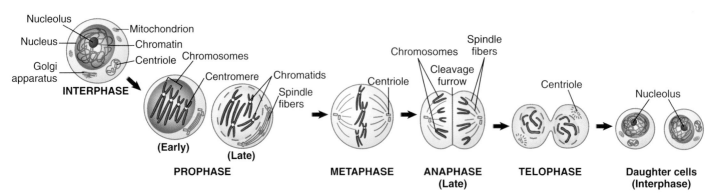

FIGURE 7.8 Deoxyribonucleic acid (DNA) molecule. Note that each side of the DNA molecule consists of alternating sugar and phosphate groups. Each sugar group is united to the sugar group opposite to it by a pair of nitrogenous bases (adenine-thymine or cytosine-guanine). The sequence of these pairs constitutes a genetic code that determines the structure and function of a cell. (From Thibodeau GA, Patton KT: *Anatomy and physiology,* ed 7, St. Louis, 2011, Mosby.)

example, insulin binds with glucose and transports the glucose into the cell. Other active transport processes (Table 7.3) include the following:

- Phagocytosis (Greek for "cell-eating"): The process that permits a cell to engulf (or surround) any foreign material and to digest it. The white blood cells in the human body often perform this function.
- Pinocytosis (Greek for "cell-drinking"): The process by which extracellular fluid is taken into the cell. The cell membrane develops a saclike indentation filled with extracellular fluid, and then closes around it and digests it.
- Sodium-potassium pump: The process of actively transporting sodium ions (Na⁺) out of cells and potassium ions (K⁺) into cells. The sodium-potassium pump maintains a lower sodium concentration in intracellular fluid than in the surrounding extracellular fluid. At the same time, this pump maintains a higher potassium concentration in the intracellular fluid than in the surrounding extracellular fluid. This active transport pump operates in the plasma membrane of all human cells and is essential for healthy cell survival.
- Calcium pump: Active calcium carriers in the membranes of muscle cells (for example) that allow the cells to force nearly all of the intracellular calcium ions (Ca^{2+}) into special compartments or out of the cell entirely. This is important because a muscle cell cannot operate properly unless the intracellular Ca^{2+} concentration is kept low during rest.

Active transport processes require cellular energy to move substances from a low concentration to a high concentration. In contrast, passive transport processes—the movement of small molecules across the membrane of a cell by diffusion—do not require cellular energy and move substances from a high concentration to a lower concentration.

Passive Transport Processes

The primary passive transport processes (Table 7.4) include the following:

- Diffusion: A process in which solid particles in a fluid move from an area of higher concentration to an area of lower concentration, resulting in an even distribution of the particles in the fluid (Fig. 7.9).
- Osmosis: The passage of water across a selectively permeable membrane, with the water molecules going from the less concentrated solution to the more concentrated solution (Fig. 7.10).

Table 7.3	Active Transport Processes*	
Description		**Example(s)**
Ion Pump Movement of solute particles from an area of low concentration to an area of high concentration (up the concentration gradient) by means of a carrier protein structure	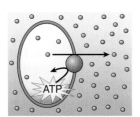	In muscle cells, pumping of nearly all calcium ions to special compartments or out of the cell
Phagocytosis Process that permits a cell to engulf or to surround any foreign material and to digest it	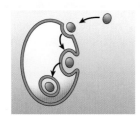	Trapping of bacterial cells by phagocytic white blood cells
Pinocytosis Movement of fluid and dissolved molecules into a cell by trapping them in a section of plasma membrane that pinches off to form an intracellular vesicle; type of endocytosis	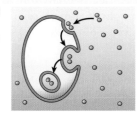	Trapping of large protein molecules by some body cells

*The energy required for active transport processes is obtained from adenosine triphosphate (ATP). ATP is involved in all active transport processes. *(From Thibodeau GA, Patton KT:* Structure and function of the body, *ed 15, St. Louis, 2016, Mosby.)*

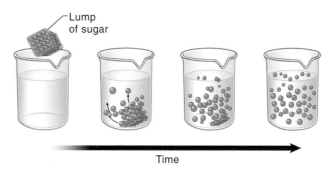

FIGURE 7.9 Diffusion. The molecules of a lump of sugar are very densely packed when they enter the water. As sugar molecules collide frequently in the area of high concentration, they gradually spread away from each other toward the area of lower concentration. Eventually the sugar molecules are evenly distributed. (From Patton KT, Thibodeau GA: *Anatomy and physiology,* ed 9, St. Louis, 2016, Mosby.)

Table 7.4   Passive Transport Processes

Description		Example(s)
Diffusion		
Movement of solute particles through a membrane from an area of high concentration to an area of low concentration (down the concentration gradient)	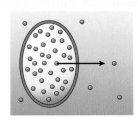	Movement of carbon dioxide out of all cells; movement of sodium ions into nerve cells as they conduct an impulse
Osmosis		
Diffusion of water through a selectively permeable membrane in the presence of at least one impermeable solute	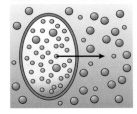	Diffusion of water molecules into and out of cells to correct imbalances in water concentration
Filtration		
Movement of water and small solute particles, but not larger particles, through a filtration membrane; movement occurs from an area of high pressure to an area of low pressure	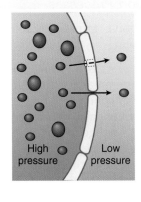	In the kidney, movement of water and small solutes from blood vessels but lack of movement by blood proteins and blood cells; begins the formation of urine

(Modified from Thibodeau GA, Patton KT: Structure and function of the body, ed 15, St. Louis, 2016, Mosby.)

- **Filtration:** The movement of water and particles through a membrane by force from either pressure or gravity. This membrane contains spaces that allow liquid to pass but are too small to be permeated by solid particles. Movement is from areas of greater pressure to areas of lesser pressure.

Tissues

Tissues are groups of similar cells that work together to perform a specific function. The body and its organs are composed of the following four main types of tissues: epithelial, connective, muscle, and nervous (Table 7.5).

Epithelial Tissue

Epithelial cells are packed closely together and contain no blood vessels. Epithelial tissue covers the outside of the body and some of the internal structures. The four types of epithelial tissue are (1) simple squamous, (2) stratified squamous, (3) simple columnar, and (4) stratified transitional (see Table 7.5).

Epithelial tissue serves several important functions in the body, including the following:

- *Protection:* By covering the body and many of its organs, epithelial tissue serves as a protective barrier against invasion of organism such as bacteria.
- *Absorption:* Certain specialized epithelial cells can absorb material in the body (e.g., the lining of the small intestine can absorb digested nutrients).
- *Secretion:* Mucus is secreted in areas such as the respiratory and digestive tracts.

Connective Tissue

As the name suggests, connective tissue "connects," or joins, tissues or structures of the body, and it also supports and protects them. Connective tissue is the most abundant and widely distributed tissue in the body. It exists in various forms: thin and delicate, tough and cordlike, or liquid (blood). Mast cells, plasma cells, and white blood cells are found in connective tissue; red blood cells are not unless blood vessels have been injured. Unlike the closely packed epithelial tissue, the connective tissue cells are spaced out and surrounded by intercellular fluid, which is composed of protein complexes and tissue fluid. Some of the most important forms of connective tissue are loose fibrous (areolar) connective tissue, adipose (fat) tissue, fibrous connective tissue, bone, cartilage, blood, and hematopoietic tissue (see Table 7.5).

Muscle Tissue

Muscle tissue is composed of cells that contract in response to an electrical signal from the brain or the spinal cord. The three types of muscle cells are (1) skeletal (striated, voluntary), (2) cardiac (striated, involuntary), and (3) visceral (smooth, involuntary) (Fig. 7.11).

Skeletal muscle cells are striated (have a striped appearance) and attach to bones to produce voluntary movement. Skeletal muscle is also known as voluntary muscle because a person has control over skeletal muscle contractions (see Fig. 7.11A).

Cardiac muscle cells are striated with fibers that branch to form many networks, or webs. These networks are found only in the walls of the heart, and the regular contractions of cardiac muscle produce the heartbeat. In general, cardiac muscle cells have involuntary action;

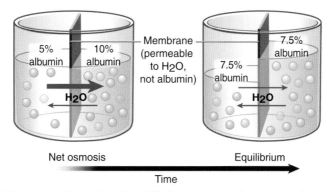

FIGURE 7.10 Osmosis. Osmosis is the diffusion of water through a selectively permeable membrane. The membrane shown in this diagram is permeable to water but not to albumin. Because there are relatively more water molecules in 5% albumin than in 10% albumin, more water molecules osmose from the more dilute into the more concentrated solution (as indicated by the large arrow in the diagram on the *left*) than osmose in the opposite direction. The overall direction of osmosis, in other words, is toward the more concentrated solution. Movement across the membrane continues until the concentrations of the solutions equalize. (From Thibodeau GA, Patton KT: *Anatomy and physiology*, ed 7, St. Louis, 2011, Mosby.)

Table 7.5   Tissues

Tissue	Location	Function
Epithelial		
Simple squamous	Alveoli of lungs	Absorption by diffusion of respiratory gases between alveolar air and blood
	Lining of blood and lymphatic vessels	Absorption by diffusion, filtration, and osmosis
Stratified squamous	Surface of lining of mouth and esophagus	Protection
	Surface of skin (epidermis)	Protection
Simple columnar	Surface layer of lining of stomach, intestines, and parts of respiratory tract	Protection; secretion; absorption
Stratified transitional	Urinary bladder	Protection
Connective*		
Areolar	Between other tissues and organs	Connection
Adipose (fat)	Under skin	Protection
	Padding at various points	Insulation; support; reserve nutrients
Dense fibrous	Tendons; ligaments	Flexible but strong connection
Bone	Skeleton	Support; protection
Cartilage	Part of nasal septum; covering articular surfaces of bones; larynx; rings in trachea and bronchi	Firm but flexible support
	Disks between vertebrae	
	External ear	
Blood	Blood vessels	Transportation
Hematopoietic	Liquid matrix with dense arrangement of blood cell–producing cells located in red bone marrow	Blood cell formation
Muscle		
Skeletal (striated voluntary); see Fig. 7.11A	Muscles that attach to bones	Maintenance of posture, movement of bones
	Eyeball muscles	Eye movements
	Upper third of esophagus	First part of swallowing
Cardiac (striated involuntary); see Fig. 7.11B	Wall of heart	Contraction of heart
Smooth (nonstriated involuntary or visceral); see Fig. 7.11C	In walls of tubular viscera of digestive, respiratory, and genitourinary tracts	Movement of substances along respective tracts
	In walls of blood vessels and large lymphatic vessels	Changing diameter of blood vessels
	In ducts of glands	Movement of substances along ducts
	Intrinsic eye muscles (iris and ciliary body)	Changing diameter of pupils and shape of lens
	Arrector muscles of hair follicles	Erection of hairs (gooseflesh)
Nervous		
	Brain; spinal cord; nerves	Irritability; conduction

*Connective tissues are the most widely distributed of all tissues.

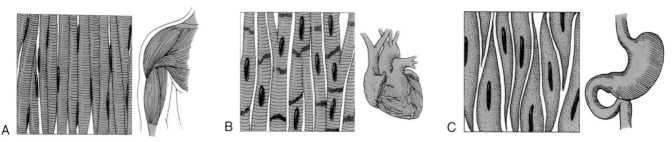

FIGURE 7.11 Types of muscles. A, Skeletal muscle. B, Cardiac muscle. C, Smooth muscle.

that is, a person cannot contract them at will (see Fig. 7.11B).

Smooth (visceral) muscle cells are nonstriated and appear in the viscera, or internal organs, such as the stomach and the intestines as well as in the walls of blood vessels and the uterus. Contractions of smooth muscle propel food and fluid through the digestive tract and help regulate the diameter of blood vessels. Contraction of smooth muscle in the tubes of the respiratory system, such as the bronchioles in the lungs, can impair breathing and result in asthma attacks and labored respiration. In general, smooth muscles are involuntary, but some control can be exerted through the use of biofeedback techniques (see Fig. 7.11C).

Nervous Tissue

Nervous tissue allows rapid communication between the brain or spinal cord and body structures and allows control of body functions. Nervous tissue is composed of two types of cells: neurons and glial cells. The neurons are the nerve cells and transmit impulses or messages. They are the system's functional or conducting units. The glial cells are connecting and supporting cells; they support and nourish the neurons. Each neuron has three parts: (1) dendrites, which carry impulses toward the cell body; (2) a cell body; and (3) an axon, which carries impulses away from the cell body.

Membranes

Membranes are thin sheets of tissue that serve many functions in the body. They cover body surfaces, line and lubricate hollow organs, and protect and anchor organs and bones. The two major types of membranes are epithelial and connective tissue membranes.

Epithelial Membranes

Epithelial membranes are usually composed of a thin layer of epithelial cells with an underlying layer of connective tissue for strength. Epithelial membranes are divided into two subgroups: mucous membranes and serous membranes.

Mucous Membranes

Mucous membranes secrete mucus (a thick, slippery material), which keeps the membranes moist and soft and protects against bacterial invasion. Mucous membranes line the body surfaces that open to the outside environment. Examples include the nose; the mouth; and urinary, respiratory, gastrointestinal, and reproductive tracts. The type of epithelium in the mucous membrane varies, depending on its location and function. The esophagus, for example, contains a tough, abrasion-resistant, stratified squamous epithelium. A thin layer of simple columnar epithelium covers the walls of the lower segments of the digestive tract.

In addition to protection, the mucus produced by mucous membranes also serves other purposes. Examples include mucus in the digestive tract, which lubricates food as it moves through the digestive tract, and mucus secreted in the respiratory tract that serves as a defense mechanism by trapping microorganisms and preventing their invasion into the respiratory system.

Serous Membranes

Serous membranes secrete a thin, watery fluid that prevents friction when organs rub against one another. These membranes line the body surfaces that do not open to the outside environment. Examples include the lungs (pleura), the intestines (peritoneum), and the heart (pericardium). Like epithelial membranes, serous membranes are composed of two distinct layers of tissue: (1) the epithelial sheet, a thin layer of simple squamous epithelium, and (2) the connective tissue layer, a very thin sheet that holds and supports the epithelial cells.

The serous membrane that lines body cavities and covers the surfaces of organs in those cavities is actually a single, continuous sheet covering two different surfaces. The **parietal** membrane lines the wall of the cavity, whereas the **visceral** membrane covers the surface of the viscera (organs within the cavity).

Connective Tissue Membranes (Synovial Membranes)

Connective tissue (or synovial) membranes are smooth and slick and secrete synovial fluid (a thick, colorless lubricating fluid). Synovial membranes line the joint spaces and prevent friction between the ends of the bones, allowing free movement of the joints. Synovial membranes also line small, cushion-like sacs called bursae, which are found between some moving body parts. Unlike serous and mucous membranes, connective tissue membranes do not contain epithelial components.

Organs and Systems

When several kinds of tissues are united to perform a more complex function than any tissue alone, they are called organs. Examples are the heart, stomach, and kidneys. These organs working together for the same general purpose make up organ systems, which maintain the whole body. Systems perform a more complex function than any one organ can perform alone (Table 7.6).

Delegation and Documentation Box 7.1

- When documenting a part of the body, be sure to use the anatomical location if possible. For example, when placing heat to the abdomen, specify which quadrant of the abdomen the heat is placed on.
- State whether you are referring to the anterior (front) of the body or the posterior (back) of the body. This helps provide clarity. For example, when placing an ice pack on a lower leg, refer to either the anterior lower leg or the posterior lower leg.

Table 7.6 Organ Systems and Their Functions

Structure	Function
Integumentary System	
Skin	Protection
Hair	Regulation of body temperature
Nails	Synthesis of chemicals
Sense receptors	Sense organ
Sweat glands	Regulation of body temperature
Oil glands	Protects hair and skin
Skeletal System	
Bones	Support
Joints	Movement (with joints and muscles)
	Storage of minerals
	Blood cell formation
Muscular System	
Voluntary or striated muscles	Movement
Involuntary or smooth muscles	Maintenance of body posture
	Production of heat
Nervous System	
Brain	Contains body's control center
Spinal cord	Responsible for all the coordination of body's activities
Nerves	Communication
Sense organs	Integration
	Control
	Recognition of sensory stimuli
	System functions by production of nerve impulses caused by stimuli of various types
	Control is fast acting and of short duration
Endocrine System	
Pituitary gland	Secretion of special substances (hormones) directly into the blood
Pineal gland	
Hypothalamus	Same as nervous system—communication, integration, control
Thyroid gland	Control is slow and of long duration
Parathyroid glands	Examples of hormone regulation: growth, metabolism, reproduction, and fluid and electrolyte balance
Thymus gland	
Adrenal glands	
Pancreas	
Ovaries (female)	
Testes (male)	

Continued

Table 7.6	Organ Systems and Their Functions—cont'd

Structure	Function
Cardiovascular (Circulatory) System	
Heart	Transportation for nutrition, water, oxygen, and wastes
Blood vessels	Regulation of body temperature
	Immunity (body defense)
Lymphatic System	
Lymph nodes	Protection
Lymphatic vessels	Maintains body's internal fluid environment by producing,
Thymus	filtering, and conveying lymph
Spleen	Production of various blood cells
Tonsils	Transportation
Respiratory System	
Nose	Exchange of waste gas (carbon dioxide) for oxygen in the lungs
Pharynx	Area of gas exchange in the lungs called alveoli
Larynx	Filtration of irritants from inspired air
Trachea	Regulation of acid-base balance
Bronchi	
Lungs	
Digestive System	
Primary Organs	
Mouth	Mechanical and chemical breakdown (digestion) of food
Pharynx	Absorption of nutrients
Esophagus	Undigested waste product that is eliminated is called feces
Stomach	
Small intestine (duodenum, jejunum, ileum)	
Large intestine (ascending, transverse, descending, sigmoid)	
Rectum	
Anal canal	
Accessory Organs	
Teeth	Appendix is a structural but not a functional part of the digestive
Salivary glands	system
Tongue	
Liver	
Gallbladder	
Pancreas	
Appendix	
Urinary System	
Kidneys	Clearing or cleaning blood of waste products; waste product
Ureters	excreted from the body is called urine
Urinary bladder	Electrolyte balance
Urethra	Water balance
	Acid-base balance
	Urethra has urinary and reproductive functions (in the male)
Reproductive System	
Male	
Gonads (testes)	Survival of species
Genital ducts (epididymis, vas deferens, ejaculatory duct, urethra)	Production of sex cells (sperm)
Accessory glands (prostate, seminal vesicles, Cowper's glands)	Transfer of sperm to female sex cells
Supporting structures (penis, scrotum)	Fertilization of female sex cells
	Production of sex hormones
Female	
Gonads (ovaries)	Survival of species
Accessory organs (uterus, fallopian tubes [oviducts], vagina)	Production of sex cells (ova)
External genitalia (vulva)	Development and birth of offspring
Mons pubis	Nourishment of offspring
Labia majora	Production of sex hormones
Labia minora	
Clitoris	
Accessory glands (Skene's glands, Bartholin's glands)	
Mammary glands (breasts)	

GROWTH AND DEVELOPMENT

The United States is in an era of increasing interest in health and well-being. Many improvements have contributed to better health and longer life. Improved sanitation, medications, immunizations, exercise, and nutrition help people stay healthy and live longer. In the coming decades, an increasing portion of the population will occupy the category of "older adult." Many factors have been identified as predictors of living long, including health, happiness, avoidance of tobacco products, and job satisfaction. The exact number of years a person will live is not possible to predict, but estimations can be made. This estimate is referred to as the life expectancy.

Life expectancy is the number of years an individual will probably live, based on the average for others with similar characteristics. Life expectancy in the United States in the beginning of the 20th century was 47.3 years. This has increased in the past 100 years. The life expectancy for the year 2015 in the United States is 78.9 years, with the life expectancy for men 76.4 years and for women 81.4 years. Despite the increases in longevity, room for improvement still exists. Many countries have life expectancies greater than that of the United States, such as the 2012 life expectancy in Monaco with 89.68 years, Japan with 83.91 years, and Australia with 81.9 years (U.S. Census Bureau, 2012; CIA, 2012).

Within the United States, differences in life expectancy are found in different segments of the population. For example, females outlive males by an average of 5 years. Other factors also influence life expectancy. Those with household incomes of greater than $25,000 live 3 to 7 years longer, depending on gender and race, than those in households with incomes of less than $10,000.

Infant mortality rate refers to the number of childhood deaths that occur before age 1 year. This number affects overall life expectancy statistics. The infant mortality rate of African Americans is more than double that of white infants. There is a great need for education and access to preventive healthcare for pregnant women of all ages and races.

Other factors also influence the life expectancy for different groups (Hoyert and Xu, 2012). According to research attributed to Healthy People 2020, the four overarching goals for the public in the United States during the next 10 years are (1) to attain high-quality, longer lives free of preventable disease, disability, injury, and premature death; (2) to achieve health equity, eliminate disparities, and improve the health of all groups; (3) to create social and physical environments that promote good health for all; and (4) to promote quality of life, healthy development, and healthy behaviors across all life stages (HHS, 2012). To motivate action toward change and progress, Healthy People 2020 is organized around a list of 12 leading health indicators (Table 7.7).

Table 7.7	Healthy People 2020 Health Indicators
Leading Health Indicators	**Goal of Taking Action**
Access to health services	Improve access to comprehensive, quality health services
Clinical preventive services	Aid in weight control Enhance well-being
Environmental quality	Promote health for all through a healthy environment
Injury and violence	Prevent unintentional injuries and violence, and reduce their consequences
Maternal, infant, and child health	Improve the health and well-being of women, infants, children, and families
Mental health	Improve mental health through prevention and by ensuring access to appropriate, quality mental health services
Nutrition, physical activity, and obesity	Promote health and reduce chronic disease risk by consuming a healthy diet as well as achieving and maintaining a healthy body weight
Oral health	Prevent and control oral and craniofacial diseases, conditions, and injuries, and improve access to preventative services and dental care
Reproductive and sexual health	Promote healthy sexual behaviors, strengthen community capacity, and increase access to quality services to prevent sexually transmitted diseases and their complications
Social determinants	Create social and physical environments that promote good health for all
Substance abuse	Reduce substance abuse to protect the health, safety, and quality of life for all, especially children
Tobacco	Reduce illness, disability, and death related to tobacco use and secondhand smoke exposure

(From U.S. Department of Health and Human Services: Healthy People 2020, Washington, D.C., 2010, U.S. Department of Health and Human Services.)

Health Promotion Across the Life Span

Development is a lifelong process that begins at conception, the beginning of pregnancy, and ends with death. Middle adulthood and late adulthood have been recently recognized as having equal importance as the earlier stages of development. Development is influenced by a series of interacting events, including personal behaviors, genetics, and the environment. Experiences that an individual has affect future development. Life span development studies examine the changes in the life cycle of an individual and the impact of these factors on the growth and development of individuals.

Life span development is made up of eight stages; their approximate ages are as follows:

- Infancy: birth to 1 year
- Toddler: 1 to 3 years

- Preschool: 3 to 5 years
- School age: 6 to 12 years
- Adolescence: 13 to 19 years
- Early adulthood: 20 to 40 years
- Middle adulthood: 40 to 65 years
- Late adulthood: 65 years and above

Each stage of the life span is unique and has certain features that separate them from other stages. Not all people experience the same milestones during the ages listed. Some may have delayed development or accelerated achievement of skills or behaviors. The guidelines are generalized. The goal of studying the life span is to enable better understanding and improved interaction and communication with individuals at various stages of development. In particular, given the significant growth of the population in the older age group, we must become more aware of the unique characteristics, needs, and problems of the older adult that pose challenges in the delivery of safe healthcare.

Growth and Development

Living beings experience continuous changes throughout the life span. Some changes are physical, such as the replacement of cells, tissues, and fluids. Other changes involve cognition, communication, emotions, behavior, and feelings.

Growth refers to an increase in size and may involve the entire being or parts within. Development refers to function and the gradual process of change and differentiation, from simple to complex. Development proceeds as an orderly, sequential series of changes. Two directional terms important to understanding growth and development are *cephalocaudal* and *proximodistal*. Cephalocaudal is defined as growth and development that proceed from the head toward the feet. The infant's head is large as compared with the rest of its body; gradually the body catches up. Proximodistal refers to growth and development that originate in the center of the body and move toward the outside. For example, the infant gains control of the shoulders before developing control of the hands and fingers.

The principles of growth and development may be summarized as follows:

- Growth and development proceed at a highly individualized rate that varies from person to person. Do not expect two people to react in the same manner to the same stimuli.
- Growth and development are continuous and interdependent processes characterized by spurts of growth and periods of rest.
- Growth and development proceed from the simple to the complex in a predictable sequence of progressive changes.

- Growth and development vary for specific structures at specific times. In other words, not all organs grow and develop at the same rate; for example, the ovaries in the female and the testes in the male do not mature until puberty.
- Growth and development are a total process that involves the whole person. The person grows physically, socially, mentally, and emotionally. Types of growth are interrelated.

Injury & Illness Prevention Box 7.1

- Infants' heads are larger in proportion to their body. Always protect an infant's head and neck to decrease the chance of head injuries.
- All persons should wear helmets to protect their head from injury when riding bicycles.

Delegation and Documentation Box 7.2

- When documenting measurements of children and adults, accuracy is very important. Use the same equipment on the same patient each time if possible.
- Know the proper technique for measuring height and weight. Height should be obtained without shoes on, for a more accurate reading. Weight should be obtained with as few clothes on as possible to decrease the variability, or fluctuation, in numbers.

Patterns of Growth

Growth patterns appear to be genetically controlled. This means that how the person is formed may play a part in how he or she grows. If one of the parents is tall, then there is a chance that the children will be tall as well. Nutrition, heredity, and environment play an important role in the patterns as well. The blueprint for all inherited traits is contained in the chromosomes (threadlike structures in the nucleus of a cell that function in the transmission of genetic information). At conception, the individual has a complex set of biologic potentials that involve characteristics such as height; skin, hair, and eye color; and talents and interests, to name a few. Only identical twins have the same combinations of chromosomes (karyotype). The process of division, transmission, and mixing of chromosomes accounts for the variations in distinctive family traits or, in contrast, their continuity. With the exception of identical twins, each person has his or her own unique set of chromosomes.

Beginnings

Development begins with conception (fertilization), or the union of the sperm and ovum (egg), which combines the genetic material of both parents. This combination of genetic material and environmental influences produce the unique individual.

After fertilization, the zygote (the developing ovum from the time it is fertilized until, as a blastocyst, it is implanted in the uterus) contains 23 pairs of chromosomes, for a total of 46 chromosomes. One of each pair has been contributed by the mother and one by the father. The first question many parents ask after the birth of their baby is whether the child is a boy or a girl. The sex chromosomes, one of the chromosome pairs, determine the gender of the baby. The ovum always carries an X chromosome, whereas the sperm sometimes carries an X and sometimes a Y chromosome. The presence of a Y chromosome in the sperm that fertilizes the ovum means that the baby will be male.

In some instances, environmental factors play a role in contributing to certain diseases or defects in the unborn. A teratogen is a substance, agent, or process that interferes with normal prenatal development, causing the formation of one or more developmental abnormalities in the fetus. Drugs, alcohol, viruses, and cigarette smoke are just a few of the known harmful substances that are best avoided during pregnancy. A possible 5% to 25% of unfavorable outcomes in all pregnancies are estimated to be attributable to smoking. Smoking is also suggested to increase the incidence of low-birth-weight babies.

Ethical Considerations

Genetic testing provides expecting parents with information about whether they are carriers of genes associated with certain inherited diseases. Genetic testing may be suggested for couples based on several factors, including age, medical history, and ethnicity. This can be done before they become pregnant or after. Test results can provide families information to use for future decision making. Decisions may be difficult for families, and supportive services should be made available. A genetic counselor can review the test results and provide information regarding the likelihood of genes being passed on to a child (Centers for Disease Control and Prevention [CDC], 2011).

THE FAMILY

The family is the basic unit of society. Families are composed of two or more individuals united by marriage, blood, adoption, emotional bonds, and social roles. The individuals of the family share emotional ties that usually persist over their entire lifetime.

Signs of several significant changes in American families are evident today. The factors that have contributed to the changed family are listed in Box 7.1. As a

Box 7.1	Changes That Have Affected Modern Families

- Economic changes, which resulted in an increase in the number of women in the workforce
- The feminist movement
- More effective birth control
- Legalization of abortion
- Postponement of marriage and childbearing
- Increase in divorce rate

result of these influences, family roles and lifestyles have changed to meet society's needs.

Types of Families

Regardless of the type of family, certain basic functions are inherent to the family unit. These basic functions include protection, nurturance, education, sustenance, and socialization. Ideally, unconditional affection, acceptance, and companionship are guaranteed to each family member. The family attempts to meet the individual's needs for growth and development, and in doing so, it helps support personal fulfillment and strengthen each individual's self-esteem.

The family is the first socializing agent for teaching children society's expectations and limitations. As a part of that socialization, the family is responsible for ensuring that the child receives a formal education. The family is also responsible for instilling morals, values, and ideals into the children. These roles and functions of families are not necessarily stable or constant but are vulnerable to change. For example, the birth of a baby or the death of a family member makes rearrangement of family roles and structures necessary. See Box 7.2 for types of families and Box 7.3 for qualities of functional families.

Nuclear Family

For most of history, the nuclear family was thought of as the so-called "normal family." The nuclear family is a family unit that consists of parents and their biologic offspring, or children. This does not include families who have adopted children. This family type had gender-based roles assigned to its members (Torbati, 2010). For example, the man of the house was known as the breadwinner, or the one who worked outside of the home and brought home the paycheck.

Today, the nuclear family is looked at as a traditional model. This type of family is on the decline in America; it comprised only 46% of households in 2013 (http://www.pewresearch.org/fact-tank/2014/12/22/less-than-half-of-u-s-kids-today-live-in-a-traditional-family/).

Box 7.2	Types of Families

Nuclear
- Consists of married man and woman and their children
- Lives in independent household

Extended
- Consists of nuclear plus additional family members living in same household
- Provides a sharing of responsibilities

Single-Parent
- Occurs by divorce, death, separation, abandonment, or choice
- More common in recent years
- Typically, one adult performs roles of two people

Blended (Reconstituted)
- Occurs when adults from previous marriages remarry and combine children within new household

Social Contract and Cohabitation
- Made up of man and woman living together without legal commitment but sharing roles and responsibilities

Homosexual
- Involves homosexual partners living together with shared responsibilities

Adoptive
- Consists of usually traditional nuclear family members, husband, wife, and adoptive child

Grandfamilies
- Children living in households headed by their grandparents
- Biological parents may or may not be involved in the child's care

Foster
- Responsible for care, supervision, and nurturing of children in their charge

Box 7.3	Qualities of Functional Families

- Sense of commitment toward promoting the members' well-being
- Sense of appreciation and encouragement for tasks accomplished
- Directed effort toward spending quality time with individual members
- Sense of purpose that encourages progress during good or difficult times
- Sense of harmony between members of the family
- Effective communication between individuals
- Established values, rules, and beliefs
- Variety of different coping techniques to enhance functioning
- Use of effective problem-solving measures and the use of a variety of options
- Positive outlook
- Ability to be flexible and adapt to changes
- Use of varied resources to facilitate coping skills

The modern-day nuclear family usually consists of a husband and wife with or without children living in an independent household setting. In the past, one parent, usually the father, was the breadwinner, or the person who worked and brought home the income for the family. Today, these roles have been redefined in their structure and function. In many families, both parents work and share equally in the financial support and the roles and responsibilities of the family unit.

Extended Family

The extended family consists of the nuclear or traditional family and additional family such as grandparents, grandchildren, aunts, and uncles who live in the same household. A sharing of support, roles, and responsibilities is common to this family structure. This family type constitutes the basic family structure in many societies. Some cultural groups such as Asians and Hispanics choose to live as extended families more so than the nuclear family. This type of family structure can provide extra resources, such as multiple sources of income, as well as multiple options for childcare.

Single-Parent Family

The single-parent family exists today by choice or as the result of death, divorce, separation, or abandonment. More than 40% of single-parent families are the result of divorce (http://www3.uakron.edu/schulze/401/readings/singleparfam.htm). The head of the household may be male or female. This type of family unit also results when an unwed parent lives alone or a single person adopts or gives birth to a child. The single parent has the sole responsibility of carrying out the functions that are typically shared by two members. This family type can be stressful for the parent because of the increased obligations, both financial and emotional.

Blended (Reconstituted) Family

The blended (reconstituted) family (also called the stepfamily) arises when adults remarry and bring together children from previous marriages. This type of family potentially presents many types of stresses. Losses resulting from death or divorce sometimes cause both adults and children to be fearful of love and trust. Children may have loyalties to the other parent, which results in difficulties achieving a bond with the new stepparent. Jealousies may arise as efforts are made to unite the stepchildren into a single family. Sometimes the two sets of parents do not get along, which increases the stressors for the children.

Social Contract Family and Cohabitation

The social contract family style is also referred to as cohabitation. It involves an unmarried couple living together and sharing roles and responsibilities. This type of family is on the rise (http://family-studies.org/the-rise-of-cohabitation/).

Homosexual Family

The homosexual family is composed of a same-sex couple. Homosexual adults form family units. The members share bonds of emotional commitment and roles of child rearing. Many of these family structures consist of biological, adopted, or foster children. Regardless of the specific family structure, all families share common parenting concerns and responsibilities.

Adoptive Family

The adoptive family is a family unit with adopted children. Each year, approximately 120,000 children are adopted in the United States (AACAP, 2011). Adoption may be time-consuming, anxiety provoking, and expensive. The couples who adopt children may have experienced years of infertility and related treatments. Those families created by adoption achieve the same fulfillment associated with parenting as those families created by natural procreation.

Grandfamilies

Grandfamilies refer to families with children under the age of 18 years who live with or in the custody of grandparents. This group represents a growing demographic. In 2013, an estimated 7.8 million children were a part of this growing trend in which children lived within households headed by grandparents. Some of these families had birth parents living in this arrangement as well. For 2.8 million children, the grandparent is the primary custodial care provider. Unfortunately, 21% of these families live below the poverty line. More than 28% of children in foster care are placed in kinship situations. The reasons for the increase in grandfamilies include substance abuse, mental illness, military deployment, incarceration, and parental death (Generations United, 2016; www.gu.org).

Foster Family

The foster family results when the biological parents are unable or unwilling to provide adequate, safe care for their children. Children placed in foster care are typically placed there by the court system. The reasons for placement traditionally involve abuse or neglect. Individual circumstances determine the amount of time for the placement. Ideally, the parents are able to achieve stability and are allowed to again care for their children, thus protecting the parental bond. A significant number of foster care placements (26%) involve children placed with family members. Although there has been a national decline in the number of children entering the foster care system, unfortunately, many children will never return to the care of their biological parents; they face living in the foster care system until they "age out" as they reach legal adulthood. In 2014, more than 415,000 children were living in foster care (Child Trends, 2016).

Causes of Family Stress

Various stressors affect the family unit. Chronic illness, abuse, and divorce are some of the most common factors. Stress, when it occurs, affects everyone, at all ages. Like adults, children often have feelings of stress. Stress in childhood results from either internal or external pressures or from a combination of both. At very early ages, stress sometimes results when the infant's needs are not met. Toddlers often perceive stress when they are separated from their mothers. School-aged children sometimes feel stress from pressures in school or from parental expectations. Even social interactions at this stage have the potential to be somewhat difficult and stressful. Parents need to observe and listen to their children and be watchful for signs of stress (Box 7.4). They must be ready to help their children deal with stress. One way to help is to anticipate what holds stress potential and to prepare children ahead of time. For example, if the child is starting a new school, the parents should talk about it before the day of the event. Allow children to express their feelings. Children must know that having uneasy feelings is all right. Children need to have someone validate their feelings. Talking about what is causing the child's uneasy feelings helps minimize the child's discomfort and helps bring about possible solutions.

Box 7.4   Common Signs of Stress in Children

- Mood swings
- Acting-out behavior
- Change in eating or sleeping patterns
- Frequent stomachaches, headaches, or other unexplained somatic symptoms
- Excessive clinging to parents
- Thumb-sucking
- Bedwetting
- Return to behavior typical of an earlier stage of development

Chronic Illness

Chronic physical or emotional illness of the parent or the child affects all family members. Factors such as financial resources, family stability, and the adequacy of the support system determine an individual's ability to cope with a family member's chronic illness.

Working Mothers

Alternative family patterns are more common, and today's families often experience change and have to adjust to new circumstances. Changes to the family's composition and economic factors have resulted in more women in the labor force. Working mothers are considered common today. Aside from the financial rewards, many believe that working mothers create a wider range of valid role models for young children (Cooper and Gosnell). Many working mothers compensate for the time they are not with their child by establishing quality time during their limited at-home time. Some fathers opt to assume primary child care responsibilities. Certainly, when both parents work outside the home, caregiving arrangements have to be considered. Child care is sometimes available; some of the various forms include in-home care by a relative or paid caregiver and out-of-home care in an organized or group setting. The federal government and most states have regulations that control and regulate staff size and safety issues concerning daycare centers. In choosing a daycare center, look for the following: a balance of age-appropriate educational structure and an open environment, ample space with a variety of materials and activities, small class size with appropriate staff-to-child ratio, an environment that fosters active staff involvement, positive encouragement, and high-quality care in a safe environment.

Abuse

Abuse refers to physical, emotional, financial, and verbal abuse; sexual assault; and neglect. Approximately 702,000 American children are victims of child abuse each year. In many families, abuse is pervasive. A parent with ineffective coping skills has difficulty maintaining family wellness and safety (U.S. Department of Health and Human Services, Administration for Children and Families, Administration on Children, Youth and Families, Children's Bureau, 2014). Further, certain objective and measurable factors are related to family violence. They include financial strain, social isolation, low self-esteem, and history of abuse. The presence of several of these risk factors raises the risk that an individual will resort to abuse. The following are some common characteristics of parents who abuse their children: they were abused themselves as children; they are often loners; they are harsh, strict, and punitive; they have unreasonable expectations; and they are immature, lack self-control, and

have low self-esteem. Early recognition, prompt reporting, and preventive measures are called for to help detect and end all forms of abuse and neglect.

Divorce

Divorce is widespread; it continues to affect more than 1 million children annually. The effects of divorce on children are varied and complex. One of the factors is the age of the child at the time of the divorce. Younger children often feel abandoned and believe that they are no longer loved by both parents. Other factors that sometimes affect the child are the bitterness and conflict surrounding the divorce, the child's prior relationship with the absent parent, the effects of the divorce on the custodial parent, and the postdivorce relationship of the parents. Many children have reconciliation fantasies for extended periods after the divorce is finalized. Changes in one parent's status create changes in emotional milieu, family role, finances, lifestyle, and often the home neighborhood (Box 7.5).

STAGES OF GROWTH AND DEVELOPMENT

The following sections discuss development by age group. It is necessary to take a look at a few aspects of development across a larger arc, however, to fully appreciate the scope of human growth and development.

Psychosocial Development

Erik Erikson, an American psychoanalyst, viewed the life cycle as a series of developmental stages, each accompanied by a developmental task or challenge. Table 7.8 provides an overview of Erikson's stages of psychosocial development. Many of the subsections that follow include stage-appropriate characterization according to Erikson's framework.

Communication and Language

Humans have the ability to learn language. They are born with the mechanism and the capacity to develop

Box 7.5	Tips for Divorcing Parents

- Encourage children to talk about their feelings.
- Do not use children as pawns or "go-betweens."
- Never speak negatively about the ex-spouse in front of children.
- Seek professional help if children need additional support.

Table 7.8	Erikson's Stages of Psychosocial Development		
Stage	**Approximate Age (Years)**	**Developmental Task**	**Outcomes**
1. Infancy	Birth to 1	Basic trust vs. mistrust	Infants learn to either trust or not trust that significant others will properly care for their basic needs, including nourishment, sucking, warmth, cleanliness, and physical contact.
2. Toddler	1 to 3	Autonomy vs. shame and doubt	Children learn to be either self-sufficient in many activities (including toileting, feeding, walking, and talking) or doubt their own abilities.
3. Preschool	4 to 6	Initiative vs. guilt	Children want to undertake many adult-like activities, sometimes going beyond the limits set by parents and feeling guilty because of it.
4. School age	7 to 11	Industry vs. inferiority	Children eagerly learn to be competent and productive or feel inferior and unable to do any task well.
6. Adolescence	12 to 19	Identity vs. role confusion	Adolescents try to figure out "Who am I?" They establish sexual, ethnic, and career identities or are confused about what future roles to play.
7. Young adulthood	20 to 44	Intimacy vs. isolation	Young adults seek companionship and love with another person or become isolated from others.
8. Middle adulthood	45 to 65	Generativity vs. stagnation	Middle-aged adults are productive, performing meaningful work and raising a family, or become stagnant and inactive.
9. Late adulthood	65+	Ego integrity vs. despair	Older adults try to make sense out of their lives, either seeing life as meaningful and whole or despairing at goals never reached and questions never answered.

speech and language skills. During infancy, the unique ability of the brain to sort out basic sounds and to extract from sentences the most meaningful elements becomes apparent. During early childhood, the brain's language-acquisition ability becomes even more sophisticated. Parents and other caregivers have an enormous potential to influence the infant's intellectual and language development. Infants do not speak spontaneously. Interaction with the environment provides a means for them to acquire these skills. Speech requires intact physiologic functioning of (1) the respiratory system, (2) the speech control centers in the cerebral cortex, and (3) the articulation and resonance structures of the mouth and nasal cavities. In addition, to be able to speak requires (1) the ability to hear, (2) intelligence, (3) a need to communicate, and (4) stimulation. The rate of speech development varies from child to child and is directly related to the ability of their brain to function and intellectual development. All children go through the same sequence of stages in language and speech development in early childhood unless abnormal conditions are present (Table 7.9).

The basic sequence of language is as follows:

- *At 3 months, babbling.* When infants babble, they typically explore all the possible sounds they are able to make by enhancing the force of the air stream as it passes their vocal cords and by varying the positions of their tongue and mouth.
- *At 1 year, recognition of words.* Between age 1 and 2 years, infants generally acquire the ability to produce holophrases (one-word sentences that convey a complete message ["up"]). Infants learn to expand their holophrases by attaching them back-to-back to other nouns or verbs. They thus form two-word sentences ("mommy milk," "daddy come"). Early speech is often referred to as telegraphic speech because, as in telegram messages, the articles, pronouns, prepositions, and conjunctions are omitted. In organizing and coding language, infants acquire an understanding of the most meaningful units of speech. No one teaches infants to use nouns and verbs first. They learn this sequence on their own.
- *At preschool age, acquisition of structure of native language.* The language explosion that occurs during the preschool years is most obvious in the growth of vocabulary, from 50 words at 18 months to 200 words at age 2 years to between 8000 and 14,000 words at age 6 years. From age 2 to 6 years, the average child learns between 6 and 10 words per day. Preschoolers have an outstanding ability to learn language. Most researchers regard early childhood as a crucial period for language learning.
- *At 6 years, ability to speak and understand new words and sentences.* Even compared with the preschool years, language development from 6 years on is remarkable, although much more subtle, as children consciously come to understand more about the many ways language can be used. This understanding gives them greater control in their comprehension and use of language and, in turn, enhances the range of their cognitive powers generally.

A common rule of thumb about the evolution of early speech acquisition is that the number of words in an average response usually corresponds to the chronologic

	Table 7.9	Normal Language and Speech Development During Early Childhood

Age (Years)	Normal Language Development	Normal Speech Development	Intelligibility
1	Says two or three words with meaning Imitates sounds of animals	Omission of most final and some initial consonants Substitution of consonants *m, w, p, b, k, g, n, t, d,* and *h* for more difficult sounds Use of unintelligible jargon peaks at age 18 mo	Usually no more than 25% intelligible to unfamiliar listener
2	Uses two-word or three-word phrases in context Has vocabulary of about 300 words and uses "I," "me," and "you"	Use of consonants *m, w, p, b, k, g, n, t, d,* and *h* with vowels, but inconsistently and with much substitution Omission of final consonants Articulation lags behind vocabulary	At age 2 yr, 65% intelligible in context
3	Says four-word or five-word sentences Has vocabulary of about 900 words Uses "who," "what," and "where" in asking questions Uses plurals, pronouns, and prepositions	Mastery of *b, t, d, k,* and *g; r* and *l* may still be unclear; omission or substitution for *w* Repetitions and hesitations common	At age 3 yr, 70% to 80% clear
4 to 5	Has vocabulary of 1500 to 2100 words Able to use most grammatical forms correctly, such as past tense of verb with "yesterday" Uses complete sentences with nouns, verbs, prepositions, adjectives, adverbs, and conjunctions	Mastery of *f* and *v;* possible distortion of *r, l, s, z, sh, ch, y,* and *th* Little or no omission of initial or last consonant	Speech is totally intelligible, although some are still imperfect
6 to 7	Has vocabulary of 3000 words Comprehends "if," "because," and "why"	Mastery of *r, l,* and *th;* possible continuing distortion of *s, z, sh, ch,* and *j* (usually mastered by age 7.5 to 8 yr)	Speech is totally intelligible

age of the child. For example, a 2-year-old might say, "Me do"; a 3-year-old might add a word, "Me do it"; and a 4-year-old might say, "Let me do it."

Girls advance more rapidly in language development than do boys. Firstborn children develop language earlier than do later-born children, and children of multiple births (twins, triplets) develop language later than children of single births.

Infancy: 1 to 12 Months

Physical Characteristics

An infant's physical development happens so rapidly that size, shape, and skills seem to change daily. Growth, which proceeds in a cephalocaudal and proximodistal sequence, is rapid during the first 6 months of life. Infants are expected to gain about 1.5 pounds per month until 5 months, and infants usually double their birth weight by 4 to 6 months. By the time the baby is 1 year of age, the birth weight has tripled (average weight is 21.5 pounds). Most of the weight gain in the first months of life is in the form of fat, which provides insulation and a source of nourishment to draw on if teething or other problems decrease food intake for a few days. After 8 months, weight gain includes more bone and muscle.

Height (length) increases by about 1 inch per month for the first 6 months. By 12 months of age, the infant's birth length has increased about 50%; the typical length is 30 inches (75 cm).

Vital Signs

Infants are subject to wide variations in body temperature related to activity levels and state of health. Apical rates slow down in infancy. At 2 months, the average apical rate is about 120 beats per minute. Count the apical pulse for a full minute, noting variations in rate, volume, and rhythm. Respiratory rates also decrease during infancy; these rates are related to activity level. Average resting respiratory rate for the 12-month-old is about 30 breaths per minute. Blood pressure readings gradually increase to 90/60 mm Hg at 12 months.

Dentition

Teething begins at about 5 to 6 months of age. Signs of teething—irritability, edematous red gums, excessive drooling, and change in stooling—begin 3 to 4 weeks before the appearance of the tooth (Box 7.6). Dental decay can begin at any time after tooth development. Oral hygiene for the young infant consists of offering sips of clear water and wiping and massaging the infant's gums.

Healthcare professionals will advise parents to begin tooth brushing after the first teeth appear; this element of dental hygiene is important to continue throughout the life span. In areas without added fluoride in the water, parents should be recommended to use fluoride toothpaste. To prevent bottle-mouth syndrome, health-care professionals will teach parents to avoid putting anything but water in the infant's night bottle. Sugar in milk, formula, and juice causes severe decay and destruction of the tooth enamel. Parents will be discouraged from propping the bottle up and then leaving the child alone. This practice potentially leads to aspiration, or choking. Furthermore, holding the infant during

feeding provides warmth, comfort, and bonding, all vital factors in providing a feeling of love and security.

Motor Development

At 2 months, the infant is able to hold the head up while in the prone position. By 4 months, the infant has the ability to hold the head up steadily to a 90-degree angle while in the prone position. At 6 months, most infants are able to balance the head quite well. By the end of 7 months, infants have acquired the ability to sit up steadily without support.

Locomotion

Crawling, an early form of movement, is a motion made with the infant's abdomen touching the floor (Fig. 7.12E). A more advanced form of locomotion is creeping. The infant accomplishes this by resting the weight on the hands and knees. Infants sometimes crawl at 7 months and creep at about 9 months. Creeping appears after age 9 months in most children (Fig. 7.12F). Standing with support and walking follow at about 8 months to 15 months (Fig. 7.12D).

Box 7.6	Primary Dentition Schedule

- *6 months:* Teething begins with eruption of two lower central incisors
- *7 months:* Eruption of upper central incisors
- *9 months:* Eruption of upper lateral incisors
- *11 months:* Eruption of lower lateral incisors
- *12 months:* Approximately 6 to 8 teeth present
- *24 months:* Approximately 16 teeth present
- *30 months:* Completion of primary dentition; 20 teeth present

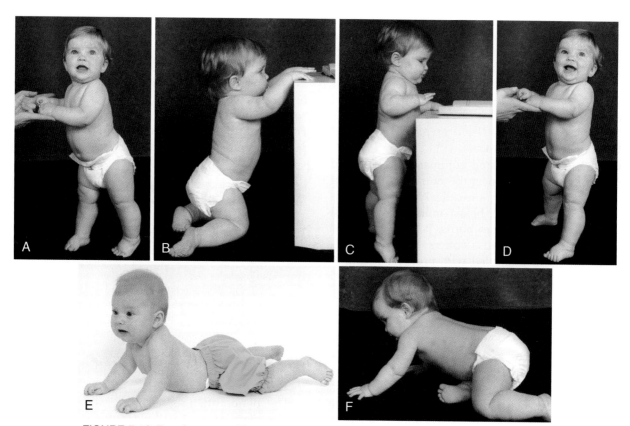

FIGURE 7.12 Development of locomotion. A, Infant bears full weight on feet by 7 months. B, Infant can maneuver from sitting to kneeling position. C, Infant can stand holding onto furniture at 9 months. D, While standing, infant takes deliberate step at 10 months. E, Infant crawls with abdomen on floor and pulls self forward, and then, F, creeps on hands and knees at 9 months. (Photos by Paul Vincent Kuntz, Texas Children's Hospital, Houston. From Wong DL: *Whaley & Wong's nursing care of infants and children,* ed 5, St. Louis, 1995, Mosby.)

Psychosocial Development

Erikson defined the task of the infant as *basic trust* versus *mistrust*. The responsiveness of others to the needs of the infant helps establish the basis of trust. Infants obtain gratification when their basic needs are fulfilled. Infants whose needs are not met develop a sense of dissatisfaction or mistrust. (See Table 7.8 for an overview of Erikson's stages of psychosocial development.)

By age 3 months, most infants respond differently to their parents or primary caregiver than they do to other people. By age 4 months, many infants are able to identify the voices of the most familiar people in their lives. Smiling occurs in response to different people and events. At the sight of their parents or primary caregivers, infants smile and begin to vocalize.

Beginning at approximately 8 months of age, infants show anxiety when they are separated from their primary caregiver. They develop shyness and a fear of strangers. The infant may cling and protest any separation from the primary caregiver. By age 9 months, most children show alarm at the presence of a stranger. Parents and child develop a form of synchrony (happening at the same time; moving or operating at the same rate). Infants who develop a secure early attachment are thought to later have the confidence to seek out future relationships. Studies on children aged 15 to 30 months who had good attachment relationships showed that they experienced a predictable behavior pattern after separation, known as separation anxiety.

Health Promotion

Nutrition

Both human breast milk and commercially prepared formula are options that meet the nutritional needs of the infant. Although today's excellent infant formulas approximate human milk, breast milk is still almost always the best food for newborns. It has been called "ultimate health food" because it offers so many benefits. However, infants who are fed with properly prepared formula and raised with love also grow up healthy and well adjusted. Breast milk or formula is the only food most babies need until they are about 4 to 6 months of age. The American Academy of Pediatrics (2012) recommends exclusive breastfeeding for the first 6 months of a baby's life.

Most experts agree that newborns should be fed on a demand schedule. Early in life, this practice may mean that babies are fed as often as every 2 hours. In the beginning, nursing mothers often start nursing for 10 to 15 minutes on each breast and then lengthen the feeding time as demanded by the infant. When infants suckle more slowly or appear uninterested in either the breast or the bottle, it is a good indication that they have had enough. The baby should have four to six wet diapers per day by the fourth day after birth. A baby who is breastfeeding should have at least two to three seedy stools each day. Breast milk is readily digested by the baby, which may result in a bowel movement shortly after each feeding. Signs of underfeeding include lack of satisfaction; a cranky, fussy baby; little weight gain; and persistent wrinkling of the skin. Signs of overfeeding include vomiting after feeding and frequent watery stools. Full-term infants have enough stored iron to last for at least the first 5 to 6 months of life. After this time, iron supplements or food sources are options to replenish the diminishing supply. Certain foods are generally accepted as best avoided in the first 6 months of life. Those foods include citrus fruits, egg whites, and wheat flour, all of which are frequently identified as allergy-producing substances.

Much controversy exists regarding the best time to introduce solid foods into the infant diet. Many physicians believe that very early introduction of solids leads to a variety of problems. A description of how to first introduce these foods into the infant diet is simpler than the decision of when to introduce solid food. The rules for solid foods include the following:

- Introduce only one new food at a time, allowing several days between new foods.
- Introduce cereals first, fruits and vegetables next, and meats last.
- Avoid mixing foods to allow the infant to develop interest in different foods and tastes.

Never leave infants alone while they are eating because infants choke easily. Avoid giving older infants round, hard foods that are easily caught in the throat. Foods that have high potential to cause choking include popcorn, grapes, raisins, hot dogs, and chicken nuggets.

Injury & Illness Prevention Box 7.2

- Never warm a bottle of milk using a microwave. It can cause harmful burns to a baby's mouth and can destroy the nutrients in the milk.
- Babies should not be put to bed with bottles. This can cause choking. Parents or caregivers should hold the baby while feeding them the bottle.
- Avoid giving infants and toddlers foods that are easily choked on. Cutting the food across the middle or down the middle will aid in decreasing the diameter of the food.

This period often serves as an excellent time to look at the type of foods the whole family is eating. Limiting the amount of sodium, fats, and sugar in the family diet is best. Lifelong eating habits are largely established early on in these toddler years. The entire family should be offered plenty of fresh fruits, vegetables, lean meats, and whole grains.

In warmer weather, fevers, prolonged vomiting, and diarrhea place infants at higher risk for dehydration because of their small fluid volume. Infants must receive adequate breast milk or formula. Infants do not need additional fluids during the first 4 months of life. By age 8 to 9 months, most babies master eating mashed or junior foods. Self-feeding of finger foods allows the infant further opportunity for exploration. By 9 months of age, the process of weaning should begin. This is usually a gradual process, with a training cup substituted for one bottle at a time, usually starting with the lunchtime feeding.

Sleep, Play Activity, and Safety

Newborns and infants sleep 18 hours out of 24. These sleep periods usually consist of short, nap-like periods. Infants are normally restless and make noises during these periods. Toward the end of the first 3 months, definite sleep patterns emerge, and nap and wake periods are clearly established. By the end of the first year, infants usually sleep 12 hours at night and take one nap during the day. Persistent crying during usual sleep or nap periods often signals discomfort or illness and calls for investigation.

A concern for parents of young infants is sudden infant death syndrome (SIDS). This disorder produces sudden, abrupt death with no identifiable warning signs. Formerly known as crib death, it appears to peak 2 to 3 months after birth. Steps to reduce the incidence of SIDS are outlined in the Injury & Illness Prevention Box 7.3.

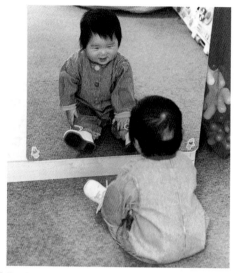

FIGURE 7.13 Nine-month-old infant enjoying own image in a mirror. (From Hockenberry MJ, Wilson D, Winkelstein ML, et al.: *Wong's nursing care of infants and children,* ed 10, St. Louis, 2015, Mosby.)

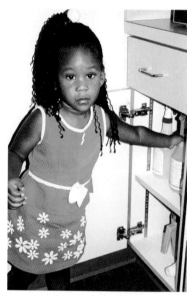

FIGURE 7.14 Children are most likely to ingest substances that are on their level, such as cleaning agents stored under sinks, rat poison, plants, and diaper pail deodorants. (From Hockenberry MJ, Wilson D, Winkelstein ML, et al.: *Wong's nursing care of infants and children,* ed 10, St. Louis, 2015, Mosby.)

Injury & Illness Prevention Box 7.3

Safety Alert: Steps to Reduce the Incidence of SIDS

1. Back to sleep: place infants on their back to sleep.
2. Avoid exposure to cigarette smoke.
3. Avoid use of soft bedding or pillows.
4. Keep room well ventilated.
5. Breastfeed if possible.
6. Maintain regular medical checkups for infants.

Play is important for learning. Play that captures the pleasures of using the senses and motor abilities is called sensorimotor play (Fig. 7.13). Early play items include turning mobiles, mirrors, colorful shapes, and toys of different textures. As hand coordination improves, other items, such as rattles and shapes, become useful play objects. Toward the end of the first year, stacking items, blocks, and puzzles encourage developing motor skills. Music is useful to soothe the infant or to stimulate awareness of sounds and rhythms. Play style during infancy is described as solitary play, which means that the infant plays alone and does not interact with or need other children to play. Allowing adequate freedom of movement helps enhance good development of muscles and bones. Young infants need room to stretch and kick. Care should be taken to prevent injury during this early stage of development. Do not push children to sit or walk before adequate muscle strength is achieved.

Accidents are the leading cause of injury and death in infants and young children. Safety precautions are essential to institute immediately at the birth of the child (Fig. 7.14). The Injury & Illness Prevention Box 7.4 lists safety rules for infants and young children.

Box 7.7	Developmental Tasks of Infancy

- Establishes trusting, meaningful relationships
- Recognizes primary caregiver
- Develops attachment behavior
- Learns to recognize objects
- Develops exploration skills
- Develops communication skills by beginning vocalization, developing nonverbal communication system, and imitating simple vocalizations
- Develops muscular control, eye-hand coordination, and object manipulation
- Develops mobility: crawling, creeping, cruising, walking
- Establishes patterns of living: eating, sleeping, elimination habits
- Begins to develop independent living skills: self-feeding, walking, undressing, communication of needs

Infancy is also a time of daily changes. Goals for the developmental tasks of infancy are shown in Box 7.7.

Toddler: 1 to 3 Years

Physical Characteristics

Rate of growth in the toddler years is slower than in infancy but follows the same general principles. It is orderly. It proceeds from head to foot, from the center outward, and from general to specific movements.

One of the most striking changes from infancy is the upright stance of the toddler. The chubby look of infancy is gone by 12 to 15 months. In the beginning of this stage, the toddler's body proportions result in a top-heavy appearance. By the end of this period, however, rapid growth of the extremities and slowed growth in the trunk produce a more proportionate body appearance (Fig. 7.15). A protruding abdomen produces a potbelly appearance, which disappears as the abdominal muscles strengthen. By age 2.5 years, all 20 deciduous teeth are present. Parents should begin routine dental examinations and tooth brushing during this period.

Vital Signs

During the toddler period, the pulse ranges from 90 to 120 beats per minute. Blood pressure averages 80 to 100 mm Hg systolic and 64 mm Hg diastolic. Body temperature ranges between 98° and 99° F (36.6° and 37.2°C). Respiration slows to 20 to 30 breaths per minute.

Neuromuscular Development

Many gross motor skills emerge in this period, including walking, climbing stairs (2 years), and hopping (3 years). The toddler develops running, pulling, and

---

Injury & Illness Prevention Box 7.4

Safety Alert: Safety Rules for Infants and Young Children

- Never leave an unsupervised infant on an elevated surface.
- Never leave an infant unattended in a high chair, stroller, walker, or any other device.
- Secure stairways and exits.
- Keep crib sides up and set mattress at lowest setting.
- Never leave infants or young children unattended in a bath for even a few seconds.
- Keep windows locked and secured with child guards.
- Never use plastic bags or coverings on mattresses or near infant's playthings.
- Avoid the use of pillows with small infants.
- Infant cribs must meet U.S. Consumer Product Safety regulations to prevent strangulation between crib bars.
- Remove wires and dangling electric cords from the crawling child's reach. Cover outlets with protective caps.
- Inspect all toys carefully for long strings and small removable parts.
- Use pacifiers that have one-piece construction.
- Do not allow children to play with balloons.
- Avoid giving infants and young children hard candies, nuts, popcorn, and other foods that are easily aspirated.
- Lock all poisons and medicines out of the reach of infants and young children (see Fig. 7.14).
- Avoid drinking hot fluids while holding an infant.
- Check temperature of foods and formula before feeding.
- Turn pot handles toward back of stove and remove burner knobs if within child's reach.
- Avoid smoking near infants and children to prevent burns and smoke inhalation.
- Keep infants and children away from hot surfaces, stoves, fireplaces, and barbecues.
- Use flame-retardant sleepwear.
- Never say that medication is candy to facilitate administration.
- Keep poison control hotline phone number accessible.
- Keep plants out of child's reach.
- Use plastic rather than glass eating and drinking utensils.
- Inspect toys and household items for sharp points.
- Inspect for chipped lead-based paint on surfaces painted before 1978 (production of lead paint for consumer use was banned in 1978).
- Keep knives and forks away from young children.
- Supervise infants and children playing around animals and pets.
- Always use safety seats and restraints when transporting infants and young children.

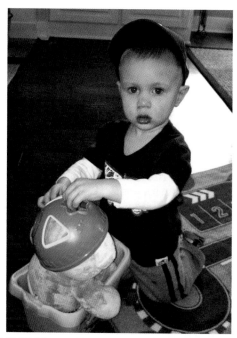

FIGURE 7.15 The toddler with proportionate body appearance. (From Cooper K, Gosnell K: *Foundations of nursing*, ed 7, St. Louis, 2015, Mosby.)

holding-on-tight skills, exploring the world in ways previously impossible. This time is also when the fine motor skills begin to be acquired, such as beginning to scribble (2 years) and copying a circle (3 years).

Toilet Training

Children do not reach the physiologic or psychological maturity necessary to begin toilet training until 18 to 24 months of age. Children need to reach maturity to have neuromuscular control, the cognitive ability to understand what is expected of them, and the language skills to express their needs. Bowel control is achieved first. Bladder control begins at the same time but takes longer to achieve. Nighttime control is usually achieved after daytime control is established. Advise parents and caregivers to expect setbacks and accidents, particularly during times of stress or illness. Do not focus on accidents; never make the child feel bad for having an accident. Praise their success and ignore their accidents. If praise is given for toileting successes and accidents are cleaned up without negativism, the toddler gains a sense of self-control, inner goodness, and pride. However, if the toddler is punished and made to feel foolish, a sense of shame develops. If the toddler is kept in diapers and given no opportunities to control the urges, a sense of doubt is fostered. Feelings of shame and doubt are not healthy personality attributes.

Psychosocial Development

The toddler is an uninhibited, energetic little person who always seeks attention, approval, and achievement

Box 7.8	Basic Principles of Discipline

- *Consistency:* Apply rules uniformly.
- *Follow-through:* Say and do what you mean.
- *Positive modeling:* Practice role model–approved behavior.
- *Promptness:* Administer any punishment in a nonhostile manner immediately after incident occurs.
- *Trust:* Express trust in the child.
- *Prevention:* Remove temptation.
- *Reinforcement:* Offer positive reinforcement for acceptable behavior.

of personal goals. Sometimes the toddler is cuddly and loving; at other times, biting, hitting, or pinching prevails. The toddler only slowly realizes that everything desired cannot be had and that some behaviors annoy others. The toddler tries to be independent, yet becomes easily frightened and runs to the caregiver for protection, security, reassurance, and approval.

Erikson views the toddler as struggling with autonomy (self-control) as opposed to shame and doubt. With newfound skills of independence, walking, talking, self-feeding, and beginning toilet training, the toddler is struggling to be independent. Characteristic of this search for autonomy is the toddler's use of the word "no," which gives a sense of control. The toddler possesses endless energy, yet often falls asleep almost while still in motion. As toddlers struggle for independence, they frequently display possessiveness and a desire to have things go their way. Ritualistic behavior and repetitive rituals are self-consoling behaviors at this stage. Toddlers enjoy the same story, the same routine, and the same foods at each meal. Rituals decrease their anxiety by helping them know what to expect. When healthcare providers follow a hospitalized child's usual rituals, the toddler feels safer and more secure in the strange environment.

Temper tantrums are common and are the result of frustration. A combination of wanting things "my way," the inability to communicate feelings, and the lack of impulse control are perhaps behind outbursts of temper. This type of negativism is best ignored unless the child or others are in danger of harm. Toddlers need many experiences of being able to choose among alternatives (to play inside or outside, to wear green pants or red pants). However, advise caregivers to make use of questions and offer alternatives for children only in situations in which either choice is acceptable. When a particular behavior is necessary (such as going to bed, holding hands to cross a street, letting go of another child's hair), it is better not to offer a choice. Erikson stressed that young children do not have the wisdom to know what behaviors are acceptable or unacceptable, healthy or unhealthy.

Discipline is a necessary means of teaching limit setting and impulse control. Basic principles of discipline are listed in Box 7.8. Toddlers seek attention, approval, and love as they struggle for independence.

Cognitive and Intellectual Development

Toddlers are constantly absorbing new ideas, widening their cognitive world, and expanding memory. Activities can be connected to past events or memories. The toddler's concept of time is limited to the present. The child's thinking is egocentric at this stage. Toddlers are often demanding, wanting things to go their way.

Communication and Language

The cognitive and language development of toddlers makes it possible for them to express their wishes. Commonly used words at this age are "no" and "me." Toddlers use these words in an attempt to exert their will and to take on new challenges.

During the toddler period, the child identifies objects by use. At 2.5 years of age, the toddler's vocabulary consists of about 450 words and 2-word sentences that include a noun and verb (e.g., "Me run."). By 3.5 years of age, the child is able to answer questions and use brief sentences, and even recite television commercials. The 3-year-old's vocabulary is approximately 900 words. Children's vocabulary can be greatly increased when they are regularly read to by their parents and caregivers. This activity also promotes bonding.

Health Promotion

Nutrition

Good nutrition requires that the toddler's daily diet consists of one serving from the meat group; two or more servings of vegetables; and at least two servings of fruit, cereal, or breads. The U.S. Department of Agriculture's guidelines (www.choosemyplate.gov) should be followed. The toddler needs 2 cups of food from the dairy group per day. Too few solid foods can lead to iron deficiency. Most children are more likely to eat foods with which they are familiar; therefore gradual introduction of new foods is advisable. Bite-sized pieces, finger foods, and smaller portions are generally more acceptable. Foods with a high risk for choking, such as hot dogs, grapes, carrots, and small candies, should not be given to toddlers. Early introduction to foods that are known allergens, such as wheat, egg whites, nuts, and chocolate, should be avoided (Nix, 2013). Idiosyncratic eating patterns are common at this stage. Toddlers need less food per unit of body weight than they did during infancy. A general guideline for serving size is 1 tablespoon of each solid food for each year of age. Parents need to be informed that during illness, brief periods of anorexia are usually not serious.

Sleep, Play Activity, and Safety

Toddlers need to release a high level of energy in daily growth, play, and exploration. Adequate rest and sleep are essential for maintaining optimal wellness. The toddler needs 12 hours of sleep each night plus a daytime nap. Suggestions helpful in promoting healthy sleeping patterns include limiting stimulation before sleep time, using quiet-time activities before sleep, allowing a favorite bedtime toy, telling a specified number of stories, and establishing and maintaining bedtime rituals. Box 7.9 lists guidelines for bedtime preparation.

Play improves muscle coordination, balance, and muscle strength. The toddler's play style, described as parallel play (Fig. 7.16), refers to the need that toddlers have to play alongside of, but not with, their peers. Unable to share and interact with their peers at this stage, they play side by side with similar toys in similar ways, but without interacting. Toddlers thrive on activities that keep them on the go. Running, jumping, and climbing activities help toddlers to develop bones and muscles. This age group's natural curiosity about how things work encourages them to explore. Play groups help encourage the shy or reluctant child to participate and try new activities.

More than half of all childhood deaths are caused by accidents, many of which are motor vehicle accidents. About 90% of the accidents that occur in the home are

Box 7.9	Guidelines for Bedtime Preparation

- Reduce activity level before bedtime.
- Establish a simple ritual (e.g., bathroom, story time, goodnight song).
- Make bedtime a pleasurable experience.
- Familiarize children with a nightly routine.
- Reassure children that they are not alone.
- Use a night light.
- Expect disruptions or setbacks during and after illness and stress or after stimulating activities.

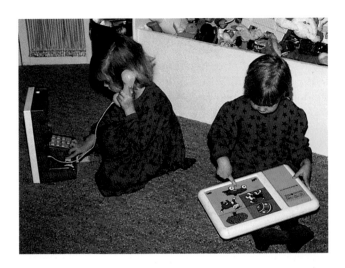

FIGURE 7.16 Parallel play. (From Hockenberry MJ, Wilson D, Winkelstein ML, et al.: *Wong's nursing care of infants and children,* ed 8, St. Louis, 2007, Mosby.)

Box 7.10	Developmental Tasks of the Toddler

- Recognizes self as a separate person; tolerates separation from primary caregiver, expresses own ideas and needs
- Develops increased attention span
- Begins to develop communication skills
- Begins to develop self-control skills
- Masters toilet-training basics
- Achieves independent mobility
- Develops independent skills of daily living: feeding, dressing, toileting, and managing simple tasks

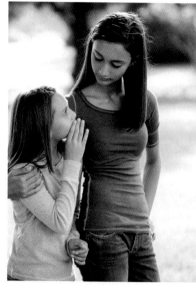

FIGURE 7.17 Siblings establishing a bond. (Copyright Thinkstock Photos.)

believed to be preventable. Prevention methods must include both supervision and education.

The developmental tasks of toddlers are summarized in Box 7.10.

Preschool: 3 to 5 Years

Physical Characteristics

Physical development during early childhood occurs on many fronts. The most obvious are the striking changes in size and shape; the most important—maturation of the nervous system and mastery of motor skills—are the least obvious.

Growth during the preschool period tends to be slow and steady. The preschooler looks taller and thinner than at earlier stages as the toddler's protuberant abdomen is gone (the abdominal muscles strengthen, and the child loses the potbelly appearance). Average weight gain is less than 5 pounds per year. Linear growth is about 2 to 2.5 inches per year. Height of the 4-year-old is usually double the birth length. The gait of the preschooler becomes steadier. The preschooler is more capable of focusing and refining activities, and the body grows slimmer, stronger, and less top heavy. Because of these developments, gross motor skills (large body movements such as running, climbing, jumping, and throwing) improve dramatically. Tasks such as tying shoelaces, cutting food with a knife and fork, and putting together a puzzle prove more difficult because of the preschooler's undeveloped fine motor skills (skills that involve small body movements); these are much harder for them to master than gross motor skills. Development of fine motor skills is important to encourage. The scribbling of the young child is comparable with the babbling of the infant. Both are ways to obtain practice with the means to later mastery of essential communication skills. Providing pencils, crayons, markers, and paper is as important as providing things to climb, objects to throw, and places to run.

Vision in the younger preschooler is described as farsighted. Vision improves during this period, and most children achieve 20/30 visual acuity by age 4 years. A yearly check of preschool children's vision is recommended. Sometimes amblyopia, a condition commonly known as lazy eye, is detected during a simple eye examination. Corrective measures, such as patching the good eye, usually strengthen the lazy eye and are necessary to prevent blindness. By age 6 years, the child begins to lose the deciduous teeth.

Vital Signs

Heart rate for the preschooler ranges between 70 and 110 beats per minute. Respiratory rate slows down to about 23 breaths per minute at rest. Blood pressure averages 110/60 mm Hg. Temperature ranges from 97° to 99° F (36.1° to 37.2° C), depending on the method used for measurement.

Psychosocial Development

Children learn to function independently; they subsequently use imagination to creatively explore new experiences. Erikson describes the task of the preschooler in terms of initiative versus guilt. Preschoolers search for and create fantasies about the different kinds of people they would like to become. They pretend to be grown up and try out a variety of roles. During the preschool period, the child's superego (conscience) functions as a censor of behavior. The dilemma of the preschooler, according to Erikson, is to test initiative without creating an overwhelming sense of guilt. Typical development of the preschooler includes gender identification. At this time, the child commonly stereotypes roles and shows marked interest in sexual differences. Strong sibling bonding is established (Fig. 7.17).

Cognitive and Intellectual Development

Preschool children see things as absolutes, in terms of white and black. All things are to the preschool child either good or bad. During the preschool stage, time is associated with weekly and seasonal events. Magical thoughts are typical of the child of this age, who believes that wishes have the power to make things happen. As a result, the preschool child sometimes feels powerful—and responsible for events that occur. Because of the belief that a wish has caused serious harm or even death to a loved one, the preschooler at times feels guilty. The occasional "white lies" or untruths of this period usually reflect some of the child's fantasies. During this stage of development, the child needs trustworthy guidance to distinguish truth from fantasy. At this stage, the child is more vulnerable to certain fears, probably fallout from the typically vivid imagination. Excessive exposure to inappropriate television content and other media has the potential to further distort reality testing. Common fears that manifest at this stage include fear of thunder, lightning, the dark, pain, abandonment, and monsters.

Communication and Language

By age 3 years, children are able to carry on a conversation. Pronunciation problems continue into the school years. Language becomes more adult-like. If the child is not talking by age 3 years, evaluation by a physician for possible hearing loss or other pathologic speech disturbances is necessary. Advise parents to continue to read to their child to help expand language ability and comprehension and to continue to foster positive child–caregiver relationships.

Health Promotion

Nutrition

Because body systems and muscles are still growing steadily, the preschool child continues to need high levels of protein. Dietary calcium and phosphorus are important to both toddlers and preschool children because of the increasing mineralization of their teeth and bones. Food habits, likes, dislikes, and appetites vary greatly from child to child. Some physicians recommend supplementary vitamins. Vitamins, like any other medication, are not intended and do not have the capacity to take the place of good eating habits (see Chapter 19).

A body mass index (BMI) at or above the 85th percentile and lower than the 95th percentile for children of the same gender and age is considered overweight. A BMI at or above the 95% percentile for children of the same gender and age is considered obese (CDC, 2012). Most cultures hold strong views regarding obesity, which results in emotional consequences for an obese child. Control of weight is an important parental concern because it helps prevent serious health issues later in life. Overweight infants are more likely to become overweight later in life. Genetic factors may predispose individuals to obesity. Children often adopt the eating habits of parents. Make suggestions to parents of ways to help with their children's weight control: model good eating behaviors, provide healthy food, and encourage physical activity.

Sleep, Play Activity, and Safety

Preschoolers often resist nap periods but still need 11 to 12 hours of sleep at night. Rest periods offered during the day enable children to reenergize and carry out the rest of their daily activities.

Play style for the preschool child becomes cooperative. The child begins to share, take turns, and interact with playmates (Fig. 7.18). Preschoolers enjoy pretending to carry out activities such as cooking, shopping, and driving. Through dramatic play, the child tries on different roles and identifies with adult models. Not only is it fun for two or more children to cooperate in creating their own scenario, but it also helps their social development to try out social roles, express their fears and fantasies, and learn to cooperate. Experiences with imaginary playmates are not uncommon in this age group. Children often feel a sense of control over what happens in their "imaginary world" and slowly learn to deal with reality through practice and experimentation.

Children during the preschool period are becoming more coordinated and want to begin participating in more organized games. By age 4 to 5 years, children learn to ride a bicycle with training wheels. They need guidance because they have difficulty maneuvering the bicycle, and their judgment and awareness of safety

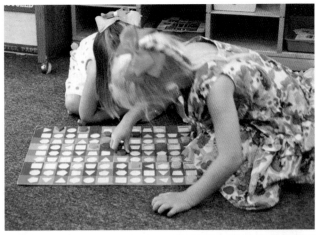

FIGURE 7.18 Playmates. (From Perry SE, Hockenberry MJ, Lowdermilk DL, et al.: *Maternal child nursing care*, ed 5, St. Louis, 2014, Mosby.)

issues is limited (see Injury & Illness Prevention Box 7.5 for safety and injury prevention tips for preschool children). Swimming, skating, and dancing are activities that children in this age group often begin to learn and enjoy. Activities of this nature should be fun for the child. It is not beneficial or appropriate for children to be pressured to participate in activities that they do not like or enjoy.

Injury & Illness Prevention Box 7.5

Safety Alert: Safety Tips and Injury Prevention for Preschool Children

- Use proper equipment that fits the child.
- Never leave children alone in pools of water. Teach children not to touch or go near pool drains.
- Inspect protective equipment, such as bicycle helmets, for potential hazards.
- Use protective sunscreen.

All the safety precautions described previously apply to the preschool child and the infant and toddler. Children need to know how to use the phone in case of an emergency.

Discipline and limit setting are needed and are as important to the child as are love and security. Necessary guidance includes offering alternative ways of expressing feelings and meeting needs (Box 7.11).

The preschool period is a time of learning to function independently and exploring the imagination. Box 7.12 shows the developmental tasks of preschoolers.

School Age: 6 to 12 Years

Physical Characteristics

During the school-age period, the growth pattern is usually gradual and subtle. The most obvious growth is in the long bones of the extremities and in the development of the facial bones. As a result of this bone growth, some children report "growing pains," particularly at night. Persistent pains call for evaluation by a physician to rule out any underlying pathologic condition. From age 6 to 12 years, height and weight increase by about 2 inches and 4.5 to 6.5 pounds, respectively, per year for both boys and girls.

Motor skills in boys and girls develop with some differences; boys often become stronger, and girls more graceful and accurate.

The child's posture becomes straighter. The causes of poor posture range from fatigue to emotional states or even minor skeletal defects. Ensure that school-aged children are routinely screened for scoliosis (abnormal lateral curvature of the spine). Muscle mass and strength gradually increase, and the body loses the "baby fat" appearance of earlier childhood. Both gross motor and

---

Box 7.11 Steps for Discipline and Limit Setting

- Define acceptable as opposed to unacceptable behaviors.
- Set limits: "I will not let you hurt anyone."
- Be consistent: keep the same rules, and enforce them reliably.
- Recognize escalating emotions and intervene: "I can see you are upset; let's go over there and sit down."
- Suggest "time out."
- Choose punishment that "fits" wrongdoing, and enact it in a timely way (and in a nonhostile manner).
- Praise and reinforce positive behavior: "I like the way you … ."
- Always start over with a clean slate.
- Stay calm; avoid arguing.
- Avoid putdowns: "You are acting like a bad boy."
- Remember to listen to the child.

Box 7.12 Developmental Tasks of Preschoolers

- Develops stronger sense of self; is able to express own needs, ideas, and feelings; has capacity to postpone immediate gratification
- Attains greater attention span; listens more attentively
- Develops and refines gross motor skills and fine motor skills
- Recognizes gender identification
- Begins to work and play more cooperatively with others
- Improves communication skills
- Develops self-control skills; learns socially acceptable ways of expressing anger, frustration, and disappointment; obeys simple rules; develops self-awareness and sense of self-protection
- Seeks information, asks questions, learns values and beliefs of the family

---

fine motor development continue to be refined during the school-age years.

Vision improves, and most children have 20/20 vision at this stage. Regular vision testing is advisable throughout the school years.

Vital Signs

Heart and respiratory rate steadily decrease, whereas blood pressure increases. Normal pulse rate is between 55 and 90 per minute, respiratory rate is 22 to 24 per minute, and blood pressure is 110/65 mm Hg.

Dentition

Permanent teeth develop rapidly. The American Dental Association (2013) recommends that children have their first dental visit within 6 months after the first tooth appears but no later than the child's first birthday. Dental checkups should continue every 6 months throughout childhood.

Psychosocial Development

Entrance into school challenges the child and creates demands for new social and cognitive skills. The child becomes more independent and participates in a broader world of peers and new experiences. School-aged children become increasingly aware of rules and socialization skills and expectations. The beginning abilities to compromise and compete are challenges that face this age group.

Erikson identified the task of the school-age years as *industry* versus *inferiority*. After the child realizes that the school-age years as "there is no workable future within the womb of his family," says Erikson, the school-aged child "becomes ready to apply himself to given skills and tasks." Children develop their own goals and direct their efforts toward mastery of these goals. As children discover their talents and accomplishments, they gain self-confidence and a sense of purpose. During these years, the child learns to work and masters skills that produce satisfaction as the result of that work. Successful mastery of learning in school leads to strengthening and stabilizing the child's sense of self. According to Erikson, as children busily try to master the skills valued in their culture, they develop views of themselves as either competent or incompetent—as either industrious and productive or inferior and inadequate.

Input from the outside is a key influence on which direction the child's self-concept will take. If the environment inadequately supports a child's pursuits, the stage perhaps is set for the development of feelings of inferiority and the lack of self-confidence. The good school setting is a pleasant, comfortable environment. Teachers and caregivers need to use praise, encouragement, and rewards to positively reinforce the school-aged child's efforts. Teachers also have to be positive role models. School helps the child learn new routines and establish important social relationships (Fig. 7.19).

Cognitive and Intellectual Development

Between age 7 and 11 years, children usually come to understand logical principles—again, as long as the principles can be applied to concrete, specific cases. They distinguish purpose from behavior and outcome and are able to focus on more than one aspect of a task. Children in this age group have begun to develop logical socialized thought. They view the world more realistically than they did at younger ages, and they are capable of understanding the views of others. Movement is away from fantasy as the child realizes that a physical

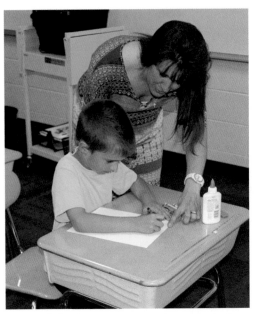

FIGURE 7.19 School represents an important change in a child's life, and teachers exert a significant influence on the child. (From Cooper K, Gosnell K: *Foundations of nursing,* ed 7, St. Louis, 2015, Mosby.)

Box 7.13	Developmental Tasks of the School-Aged Child

- Develops a sense of belonging with family and peers
- Develops work habits and learns to organize, set, and reach goals; evaluate work; and accept criticism
- Learns competence in reading, writing, calculation, grammar, and communication
- Refines fine motor and gross motor coordination

cause is behind an event. The child's developing cognitive skills serve as a motivator for learning how to work. A supportive learning environment often enhances the child's approach to problem solving and helps lead to success.

The school-aged child experiences gradual and subtle growth changes while learning new social and cognitive skills. Box 7.13 contains a list of the developmental tasks of the school-aged child.

Communication and Language

Most 6-year-olds have a good command of sentence structure. The child's vocabulary has become larger and includes slang and swear words, which many children enjoy using for the effect they create. Fine motor development continues and, combined with growth in cognitive and communication skills, produces refinements in written language and musical abilities. By age 7 years, the hands of the child have become steadier. Printing becomes clearer and smaller. Between age 8 and 10 years, the hand becomes more efficient, which enables the child to write rather than print. The 10-year-old to 12-year-old child has the capacity to accomplish complex, intricate, fine-quality handcrafts and sometimes begins piano, violin, or guitar lessons.

Health Promotion

Nutrition

Total metabolic needs are largely determined by the energy expenditure of each individual child. The sedentary, quiet child who prefers fine motor activities needs fewer calories than the child who is more oriented to athletics or is more physically active. The recommended daily intake of food is listed at the ChooseMyPlate website (www.choosemyplate.gov).

Building on toddler-age and preschool-age foundations, strong dietary habits and food preferences are laid down during the school-age period. Cultural influences, family habits, and peer pressure are all critical factors in how a child's food habits develop. Obesity during this period is closely correlated with obesity in adult years; therefore the child's weight needs to be maintained within normal limits. In middle childhood, obese children are teased, picked on, and rejected. They know that they are overweight, and they often hate themselves for it. Obese children usually have fewer friends than other children. The best way to get children to lose weight is to increase their physical activity. Indeed, inactivity is possibly as responsible for childhood obesity as overeating. Diets high in saturated fat increase a child's risk for high blood cholesterol and earlier occurrence of heart disease unless steps are taken to lower these levels.

Sleep, Play Activity, and Safety

Fatigue, irritability, inattention, and poor learning are often signs of inadequate sleep. The 6-year-old needs about 12 hours of sleep at night. By 12 years of age, the child usually needs about 10 hours of sleep. Some children have frequent nightmares that disrupt their sleep. Stress, violence on television, and overtiredness all have the potential to contribute to a child's nightmares. Relaxation techniques such as quiet music, story time, and bathing often help the child relax before sleep.

School-aged children need adequate exercise to enhance muscle development, coordination, balance, and strength. In addition, music, craft projects, board games, appropriate television, and video games are all enjoyed by the school-aged child. Privacy and a place for their belongings are important at this age. The school-aged child is often a willing worker and enjoys being paid for small jobs. Collection and hoarding of "treasures" among their belongings are a part of this stage of development.

Many children during the school years become involved with competitive or team sports (Fig. 7.20).

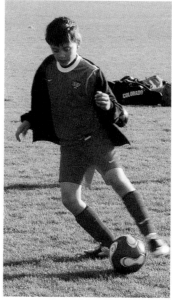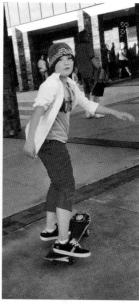

FIGURE 7.20 Activities engaged in by school-aged children, such as soccer and skateboarding, vary according to the child's interest and opportunity. (From Cooper K, Gosnell K: *Foundations of nursing*, ed 7, St. Louis, 2015, Mosby.)

Children of this age show interest and loyalty to peers of the same gender. They learn to follow the rules of games. Some are able to benefit from team competitiveness and use it to motivate themselves to excel. Others shy away from competition and become disinterested or develop feelings of inadequacy and disappointment.

Accidents are still the leading cause of death in this age group. Impulsiveness, poor judgment, curiosity, and incomplete control over motor coordination are some of the factors that increase the school-aged child's risk of accidents.

Television, as well as social media, often exerts a powerful influence on a child's development. One concern about television and social media today is the increased amount of violence it portrays. Some children have actually been bullied through use of social media. There have been documented suicides in children and adolescents that have occurred partly as a result from being bullied on social media sites. Many believe that a good deal of available television content offers the child a potent model for aggressive behavior. Ways to reduce the negative influence of television include (1) limit the amount of time children watch television, (2) screen programs for content and age appropriateness, and (3) watch programs with children and discuss the content. Screen time should be limited for children each day so that the eyes and brain are not overstimulated. This includes, but is not limited to, television, tablets, electronic gaming devices, such as Xbox™ and Wii™, as well as use of computers.

Preventing school violence is another critical issue these days. School violence is defined as anything that physically or psychologically injures schoolchildren or damages school property. Today, school violence appears to have increased in many locations. Two factors that are possibly contributing to this increase are an increased availability of weapons and a breakdown of communication. Experts agree that children need resources to help them deal with the daily stressors that they face. Many children today spend less time with parents and more time in front of a television and on the Internet watching or playing violent shows and games. The average American child witnesses 200,000 violent acts on television by age 18 years (KidsHealth, 2016). Parents need to be aware of the effects of television violence on children. Children who view violent acts are more likely to show aggression but are also fearful that something bad will happen to them. Children need to feel comfortable discussing their feelings and concerns with parents and teachers and must be able to use these discussions to learn how to recognize whether they are in danger and whether others are exhibiting signs of troubled behavior. Encourage parents to ask questions about their child's feelings and their school activities every day. If children have difficulty talking to parents or answering their questions, advise parents to seek professional help. A key responsibility of parents is to stay involved and be active participants in their child's daily affairs.

Children need to be taught constructive ways to handle their impulses; otherwise they are more likely to resort to unacceptable ways of channeling their feelings. One possibility is that they will look for revenge, which perhaps makes them feel in control and powerful. Although many children have access to weapons, most of them do not engage in violent behavior. However, we need to work to inhibit violent tendencies and to look for ways to prevent the few who do act out their feelings in violent ways from causing harm to others (see Injury & Illness Prevention Box 7.6). The first step in preventing a tragedy is recognizing the behavioral tendencies that have the potential to lead to violence or other problem behavior. Give children the guidance and encouragement they need to recognize and report the signs of troubled behavior if they notice them in a friend or classmate without feeling that they have deceived the other person or let the other person down (Box 7.14).

Gun safety is a must regardless of how one feels about guns. Gun enthusiasts, collectors, and law enforcement agents all are obliged to ensure the safety of others. Most children and many adults have a fascination with guns. Even when children and adults are taught gun safety, some exhibit unsafe behavior when the opportunity arises. Even toy guns create the potential for dangerous situations. Parents and individuals with weapons in the home are under the obligation to take adequate steps to prevent accidents and injury from their weapons. Knowledge of how to handle a gun is not sufficient to protect the owner's family and others from injury.

Box 7.14	Common Signs of Troubled Childhood Behavior

- Problems getting along with peers
- Difficulty accepting authority and resistance to direction
- Outbursts of uncontrolled behavior
- Bullying tendencies
- Frequent victimizing or teasing
- Social isolation
- Poor school performance
- Violence to pets or other living creatures
- Preoccupation with weapons
- Verbal expression of threatening behavior or revenge

Injury & Illness Prevention Box 7.6

Safety for Parents With Children in Schools

- Secure weapons in homes.
- Develop a zero-tolerance program with school officials.
- Work with a parent–teacher association (PTA) to make schools safe.
- Determine with school officials an emergency and security plan.
- Maintain open lines of communication between child and parent and school officials.

Injury & Illness Prevention Box 7.7

Safety Alert: Gun Safety Rules

For Children
- Stop and DO NOT TOUCH any gun, real or toy.
- Leave the area if a gun is found.
- Report any gun to an adult.

For Adults
- Never store ammunition with the gun.
- Keep the gun in a locked location out of reach of children.
- Lock the ammunition in a separate location from the gun.
- Lock gun-cleaning supplies, which are often poisonous.

Ammunition must be removed from firearms, and guns must be locked away securely and apart from ammunition, which is properly kept secured in another, separate locked area. In addition, and most importantly, children of all ages must be taught what to do if they find a gun (see Injury & Illness Prevention Box 7.7).

Adolescence: 12 to 19 Years

Physical Characteristics

The term *adolescence* covers the transition period from childhood to adulthood. Adolescence begins at puberty;

accompanying the pubertal changes are corresponding changes in the personality. *Puberty,* the period of life at which the ability to reproduce begins, entails the maturation of the reproductive system, including all the primary and secondary sexual developmental changes. Primary changes occur in the organs related to reproduction (ovaries, breasts, uterus, testes, and penis). Secondary sexual changes occur in other parts of the body (development of pubic and facial hair, voice changes, and fat deposits). Adolescence literally means "to grow into maturity" and is generally regarded as the psychological, social, and maturational process initiated by pubertal changes.

Adolescence is characterized as the second major period of rapid growth. Females grow 2 to 8 inches (5 to 20 cm), whereas males grow 4 to 12 inches (10 to 30 cm). During this adolescent period, females gain 15 to 55 pounds (7 to 25 kg), and males gain 15 to 65 pounds (7 to 30 kg). Females develop more body fat, and males develop more muscle tissue. After puberty, men average 50% muscle and 16% fat, whereas women average 40% muscle and 27% fat. Muscle strength and muscle mass increase in the male, which causes the average male to have more muscle strength. Exercise facilitates the size, strength, and endurance of each adolescent.

In the female, menarche (the first menstrual period) signals the beginning of adolescence; sperm production signals the beginning of adolescence in the male. Girls develop larger breasts, a narrower waist, wider hips, and a lower center of gravity. Boys develop broader shoulders, narrower hips, and larger limbs. Both boys and girls experience voice changes. Girls' voices become fuller and richer because of the lengthening of their vocal cords. Boys' voices become lower and louder. The deeper male voice results from enlargement of the larynx (the Adam's apple) and lengthening of the vocal cords.

Sexual interests increase markedly in vigor and intensity and are usually focused on members of the opposite sex. New problems arise as adolescents find social disapproval and prohibitions arising in their own conscience that conflict with intense sexual drives.

Vital Signs

Average pulse rate is 70 beats per minute. Respiratory rate averages 20 breaths per minute. Blood pressure increases to 120/70 mm Hg.

Psychosocial Development

Exactly when adolescence begins is different in each individual. Some begin adolescence at an early age; others develop later. Regardless of the exact age of onset, we usually perceive the nearing of this stage by recognizing the onset of distinct behavioral changes. A mother may notice that her 11-year-old daughter has become quiet about school and activities, no longer wanting her mother's opinion or listening ear. Her daughter is now spending most of her time at home in her room with the door closed. A father may enjoy his son's musical talents and his band's energy and success, although the two might butt heads over the taste of their lyrics and the sound level.

The period of adolescence is frequently described as difficult and involving a stormy search for oneself. Confronting every adolescent are a changing body, sexual demands, responsibilities, expectations, and questions about values and beliefs. The search for identity amid a world of social pressures creates a painful struggle. Erikson described the developmental task of adolescence as establishing a sense of identity. He proposed the conflict of identity versus role confusion as characteristic of adolescence. The search for a sense of identity, he believed, reaches crisis proportions at this time. Not only does the adolescent need to adjust to a sexually mature body, but also all previous conflicts (trust vs. mistrust, autonomy vs. doubt, initiative vs. guilt, and industry vs. inferiority) have to be resolved yet again in light of the newly sensuous self. The period of adolescence requires major reorganization of the personality, resolution of childhood insecurities, and acceptance of adult responsibilities. The value of peers is usually significant to the adolescent (Fig. 7.21). Peers influence preferences of dress, speech, and leisure activities. The peer group is often the milieu to learn and test developing interpersonal skills. Many adolescents use conforming behavior to win praise and acceptance by peers. If handled properly, adolescence is often a great period of accomplishment and creativity (Box 7.15).

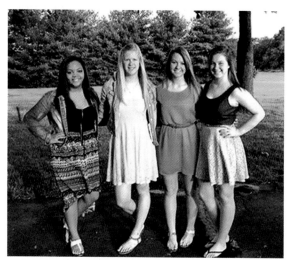

FIGURE 7.21 The peer group provides the adolescent with a sense of belonging. (From Cooper K, Gosnell K: *Foundations of nursing,* ed 7, St. Louis, 2015, Mosby.)

Box 7.15   Parenting Tips During Adolescence

- Educate yourself and your adolescent.
- Maintain open communication.
- Choose your battles.
- Set realistic expectations.
- Set good examples for behavior.
- Honor individuality.
- Respect privacy.
- Try to remember your own experiences during this stage.
- Set appropriate rules and regulations.
- Be consistent.
- Stay involved; meet your child's friends and acquaintances.
- Be active in school and after-school activities.

Cognitive Development

Adolescents become capable of reasoning and formal logic. At this time, thoughts may be influenced more by logical principles than by personal perceptions and experiences. The adolescent thinks beyond the present. Without having to focus exclusively on the immediate situation, the adolescent is able to imagine the possible: a sequence of events that might occur, such as college and occupational possibilities; how things might change in the future, such as relationships with parents; and the possible consequences of actions they are considering, such as dropping out of school.

Moral Development

As children move through the stages of cognition and logical thinking, they also progress through stages of moral development. As with other developmental processes, moral development approaches or achieves adult levels during adolescence.

In some ways, adolescence is an uncomfortable in-between phase. Old principles are challenged, but new and independent values do not emerge immediately. As a consequence, young people find themselves searching for a moral code that preserves their personal integrity and guides their behavior, especially in the face of strong pressure to violate the old values. They face many decisions involving moral dilemmas.

Health Promotion

Nutrition

The rate of body growth and the adolescent's increased basal metabolic rate require an increase in the individual's caloric needs. At peak growth, females may need as much as 2600 calories per day and males as much as 3600 calories per day. Many factors affect the individual's dietary habits, including cultural background, family habits, work schedules, school, concern about weight gain, peer influence, and lack of knowledge concerning correct food choices. Protein needs are increased as a consequence of the rapid growth of this period. Advise adolescents to obtain 12% to 16% of their total daily food intake from protein.

The adolescent diet is most likely to be deficient in calcium, iron, and zinc. The need for these minerals during the period of rapid growth is substantially increased—calcium for skeletal growth; iron for expansion of muscle mass and blood volume, soft tissue growth, and the rapid growth demands of the expanding red blood cell mass; and zinc for the generation of both skeletal and muscle tissue. Adolescent boys have greater muscle mass, but adolescent girls have an additional iron loss from menstruation. Consequently, the need for iron is equivalent in both sexes. Increased amounts of milk are usually required to supplement the average diet to ensure an adequate calcium intake during this time. The adolescent is advised to follow the guidelines at the ChooseMyPlate website.

Sleep, Play Activity, and Safety

The adolescent needs to pace activities to allow for adequate rest. The adolescent often requires increased hours of sleep to restore energy levels. During puberty and adolescence, caution must be taken to prevent injuries related to exercise and sports. Injuries sometimes occur at this time in connection with the adolescent's growth spurt. Growth spurts cause the bones to grow more quickly than the muscles and tendons, which causes the muscles and tendons to become short and tight. Sports-related injuries may result from these factors. Teaching youngsters to perform appropriate warm-up and stretching exercises before starting any strenuous sport can lessen the risk of injury (see Injury & Illness Prevention Box 7.8). Participating in organized sports at this age helps adolescents learn to work with others, meet challenges, and set personal goals. Parents have an opportunity to encourage children to exercise by setting an example and practicing good, healthy behaviors for themselves. Having parents involved on the sidelines supporting their adolescent's efforts potentially enhances self-esteem.

Injury & Illness Prevention Box 7.8

Sports-Related Safety Tips

- Use safety helmets.
- Use properly fitting equipment.
- Play on properly maintained surfaces.
- Perform warm-up exercises before sports practice.
- Avoid overuse of muscles.
- Insist on adequate supervision.
- Obtain proper training.
- Treat existing injuries and prevent re-injury.

Accident prevention is vitally important during this stage of development. The greatest number of deaths in this age group is attributable to accidents. Driver's education, water safety training, education about safe sex practices, and drug education are necessary to inform adolescents of the risks and dangers inherent in these activities. Injury & Illness Prevention Box 7.9 lists safe sex practices that are crucial to emphasize early in adolescence, with special emphasis on abstinence.

Injury & Illness Prevention Box 7.9

Safety Alert: Guidelines for Practice of Safe Sex

- The safest sexual practice is abstinence, or not having sex.
- Be familiar with your sexual partners. Ask about their sexual lifestyle before you engage in sexual relations.
- Avoid engaging in sexual relations with intravenous drug users or with individuals who have had multiple sex partners.
- Use a latex condom as the best type of protection from infection.
- Condoms should be inspected for tears before use. Avoid lengthy storage and exposure to excessive heat.
- Fit the condom over the erect penis, leaving a small space at the end for the collection of semen.
- Hold the upper end of the condom when withdrawing from the vagina to prevent slippage.
- Avoid sexual relations with individuals who have genital lesions or unusual drainage; this includes oral sex.
- Be aware that the risk of human immunodeficiency virus (HIV) infection is increased with oral sexual practices. Anal intercourse requires additional education for safe practice.

Emotional Health

Adolescence is, as described previously, a period of maturation that covers the transition from childhood to adulthood (Box 7.16). In part as a result of the complexity of the tasks that face them, adolescents go through different moods that are common in this period. At times they are outgoing and gregarious and active participants in family matters. They offer their opinions and seem to ignore others. There are also times when they are moody and loners who seem not to want any part of family activities. Such mood swings generally occur at this stage. Families should recognize and distinguish normal moodiness from signs of depression. Depression is defined as a mood disturbance characterized by feelings of sadness, despair, and hopelessness. People who are depressed are often unable to improve their condition without help from professional therapy. Teach parents, teachers, and healthcare workers to recognize the common signs of depression. Early detection and intervention is crucial when dealing with depression because

---

Box 7.16 Developmental Tasks of the Adolescent

- Recognizes individuality
- Accepts strengths and weaknesses
- Develops own value system
- Assumes responsibility for own behavior
- Develops philosophy of life
- Adapts to somatic changes (changes that affect the body)
- Acquires skills necessary for adult living
- Refines social skills
- Develops independent living skills

Box 7.17 Signs of Depression and Indicators of Suicide Risk

- Change in appetite
- Change in mood (sadness, hopelessness)
- Inability to concentrate
- Loss of interest in activities
- Change in sleep habits (either always sleeping or unable to sleep)
- Talk of suicide
- Preoccupation with death or dying
- Giving away of possessions

---

this leads to higher success rates. Untreated depression can lead to suicide (Box 7.17). Advise parents to seek professional help if their child expresses feelings of marked depression. All threats must be taken seriously, and it is imperative to be alert to sudden changes in behavior, such as a change from extreme sadness to manic behavior. This mood swing potentially signals a decision to carry out the person's suicide plan.

Early Adulthood: 20 to 40 Years

The transition to adulthood in the United States is marked by events such as taking on financial responsibilities, making career choices, beginning social relationships, entering marriage, and becoming a parent. All the challenges and accomplishments of the earlier developmental stages have helped prepare the individual for the responsibilities of adult maturity. Fantasies of what adulthood entails usually give way to more realistic expectations and hopes.

Early adulthood, the period of optimal physical condition, is marked by big changes in lifestyle. Box 7.18 contains a list of the developmental tasks of early adulthood.

Physical Characteristics

The body during early adult years is at its best level of functioning. The typical young adult is a fine physical

Box 7.18	Developmental Tasks of Early Adulthood

- Achieves independence, both financial and social
- Maximizes personal worth and identity
- Develops meaningful and satisfying social relationships
- Assumes responsibilities and independent decision making
- Learns to balance personal needs and societal expectations
- Accepts self and others
- Distinguishes physical attraction from love and permanent commitment
- Decides on a marriage, career, and children

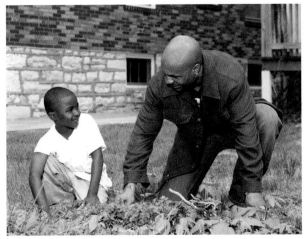

FIGURE 7.22 Father and child bonding. (From Sorrentino SA, Remmert LN: *Mosby's textbook for nursing assistants,* ed 8, St. Louis, 2012, Saunders.)

specimen. During the middle twenties, most body functions are fully developed, and muscular strength, energy, and endurance are now at their peak.

Physical appearance is influenced by heredity, environment, and general state of wellness. Females usually reach their maximal height at about 16 to 17 years of age. Males continue to grow until 18 to 20 years of age. Between age 30 and 45 years, height is stable, and then it begins to decline because of settling of spinal disks. Often, an increase in fatty tissue causes weight gain, a decrease in muscle strength, and a stabilization of reaction time. The senses are also at their sharpest during young adulthood. Visual acuity is keenest at about age 20 years and does not begin to decline until about age 40 years.

Diet plays an important role, as it does throughout the developmental stages. Both heart disease and cancer are major concerns in the adult years. Proper diet and exercise often has a decisive impact on the control of heart disease, which is caused by increased cholesterol deposits occluding the walls of blood vessels. Likewise, low-fat, high-fiber, and low-cholesterol diets are recommended as preventive measures against cancers of the breast, the stomach, and the intestine. Other lifestyle habits such as the use of tobacco, drugs, and alcohol affect the adult's health status (Injury & Illness Prevention Box 7.10).

Injury & Illness Prevention Box 7.10

Health Promotion Recommendations for a Healthy Lifestyle

- Follow the guidelines at www.myplate.gov
- Drink adequate fluids.
- Avoid smoking and drugs.
- Consume little or no alcohol.
- Maintain optimal weight.
- Participate in a scheduled program of daily exercise.
- Obtain adequate restorative sleep.
- Practice stress reduction.
- Enjoy leisure activities.

In the past few decades, attention to physical fitness has become more popular, with benefit to general welfare. Regular, paced exercise increases heart and lung capacity, lowers blood pressure, helps control weight, enhances body function, and improves emotional health.

By adulthood, men and women have reached their sexual maturity. Sexual drive continues for both men and women throughout adulthood.

Psychosocial Development

Dual-career families have grown out of the economic realities of our times, as well as women's interest in pursuing careers. The feminist movement has resulted in many positive social changes. Both the home and the workplace show the effects of these changes and the dual-career lifestyle.

Another important option for this age group is the decision to start a family (Fig. 7.22). If they choose to start a family, another issue is how many children to have. Further thought is needed regarding considerations such as financial means, safety, family support, housing, the relationship to members of the extended family, and the roles and responsibilities of the nuclear family unit. Young adults who establish a family today need to have open communication about self-development, which includes issues of dual careers, child-rearing practices, and domestic duties within the home.

Family development and harmony are major goals for many young adults, both male and female. Although family size and structure have undergone dramatic changes in the past decades, concerns about individual members' health and safety continue to form a primary focus within the family as a unit. Family life is influenced by the characteristics of individual family members. Typically, healthy family adjustment is associated with the age of the individuals, job security, the family's and the individuals' places in the community, and healthy patterns of living (good nutrition, personal cleanliness, physical fitness). Therefore the physical and mental health of one family member affects all family members.

Erikson identified *early intimacy* versus *isolation* as the developmental task of adulthood. Intimacy is the ability to develop one's deepest hopes and concerns in connection to another person. One aspect of intimacy is the capacity to accept the closeness of another person. Intimacy leads to commitment, sharing, and compromise. The "virtue" that develops in young adulthood is the virtue of love, or the mutuality of devotion between partners who have chosen to share their lives. As young adults resolve conflicting demands of intimacy, competitiveness, and distance, they develop an ethical sense, which Erikson considers the mark of the adult. The opposite of intimacy, the distancing of oneself from intimate relationships, is the negative resolution of the task of this life stage and leads to isolation and self-absorption.

Health Promotion

Nutrition

Fewer total numbers of calories are needed when compared with the amount needed in adolescence because the adult has completed biophysical growth. Calories are needed to maintain body functioning for cell replacement and repair and for provision of energy. Calorie needs vary based on age, gender, size, physical activity, metabolism, and levels of stress.

Rest and Sleep

Most adults function well with 7 to 9 hours of restorative sleep. Adults do not commonly schedule daytime naps to prevent fatigue; however, they can increase their productivity by obtaining adequate rest during the day. Adequate rest is essential for the pregnant woman to ensure the health of both herself and her unborn baby.

Physical and Dental Examinations

Annual physical and dental examinations are recommended. A routine testicular examination for the male and an annual Papanicolaou (Pap) smear for the female are essential for early detection of cancer. The American Cancer Society recommends that women have a mammogram at age 40 years, and every 1 to 2 years annually thereafter. At age 50 years, annual mammograms are recommended. Beginning at age 40 years, men are advised to obtain a yearly physical examination that includes a digital rectal examination, and beginning at age 50 years, a prostate-specific antigen (PSA) study should be included to screen for prostate cancer. Routine dental examinations should be scheduled for adults every 6 months. Eye examinations are necessary every 2 years unless otherwise indicated.

Safety

Accidents are the leading cause of disability and death in this age group. Injuries commonly result from work, vehicle, and sports accidents and from violence.

Middle Adulthood: 40 to 65 Years

The middle adulthood period is designated as occurring between 40 and 65 years of age. Most individuals of this age group enjoy a healthy body. Some changes result in a gradual shift of balance away from peak performance. The extent of these changes is directly related to diet, heredity, exercise, rest, mental outlook, stress, and disease.

Middle adulthood is characterized by shifts in responsibilities and physical adjustments. According to Erikson, the main task for middle adulthood is generativity versus self-absorption or stagnation. If an individual is unsuccessful at meeting this task, he or she may become self-absorbed or stagnate. Box 7.19 contains a list of the developmental tasks of middle adulthood.

Physical Characteristics

Bone mass decreases as skeletal growth cells are depleted. This bone loss leads to an increased risk of osteoporosis. Women lose calcium from bone tissue after menopause. Men also lose calcium from bones, but at a more gradual rate than women, and their risk of osteoporosis is lower. Slight changes in height continue to occur as a result of the compression of the spinal vertebrae and the hardening of collagen fibers. A decrease in muscle fibers results in a reduction of muscle mass. Heredity, nutrition, and exercise patterns account for much of the individual variation commonly seen. Changes in muscle strength are perhaps related more to level of activity than to age. A redistribution of body weight leads to changes in body shape and contour. A

Box 7.19   Developmental Tasks of Middle Adulthood

- Balances goals and realities and redirects energies as necessary
- Extends caring and concern beyond immediate family (to neighborhood, community, society)
- Develops career and job satisfaction
- Adapts to physical changes
- Establishes new roles and relationships with spouse, children, grandchildren, and parents

decrease in basal metabolism and less activity often necessitate calorie reductions to prevent weight gain.

Basic neurologic functioning remains at a high level during this age period.

Noticeable changes in vision occur as a result of presbyopia (a defect in vision in advancing age that involves loss of accommodation or the recession of the near point caused by loss of elasticity of the crystalline lens and the ensuing change in close vision).

Other sensory changes may include presbycusis (a normal progressive, age-associated loss of hearing acuity, speech intelligibility, auditory threshold, and pitch). These changes usually begin around age 40 years and occur more commonly in men than in women.

One of the most noticeable changes that occur during this period is in the appearance of the individual's skin. A decrease in the elastic fibers and a slight loss of subcutaneous tissue give skin a looser, more wrinkled appearance. Hair color often changes with age with the onset of graying. Graying usually begins at the temples. Hair growth and distribution sometimes changes during the middle adult years. Scalp hair tends to become thinner.

A higher incidence of periodontal (gum) disease is seen in the middle adult years. Preventive treatment programs that include fluoride usage, regular flossing, and dental cleaning are important.

Hormonal changes include the woman's declining production of estrogen and progesterone. Menopause (female climacteric) is a gradual process that takes about 5 years to complete. A woman's perception of menopause is likely to be affected by her perceptions of her general health. The period of menopausal transition is known as perimenopause. During this process, the functions of the ovaries diminish and eventually cease. Noticeable signs and symptoms of menopause typically include irregular menstrual periods, flow changes, excess fluid retention, breast tenderness, hot flashes (feeling "hot," flushing, and blushing), palpitations, night sweats, and irritability or mood swings. Some women have very few signs or symptoms related to menopause. Some women receive small doses of estrogen aimed at relieving the complications of decreased estrogen levels. Some investigators suggest that hormone replacement therapy (HRT) offers a way to reduce osteoporosis and the risk of atherosclerosis and heart disease; however, HRT is also feared to increase the risk of stroke, endometrial cancer, and breast disease and to raise blood pressure. Therefore the risks and the benefits of this treatment need to be evaluated on an individual basis. The woman is able to continue to experience positive, satisfying sexuality and sexual responses throughout her middle adult years. With any fears of pregnancy now out of the picture, many women enjoy a period of enhanced sexuality.

Possible evidence of the male climacteric includes decreased libido (sex drive), loss of body hair, and delayed erection. Men do not lose the ability to reproduce during the middle adult years. Changes in male sexual function are often more related to psychological than physiologic occurrences. A man's actual capacity to function sexually often has more to do with self-perception and mental outlook and less with the changes he experiences in body appearance, including weight gain, hair loss, and decreased muscle strength. These changes cause some men to go through what is described as a "midlife crisis." Many men are unaffected by the physiologic and psychological occurrences of the climacteric.

Psychosocial Development

According to Erikson, the developmental task of middle age is *generativity* versus *stagnation*, which means accepting responsibility for and offering guidance to the next generation. Generativity encompasses productivity, continuity, and creativity (Fig. 7.23). If this developmental task is not met, people become stagnant—inactive or lifeless. The middle adult years are a time for vocational, interpersonal, and personal fulfillment. The impulse to foster development of the young is not limited to guiding one's own children and does not cease with their maturation. Many middle-aged adults enjoyably express this desire through activities such as teaching and mentorship, a mutually fulfilling relationship that satisfies a younger protégé's need for guidance along with an older person's need for generativity.

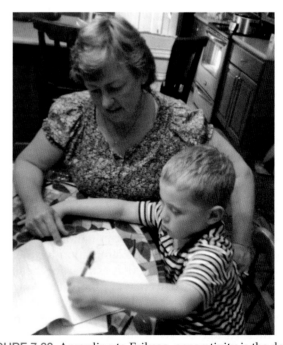

FIGURE 7.23 According to Erikson, generativity is the developmental task of middle adulthood. Nurturing and guiding the younger generation is a task people accomplish with their own children or with other children and adolescents in their family and community. (From Cooper K, Gosnell K: *Foundations of nursing*, ed 7, St. Louis, 2015, Mosby.)

Resumption of education, career growth or changes, reentry into the workforce, and involvement with community activities create a multitude of possibilities for personal growth and satisfaction during the middle adult years.

Family roles change during this stage. Children are sometimes present in the home, and sometimes not. For most caregivers, a significant change in their lives occurs with the end of daily, active responsibility for children. Relationships between spouses change, and the couple often has to regain familiarity with each other. For many, this offers the opportunity for new or renewed companionship. Survival of the marriage after children leave home possibly depends on the growth, the maturity, and the commitment of each partner. Most "empty-nest" women actually look forward to their emancipation from parenting duties, seeing it as an occasion to further develop their personal and social roles.

The role of grandparenting often begins at this developmental stage. Because it often does not have the constraints and responsibilities of childrearing, grandparenting becomes a rich and rewarding experience for many middle-aged adults. The past few decades have probably been the best time ever to be an American grandparent and to enjoy grandparenting as a joyful experience. Grandparents now have the longest, healthiest life spans ever recorded, the best social services, and the most independence. Many still hover just above the poverty line, and some are below it; however, many grandparents are prosperous. Many of today's grandparents have lots of grandchildren to enjoy. Many American grandparents are not involved in the upbringing and disciplining of their grandchildren, preferring a "norm of noninterference." Grandparents often refrain from giving their grown children childrearing instruction, even when they do not like something they see going on with their grandchildren. Most contemporary grandparents value their independence; many are unwilling to exchange their hard-won and long-awaited lifestyles for another round of the hard, often frustrating work of raising children.

On the other hand, most adults are not prepared for the increased responsibility of caring for aging parents. Economic stress and emotional pressure are both associated with the role reversal sometimes known as "parenting the parent." Studies have indicated that a midlife daughter is most likely to be involved in elder care with her parents and her husband's parents.

Health Promotion

Nutrition

Many adults exhibit a slowdown of activities in their middle adult years; therefore they need fewer calories than they did in their teens and twenties. The Centers for Disease Control and Prevention (CDC) reports that 70.7% of Americans aged above 20 years are overweight or obese, which is defined as being 20% over the desirable weight for one's gender, height, and body build (www.cdc.gov, 2013–2014). Inadequate calorie intake, or undernutrition, is also becoming more common. In some cases, this is the result of poverty; however, in many cases, it is a result of self-imposed dieting. A good diet with supplemental vitamins and minerals combined with regular exercise often helps lessen the effects of menopause.

Positive lifestyles with regular exercise are important to maintain healthy joints and bones. Activities that are stress reducing, such as walking, swimming, golf, and tennis, also have the potential to enhance calcium utilization. Premenopausal women need to obtain about 1000 to 1200 mg of dietary calcium per day. The diet also should be rich in phosphorus and magnesium. A diet rich in green leafy vegetables, fresh fruits, whole-grain cereals or breads, and dairy products helps support healthy bones. A reduced intake of fat is recommended; most of it should come from unsaturated fats such as soy, sunflower, corn, or safflower oil. High blood levels of saturated fats and cholesterol contribute to atherosclerosis, coronary heart disease, and cancer.

Physical and Dental Examinations

The person in middle adulthood needs an annual physical examination and biannual dental examinations. Preventive American Cancer Society guidelines (www.cancer.org) should be followed.

Sleep and Rest

The adult in this age group sleeps less and experiences more nighttime awakenings than does the younger adult. In somewhat circular fashion, the subsequent need for additional daytime rest sometimes lessens the number of nighttime hours of sleep necessary.

Late Adulthood: 65 Years and Older

Older adults represent a rapidly growing segment of the population, and we all should prepare for and understand the aging process (Box 7.20). There are many

Box 7.20	Developmental Tasks of Late Adulthood

- Accepts own life
- Recognizes accomplishments
- Finds satisfaction with new roles, relationships, and leisure time
- Maximizes independence and maintains high level of involvement
- Accepts own mortality and prepares for death

approaches to examining the experience of growing old. Aging is a normal condition of human existence and has been studied from sociologic, physiologic, and psychological perspectives. Throughout the life span, all these aspects of the human experience are interrelated. Gerontologists, who study the older adult and the aging process, note that many 70-year-olds today act and think as 50-year-olds did as recently as the 1960s.

The fact remains that everyone ages. The physiologic changes are not universal, however, or even necessarily inevitable, and the changes are often amenable to many interventions and treatments. An individual's adjustment to aging is a uniquely complex process. How an individual responds to the age-related changes visible in the mirror has much to do with the person's self-esteem. Successful aging depends on the individual's capacity to cope and ability to change. The process of aging affects the individual, the family, and society at large.

The sociologically relevant issues of aging have to do with work, retirement, social security, and healthcare. As more and more people reach late adulthood, society must recognize and value these individuals' knowledge, skills, and contributions. Arrangements and plans for the future that are addressed and encouraged in the early adult years help prepare, support, and enhance adjustments once they are necessary. Implementation of flexible services and financial assistance programs helps people fulfill their goals.

The response to getting older is often also related to lifelong health habits, diet, and exercise patterns. Family, love, friendships, and intimate relationships are additional factors important to survival and well-being (Fig. 7.24). These relationships are crucial to people's happiness whatever the age. Love relationships vary in intensity and meaning in adulthood. Early on, these relationships usually have an intense physical basis, which leads to intimacy, respect, and commitment. Although intense sexual drive decreases with age, sexual behavior remains an important part of many adult relationships.

Ageism

Ageism, a form of discrimination and prejudice against the older adult, is an unfortunate reality. Like racism and sexism, ageism works to prevent people from being as happy and productive as they otherwise have the ability to be. It is passed on from generation to generation by the process of socialization. Society today must relinquish old stereotypes about the older adult and learn to affirm the positive aspects of aging. It is a mistake to view aging only as a decline; it involves growth as well. Box 7.21 provides a brief list of true-false statements that helps clarify beliefs on aging.

The number of older people has grown steadily in the past century. According to the U.S. Census Bureau (2012), 38.6 million people, or about 13.3% of the population, are older than 65 years. By 2030, almost 72 million people will be 65 years or older (U.S. Census Bureau, 2012).

Every year another group of adults reaches late adulthood. Late adulthood is defined as age 65 years and older. It can be further subdivided into "young older adult" (age 65 to 74 years), "middle older adult" (age 75 to 84 years), and "old older adult" (older than 85 years). This population is constantly changing as new individuals enter the group and others leave through death. Each person has a unique personal history that reflects many influences. Box 7.22 lists keys to successful aging. The fastest growing segment of the U.S. population is the group aged 85 years and older.

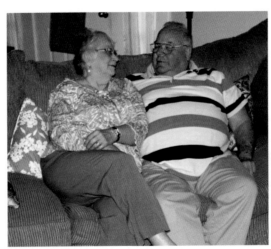

FIGURE 7.24 According to Erikson, generativity versus stagnation is the developmental task of older adulthood. A loving relationship with a spouse is an example of a positive influence during this stage of life. (From Cooper K, Gosnell K: *Foundations of nursing*, ed 7, St. Louis, 2015, Mosby.)

Box 7.21	Your Beliefs on Aging

True or False?

____ 1. All older people become senile.
____ 2. Most older people live in a nursing home or other institutional setting.
____ 3. Most older people are isolated from their families.
____ 4. Most older people have no interest in or capacity for sexual relationships.
____ 5. Older workers are less productive than younger workers.
____ 6. Intelligence declines in old age.
____ 7. Older people do better to cease exercising and just rest.
____ 8. Marked personality changes occur in the older person.
____ 9. Older people naturally become inflexible and demanding.

NOTE: All of these statements are false.

Physical Characteristics

Aging is a complex process that affects cells, tissues, and organs. Like growth and development, aging occurs at a highly individualized rate. A gradual reduction in the number of aging cells and a change in the composition of aging cells occur. A slow increase in body weight usually is seen until 45 to 50 years of age, and then a gradual decline begins. Body fat content and distribution differ in men and women. The accumulation of adipose tissue in females is typically found over the chest, the waist, the hips, and the thighs. Adipose tissue in the male is deposited mostly in the waist, the chest, and the lower abdomen.

Loss of height begins after age 50 years. Most of the noticeable decrease in trunk length is a result of the increase in spinal curvature caused by a slight thinning of the intervertebral disks. In addition to the shortening of the spine, certain abnormal postures and contours are noted. Kyphosis, an exaggeration of the thoracic curvature, may increase with aging. This sometimes leads to a barrel-chest appearance, which possibly affects the position of the diaphragm and reduces the effectiveness of inspiration. These and other postural changes have the potential to affect body posture, mobility, gait, and respiratory efficiency. Common age-related changes specific to each body system are listed in Table 7.10, along with suggested nursing interventions to minimize the effect of these changes.

Box 7.22   Keys to Successful Aging

- Practice pleasurable activities.
- View life as meaningful.
- Maintain a positive self-image.
- Accept responsibility for the past.
- Be optimistic.
- Remain motivated to maintain or expand intellectual capacity.
- Participate in a planned exercise program.

Table 7.10   Common Age-Related Changes

System	Normal Changes	Suggested Nursing Interventions
Musculoskeletal System		
Bones, muscles, joints, and connective tissue	Mineral salts move from bones to blood, making bones more porous; tendons, ligaments less elastic; increase in joint stiffness with less range of motion; varying degrees of increase of flexion at wrists, hips, knees, producing less joint mobility, agility, and endurance; thinning of vertebral disks	Maintain mobility. Encourage exercise (with physician's guidance). Encourage passive and active exercises. Avoid fatigue. Use assistive aids when indicated.
Nervous System		
	Fewer, smaller neurons (nerve cells), slowed reaction time, decrease in tactile sensitivity, decrease in pain perception, altered motor coordination	Allow adequate time to complete activities. Be alert to danger of and prevent burning and chilling related to diminished sensitivity. Encourage position changes; inspect skin daily.
Special Senses		
Taste and smell	Decline in taste and smell perception	Use smoke detectors. Serve attractive, colorful food.
Vision	Decreased tear production, increase in lens density; presbyopia (farsightedness; loss of elasticity of lens); yellowing of lens; slowing of accommodation (reaction to changes in light and distance); narrowing of visual field; decrease in depth perception	Encourage annual eye examinations. Use more diffuse lighting. Use bright colors (red, yellow). Place articles within visual field. Use night lights.
Hearing	Presbycusis (increased difficulty hearing high-pitched sounds); increase in degenerative changes within ear structure; increase in buildup of wax production	Speak slowly, clearly. Face individual. Do not shout. Speak in lower tones. Control background noise. Encourage use of aids if available.
Respiratory System		
Ribcage	Increase in calcification of thorax; respiratory muscles weaken, producing diminished respiratory efficiency; maximum breathing capacity reduced; more susceptible to respiratory infection; easily fatigued	Allow for rest periods. Encourage coughing and deep breathing.
Lungs	Alveoli (air sacs) thinner, smaller, with decreased alveolar surface for gaseous exchange; decreased cough reflex action; decreased ciliary action, reduced maximum breathing capacity	Maintain adequate exercise and nutrition. Encourage regular physical examinations. Avoid overexertion and allow for rest between activities. Discourage smoking. Obtain streptococcal pneumonia (pneumococcal) vaccine.

Continued

Table 7.10	Common Age-Related Changes—cont'd	

System	Normal Changes	Suggested Nursing Interventions
Cardiovascular System		
	Fewer blood cells produced; loss of elasticity and narrowing of blood vessels, with an increase in blood pressure; valves thicker, more rigid; heart needs more time to return to resting state; decreased cardiac output	Encourage regular, paced exercise with adequate rest periods. Maintain low-fat, low-sodium diet. Obtain regular physician examinations.
Integumentary System		
Skin	Paler, thinner, irregularly pigmented; decrease in moisture; decrease in sweat and sebaceous gland activity; less elastic, more wrinkling; loss of subcutaneous fat; skin more fragile and prone to injury	Inspect skin for impairment or signs of pressure. Change position frequently. Wash with water and mild soap as needed. Rinse thoroughly and pat skin dry. Use lotions to replenish moisture. To maintain body warmth, provide adequate clothing.
Reproductive System		
Female	Fallopian tubes atrophy and shorten; ovaries smaller, thinner; uterus, cervix smaller; vagina less elastic, more alkaline, drier; reproductive capacity ceases	Suggest use of vaginal lubricants if indicated. Instruct person to have annual mammogram and vaginal examination with Papanicolaou test.
Male	Increased size of prostate; decreased testosterone levels; decreased circulation, and decreased rate and force of ejaculation	Instruct person to have annual prostate examination and prostate-specific antigen (PSA) test.
Endocrine System		
	Slowing of thyroid gland activity; decreased basal metabolic rate; decreased hormone production that affects other systems	Recommend annual physical examination with thyroid function testing.
Urinary System		
	Fewer cells in kidney, decreased renal blood flow; less effective filtration; decreased bladder elasticity and capacity; need for more frequent voiding	Observe for signs of urinary tract infections. Observe closely for adverse drug reactions. Observe male for signs of benign prostatic hypertrophy causing impairment of urinary flow.
Hair		
	Increase in graying; balding and changes in thickness of hair occur; changes in distribution of body hair	
Nails		
	More fragile, brittle; appear dull, opaque yellow or gray in color; toenails thicken	Have toenails trimmed by podiatrist as indicated.
Gastrointestinal System		
	Decreased saliva production; decreased chewing efficiency; decreased esophageal motility; total capacity of stomach reduced; decreased gastric enzyme secretion; liver smaller; less absorption of nutrients; slowing of peristalsis	Ensure adequate fluid intake. Encourage annual dental checkups. Offer five or six small daily meals, rather than three large ones. Assess for indigestion. Encourage regular toileting habits.

Psychosocial Development

Years of living along with successes, failures, strengths, weaknesses, and all the early experiences influence the emotional stability of older adults. Despite the physiologic changes associated with the aging process, the older years should be viewed as a time of satisfaction and pleasure. Many older adults choose to work after age 65 years. These activities provide interest, intellectual stimulation, and added income (Fig. 7.25). Older people need to recognize their changing capabilities and begin a process of adjustment.

Erikson described the challenge of late adulthood as *ego integrity* versus *a sense of despair*. The task here is to evaluate one's life and accomplishments and find satisfaction and meaning in life. The process of reminiscing with others often serves to further validate the meaning and importance of the individual's life. Those who can believe that their lives have been well spent and are satisfied with their decisions and achievements have mastered this task of integrity. This allows the person to continue life with a sense of dignity and peacefulness. Adults who are dissatisfied with their accomplishments often experience conflict and despair.

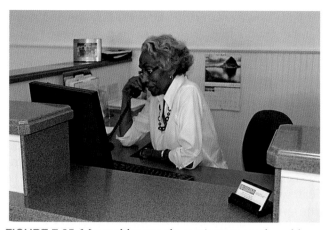

FIGURE 7.25 Many older people continue to work and learn after the traditional retirement age. (From Cooper K, Gosnell K: *Foundations of nursing,* ed 7, St. Louis, 2015, Mosby.)

Dissatisfaction contributes to a feeling of restlessness and a sense of panic that time is "running out." Often the individual feels the need for more time and a chance to do things over again differently.

Many other factors also affect the older adult's adjustment to this stage of life. Retirement is a major adjustment for the older adult. Health and financial resources are critical elements in determination of life satisfaction after retirement. In general, society is relatively unprepared for the phenomenon known as retirement. Retirement creates many changes—some welcome, some not. Examples are changes in roles, self-esteem, support systems, life patterns, and leisure time. Retirement brings more time to spend as one wishes; therefore individuals need to plan and discuss their hopes and expectations for the retirement period. Planning for retirement helps identify activities that will be meaningful and promote self-esteem and a sense of usefulness to both oneself and society.

Family Roles

For many individuals, the older years become a time to explore feelings about parenting and grandparenting. Grandparenting today, as discussed previously, is often very different from the role of grandparenting three or four decades ago. Today's grandparent often works and remains highly active. For some grandparents, caring for grandchildren has become a full-time responsibility that leads to multiple stresses. Raising grandchildren has the potential to create financial stress, cause a decrease in living space, and limit roles. Events that affect children such as divorce, abandonment, unemployment, death or illness, and incarceration are some of the factors that have contributed to the increased numbers of grandparents raising grandchildren on a full-time basis. Support groups, community resources, and other organizations are some of the resources that assist grandparents in their grandparenting roles.

During this stage, couples may need to adjust to increased time together; couples often enjoy the increase in companionship and closeness. Maintaining old friendships and exploring ways to form new ones, along with continuing strong family ties, are means to help soften the losses that are frequently experienced during this period.

The death of a spouse is traumatic at any age. In the older years, it is more common for women to become widows than men. Children and a strong social network often play important roles in supporting the surviving spouse. The experience of being widowed goes beyond ending a partnership. Role changes, changes in lifestyle, and access to fewer financial resources are just some of the adjustments that are called for when a spouse dies. Some older people find remarriage to be a solution to the challenge of being widowed and discover the companionship, love, and security they seek.

Cognitive and Intellectual Development

Evidence suggests that older adults in good health and in nurturing environments have the capacity to maintain or increase their level of functioning, particularly in their areas of interest or specialization. Several factors are important to continued cognitive functioning: level of education, work roles, personality, health, lifestyle, and the relevancy or associated meaning of the tasks one is called on to perform. Some "practical" abilities may decline with age, whereas others may remain stable or improve with age.

Memory

Some older adults notice changes in memory. Such benign forgetfulness is far more common than the forgetfulness associated with Alzheimer's disease. As adults advance in years, there appears to be a greater loss of recent memory over remote memory. An older individual perhaps forgets what was served for breakfast 2 hours earlier and yet may remember in great detail the events of a wedding many decades ago. Older people are slower than younger people but often are more accurate in what they remember and do. Many people believe that this is deliberate: the older person is more willing to sacrifice speed for accuracy.

Health Promotion

Health promotion rests on the belief that individuals are able to have a strong influence on their health status. Environment, social patterns, diet, exercise, and personal habits are all factors that determine a person's state of health. Healthcare workers must clarify the common misconceptions about health and aging. It is essential to emphasize that people of all ages can benefit from living a healthy lifestyle, even in their later years.

Advise older adults to receive both pneumococcal and influenza vaccines yearly. Individuals who have compromised immune systems, who have a history of an allergy to eggs or egg products, or who have had a severe reaction to a previous vaccine should check with their physician before immunization.

Nutrition

Adequate nutrition plays a significant role in health maintenance and contributes to the older person's quality of life. Activities related to food and diet include transportation for food purchase, meal planning, and meal preparation. The task of providing older individuals with assistance for these activities often falls on family members. Older adults need a diet of foods of higher quality and lower quantity that provide the basic necessary nutrients. Although caloric needs are highly individualized, older adults are in general less active and have more adipose tissue and less body mass and therefore often need less daily caloric intake. Diets that are low in saturated fats and carbohydrates and high in fiber are usually recommended. Common concerns related to the adequacy of the older adult's diet are poor oral health, lack of appetite, food intolerances, and constipation. Proper nutritional assessment and counseling help identify problems and useful interventions. To ensure dietary compliance, take long-standing habits and cultural influences into consideration when introducing any dietary changes.

Various psychosocial factors also have the potential to affect the older person's diet. The choice of foods purchased and included in the diet sometimes comes down to economic factors. Loneliness also contributes to inadequate dietary intake for some people. If people are not able to shop for and prepare meals, their diets are likely to become less than desirable. Another crucial component in the older person's diet is adequate fluid intake. Advise older adults to maintain a minimum daily intake of 1500 ml/day. Often, an older person avoids fluids out of a fear of incontinence and a lack of thirst.

Activity

Throughout the life span, evenly paced, satisfying exercise is crucial to general well-being. Exercise has benefits for cardiovascular functioning, lowering blood pressure while enhancing oxygen utilization and maintaining joint mobility. Exercise to the point of exhaustion is misguided; always recommend a rest period after exercise to recuperate and restore the body to its maximum level of functioning.

Sleep

Older individuals need more rest but less actual sleep. The incidence of accidents that occur during nighttime awakenings is increased, and safety concerns must be dealt with. Use of nightlights and reduced excess furniture and clutter are some methods of decreasing the risk of nighttime injury. Sleep for the older person is often affected by medications, alcohol, caffeine, stress, and environmental noise and temperature.

Safety

Most accidents are preventable (see Injury & Illness Prevention Box 7.11). The key to prevention is knowledge and recognition of and attention to the factors that contribute to the increased risk for accident or injury. Diminished sight and changes in posture or balance sometimes expose the older person to the risk of falls. A single fall has the potential to produce an injury that necessitates a long period of immobilization, thus diminishing the person's independence and self-esteem.

Injury & Illness Prevention Box 7.11

Safety Alert: Safety Tips for the Older Adult

- Minimize clutter and excess furniture in rooms and hallways.
- Remove scatter rugs.
- Use handrails on stairs.
- Install grab bars in showers and bathrooms.
- Use nightlights.
- Get up slowly from a lying-flat position.
- Use caution in going from well-lighted areas to darkened areas or vice versa.
- If self-medicating, use dispensing aids to decrease the risk of error.
- Wear properly fitting shoes and clothing.
- Allow enough time; do not rush or hurry.

CHAPTER SUMMARY

Anatomy is the study, classification, and description of structures and organs of the body. Physiology explains the function of the various structures and how they interrelate. The normal anatomical position of the body is standing up with the face and palms of the hands forward. To study the body, you can divide the body into three imaginary planes: sagittal, coronal (frontal), and transverse. Organization is a fundamental characteristic of body structure. Cells are considered to be the smallest living units of structure and function in the body. They are extremely complex. The body is made up of four main types of tissues: epithelial, connective, muscle, and nervous tissue. The major systems of the body are integumentary, skeletal, muscular, nervous, endocrine, cardiovascular (circulatory), lymphatic, respiratory, digestive, urinary, and reproductive.

Development is a lifelong process that begins at conception and ends at death. All types of families serve similar basic functions: protection, nurturance, education, sustenance, and socialization of their members. Growth patterns suggest rapid growth during infancy, continued growth during toddler and preschool years, and slowed but steady growth during the school years, followed by a rapid surge of growth during puberty and adolescence. Erikson identified a central task that needs to be resolved at each stage of the life span: infancy, toddler, preschool, school age, adolescence, early adulthood, middle adulthood, and late adulthood.

Accidental injuries are a major cause of death during infancy, childhood, and adolescence. Consistent discipline and supervision are needed throughout childhood.

Peer relationships become significant at school age. Adolescence is the transitional period between childhood and adulthood. Adulthood is marked by significant events: career decisions, marriage, new social relationships, and financial concerns. Certain physical changes become evident during middle age, including graying of hair and vision changes.

Menopause and hormonal changes characterize the reproductive changes of the middle-aged female.

Roles undergo change during middle adulthood, including nuclear family roles, relationships with grown children, grandparenting, and possibly career changes. Late adulthood is marked by a gradual slowing of the body's functioning. Several significant physical changes become evident in the older adult. Family changes and an increased awareness of one's mortality are common adjustments called for by the aging process.

Life review and acceptance of one's strengths and weaknesses are necessary aspects of the aging process. Aging, like growth, is a highly individualized process.

Case Scenario

As the patient care technician working in a pediatric office, you are asked to obtain the height and weight of a 2-year-old who is being seen for a regular health visit. The child appears to have a pot belly and a large head. The mother verbalizes concern to you that something is wrong with her child. How should you respond? Should you explain to her why the child has a large head and round belly? Why or why not?

REVIEW QUESTIONS

1. The trachea, the heart, the blood vessels, and the lungs are located in which body cavity?
   a. Dorsal
   b. Abdominopelvic
   c. Ventral
   d. Pelvic

2. The student nurse correctly identifies _____ as when a person's body is maintaining a balanced state within its internal environment.
   a. Homeostasis
   b. Mitosis
   c. Lysosomes
   d. Protein synthesis

3. What process has occurred when the patient inhales oxygen and it passes through the lungs and into the bloodstream (area of higher concentration to an area of lower concentration)?
   a. Phagocytosis
   b. Pinocytosis
   c. Osmosis
   d. Diffusion

4. What type of tissue is composed of cells that contract in response to a message from the brain or spinal cord?
   a. Epithelial
   b. Connective
   c. Membrane
   d. Muscle

5. The student nurse demonstrates knowledge of basic human anatomy and physiology with which statement?
   a. "Mucous membranes line many organs, open to the outside environment, and are part of the body's defense mechanism against invasion of microorganisms."
   b. "Serous membranes line many organs, open to the outside environment, and are part of the body's defense mechanism against invasion of microorganisms."
   c. "Striated smooth muscle lines many organs, open to the outside environment, and are part of the body's defense mechanism against invasion of microorganisms."
   d. "Visceral, involuntary smooth muscle lines many organs, open to the outside environment, and are part of the body's defense mechanism against invasion of microorganisms."

6. When the body recognizes a foreign body invasion and responds by engulfing or surrounding the foreign material and digesting it, the nurse is accurate in identifying this process as what?
   a. Mitosis
   b. Pinocytosis
   c. Phagocytosis
   d. Filtration

7. When a group of several different kinds of tissues is arranged to perform a special function, the patient care technician correctly uses which term to describe it?
   a. Cell
   b. Organ
   c. Tissue
   d. System

8. What are the two major cavities of the body?
   a. Thoracic and abdominal
   b. Abdominal and pelvic
   c. Dorsal and ventral
   d. Anterior and posterior

9. What structure divides the thoracic cavity from the abdominal cavity?
   a. Mediastinum
   b. Diaphragm
   c. Lungs
   d. Stomach

10. The patient care technician is aware that the first socializing agent for the child is
    a. daycare.
    b. family.
    c. school.
    d. play groups.

11. A 4-year-old child is working on which of Erikson's developmental tasks?
    a. Trust versus mistrust
    b. Industry versus inferiority
    c. Autonomy versus shame and doubt
    d. Initiative versus guilt

12. Which statement most accurately describes growth during the school-age period?
    a. Growth occurs at a rate similar to that during infancy.
    b. Growth is slow and consistent.
    c. Growth is mainly in the body's upper region.
    d. Growth is more rapid than during the preschool period.

13. An 8-year-old loves to draw and do craft projects. Her need for praise and encouragement for her work efforts demonstrates her development of which of Erikson's tasks?
    a. Autonomy
    b. Initiative
    c. Industry
    d. Identity

14. Peak physical strength and endurance occurs during which period of life?
    a. Adolescence
    b. Early adulthood
    c. Middle adulthood
    d. Late adulthood

15. What term accurately describes the principle that growth begins at the head and moves toward the lower extremities?
    a. Integrated
    b. Proximodistal
    c. Cephalocaudal
    d. Differential

16. To counteract the effect of aging, _____ helps to increase the flow of _____.
    a. Rest; blood
    b. Sleeping; oxygen
    c. Exercise; oxygen
    d. Carbohydrates; oxygen

Pain Management, Comfort, Rest, and Sleep

LEARNING OBJECTIVES

1. List 10 possible causes of discomfort.
2. Discuss McCaffery and Pasero's description of pain.
3. Identify subjective and objective data in pain assessment.
4. Discuss the concept of pain assessment as the fifth vital sign.
5. Discuss the synergistic impact of fatigue, sleep disturbance, and depression on the perception of pain.
6. Identify pain scales used to identify intensity of pain.
7. List several methods for pain control.
8. Discuss the differences and similarities between sleep and rest.
9. Discuss the sleep cycle, differentiating between non–rapid eye movement and rapid eye movement sleep.
10. List six signs and symptoms of sleep deprivation.

KEY TERMS

acute pain Pain that is intense and of short duration, usually lasting less than 6 months

chronic pain Pain lasting longer than 6 months

non–rapid eye movement Phase of sleep necessary for body tissue restoration and healthy cardiac function

noxious Injurious to physical health

patient-controlled analgesia A portable, computerized pump with a chamber for a syringe that allows patients to self-administer medication when they feel that they need it

rapid eye movement Phase of sleep that is believed to be functionally important, more vivid, and elaborate, allowing a person to clarify emotions and prepare the mind for events of the next day.

referred pain Pain that is felt at a site other than the injured or diseased organ or part of the body

synergistic A relationship in which the actions of two or more substances or organs achieve an effect that cannot be achieved by an individual substance or organ

transcutaneous electric nerve stimulation A pocket-sized, battery-operated device that provides a continuous, mild electric current to the skin via electrodes that are attached to a stimulator by flexible wires

visual analog scale A pain scale used when the patient marks a spot on a horizontal line to indicate pain intensity (intensity increases as the line moves from left to right).

To comfort means to give strength and hope, to cheer, and to ease the grief, pain, or trouble of another. Promoting physical and psychological comfort is a vital aspect of nursing care. Many healthcare providers refer to pain as the fifth vital sign and recommend its assessment and management in much the same manner the traditional vital signs are regarded. Although the patient care technician does not administer any types of pain medication, they may assist the patient with alternative methods to manage their comfort, and should therefore have an understanding of what it means to have discomfort.

Many factors contribute to a patient's lack of comfort, which manifests in many forms, including the following:

- Anxiety
- Constipation
- Constricting edema (swelling that is very tight)
- Depression
- Diaphoresis (excess sweating)
- Diarrhea
- Distention (bloating)
- Dry mouth
- Dyspnea
- Fatigue
- Fear
- Flatus (gas)
- Grief
- Headache
- Hopelessness
- Hyperthermia
- Hypothermia
- Hypoxia (decreased oxygen to the tissues)
- Incontinence
- Muscle cramping
- Nausea
- Pain
- Powerlessness
- Pruritus (itching)
- Sadness
- Thirst
- Urinary retention
- Vomiting

It is important to explore the patient's concept of what gives them comfort. By actively listening to the patient, the nurse is better prepared to plan nursing interventions and delegate certain appropriate interventions to the patient care technician. Knowing the possible elements of patient discomfort allows for recognition of discomfort signals even when the patient is not able to verbalize, as in the case of a patient who is aphasic (unable to speak) or one who is semicomatose. The nurse should be diligent in efforts and pursue all the methods to relieve patients' discomfort. If interventions are not successful, the nurse will seek out and apply alternative interventions. As the patient care technician, you may responsible for assisting with these alternative interventions. An example would be the application of hot and cold therapy.

PAIN

Nature of Pain

Pain is a complex, abstract, personal subjective experience. It is an unpleasant sensation caused by noxious (injurious to physical health) stimulation of the sensory nerve endings. It serves as a warning to the body inasmuch as it often occurs where there is actual or potential tissue damage. Pain is often a cardinal symptom of inflammation and is important to aid in the diagnosis of many disorders and conditions. Pain is also possible when there is no tissue damage, such as the emotional pain of grief at the death of a loved one or the pain of migraine headaches. Pain causes fatigue and decreases the patient's ability to cope physically, emotionally, and mentally. Pain has the potential to be totally debilitating and is one of the most common reasons that patients seek out a healthcare provider.

Pain is subjective, which means it is what the patient says it is. The interpretation and significance of pain depends on an individual's learned experiences and involves psychosocial and cultural factors. The defining characteristic of pain is the verbal or nonverbal communication by the patient of the presence of pain (Box 8.1). McCaffery and Pasero's (2003) description of

Box 8.1	Behavioral Characteristics of Patients in Pain

The patient with pain exhibits the following behaviors:
- Is self-protective; guards (places hands over) the painful area
- Has narrowed focus; cannot think of anything but the pain; has reduced attention span
- May withdraw from social contact; may avoid conversation or social contacts
- Has impaired thought processes
- Demonstrates distraction behavior, which includes moaning, rocking, crying, pacing, restlessness, or seeking out different activities or possibly other people
- Presents facial mask of pain; eyes appear dull or lusterless, fixed or rapidly changing facial movements, grimacing, teeth clenching, lip biting, or jaw tightening
- Experiences alterations in muscle tone, ranging from flaccidity to rigidity
- Exhibits diaphoresis, changes in blood pressure and pulse rate, pupillary dilation, and increased or decreased rate of respiration
- Sometimes demonstrates no outward expression of pain. Remember that lack of pain expression does not mean lack of pain. There is no specific "picture" of a patient in pain.

pain is a practical one: "Pain is whatever the experiencing person says it is, existing whenever he says it does." According to McCaffery and Pasero's description, the healthcare provider should believe every patient who says he or she has pain.

Only the person with pain, and not the healthcare provider, is the expert about that pain: its onset, duration, location, intensity, quality, and pattern, as well as the degree of pain relief obtained from therapy. Many patients do not recognize that healthcare providers are not able to tell how much pain the patients are experiencing. Individuals experiencing pain may not know how to best report their pain and its defining characteristics. Assist the patient to recognize his or her experience with the pain and to use that experience in partnership with healthcare providers to obtain better pain management. Empowering the patient to be an active partner in reporting information about the pain is an important skill.

Definitions of Pain

The most widely accepted definition of pain, adopted by the International Association for the Study of Pain and the American Pain Society, is as follows: "Pain is an unpleasant sensory and emotional experience associated with actual or potential tissue damage, or described in terms of such damage" (McCaffery and Pasero, 2003). According to this definition, pain is a phenomenon with multiple components that makes an impact on a person's psychosocial and physical functioning. A person's pain experience can be very complex. Pain is not determined by tissue damage alone. In fact, no predictable relationship exists between identifiable tissue injury and the sensation of pain. The patient's description of pain may not make sense when you try to compare it to the actual injury the patient has. It does not mean the patient is not in pain, or is in less pain than he or she verbally states. In times of high stress and trauma, patients sometimes describe pain as less severe than expected. The inability to identify tissue damage sufficient to explain the pain is not proof that the pain is of psychological origin. Regardless of age, patients typically receive comfort and a sense of well-being from gentle touch and eye contact (Fig. 8.1).

Types of Pain

There are many types of pain: mild and severe; chronic and acute; intermittent and intractable (constant); burning, dull, and sharp; precisely and poorly localized; and referred. Referred pain is felt at a site other than the injured or diseased organ or part of the body. An example of referred pain is the pain of a heart attack that in some cases is felt in the left shoulder, the left arm, or the jaw.

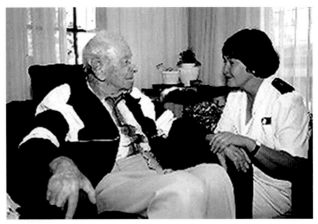

FIGURE 8.1 Eye contact and gentle touch promote comfort and well-being. (From Leahy JM, Kizilay PE: *Foundations of nursing practice: a nursing process approach*, Philadelphia, 1998, Saunders.)

Acute pain is intense and of short duration, usually lasting less than 6 months. In general, acute pain provides a warning to the individual of actual or potential tissue damage. It creates an autonomic response that originates within the sympathetic nervous system, flooding the body with epinephrine and commonly referred to as the *fight-or-flight response.* Anxiety is usually associated with the pain. Because the pain is of short duration, healthcare providers are likely to prescribe opioids and other analgesics.

Chronic pain is generally characterized as pain lasting longer than 6 months. Sometimes the pain is continuous and sometimes it is intermittent; at times, it may be as intense as acute pain. Chronic pain does not serve as a warning of tissue damage in process; rather, it signals that such damage has occurred. In rheumatoid arthritis, for example, joint pain often continues when the disease process is no longer active because of the structural damage that has already occurred in the joint. The reason for some forms of chronic pain sometimes remains unknown. Because of the prolonged time involved in chronic pain, many patients develop chronic low self-esteem, change in social identity, changes in role and social interaction, fatigue, sleep disturbance, and depression.

It is possible that fatigue, sleep disturbance, and depression act in a type of synergistic relationship in which the actions of two or more substances or organs achieve an effect that cannot be achieved by an individual substance or organ. The combination of fatigue, sleep disturbance, and depression has the potential to significantly change a person's perception of pain. Depression is associated with sleep disturbance, which in turn increases the intensity of the fatigue. As the pain continues unmanaged and unchecked, the patient becomes less aware of other events and begins to focus solely on his or her own body and mind. As the focus narrows more and more, it entraps the individual in a vicious cycle, making the pain difficult to treat. Pain-related disability, such as inability to perform activities of daily living, contributes to low self-esteem and social problems. Depression is common in patients with chronic pain. Results of a study conducted by researchers at the University of Michigan, Ann Arbor, suggested a connection between pain and an increased risk for suicide: Pain types linked most heavily to suicide were psychogenic, back, and migraine (Lowry, 2013).

Because of the general differences between acute and chronic pain, some aspects of nursing interventions for these conditions often differ. Keep in mind that the patient's perception of pain, whether acute or chronic, is real, and use appropriate measures to relieve that pain, as delegated to you by the nurse.

Controlling Pain

Requirements of the Joint Commission for Pain Control

Assessing and managing pain has long been a major nursing responsibility. In the 1992 standards manual issued by The Joint Commission (TJC) (McCaffery and Pasero, 2003), effective pain management is considered as one of the rights of a dying patient. In 1994, TJC broadened this statement to cover all patients, stating, "The management of pain is appropriate for all patients, not just dying patients" (McCaffery and Pasero, 2003). Joint Commission accreditation visits began to include a focus on what institutions were doing about pain management.

In 1997, under a grant from the Robert Wood Johnson Foundation, TJC began working collaboratively with institutions to create standards for pain assessment and treatment, with plans to conduct national quality improvement programs to help healthcare facilities meet these standards (McCaffery and Pasero, 2003). TJC now requires accredited facilities and organizations to develop policies and procedures that formalize this obligation (TJC, 2013).

The Joint Commission Standards

Under the new TJC standards, healthcare providers are expected to be knowledgeable about pain assessment and management, and facilities are expected to develop policies and procedures supporting the appropriate use of analgesics and other pain control therapies. Here are some key concepts (Acello, 2000):

- Patients have the right to appropriate assessment.
- Patients will be treated for pain or referred for treatment.
- Pain is to be assessed and regularly reassessed.
- Patients will be taught the importance of effective pain management.
- Patients will be taught that pain management is part of treatment.
- Patients will be involved in making care decisions.
- Routine and as-needed (PRN) analgesics are to be administered as ordered.
- Discharge planning and teaching will include continuing care that is based on the patient's needs at the time of discharge, including the need for pain management.

Making Pain the Fifth Vital Sign

One simple strategy to increase accountability for pain control is for an institution to make pain intensity ratings a routine part of assessment and documentation of vital signs. This suggestion was made by the American Pain Society (1995) and has been implemented in many hospitals, often simply by including pain on the vital sign record (McCaffery and Pasero, 2003). This makes any presence of pain known and raises awareness of the problem of unmanaged pain. Thanks to the work of pain and palliative care associations, more attention is being paid to pain management, and many institutions have included pain assessment as a vital sign.

When pain is assessed with the same zeal as are other vital signs, there is a much better chance of its being treated properly. Vital signs are monitored to detect changes or trends that signal a need for further assessment, diagnosis, and treatment. Considering pain a vital sign—along with pulse, temperature, blood pressure, and respiration—will ensure that it is monitored regularly. Use of a pain rating scale allows patients to clearly articulate their pain and makes them more likely to receive proper treatment.

Unrelieved pain has harmful physical effects, such as increased oxygen demand, respiratory dysfunction, decreased gastrointestinal motility, confusion, and depressed immune response. Possible emotional consequences of unrelieved pain include anxiety, depression, irritability, and an inability to enjoy life. Neglected pain erodes a patient's trust in the healthcare system and possibly leads to setbacks and increased costs in treatment. Conversely, appropriate pain management typically brings about quicker recoveries, shorter hospital stays, fewer readmissions, and improved quality of life (Mayer et al., 2001). It is important that the patient care technician communicate to the nurse if a patient reports that he or she is experiencing pain. You would not want to wait to report this information until rounding is completed. A delay in responding to someone's pain could mean a delay in them achieving any sort of pain relief.

Noninvasive Pain Relief Techniques

Pain is most effectively controlled through a combination of noninvasive pain relief measures and pharmacologic, or drug therapy. The purpose of noninvasive pain

Table 8.1	Nonpharmacologic Interventions for Pain

Interventions	Comments
Physical	
Progressive muscle relaxation	Reduces mild to moderate pain. Requires 3 to 5 min of staff time for instruction.
Massage	Effective for reduction of mild to moderate discomfort. May be firm, gentle, or light stroking of the body part involved or the opposite extremity. Requires 3 to 10 min of staff time.
Transcutaneous electric nerve stimulation (TENS)	Effective in reducing mild to moderate pain by stimulating the skin with mild electric current. Electrodes are placed over or near the site of pain. Requires special equipment. Requires an order by the healthcare provider.
Heat or cold application	Selection of heat vs. cold varies with the situation. Moist heat relieves stiffness of arthritis and relaxes muscles. Cold applications reduce acute pain associated with inflammation from arthritis or from acute injury. Requires an order by the healthcare provider.
Psychological and Cognitive	
Music	Simple relaxation. Best taught preoperatively. Both patient-preferred and "easy-listening" music are effective for mild to moderate pain.
Biofeedback	Reduces mild to moderate pain and operative-site muscle tension. Requires patient to have high level of cognitive function. Requires skilled personnel and special equipment.
Imagery	Reduces mild to moderate pain. Requires skilled personnel.
Education	Effective for reduction of all types of pain. Should include sensory and procedural information and instruction aimed at reducing activity-related pain. Requires 5 to 15 min of staff time.

Nonpharmacologic interventions for pain should be used with analgesic medication. *(From Elkin MK, Perry AG, Potter PA: Nursing interventions and clinical skills, ed 4, St. Louis, 2007, Mosby.)*

relief techniques, which are sometimes of help even when used alone, is to decrease the patient's perception of pain, as well as improve the patient's sense of control. Useful noninvasive approaches include cutaneous stimulation (heat, cold, massage, and transcutaneous electric nerve stimulation [TENS]), the removal of painful stimuli, distraction, relaxation, guided imagery, meditation, hypnosis, and biofeedback (Table 8.1). In guided imagery, the patient is encouraged to concentrate on an image that helps relieve pain or discomfort. For the best results, help the patient choose a scene that holds especially pleasant memories. Ask the patient where he or she feels the most relaxed, such as at a lake, in a forest, or in a meadow, and then encourage the patient to use sensory memories to make the image as realistic as possible. The patient care technician can assist the patient in achieving relief through nonpharmacologic pain relief measures.

Most nonpharmacologic pain relief measures are inexpensive and easy to perform, have low risk and few side effects, and frequently do not require an order by the healthcare provider. The greatest advantage of these techniques is the patients' ability to have some control over the treatment of their pain. Having options to choose from provides comfort and assurance to the patient. Although not everyone reacts successfully to these pain relief measures, it is worthwhile to attempt any of them before advancing to more invasive techniques.

Transcutaneous Electric Nerve Stimulation

A special pain relief system, transcutaneous electric nerve stimulation (TENS), entails the use of a pocket-sized,

battery-operated device that provides a continuous, mild electric current to the skin via electrodes that are attached to a stimulator by flexible wires. The electric current is adjustable. Like other forms of cutaneous stimulation, TENS is thought to work by stimulating large nerve fibers to "close the gate" in the spinal cord, thus blocking transmission of pain impulses. In addition, TENS is hypothesized to stimulate endorphin production.

TENS is typically used for patients suffering postoperative or chronic pain. It is customary to place the electrodes on or near the painful site. Be alert to the possibility that a TENS unit can interfere with the function of a cardiac pacemaker device. The nurse or patient applies the TENS unit.

Invasive Pain Relief Techniques

Invasive means anything that enters the body. Examples of invasive techniques are nerve blocks, epidural analgesics, neurosurgical procedures, and acupuncture. Certain invasive techniques offer relief for many patients with pain. However, careful patient selection and proper technique are essential because the costs and risks are potentially high.

Preventing and Managing Opioid-Induced Constipation

Opioids are a different type of narcotic that often delay gastric emptying, slow bowel motility, and decrease peristalsis. They also tend to reduce secretions from the colonic mucosa. The result is slow-moving, hard stool that is difficult to pass. At its worst, gastrointestinal dysfunction can result in ileus, fecal impaction, and obstruction. The patient care technician may need to assist with bowel elimination for the patient who is experiencing opioid-induced constipation.

Constipation is the most common side effect of opioids and the only one for which individuals do not develop tolerance. Thus it means that the healthcare team must take a preventive approach ahead of time, conduct regular assessment of bowel elimination, and manage any constipation aggressively. Factors contributing to constipation in patients who take opioids include advanced age, immobility, abdominal disease, and concurrent medications that may also have constipating side effects. Patients prescribed opioid analgesics may also be prescribed a stool softener with a mild peristaltic stimulant.

The healthcare team should instruct the patient in proper diet, fluids, and exercise, and provide for the patient's privacy and convenience. Keep in mind, however, that these aspects of bowel management are important but usually insufficient on their own to prevent opioid-induced constipation. Bulk laxatives, natural roughage, and large amounts of fluid are sometimes unable to be eaten or swallowed and ineffective. In addition, if fluid intake is inadequate, bulk laxatives, such as psyllium (Metamucil), sometimes cause fecal impaction and obstruction. Stool softeners alone are inadequate.

Administration Routes for Analgesics

Patients receive pain medication through routes that are specific for their need. The physician or advanced-practice registered nurse (RN) will make the decision as to which route the analgesic, or pain medication, should be given.

The intravenous (IV) route is best for administration of opioid analgesics after major surgery. The most appropriate opioids for pain relief for rapidly escalating, severe pain include morphine, hydromorphone, and fentanyl. For rapid onset of analgesia to treat pain that is quickly rising in intensity, these drugs are administered via the IV route. Some pain medication is given via patient-controlled analgesia, or PCA. The ability to obtain a dose when it is needed places the patient in control and eliminates the wait for medication to be given.

Intramuscular (IM) administration of opioids is associated with wide fluctuations in absorption, including delayed absorption in postoperative patients; thus it is an ineffective and potentially dangerous method of managing pain. The medication is delivered to the muscle tissue, and then must be absorbed. Furthermore, repeated IM injections are often painful and traumatic, which keeps patients from requesting medications for relief of pain; they also have the potential to cause fibrosis of muscle and soft tissue, as well as sterile abscesses. In general, therefore, the IM route, especially repeated IM administration, should be avoided.

The oral route is often the optimal route, especially for chronic pain treatment, because of its convenience, its flexibility, and the relatively steady blood levels produced. However, the IV route is usually necessary when a quick onset of analgesia is desired or when the patient is unable to take oral medication. When the pain is under control, the regimen may then be changed to oral administration of the analgesic. Oral administration is convenient and inexpensive. Its use is appropriate as soon as the patient can tolerate oral intake and is the mainstay of pain management for ambulatory surgical patients.

Patient-Controlled Analgesia

A drug delivery system called patient-controlled analgesia (PCA) allows patients to self-administer analgesics whenever needed. The PCA device is a portable, computerized pump with a chamber for a syringe (Fig. 8.2). The pump delivers a small, preset dose of IV medication, usually morphine, meperidine, hydromorphone, or fentanyl. To receive a dose, the patient pushes a button on a cord attached to the pump. A timer prevents the system from delivering more than a specified number of doses every hour, to prevent overdose. Each dose may be as low as 1 ml or 1 mg of morphine every 6 to 12 minutes. It has a locked safety system that prevents tampering.

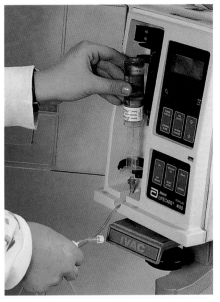

FIGURE 8.2 Patient-controlled analgesia (PCA) pump with syringe chamber. (From Potter PA, Perry AG: *Fundamentals of nursing: concepts, process, and practice,* ed 6, St. Louis, 2005, Mosby.)

PCA is based on the idea that only the patient can feel the pain and only the patient knows how much analgesic will relieve it. By allowing patients to determine the need for doses, PCA addresses the significant variations in analgesic requirements between individuals. The patient care technician does not administer, monitor, or discontinue the PCA because there is always a drug involved, which must be carefully calculated, wasted, and documented by the RN.

When caring for the patient who uses the PCA delivery system, it is the responsibility of the nurse to assess the IV site and the PCA device for proper functioning and correct drug dosing. The nurse may have the patient care technician closely monitor vital signs for signs of respiratory depression. The patient's level of orientation should be evaluated for signs of oversedation. The amount of medication being used is recorded every shift or per agency policy and is documented by the RN.

Pain Interventions

The following measures are performed to assist in pain control and comfort:

- Tighten and straighten wrinkled bed linens.
- Reposition drainage tubes or other objects on which patient is lying.
- Place warm bath blankets if the patient is cold.
- Check tape to prevent pulling on skin.
- Position patient in anatomic alignment.

Pain Rating Scales

Several research studies have focused on the development of tools to specifically assess the patient's pain perception. Pain is a subjective experience, and nurses face difficulty when attempting to measure and evaluate this experience for the patient. Pain rating scales aid with this assessment.

Visual analog scales and numerical scales are commonly used to qualify the intensity of the pain experience (Fig. 8.3). With the **visual analog scale,** the patient marks a spot on a horizontal line to indicate pain intensity (intensity increases as the line moves from left to right). The most frequently used numerical scale is 0 to 10; the patient chooses the pain rating, with 0 being no pain and 10 being the worst pain imaginable. A visual scale with numerical ratings combines both, providing a description and facial expressions with assigned numbers from 0 to 10 (see Fig. 8.3). For clinical assessment, any of these scales is adequate and appropriate. It is important that the same scale always be used with the same patient. All personnel in a given healthcare setting also need to use the same scale.

A good pain scale is easy to use and not time-consuming. If a patient is able to read and understand a scale easily, the description of pain is more accurate. If the patient wears a hearing aid or glasses, be sure that they are worn when the patient is answering pain assessment questions or marking a pain scale. Several pain scales have been developed to assess pain in children. Wong and Baker developed the FACES pain rating scale (Fig. 8.4). Most patients require a pain level of 4 or less to function well.

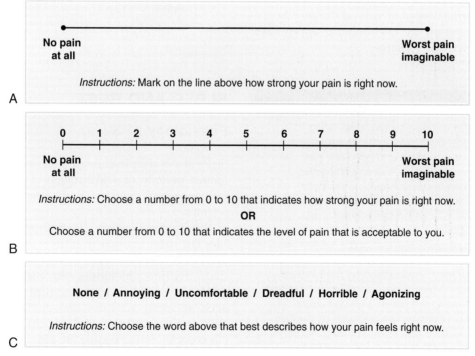

FIGURE 8.3 Sample pain scales. A, Visual analog. B, Numerical. C, Verbal descriptive. (From Potter PA, Perry AG: *Fundamentals of nursing: concepts, process, and practice,* ed 6, St. Louis, 2005, Mosby.)

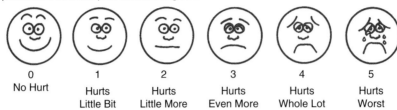

MY PAIN RATING SCALE*

Please keep a record of how well your child's pain medicines are working. Rate your child's pain before and after pain medicine is given.

0	1	2	3	4	5
No Hurt	Hurts Little Bit	Hurts Little More	Hurts Even More	Hurts Whole Lot	Hurts Worst

Explain to your child that each face is for a person who has no hurt (pain) or some or a lot of hurt (pain). Point to each face and say the words under the face. Ask the child to pick the face that best describes how much hurt he (or she) has. Record the number of that face in the Pain Rating column. If your child's pain is above 2, or if you have other concerns with pain, let your nurse or physician know.

Date and time	Pain rating	Medicine I took	Side effects, such as drowsiness or upset stomach

FIGURE 8.4 Wong-Baker FACES pain rating scale. Explain to the patient that each face is for a person who feels happy because he has no pain or sad because he has some or a lot of pain. (Copyright Wong FACES Pain Scale. IN Hockenberry MJ, Wilson D: *Wong's essentials of pediatric nursing*, ed. 8, St. Louis, 2009, Mosby.)

- Check temperature of hot and cold applications, including bath water.
- Lift—do not pull—patient up in bed; handle gently.
- Position patient correctly on bedpan.
- Avoid exposing skin or mucous membranes to irritants (e.g., diarrheal stool or wound drainage).
- Prevent constipation by encouraging appropriate fluid intake, diet, and exercise.

Health Promotions Promoting Comfort

- Measures that promote a sense of well-being to minimize or avoid discomfort include warm baths, thorough personal hygiene, and adequate rest.
- Pain has the potential to disable and immobilize a person enough to impair the ability to perform self-care activities. This results in social isolation, depression, and changes in self-concept. Help patients and families learn to discuss their feelings about the loss of function and to find ways to cope with pain and the lifestyle it imposes.
- When a patient has chronic, disabling pain, instruct family members on proper positioning techniques and methods of assisting the patient with ambulation.
- A number of nonpharmacological or complementary therapies are used for pain relief, including massage, guided imagery, music, biofeedback, meditation, hypnosis, exercise, therapeutic touch, acupuncture, and relaxation techniques.

Delegation and Documentation Box 8.1

- To assess pain is a nursing skill and should not be performed by the patient care technician.
- All medications are administered by the RN or LPN.
- Nonpharmacological or complementary therapies such as giving a backrub and providing for soft music are included within the scope of the patient care technician responsibilities.

SLEEP AND REST

Physiology of Sleep

Sleep is a cyclic physiologic process that alternates with longer periods of wakefulness. The sleep-wake cycle influences and regulates body functions and behavioral responses.

People experience cyclic rhythms as part of everyday life. The most familiar rhythm is the 24-hour day-night cycle known as the *diurnal* or *circadian rhythm*. All circadian rhythms, including the sleep-wake cycle, are affected by light and temperature and external factors such as social activities and environmental stressors. Each individual has a biologic clock that synchronizes sleep cycles. Some people are able to fall asleep at 8 PM, whereas others go to bed at midnight or early in the morning. Different people also function best at different times of the day.

The biologic rhythm of sleep frequently becomes synchronized with other body functions. Normal variations in body temperature, for example, are correlated with sleep patterns. When the sleep-wake cycle is disrupted (e.g., by working rotating shifts), other physiologic functions typically change as well. For example, some affected persons experience decreased appetite and lose weight. Failure to maintain one's usual sleep-wake cycle is likely to adversely affect a person's overall health (Potter and Perry, 2009). It is important as a patient care technician that you support a person's need for sleep each night if possible. Clustering your care is one way to assist with this. Clustering your care means that you complete as many tasks as possible when you enter the person's room, instead of coming in multiple times to complete tasks individually.

Sleep Cycle

Sleep involves two phases: rapid eye movement (REM) and non–rapid eye movement (NREM) (Box 8.2). NREM sleep is further divided into four stages through which a sleeper progresses during a typical sleeping cycle. The sleeping stages are highly individualized, meaning that they can vary from one person to the next (Fig. 8.5).

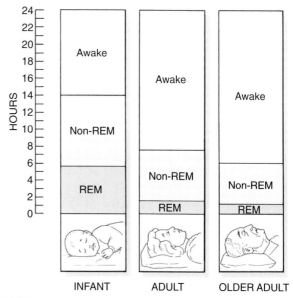

FIGURE 8.5 Sleep-wake cycles across the life span. *Infants:* Approximately 40% of total sleep time is spent in rapid eye movement (REM) sleep. *Adults:* 20% of total sleep time is spent in REM sleep. *Older adults:* Total sleep time is slightly reduced; REM sleep continues to make up 20% of total sleep time. (From Cooper K, Gosnell K: *Foundations of nursing,* ed 7, St. Louis, 2015, Mosby.)

Box 8.2   Stages of Sleep

Non–Rapid Eye Movement (NREM) Sleep
Stage 1
- Lightest level of sleep
- Lasts a few minutes
- Decreased physiologic activity, beginning with a gradual fall in vital signs and metabolism
- Person is easily aroused by sensory stimuli such as noise
- If person awakes, feels as though daydreaming has occurred
- Reduction in autonomic activities (e.g., heart rate)

Stage 2
- Period of sound sleep
- Lasts 10 to 20 minutes
- Relaxation progresses
- Arousal is still easy
- Body functions are still slowing

Stage 3
- Initial stage of deep sleep
- Lasts 15 to 30 minutes
- Arousal is difficult; movement is rare
- Muscles are completely relaxed
- Vital signs decline but remain regular
- Hormonal response includes secretion of growth hormone

Stage 4
- Deepest stage of sleep
- Lasts approximately 15 to 30 minutes
- Arousal is very difficult
- If sleep loss has occurred, sleeper spends most of night in this stage
- Restores and rests the body
- Vital signs are significantly lower than during waking hours
- Sleepwalking and enuresis are possible
- Hormonal response continues

Rapid Eye Movement (REM) Sleep
- Stage of vivid, full-color dreaming consistent with sensory experiences (less vivid dreaming sometimes occurs in other stages)
- First occurs approximately 90 minutes after sleep has begun, thereafter occurs at end of each NREM cycle
- Duration increasing with each cycle and averaging 20 minutes
- Typified by autonomic response of rapidly moving eyes, fluctuating heart and respiratory rates, and increased or fluctuating blood pressure
- Loss of skeletal muscle tone
- Responsible for mental restoration
- Stage in which sleeper is most difficult to arouse

Normally an adult's routine sleep pattern begins with a presleep period during which the person is aware only of a gradually developing drowsiness. This period normally lasts 10 to 30 minutes, but if a person has difficulty falling asleep, it can last an hour or longer.

As adults fall asleep, they progress through the four stages of NREM sleep. At the end of the fourth stage, they come out of a deep sleep, go back to stage 2, and then enter a period of REM sleep. A person reaches REM sleep in about 90 minutes (average). Each person differs, but a typical night's sleep consists of four to six such cycles.

Dreams occur during both the NREM and REM stages. The dream of REM sleep is believed to be functionally important, more vivid, and elaborate, allowing a person to clarify emotions and prepare the mind for events of the next day.

NREM sleep is necessary for body tissue restoration and healthy cardiac function (McCance and Huether, 2009; Potter and Perry, 2009). A person's biologic functions slow during NREM sleep. For example, a healthy adult has a heart rate of 70 to 80 beats per minute during the day; however, during sleep the heart beats at 60 beats per minute or less. Respirations and blood pressure are also decreased during sleep. It is very difficult to arouse the sleeper in REM sleep.

REM sleep is important for brain and cognitive restoration. During REM sleep, there are changes in cerebral blood flow and increases in cortical activity, oxygen consumption, and epinephrine release, which are beneficial to memory storage and learning (McCance and Huether, 2009).

A patient at rest feels mentally relaxed, free from worry, and physically calm. A patient at rest is free from physical or mental exertion. Everyone has his or her own method of obtaining rest and is usually able to adjust to new environments or conditions that affect the ability to rest.

Rest is important in healing the body of both physical and psychological illness. Patients are often prescribed bed rest. This treatment confines patients to bed to decrease physical or psychological demands on the body. Bed rest does not necessarily mean that a patient is resting; it just means that they have to stay in their bed. Emotional or metabolic stressors naturally cause the patient to be restless.

Sleep is a state of rest that occurs for a sustained period. The reduced consciousness during sleep provides time for repair and recovery of body systems for the next period of wakefulness. The theory that sleep is associated with healing suggests that achieving optimal sleep quality is important for patients' recovery. Sleep restores a person's energy and feeling of well-being.

The routines of healthcare facilities easily disrupt the rest and sleep habits of patients (Box 8.3). The extent of the change depends on the seriousness of the illness, as well as the environment in which the patient is placed. Intensive care units tend to be noisier units. It is important to remain aware of the patient's need for rest. Without it, the patient becomes fatigued and irritable and has a decreased ability to cope with stressors.

Box 8.3   Factors Affecting Sleep

Physical Illness
- Pain and physical discomfort result in difficulty falling or staying asleep.
- Chronic pain sometimes has a circadian rhythm, including increasing in intensity at night, thus disrupting sleep.
- Illness frequently forces patients to sleep in positions to which they are unaccustomed.
- Respiratory diseases interfere with the rhythm of breathing and sometimes oblige a person to assume a certain position to be able to breathe easily. Both factors can disturb sleep.
- A patient with heart disease may be afraid to go to sleep at night.
- Hypertension causes early morning awakening and fatigue.
- Nocturia and restless legs syndrome disrupt sleep, causing the patient to awaken and have trouble going back to sleep during the night.
- Conditions that increase intracranial pressure or alter central nervous system physiology alter sleep patterns and sometimes cause excessive daytime sleepiness.

Anxiety and Depression
- As anxiety and depression increase, so does lack of sleep; as amount of sleep decreases, anxiety and depression increase.
- Bereaved people may experience sleep problems related to fear of intruders, loneliness, and the dreams or nightmares that occur involving the lost loved one.

Drugs and Substances
- Various drugs and substances affect the pattern and the quality of sleep.
- Hypnotic medications interfere with reaching deeper sleep stages, provide only a temporary (1-week) increase in quality of sleep, and eventually cause a "hangover" feeling during the day. Hypnotic drugs often worsen sleep apnea in older adults.
- Older adults often take several drugs, the combined effects of which disrupt sleep.
- L-Tryptophan, a protein found in foods such as milk, cheese, and meats, frequently helps induce sleep.

Lifestyle
- Daily routines such as work shifts influence sleep patterns; changing routines, as with rotating shifts,

Box 8.3 Factors Affecting Sleep—cont'd

disrupt these patterns. Only after several weeks of working a night shift does an individual's biologic clock adjust.
- Performing unaccustomed heavy work, late-night social activities, and changing evening mealtimes are activities that can disrupt sleep.

Sleep Patterns
- Sleep patterns include starting time and duration of sleep. The most significant cause of daytime sleepiness is inadequate or abnormal sleep at night.
- Everyone has an increased tendency to feel sleepy from 2 AM to 7 AM.
- When sleep patterns are disrupted, the natural tendency to sleep at certain times increases.
- Sleep patterns influence future attempts to fall asleep because of changes in circadian rhythm. Sleeping 1 hour later results in falling asleep 1 hour later the next night.

Stress
- Stress resulting from personal problems or situational crises causes tension and at times will cause a person to try too hard to fall asleep, to awaken frequently, or to oversleep.
- Stress causes release of corticosteroids and adrenalin, which leads to catabolism and sleeplessness.
- Patients with advanced cancer or chronic illness often are afraid to go to sleep for fear they might die.

- The stress of losses such as retirement or death of a loved one sometimes causes older adults to suffer delays in falling asleep, earlier rapid eye movement (REM) sleep, frequent awakening, increased total bedtime, and feelings of sleeping poorly.

Environment
- Environmental factors influence the ability to fall and remain asleep. Significant factors include ventilation, lighting, type of bed, sound level, and the presence or absence of a bed partner.
- In hospitals, unfamiliar noises and higher noise levels such as that created by wall suction, opening packages, ringing alarms, and flushing toilets can cause sleep deprivation.
- Intensive care units have high noise levels.

Exercise and Fatigue
- Exercise and fatigue in moderation usually facilitate restful sleep, but excess fatigue from exhausting or stressful work typically makes falling asleep difficult.
- Performing exercise 2 hours before bedtime allows the body to cool down and promotes relaxation.

Nutrition
- Weight gain causes longer sleep periods with fewer interruptions and later awakening.
- Weight loss sometimes causes reduction in total time spent asleep along with broken sleep and earlier awakening.

Life Span Considerations for Older Adults Regarding Sleep

- Older adults require about the same amount of sleep as younger people but are more likely to achieve it in separate episodes; they take more daytime naps and get less sleep at night.
- The sleep of an older adult is less deep. This increases the risk of early awakening and complaints of sleep disturbance.
- Sleep is likely to be disturbed in older adults with chronic health problems such as arthritis, heart failure, and chronic obstructive pulmonary disease. Adequate pain control and positioning facilitate breathing and help promote rest and sleep.
- Many older adults take medications such as diuretics and theophylline that are likely to disturb sleep. Diuretics cause a person to have to toilet more often, and theophylline often stimulates someone as caffeine might.
- Insufficient sleep may lead to memory and personality changes in older adults.
- Include nonpharmacologic comfort measures to promote rest and sleep.

Sleep Deprivation

Sleep deprivation is a problem many patients experience as a result of hospitalization. Sleep deprivation involves decreases in the amount, the quality, and the consistency of sleep. When sleep is interrupted or fragmented, changes in the normal sequence of sleep stages occur, and cycles are not completed. Cumulative deprivation gradually develops.

Safety Alert Daytime Sleepiness

- Safety precautions are important for patients and residents who awaken during the night to use the bathroom and for those with excessive daytime sleepiness.
- Set beds lower to the floor to lessen the chance that the patient or resident will fall when first standing.
- Some patients and residents who experience daytime sleepiness fall asleep while sitting up in a chair or wheelchair. Position the person so that he or she will not fall out of the chair while sleeping.

In preparing the patient for sleep, wash the patient's back if the patient is on bed rest, gently massage it, change the linens, make certain the patient is warm enough, offer an uncaffeinated beverage such as milk (if allowed), change soiled dressings, and have the patient void.

Decrease environmental stimuli by dimming the lights and decreasing the noise level. Direct the patient to assume a comfortable position, and assist if needed. A night light is a necessity for promotion of safety for the older adult. The nurse may administer a sleeping medication or analgesic as ordered if the patient cannot sleep.

CHAPTER SUMMARY

McCaffery and Pasero (2003) provided a realistic description of pain: "Pain is whatever the experiencing person says it is, existing whenever he says it does." Remember that pain is largely a subjective experience. Pain could be a protective mechanism that warns of tissue injury. There are pain scales used to objectively evaluate pain intensity and the effectiveness of pain therapies; the numerical pain scale is often used to assess a patient's pain. Considering pain as the fifth vital sign helps ensure that pain is monitored regularly. Fatigue, sleep disturbance, and depression act in a type of synergistic relationship that can markedly change a person's perception of pain.

The circadian rhythm is the 24-hour, day-night cycle known also as the diurnal rhythm. Sleep is important and necessary for the body to achieve tissue restoration. As a patient care technician, your strategies can make a difference in how the patient rests each night. Clustering care is one way the PCT can encourage a good night's rest.

Case Scenario

During the morning activities of daily living, Mr. J states, "I feel so useless. I can't even place the urinal for myself." What would be the patient care technician's most therapeutic response? Should the patient care technician place the urinal for Mr. J or require him to do it? Explain the reason for your answer.

Mr. J has not been able to rest for the past several nights. Which comfort measures could the patient care technician perform to ensure that the patient has several hours of restorative sleep?

Mr. J complains of his eyes burning and feeling dry and the lights annoying him. As a patient care technician, what measures are most likely to help relieve his symptoms?

REVIEW QUESTIONS

1. Acute pain is pain that is not new in onset, and has been going on for at least 6 months.
   a. True
   b. False

2. Which of the following can contribute to the person's discomfort?
   a. Fear
   b. Sleep
   c. Family
   d. Diet

3. Which of the following treatments can the patient care technician assist with in order to provider patient comfort?
   a. Pushing the button on the PCA for the patient
   b. Giving the patient a sleeping pill
   c. Giving the patient a backrub
   d. Placing a Foley catheter in the patient

4. What is one way the patient care technician can assist the person with getting a good night's rest?
   a. Setting the volume on the alarms in the room and hallway on loud so that you will hear them from wherever you are
   b. Leaving the overhead light on in the person's room so that he or she will always be able to see
   c. Breaking up your tasks to complete into several visits to the person's room
   d. Closing the curtains on the window and turning down the lights

5. Which phase of sleep is more important for the body?
   a. REM
   b. NREM
   c. Both are equally important.
   d. Neither are important; not everyone experiences each phase.

Safety

SECTION

3

Asepsis and Infection Control

1. Explain the difference between medical and surgical asepsis.
2. Explain how each element of the chain of infection contributes to infection.
3. List five major classifications of pathogens.
4. Identify the body's normal defenses against infections.
5. Discuss standard precautions.
6. Demonstrate the proper procedure for hand hygiene.
7. Demonstrate technique for gowning and gloving.
8. Identify principles of surgical asepsis.
9. Describe the accepted techniques of preparation for disinfection and sterilization.

KEY TERMS

antiseptic A substance that tends to inhibit the growth and reproduction of microorganisms and may be used on humans

asepsis The absence of pathogenic microorganisms

Centers for Disease Control and Prevention (CDC) An agency which provides facilities and services for investigation, prevention, and control of disease

contamination The entry of infectious materials into a previously clean or sterile environment

disinfection The use of a chemical that can be applied to objects to destroy microorganisms

endogenous Growing within the body

exogenous Growing outside the body

fomite A nonliving object that can harbor microorganisms, such as computers or chairs

healthcare–associated infection (HAI) Infections patients can get while receiving medical treatment in a healthcare facility

host An organism in which another organism is nourished and harbored

infection prevention and control The act of decreasing the spread of healthcare-associated or community-acquired infections to patients and other staff members

medical asepsis Techniques that inhibit the growth and transmission of pathogenic microorganisms

microorganisms Tiny, usually microscopic, entities capable of carrying on living processes

reservoir Any natural habitat of a microorganism that promotes growth and reproduction

spore The reproductive cell of some microorganisms, such as fungi or protozoa

standard precautions A set of guidelines designed to reduce the risk of transmission of microorganisms from both recognized and unrecognized sources of infections

sterilization Methods used to kill all microorganisms, including spores

surgical asepsis Techniques designed to destroy all microorganisms and their spores

vector A person or animal that does not become ill but harbors and spreads an organism, causing disease in others; also known as a carrier

vehicle The means by which microorganisms are carried about and transported to the next host once they have left the reservoir

In today's healthcare environment, all healthcare workers are responsible for doing their part to protect patients from infection. Some patients enter the healthcare system with an infection; others can end up with an infection from being in the healthcare setting. The goal for both the healthcare provider and for patients is to not get an infection while being treated in the healthcare setting. It is also the goal to prevent occupational exposure to infectious material, which helps reduce healthcare delivery costs.

ASEPSIS

The increased incidence of infections, which can be transmitted to others, not only in healthcare facilities but also in the home, is an issue of great concern. Microorganisms (tiny, usually microscopic, entities capable of carrying on living processes) are naturally present on and in the human body and in the environment. Many of these microorganisms are harmless (nonpathogenic) and in most individuals do not produce disease. Some are even helpful. If someone is highly susceptible to infection, the nonpathogenic microorganisms can be dangerous.

Any patient who enters a healthcare facility has a greater risk of an infection developing because of reduced immunologic function and increased chances of coming in contact with microorganisms in the healthcare setting. Increased stressors on the patient's immune system are caused by the presenting illness, exposure to disease-causing microorganisms, and portals of entry (openings) created by invasive procedures. Invasive procedures may include surgical operations or treatments such as skin lesion removal, indwelling catheter insertion, or even a skin preparation. In addition, healthcare facilities are an environment that encourages the spread of these microorganisms because of the many ill carriers seeking treatment. The patient care technician's knowledge related to infection and the application of infection prevention and control principles helps protect patients from infection. With each patient care activity, the patient care technician should ensure that infection prevention and control is part of the routine.

Infection prevention and control consists of following the policies and procedures in hospitals and other healthcare facilities to decrease the spread of healthcare-associated or community-acquired infections to patients and other staff members. During patient care activities, the patient care technician may be exposed to pathogenic microorganisms. The nurse is a chief player in the prevention of the spread of infection, which is accomplished with learning and continued observation of both routine and specialized practices of cleanliness and disinfection. The patient care technician follows the specialized practices under the direction of the nurse when providing any care to patients. These techniques aid in accomplishing asepsis (the absence of pathogenic

microorganisms). Asepsis is divided into the following two categories:

1. Medical asepsis consists of techniques that inhibit the growth and transmission of pathogenic microorganisms. Medical asepsis is also known as *clean technique* and is used in many daily activities, such as hand hygiene and changing of patient bed linens.
2. Surgical asepsis consists of techniques designed to destroy all microorganisms and their spores (the reproductive cell of some microorganisms, such as fungi or protozoa). Surgical asepsis is known as *sterile technique* and is used in specialized areas, such as the operating room, or during invasive procedures, such as urinary catheter insertion.

INFECTION

For an infection to develop, a specific cycle or chain of events must occur. The following six elements are necessary for infection and are referred to as *the chain of infection* (Fig. 9.1):

1. Infectious agent: A pathogen
2. Reservoir: Where the pathogen can grow
3. Portal of exit: Exit route from the reservoir
4. Mode of transmission: Method or vehicle of transportation, such as exudate, feces, air droplets, hands, and needles
5. Portal of entry: Entrance through skin, mucous lining, or mouth
6. Host: Another person or animal that is susceptible to the pathogen

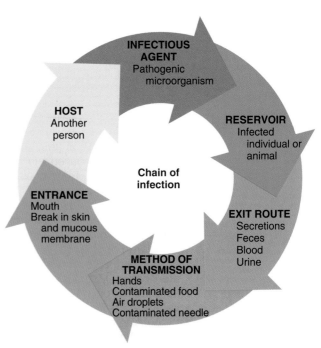

FIGURE 9.1 The chain of infection. (From Cooper K, Gosnell K: *Foundations of nursing*, ed 7, St. Louis, 2015, Mosby.)

To prevent the transmission of an infection, the cycle must be interrupted. Medical asepsis is an effective way to disrupt the chain of infection. This practice helps to inhibit (to stop or slow a process) the growth and reduce the number of microorganisms.

Infectious Agent

Pathogens can be bacteria, viruses, yeasts, fungi, and protozoa. All these microorganisms need nutrients for growth and a suitable environment in which to live. Unwashed hands, wound drainage, soiled linen, and decaying teeth provide ideal areas for pathogenic growth. The microorganism strength, the number of microorganisms present, the effectiveness of a person's immune system, and the length of exposure to the microorganisms determine the ability to produce disease. The role of the patient care technician is to provide a safe environment for the patient by working to prevent the transmission of infection.

Healthcare workers have several ways to help their patients remain free of infection. Proper disinfection (the use of a chemical that can be applied to objects to destroy microorganisms), appropriate use of an antiseptic (a substance that tends to inhibit the growth and reproduction of microorganisms and may be used on humans), proper hand hygiene, and use of surgical asepsis when indicated are all important ways to help reduce the presence of microorganisms.

Bacteria

Bacteria have many different characteristics. In addition to their three basic shapes (round, oblong, and spiral), there are many variations. Some are elongated or have pointed ends, and some are flattened on one side. Some are shaped like commas, and others appear square. Spirilla are often tightly coiled, like a corkscrew. During cell division, some bacteria remain together to form pairs, whereas others form long chains. Diagnostic testing focuses on the unique characteristics for identification of specific types of bacteria.

Bacteria can also be differentiated by their chemical compositions, the nutrients that they need to grow, and the waste products that the bacteria form. *Aerobic* bacteria grow only in the presence of oxygen, whereas *anaerobic* bacteria grow only in the absence of oxygen (Fig. 9.2, *A* and *B*). Some bacteria are capable of movement. This movement is possible because of fine, hair-like projections—flagella—that extend from the bacterial cell. This type of bacteria often resembles a jellyfish. These projections move in a wavelike fashion to propel the cell. Some bacteria have only one flagellum attached to one end of the cell, and others have many flagella surrounding the cell. Locomotion of the spirochete is achieved with a wiggling motion that involves the entire cell body.

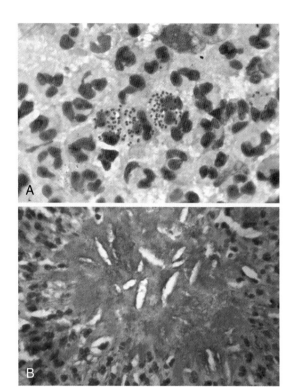

FIGURE 9.2 A, Aerobic bacteria. B, Anaerobic bacteria. (Courtesy the Centers for Disease Control and Prevention. A, Bill Schwartz; B, Dr. Richard L. Levin, Greater Southeast Community Hospital, Washington, D.C.)

Some bacteria form a specialized structure called a spore. The spore is a round body that is formed by the bacterium when conditions are unfavorable for growth of the bacterium. The spore enlarges until it is as large as the bacterial cell and is surrounded by a capsule. Eventually, the portion of the cell that surrounds the spore disintegrates. The spore remains dormant, or asleep, until environmental conditions become favorable for growth. Then, the spore germinates and begins reproducing. Characteristically, spores have a high degree of resistance to heat and disinfectants. Some bacteria have the ability to form capsules around the cell wall, which helps to protect the bacteria. A thick, sticky, slimy substance forms a capsule around the bacteria in order to keep it safe. This formation can make the bacteria particularly difficult to treat with some antibiotics. When capsules are present, antibiotic therapy is sometimes ineffective because the capsule prevents the drug from reaching the bacteria within the capsule.

Antimicrobial therapies provide a system of attack that is individualized to specific microorganisms. Specially trained laboratory personnel perform this identification. In some instances, they examine a specimen before staining it, but this method is usually less satisfactory. Most bacteria are not visible without a special staining process, in which a dye is applied to a specially prepared glass slide that contains a small amount of the material to be examined. Identification of most bacteria is possible with this simple process; however, other bacteria necessitate additional staining.

Depending on whether a color can be removed with a solvent or the color is retained after the use of the solvent, the organism is identified as *gram positive* or *gram negative*. Special staining techniques are required for bacteria that have flagella, spores, or capsules.

The patient care technician may collect specimens of body fluids and secretions suspected of containing pathogenic organisms in sterile containers and send them to the laboratory for culture and sensitivity testing. Laboratory personnel transfer the specimen to a special culture medium that promotes growth. They then study the culture and identify the pathogens. The results of the sensitivity tests assist the practitioner in determining which antimicrobial (antibiotic) medication will effectively stop the pathogens' growth. The practitioner then orders appropriate antimicrobial agents on the basis of these tests, which typically take 48 to 72 hours to complete. Different organisms require different antibiotics to be effectively destroyed.

Bacterial infections are transmitted from person to person by direct contact, by inhalation, and by indirect contact with articles contaminated with the pathogen. Some are also transmitted through the ingestion of contaminated food and drink (Fig. 9.3).

The *Streptococcus* bacterium is responsible for more diseases than any other organism, but methicillin-resistant *Staphylococcus aureus* (MRSA) has been found to be responsible for a number of serious and sometimes fatal infections. Patients with immunocompromised conditions who are admitted to healthcare facilities have an increased risk of exposure to strains of MRSA that are multidrug resistant and therefore more difficult to treat. Examples of immunocompromised conditions

include those who are undergoing treatment for cancer such as chemotherapy.

Rocky Mountain spotted fever has been found in almost every area of the United States, and its prevalence continues to increase (www.cdc.gov). It is transmitted to humans through the bite of an infected tick. Several varieties of ticks carry the disease. The ticks live on many different kinds of animals found in rural and wooded areas. They are also able to live on common house pets, such as cats and dogs. People who work in areas where ticks are known to be abundant are more likely to become infected. The tick attaches itself to the skin, and the longer it remains attached, the more likely the person is to become infected. Great care must be taken not to crush or squeeze the tick on removal from the skin.

Viruses

Viruses are the smallest known agents to cause disease. They are not complete cells. Before 1900, scientists discovered that certain agents, unlike bacteria, have the ability to pass through a laboratory filter. In addition, they were unable to observe these tiny bodies with the ordinary microscope. In 1898, Martinus W. Beijerinck called these small organisms *viruses*, and they became known as filterable viruses.

Viruses gain entrance to the body through various portals such as the respiratory tract, the gastrointestinal tract, and broken skin. Sometimes a virus can infect a susceptible host through a mosquito bite or during an accidental needle stick with a contaminated needle. Viruses are selective in the type of body cells they attack, but once they have found cells for which they have an affinity, they enter the cell and reproduce rapidly. As they multiply, they interrupt the cell activities and use the cell material to produce new virus material.

Viral infections are usually self-limiting, meaning that they run their course and then recovery occurs. One exception is acquired immunodeficiency syndrome (AIDS). Without adequate treatment with specific types of medication, the human immunodeficiency virus (HIV) reproduces and the immune system continues to be stressed to the point where it can no longer fight off even the most common infection; the patient then receives the diagnosis of AIDS.

Other viral diseases have the capacity to cause death if complications occur or if they attack individuals with extremely weak or debilitated conditions. People who are at either end of the age spectrum are also at increased risk for complications.

The common cold is caused by a virus. Symptoms of the common cold are usually relieved with the patient staying in bed and taking certain over-the-counter remedies. No medicine cures the cold; medicine only relieves the discomfort. Antibiotics do not alter the course of the vast majority of viral diseases.

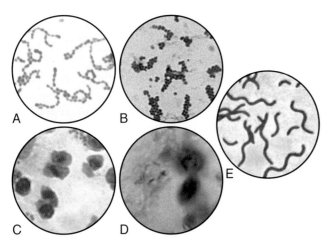

FIGURE 9.3 Some common disease-producing bacteria. **A,** Streptococci. **B,** Staphylococci. **C,** Diplococci. **D,** Bacilli. **E,** Spirilla. (Courtesy the Centers for Disease Control and Prevention. **A,** Dr. Gilda Jones; **B,** Dr. Richard Facklam; **C,** Dr. Norman Jacobs; **D,** Dr. Roger Feldman.)

Viruses are classified in various ways, either according to the diseases they cause or by the characteristics of a specific group. In the latter classification system, each subgroup often has many types or strains (Table 9.1).

Fungi

Fungal (mycotic) infections are among the most common diseases found in humans. Fungi are among the most plentiful forms of life. They belong to the plant kingdom, and although many of them are harmless, some are responsible for infections. Fungus types that many people are familiar with include the fuzzy black, green, or white growth on stale bread. Mycotic infections are diseases caused by yeasts and molds. Some are superficial and involve the skin and the mucous membranes. Most frequently, the infections involve the external layers of the skin, the hair, and the nails.

Protozoa

The protozoa are single-celled animals; in some form, they exist everywhere in nature. Some of the parasitic forms of protozoa are found in the intestinal tract, the genitourinary tract, the respiratory tract, and the circulatory system of humans and other animals. Protozoa are responsible for malaria, amebic dysentery, and African sleeping sickness (see Table 9.1).

Reservoir

To thrive, organisms need a proper atmosphere. Characteristics of an environment that supports organism growth include an available nutrient source, oxygen, water, light, and desirable temperatures and levels of acidity or alkalinity. Any natural habitat of a

Table 9.1	Common Pathogens, Reservoirs, and Infections or Diseases	
Organism	**Primary Reservoir**	**Infection or Disease**
Bacteria		
Staphylococcus aureus	Skin, hair, anterior nares	Wound infection, pneumonia, food poisoning
β-Hemolytic group A streptococci	Oropharynx, skin, perineal care	Strep throat, rheumatic fever, scarlet fever, impetigo
β-Hemolytic group B streptococci	Adult genitals	Urinary tract infection, wound infection, neonatal sepsis
Escherichia coli	Colon	Enteritis
E. coli serotype O157:H7	Colon—food and water	Hemolytic-uremic syndrome (HUS)
Neisseria gonorrhoeae	Genitourinary tract, rectum, mouth, eye	Gonorrhea, pelvic inflammatory disease, conjunctivitis
Staphylococcus epidermidis	Skin	IV line infection, bacteremia, endocarditis
Tubercle bacillus (Mycobacterium tuberculosis)	Lungs	Tuberculosis infection, tuberculosis disease
Bacillus anthracis	Infected animals or their products; bioterrorist release	Cutaneous anthrax, inhalation anthrax, gastrointestinal anthrax
Rickettsia rickettsii	Wood tick	Rocky Mountain spotted fever
Viruses		
Herpes simplex virus I and II	Lesions of the mouth, skin, adult genitals	Cold sores, sexually transmitted infections
Hepatitis A and E	Food or water, feces	Hepatitis A and E
Hepatitis B, C, D, and G	Blood, body fluids, and excretions	Hepatitis B
Human immunodeficiency virus (HIV)	Blood, semen, vaginal secretions, breast milk	HIV-positive status, HIV infection
Varicella zoster virus	Vesicle fluid, respiratory tract infections	HIV disease, varicella (chickenpox) primary infection, herpes zoster (shingles) reactivation
Fungi		
Pneumocystis jiroveci (carinii)	Intestinal tract, genitourinary tract, respiratory tract, and circulatory system of humans and animals	Pneumonia referred to as an opportunistic infection in acquired immunodeficiency syndrome (AIDS)
Candida albicans	Mouth, skin, colon, genital tract	Thrush, dermatitis, sexually transmitted diseases
Cryptococcus species	Bird feces	Pneumonia-like illness, meningoencephalitis
Protozoa		
Plasmodium falciparum	Mosquito	Malaria
Entamoeba histolytica	Intestinal tract (specifically the large intestine)	Diarrhea, colitis

IV, intravenous.

microorganism that promotes growth and reproduction is a reservoir. Many areas of the body typically host a variety of microorganisms, but the presence of these microorganisms does not always cause illness. Reservoirs include humans, animals, and environmental sources. Within the healthcare environment, infection may breed and thrive in soiled dressings and medical equipment, including stethoscopes, bedside tables, and over bed tables. A *carrier*, or vector, is a person or animal that does not become ill but harbors and spreads an organism, causing disease in others.

The patient care technician must be aware of the potential risk presented within the healthcare environment. Ensuring that cleaning is performed between patient use, promptly changing soiled materials, and properly disposing of contaminated materials is helpful in this mission (Box 9.1).

Portal of Exit

A microorganism does not have the capacity to cause disease in another host without finding a point of escape from the reservoir. Examples of exit routes in humans are any body fluids produced from the patient, such as those from the gastrointestinal, respiratory, and genitourinary systems or from an open area on the patient's body.

Using proper hand hygiene techniques, the patient care technician can help prevent the spread of microorganisms. The patient care technician should cover their nose and mouth when coughing or sneezing to prevent spread of any organism.

Mode of Transmission

A contaminated vehicle is the means by which microorganisms are carried about and transported to the next host once they have left the reservoir. Contamination means a condition of being soiled, stained, touched by, or otherwise exposed to harmful agents (e.g., the entry of infectious materials into a previously clean or sterile environment), which makes an object potentially unsafe for use. If the vehicle is a living carrier, it is called a *vector*. If the vehicle is an inanimate (nonliving) object, it is called a fomite. Some examples of fomites found in healthcare facilities are computers (many people touch the computer throughout the day), medical records and charts, stethoscopes, thermometers, bandage scissors, used tissues, drinking glasses, needles, and soiled dressings.

Transmission via this kind of common contact with a fomite or vector is known as the *indirect method of transmission*. Transmission through direct contact is also possible, such as when the patient care technician uses poor hand hygiene technique and then turns or bathes a patient.

Air currents can carry microorganisms. To help reduce the number of microorganisms in the air, the patient care technician should not shake the linens when making a bed. Use of a dampened or treated cloth when dusting can help prevent circulation of dust particles.

Box 9.1   Measures to Reduce Reservoirs of Infection

Bathing
- Use soap and water to remove drainage, dried secretions, excess perspiration, or sediment from disinfectants.

Dressing Changes
- Change wet or soiled dressings.

Contaminated Articles
- Place used tissues, soiled dressings, and soiled linen in moisture-resistant bags for proper disposal. Place dressings that can be poured, dripped, or squeezed in biohazard bags.

Contaminated Needles and Sharps
- Place syringes, uncapped hypodermic needles, and sharps such as scalpels in moisture-resistant, puncture-proof containers. Keep these in patients' rooms or treatment areas so that carrying exposed, contaminated equipment any distance is not necessary.
- Do not recap needles or attempt to break them.

Bedside Unit
- Keep table surfaces clean and dry.

Bottled Solutions
- Do not leave bottled solutions open for prolonged periods.
- Keep solutions tightly capped.
- Date bottles when opened.
- Use only as directed by the manufacturer.

Surgical Wounds
- Maintain the patency of drainage tubes and collection bags to prevent accumulation of serous fluid under the skin surface.

Drainage Bottles and Bags
- Empty and dispose of drainage suction canisters according to agency policy.
- Empty all drainage systems on each shift unless otherwise ordered by a physician.*
- Never raise a drainage system (e.g., urinary drainage bag) above the level of the site being drained unless it is clamped off.

*Closed, water-sealed chest drainage system receptacles are never emptied, but only replaced if necessary, per hospital protocol.

The floor is one of the dirtiest areas in any building. The patient care technician should not use anything that has been dropped on the floor. Linens that have been dropped on the floor should be treated as soiled and placed in the appropriate container to be sent for laundering. Supplies (such as dressings) should be discarded. Feet and furniture are the only items that belong on the floor.

Injury & Illness Prevention Box 9.1

- The floor is one of the dirtiest areas in the healthcare facility.
- Remove shoes before entering your home to prevent carrying organisms onto the floor.
- This is especially important should you have small children who live at home who crawl on the floor.
- Wash shoes periodically to remove organisms from the soles.
- Some silicone or hard rubber-soled shoes, such as Crocs®, may be top-rack dishwasher safe, and are machine washable

---

Because so many factors can promote the spread of infection to a patient, all healthcare workers who provide direct care (physical therapists, physicians, nurses) and those who perform diagnostic and support services (laboratory technicians, respiratory therapists, patient care technicians, dietary workers) must follow infection prevention and control practices to prevent or minimize the spread of infection.

Portal of Entry

Once the microorganism has exited the reservoir and has been transmitted to a susceptible host, it has to find a way to enter the host. When the host's defense mechanisms are reduced (see the section Host), the microorganism has a greater chance to gain entry to the host and produce infection. If the patient's skin is punctured with a contaminated needle, microorganisms can enter into the bloodstream. If the nurse is not careful when changing a wound dressing, contamination of the new dressing or the wound could occur and could introduce possible pathogenic microorganisms into the open wound and cause an infection.

Many of the entrance and exit routes microorganisms take are the same, and methods used to prevent or control both processes are also similar. The skin is the first line of defense. It should be kept intact, lubricated, and clean. The patient care technician should closely observe the patient's skin and report any open areas to the nurse immediately.

Accidental needle sticks are a potential hazard for all personnel who work in a healthcare facility. Any injury caused by a sharp piece of possibly dirty equipment (such as a used needle or scalpel) should be reported immediately so that procedures can be started to help prevent development of specific types of infections (such as hepatitis B and HIV). Available and appropriate waste containers are essential for safe disposal of sharp instruments. Needles should never be recapped.

An indwelling catheter or another type of drainage equipment often provides an entrance for microorganisms. The patient care technician should ensure that tubes remain connected and intact. Take care when turning, positioning, or transferring a patient to prevent any tubes from becoming tangled or pulling apart.

In the care of open areas, specific techniques can be used to prevent the entrance of microorganisms. Always wear gloves when handling soiled dressings and place the dressings in the appropriate type of waste container for disposal per facility policy.

Host

A host is an organism in which another organism is nourished and harbored. Susceptibility to an infection is defined by the amount of resistance that the host can exhibit against the pathogen. Microorganisms are constantly in contact with people, but an infection does not develop unless a person is susceptible to the microorganism's strength and numbers. As the pathogen's strength and numbers increase, the person becomes more susceptible. Factors that affect a person's immunologic defense mechanisms are described in Box 9.2.

Immunizations have proven effective in reducing susceptibility to some types of infectious diseases. These are given before a person has been exposed to a disease (to provide protection before contact) or after exposure (if the person's history indicates possible contact with an infectious microorganism). Table 9.2 lists the normal defense mechanisms against infection.

Healthcare facility policies mandate that workers be current with immunizations. Many facilities also require preventative medications and vaccines.

Box 9.2   Factors That Affect Immunologic Defense Mechanisms

- Increasing age and extreme youth
- Stress
- Fatigue
- Nutritional status
- Hereditary factors
- Disease processes
- Environmental factors
- Medical therapy
- Chemotherapy
- Radiation
- Lifestyle
- Occupation
- Diagnostic procedures
- Travel history
- Trauma

Table 9.2	Normal Defense Mechanisms Against Infection	
Defense Mechanisms	**Action**	**Factors That May Alter Disease**
Skin		
Intact multilayered surface (body's first line of defense against infection)	Provides barrier to microorganisms	Cuts, abrasions, puncture wounds, areas of maceration
Shedding of outer layer of skin cells	Removes organisms that adhere to skin's outer layers	Failure to bathe regularly
Sebum	Contains fatty acid that kills some bacteria	Excessive bathing
Mouth		
Intact multilayered mucosa	Provides mechanical barrier to microorganisms	Lacerations, trauma, extracted teeth
Saliva	Washes away particles that contain microorganisms Contains microbial inhibitors (e.g., lysozyme)	Poor oral hygiene, dehydration
Eye tearing and blinking	Provides mechanisms to reduce entry (blinking) or to assist in washing away (tearing) particles that contain pathogens, thus reducing number (dose) of organisms	Injury, exposure—splash or splatter of blood or other potentially infectious material into the eye
Respiratory Tract		
Cilia lining upper airway coated by mucus	Trap inhaled microbes and sweep them outward in mucus to be expectorated or swallowed Engulf and destroy microorganisms that reach lungs' alveoli	Smoking, high concentration of oxygen and carbon dioxide, decreased humidity, cold air
Urinary Tract		
Flushing action of urine flow	Washes away microorganisms on lining of bladder and urethra	Obstruction to normal flow by urinary catheter placement, obstruction from growth or tumor, delayed micturition Introduction of urinary catheter, continual movement of catheter in urethra
Gastrointestinal Tract		
Acidity of gastric secretions	Chemically destroys microorganisms incapable of surviving low pH	Use of antacids
Rapid peristalsis in small intestine	Prevents retention of bacterial contents	Delayed motility resulting from impaction of fecal contents in large bowel or mechanical obstruction by masses
Vagina		
At puberty, normal flora cause vaginal secretions to achieve low pH	Inhibit growth of many microorganisms	Antibiotics, excessive douching, and oral contraceptives disrupting normal flora

Inflammatory Response

Inflammation is the body's response to injury or infection at the cellular level. Inflammation is a protective vascular reaction that delivers fluid, blood products, and nutrients to interstitial tissues in the area of an injury. The process neutralizes and eliminates pathogens or necrotic (dead) tissues and establishes a means of repairing body cells and tissues. Signs of inflammation frequently include edema (swelling), rubor (redness), heat, pain or tenderness, and loss of function in the affected body part. When inflammation becomes systemic, other signs and symptoms develop, including fever, leukocytosis (increased white blood cell count), malaise (generalized discomfort), anorexia, nausea, vomiting, and lymph node enlargement.

The inflammatory response is triggered by physical agents, chemical agents, or microorganisms. Mechanical trauma, temperature extremes, and radiation are examples of physical agents. Chemical agents include external and internal irritants, such as harsh poisons or gastric acid. Microorganisms trigger this response as well, as previously discussed. The inflammatory response sometimes occurs in the absence of an infectious process.

HEALTHCARE-ASSOCIATED INFECTIONS

One in every 25 patients admitted to the hospital has development of a healthcare-associated infection (HAI)

(Centers for Disease Control, 2016). These infections were previously referred to as nosocomial infections. To be classified as an HAI, the infection develops at least 48 hours after hospitalization or contact with another type of healthcare facility. These infections pose a serious problem. Hospitals harbor microorganisms that spread easily, and this makes hospitals more likely to be places for infection. The hospitalized patient's immune system is probably already weakened from disease or invasive procedures, which makes the patient more susceptible to pathogens. Hospital-associated infections not only necessitate longer hospital stays for the patient but also increase costs for both the patient and the hospital.

An exogenous (growing outside the body) infection is caused by microorganisms from another person (e.g., an infection transmitted to the patient by a healthcare worker). An endogenous (growing within the body) infection is caused by the patient's own normal microorganisms, which become altered and overgrow or are transferred from one body site to another (e.g., microorganisms in fecal material are transferred to skin by hands and infect a wound).

Hospital-associated infections are most commonly transmitted via direct contact between healthcare workers and patients or from patient to patient. For this reason, a strong emphasis must be placed on the prevention of transmission with measures such as hand hygiene and environmental cleaning.

The patient care technician should provide the patient with a clean and safe environment. The patient care technician must also be conscientious and thorough while performing clean and sterile procedures to reduce the transmission of infection. To decrease the occurrence or duration of HAIs, many facilities have an infection prevention and control department, which investigates and establishes policies to ensure that all personnel maintain aseptic techniques while performing a procedure on a patient. These procedures include clean technique, which is used in all areas, and sterile technique, which is used in invasive procedures, such as indwelling catheter insertion.

Hospital-associated infections significantly increase healthcare costs. Extended lengths of stay in healthcare facilities increase disability, and lengthened recovery times add to the expenses the patient has to bear and to those of the healthcare facility and any funding bodies (e.g., health insurance companies, Medicare, and Medicaid). In 2008, the Centers for Medicare and Medicaid Services took a stance against hospital-acquired infections by discontinuing reimbursement for conditions such as catheter-associated urinary tract infections and bloodstream infections. This means that if a patient receives a hospital-acquired infection, they no longer have to pay for the extended treatment this infection will cause. This position encourages healthcare facilities to focus on activities that prevent hospital-acquired infections to avoid financial penalties. As a patient care technician, you can do your part to ensure that you use the best aseptic or sterile technique possible when collecting specimens or placing indwelling catheters.

Delegation and Documentation Box 9.1

- When performing straight catheterization or inserting an indwelling catheter, sterile technique is always used to remove any microorganisms from the insertion site; this limits the opportunity for a catheter-assisted urinary tract infection.
- When documenting the procedure, be sure to document that the procedure was performed under sterile technique.

Occupational Health Service

The occupational health service plays an important role in the prevention or the control of an infection in a healthcare setting by taking measures to protect the healthcare worker and patients from certain infections. Federal law requires that healthcare employers make available the hepatitis B vaccine and vaccination series to all employees who have the risk for occupational exposure.

When any needle stick occurs, the healthcare worker must report it immediately. Hepatitis B, or serum hepatitis, is the most commonly transmitted infection from contaminated needles. Healthcare agencies require workers who have had a needle stick to complete an injury report and seek appropriate treatment (Box 9.3).

Many facilities mandate that all workers and students obtain titers as proof of immunity against varicella, measles, mumps, and rubella. Titers are laboratory tests that measure the amount of an antibody in the bloodstream. If the amount of the antibody is not high enough, the healthcare agency often requires personnel to receive a vaccination or be revaccinated to prevent the disease.

STANDARD PRECAUTIONS

With the understanding that exposure to blood-borne pathogens (e.g., hepatitis B virus, HIV) can produce illness and infection came the realization that specific precautions can be used to help prevent infections. The Centers for Disease Control and Prevention (CDC), an agency of the U.S. Department of Health and Human Services, provides facilities and services for investigation, prevention, and control of disease. The CDC has conducted studies on healthcare workers with documented skin or mucous membrane exposure to blood or body fluids of infected patients (Siegel et al., 2007). The studies show that infection is much more likely to occur when healthcare workers do not use appropriate protective measures.

The CDC guidelines for transmission-based precautions in hospitals, revised in 2007, have been adopted by

Box 9.3   Vaccination and Follow-Up Care for Healthcare Workers

Hepatitis B

1. Federal law requires that healthcare employers make available the hepatitis B vaccine and vaccination series to all employees who have occupational exposure. If an employee declines the vaccine, the employee is required to sign a declination form. Evaluation and follow-up care are available to all employees who have been exposed.
2. Hepatitis B vaccinations are made available to employees within 10 working days of assignment, which means before the employee starts to provide patient care and after the employee receives education and training about the vaccine.
3. A blood test (titer) is offered in some facilities 1 to 2 months after completion of the three-dose vaccine series (check the healthcare facility or agency policy).
4. The vaccine is offered at no cost to employees. Vaccine does not require any boosters.
5. After exposure, no treatment is needed if a positive blood titer is on file. If no positive titer is on file, it is mandatory to follow the CDC guidelines.

Hepatitis C

1. If the source patient tests positive for hepatitis C virus (HCV), the employee receives a baseline test.

2. At 4 weeks after exposure, the employee is to be offered an HCV-RNA test to determine whether the employee contracted HCV.
3. If results are positive, the employee is started on treatment. (No prophylactic treatment exists for HCV after exposure.)
4. Early treatment for infection has the potential to prevent chronic infections.

Human Immunodeficiency Virus

1. If the patient tests positive for HIV infection, a viral load study is performed to determine the amount of virus present in the blood.
2. If the exposure meets the CDC criteria for HIV prophylactic treatment, or postexposure prophylaxis (PEP), it is optimally started as soon as possible, preferably within 2 hours after the exposure (CDC, 2005). All medical evaluations and procedures, including the vaccine and vaccination series and evaluation after exposure (prophylaxis), are made available at no cost to at-risk employees. A confidential written medical evaluation is available to employees who have experienced exposure incidents.

(From Centers for Disease Control and Prevention. Retrieved from www.cdc.gov; and Occupational Safety and Health Administration, Occupational Safety and Health Act of 2001. Retrieved from www.osha.gov.)

many healthcare facilities (Siegel et al., 2007). The goal of these guidelines is to interrupt the chain of infection and reduce transmission of blood-borne pathogens and other potentially infectious materials. The guidelines apply to (1) blood; (2) all body fluids, secretions, and excretions except sweat, regardless of whether or not they contain visible blood; (3) nonintact skin; and (4) mucous membranes. Standard precautions are designed to reduce the risk of transmission of microorganisms from both recognized and unrecognized sources of infections.

These precautions promote hand hygiene and use of gloves, masks, eye protection, and gowns when appropriate for patient contact.

Accurate identification of all patients infected with blood-borne pathogens is difficult. In the past, the CDC recommended that healthcare workers use "universal blood and body fluid precautions," or "universal precautions," and body substance isolation when caring for all patients. These two sets of precautions have now been incorporated into one standard set of guidelines, called standard precautions (Box 9.4).

Hand Hygiene

Hand hygiene is the single most important and basic preventive technique that healthcare workers can use to interrupt the infectious process. Box 9.5 indicates when initiation of hand hygiene is essential.

Performing hand hygiene (Procedure 9.1) provides necessary protection before the patient care technician provides care for a patient. Effective cleansing of hands with soap or detergents that contain antiseptic and water is mandatory if soiled with dirt or organic matter, or if the patient care technician has handled a contaminated item. The standard is to wash for 15 to 30 seconds with facility-approved soap, running hands under warm water (very hot water increases the risk of drying and chapping the skin). Box 9.6 contains an overview of the CDC hand hygiene guidelines, and Box 9.7 addresses the use of alcohol-based waterless antiseptics for hand hygiene. All forms of HAIs can result from improper hand hygiene and use of contaminated equipment.

The wearing of artificial fingernails and nail polish has prompted several research studies. A series of regulatory agencies, including the CDC, The Joint Commission, and the Association of periOperative Registered Nurses (AORN), has adopted position statements concerning the wearing of nails in the operating room setting. Only natural nails should be worn in the healthcare setting; these should be no longer than ¼ inch. The use of artificial and acrylic nails should be avoided because of their potential for being carriers of harmful microorganisms. Microorganisms can hide underneath the fingernail if the length is longer than ¼ inch, and make it difficult for removal during normal hand hygiene.

In addition to hand hygiene, other actions can be taken to reduce the chance of transmitting microorganisms.

Box 9.4 Standard Precautions

Hand Hygiene

- Hand hygiene is considered of utmost importance when practicing standard precautions. Hands are to be washed before patient care and after touching blood, body fluids, secretions, excretions, and contaminated items, regardless of whether gloves are worn. Perform hand hygiene immediately after gloves are removed, between patient contacts, and when otherwise indicated to prevent transfer of microorganisms to other patients or environments. Washing hands may be necessary between tasks and procedures on the same patient to prevent cross contamination of different body sites.
- Use approved soaps and alcohol-based hand sanitizers and lotions.

Gloves

- Wear clean gloves when the potential for touching blood, body fluids, secretions, excretions, and contaminated items exists. Put on clean gloves just before touching mucous membranes and nonintact skin. Change gloves between tasks and procedures on the same patient after contact with material that possibly contains a high concentration of microorganisms. Remove gloves promptly after use, before touching noncontaminated items and environmental surfaces. Perform hand hygiene immediately after removing gloves to prevent transfer of microorganisms to other patients or environment.

Mask, Eye Protection, and Face Shield

- Wear a mask and eye protection or a face shield to protect mucous membranes of the eyes, the nose, and the mouth during procedures and patient care activities that are likely to generate splashes or sprays of blood, body fluids, secretions, and excretions.

Gown

- Wear a fluid-resistant gown (a clean, unsterile gown is adequate) to protect skin and prevent soiling of clothing during procedures and patient care activities that are likely to generate splashes or sprays of blood, body fluids, secretions, or excretions or cause soiling of clothing. Select a gown that is appropriate for the activity and amount of fluid likely to be encountered. Remove the soiled gown as promptly as possible and perform hand hygiene to prevent transfer of microorganisms to other patients or environments.

Miscellaneous Guidelines

- Place used sharps, such as needles or scalpels, in a designated sharps disposal container.
- Do not purposefully bend, break, or recap needles.
- Place disposable wastes and articles contaminated with blood or large amounts of body fluids in a biowaste container for a trash pickup.
- Clean up spills of blood or body fluids per facility protocol (i.e., blood spill kit).
- Place all soiled linen in a laundry bag. Do not overfill the bag, to prevent contamination of the environment.
- For patients with diarrhea, strongly recommend soap and water for hand hygiene.
- For patients who are coughing, wear a face mask if within 3 feet of patient and teach patient about respiratory hygiene.
- Use mouthpieces, resuscitator bags, or other ventilation devices if resuscitation is needed.
- Healthcare workers: If you have exudative (draining) lesions, refrain from all direct patient care and from handling patient care equipment until wound is healed.
- Handle laboratory specimens from all patients as if they are infectious (refer to agency manual).
- Use private rooms for patients with communicable diseases subject to airborne transmission or patients who soil their environment uncontrollably with body substances. For certain diseases (e.g., meningococcal meningitis), personnel and family entering the patient's room are to wear masks. This is true for the first 24 hours until antibiotics have been started, and then is no longer required per the CDC. Roommates who are immune to the patient's disease or who are currently infected with the same disease are permitted to share rooms (institutional policy may vary on this specific procedure).

(From Siegel JD, Rhinehart E, Jackson M, et al.: Guideline for isolation precautions: preventing transmission of infectious agents in healthcare settings. Retrieved from www.cdc.gov/ncidod/dhqp/pdf/isolation2007.pdf.)

Box 9.5 Hand Hygiene Is Essential

- When hands are visibly soiled
- Before and after caring for a patient
- After contact with organic material, such as feces, wound drainage, and mucus
- In preparation for an invasive procedure, such as suctioning, catheterization, or injections
- Before changing a dressing or having contact with open wounds
- Before preparing and administering medications
- After removing disposable gloves or handling contaminated equipment
- Before and after using the toilet
- Before and after eating
- At the beginning and end of the shift

PROCEDURE 9.1

Performing Hand Hygiene With Soap and Water

1. Inspect hands, observing for visible soiling, breaks, or cuts in the skin and cuticles. Determine amount of contaminant on hands. Assess areas around the skin that are contaminated. Adjust the water to appropriate temperature and force. Wet hands and wrists under the running water, always keeping hands lower than elbows. Lather hands with liquid soap (about 1 teaspoon). Wash hands thoroughly with a firm, circular motion and friction on back of hands, palms, and wrists. Wash each finger individually, paying special attention to areas between fingers and knuckles by interlacing fingers and thumbs and moving hands back and forth, causing friction.

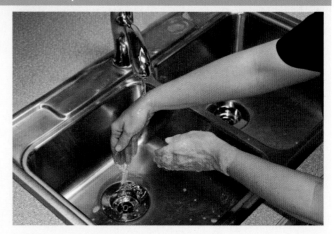

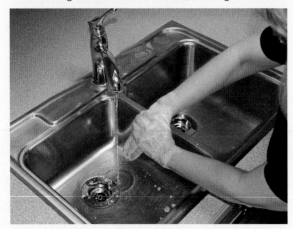

2. Wash for 15 to 30 seconds. Rinse wrists and hands completely, again keeping hands lower than elbows.

3. Dry hands thoroughly with paper towels. Start by patting at fingertips, then hands, and then wrists and forearms. If it is necessary to turn off faucets manually, use a dry paper towel. Use hospital-approved hand lotion if desired. Inspect hands and nails for cleanliness. If hands are not visibly soiled, use an alcohol-based waterless antiseptic for routine decontamination of hands in all clinical situations, unless you are caring for a patient with *Clostridium difficile* or *Candida* infection. The spores are unaffected by alcohol, so soap and water must be used in this instance.

4. If contamination occurs, it is necessary to reassess technique.

Box 9.6   Overview of CDC Hand Hygiene Guidelines

The Centers for Disease Control and Prevention (CDC) makes recommendations for hand hygiene in healthcare settings. *Hand hygiene* is a term that applies to hand washing, use of an antiseptic hand sanitizer, and surgical hand antisepsis. Evidence suggests that hand antisepsis, the cleansing of hands with an antiseptic hand sanitizer, is more effective in reducing healthcare-associated infections than is plain hand washing.

Follow These Guidelines in the Care of All Patients

- Continue practice of washing hands with either facility-approved soap or antimicrobial soap and water whenever hands are visibly soiled.
- Use an alcohol-based hand sanitizer to routinely decontaminate the hands in the following clinical situations: (if alcohol-based hand sanitizers are not available, the only alternative is hand washing.)
  - Before and after patient contact
  - Before donning sterile gloves when inserting central intravascular catheters
  - Before performing nonsurgical invasive procedures (e.g., urinary catheter insertion, nasotracheal suctioning)
  - After contact with body fluids or excretions, mucous membranes, nonintact skin, and wound dressings
  - If moving from a contaminated body site (rectal area or mouth) to a clean body site (surgical wound, urinary meatus) during patient care
  - After contact with inanimate objects (including medical equipment) in the immediate vicinity of the patient
  - After removing gloves
- Before eating and after using a restroom, wash hands with facility-approved soap and water.
- Antimicrobial-impregnated wipes (i.e., towelettes) are not a substitute for using an alcohol-based hand sanitizer or antimicrobial soap.

General Recommendations for Hand Hygiene

- Use facility-approved hand lotions or creams to minimize the occurrence of irritant contact dermatitis associated with hand antisepsis or hand washing.
- Do not wear artificial fingernails or nail polish when having direct contact with patients at high risk (e.g., those in intensive care units or operating rooms).
- Keep natural nail tips less than $\frac{1}{4}$ inch long.

Box 9.6	Overview of CDC Hand Hygiene Guidelines—cont'd

- Wear gloves when contact with blood or other potentially infectious materials, mucous membranes, and nonintact skin could occur.
- Remove gloves after caring for a patient. Do not wear the same pair of gloves for the care of more than one patient, and do not wash gloves between uses with different patients.
- Change gloves during patient care if moving from a contaminated body site to a clean body site.

(Modified from Boyce JM, Pittet D: HICPAC/SHEA/APIC/IDSA Hand Hygiene Task Force and the CDC Healthcare Control Practices Advisory Committee draft guidelines for hand hygiene in healthcare settings. Infect Control Hosp Epidemiol 23[12 Suppl]:S3–S40, 2002.)

Box 9.7	Follow These Guidelines for Alcohol-Based Hand Antisepsis

- When using an alcohol-based surgical hand product with persistent activity, follow the manufacturer's instructions. Before applying the alcohol solution, prewash hands and forearms with a nonantimicrobial soap and dry hands and forearms completely. After application of the alcohol-based product as recommended, allow hands and forearms to dry thoroughly before donning sterile gloves (see Procedure 9.6).

Each patient should be provided his or her own set of personal care articles, such as a bedpan, urinal, bath basin, water pitcher, and drinking glass, to prevent cross contamination. It helps to label the patient's items so that there is no confusion when it comes time to refill multiple water pitchers at once. Most facilities now provide a set of computer-generated patient identification labels that can be used for labeling personal care items that are carried away from the patient's bedside, such as the water pitcher.

Because microorganisms are also transmitted by indirect contact with contaminated equipment and soiled linen, these articles should be placed in special waste containers or laundry bags. These items should be kept away from the patient care technician's uniform. The risk of transmitting healthcare-acquired infections or infectious diseases among patients is high when standard precautions are not followed. Healthcare workers need to stay informed about patients who have a known source of infection and communicate the information with other healthcare workers as appropriate. By following recommendations for infection prevention and control practices, healthcare workers experience more protection from exposure and reduce the patient's risk for acquiring an HAI.

Gloving

All healthcare workers should don (put on) gloves if any possibility exists of contact with infectious material with

their hands. The CDC (Boyce and Pittet, 2002) gives the following advice regarding gloves:

- Select gloves that fit and are not too loose or hang down from the hand.
- Wear gloves only once, and then place them into the appropriate waste container for safe disposal.
- If you have not completed the patient's care but have come into contact with infectious material, change the gloves before continuing the patient's care.
- Because of the risk of perforating the gloves during use, perform hand hygiene after removing the gloves (Procedure 9.2).

Family members need to understand the importance of the use of gloves. Explain that gloves become contaminated if they touch infected material or a contaminated object.

Gowning

Patient care technicians should don a gown when preparing to provide care for a patient in isolation to help protect their clothing from becoming soiled. The gown also provides protection against unknown infectious microorganisms. Another rationale for use of a gown is protection of a patient whose immune system is inadequate. In this situation, healthcare workers and visitors wear a gown to prevent the transfer of microorganisms from themselves to the patient. It is recommended that the patient care technician discards the gown when leaving the patient's room rather than reuse it. This aids in preventing the spread of pathogens to other patients or personnel. This procedure also applies to visitors. Some gowns are made of reusable material and some are made of paper-like disposable material. If the gown is reusable, be sure to place it in the proper dirty laundry receptacle before leaving the patient's room. If the gown is disposable, discard the gown in a trash receptacle designated for contaminated materials inside the patient's room before exiting the room. This limits transmitting any microorganisms to other patients.

There are several types of isolation. Some necessitate the wearing of a gown, whereas others do not. Donning of an isolation gown is indicated in the care of patients

PROCEDURE 9.2

Gloving

Donning Gloves

1. Remove gloves from dispenser. Inspect gloves for perforations. Don gloves when ready to begin patient care. Wearing gloves with a gown does not necessitate any special technique for putting them on; wear them pulled over cuffs of gown. Change gloves after direct handling of infectious material such as wound drainage. Do not touch side rails, tables, or bed stands with contaminated gloves.

Removing Gloves

2. Remove first glove by grasping outer surface at palm with other gloved hand and pulling glove inside out and off. Place this glove in the hand that is still gloved.

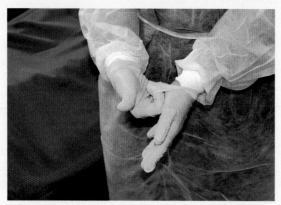

(From Cooper K, Gosnell K: *Foundations of nursing*, ed 7, St. Louis, 2015, Mosby.)

3. Remove second glove by placing finger under cuff and turning glove inside out and over other glove. Drop gloves into waste container.

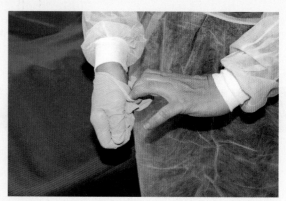

(From Cooper K, Gosnell K: *Foundations of nursing*, ed 7, St. Louis, 2015, Mosby.)

4. Perform hand hygiene.
5. If contamination occurs, it is necessary to reassess technique.

---

with diseases characterized by heavy drainage or exudate, infectious and acute diarrhea, other gastrointestinal disorders, respiratory disorders, skin wounds or burns, and urinary disorders.

Isolation gowns open at the back and have ties at the neck and the waist to keep the gown securely closed, protecting the back and the front of the patient care technician's uniform. The gown must be long enough to cover the uniform and, for added protection, have long sleeves with cuffs. To don gowns correctly, follow the procedure listed in Procedure 9.3.

Mask and Protective Eyewear

When a mask is correctly worn, it fits snugly below the healthcare worker's chin and securely over the nose and mouth, and the top edge fits below eyeglasses (this prevents fogging of glasses). Masks are available with eye shields to cover the wearer's eyes (or glasses). Goggles are another possible way to protect eyes (Fig. 9.4A). Patient care technicians should change the mask at least every 20 to 30 minutes and when it

becomes moist. Healthcare workers should not reuse the mask or allow it to dangle around their neck and then reuse it (Procedure 9.4). Masks and protective eye wear protect members of the healthcare team in the following ways:

- They protect the wearer from inhaling microorganisms that travel on airborne droplets for short distances or that remain suspended in the air for longer periods and from splashing if it should occur. Masks also prevent the mucous membranes of the nose and mouth from coming into contact with contaminants.
- They prevent the patient from inhaling pathogens if resistance is reduced or if a patient with an airborne respiratory infection is being transported to another care area.
- Eyewear shields protect the membranes and conjunctiva of the eye.

Disposing of Contaminated Equipment

Healthcare facilities accumulate large quantities of contaminated materials, some of which are disposable

PROCEDURE 9.3
Gowning for Isolation

1. Push up long sleeves, if you have them.
2. Perform hand hygiene.
3. Don gown and tie it securely at neck and waist.
4. Remove gown after providing necessary patient care.
5. Discard soiled gown appropriately.
6. Perform hand hygiene.

7. Record use of gown in isolation procedure if required by the healthcare agency. Some agencies charge a daily rate for isolation precautions. This is noted on a daily basis in the patient's record. Therefore repeated notations throughout the 24 hours are not necessary.

If contamination occurs, it is necessary to reassess technique.

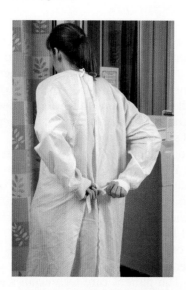

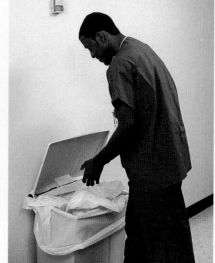

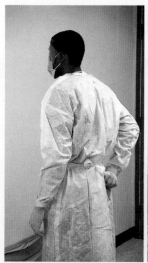

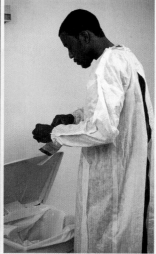

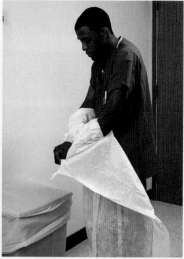

(Step 3 figure from Potter PA, Perry AG: Fundamentals of nursing: concepts, process, and practice, ed 9, St. Louis, 2017, Mosby. Steps 4 and 5 figures from Elkin MK, Perry AG, Potter PA: Nursing interventions and clinical skills, ed 3, St. Louis, 2004, Mosby.)

and some of which are reusable. It is essential to design and implement an effective way to handle this material within the facility. Some facilities manage the waste onsite, and other facilities rely on waste haulers to remove the waste. A major risk to healthcare workers and facility personnel is in the improper disposal of sharps (needles, scalpels), which are often contaminated by blood or bodily fluid. When left in linens, these sharp items have the potential to injure workers cleaning patient care areas. For prevention of this problem, all patient care areas in which sharps are ever used must be provided with puncture-proof containers into which healthcare workers place used disposable sharp items.

Handling Linen

The CDC recommends the following guidelines for handling linen:

- Place soiled linen in a laundry bag in the patient's room.
- Treat all linen as though it is infectious.

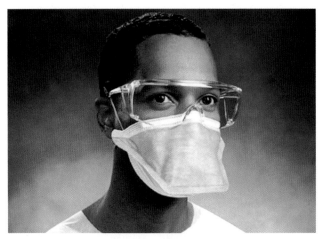

FIGURE 9.4 Nurse wearing particulate respirator mask. (From Ignatavicius DD, Workman ML: *Medical-surgical nursing across the health care continuum*, ed 8, Philadelphia, 2013, Saunders.)

Note that double bagging (placing a plastic bag that contains contaminated linen into another clean plastic bag) is no longer recommended as a universal practice, unless a cloth bag is being placed in a plastic bag. In most cases, a single bag is adequate if it is possible to place the contaminated articles in the bag without contamination of the outside of the bag.

Isolation Technique

The CDC issued isolation guidelines, in addition to standard precautions, that contain a two-tier approach (Siegel et al., 2007). The first tier recommends precautions designed for healthcare workers to use when caring for all patients in healthcare facilities regardless of their diagnosis or presumed infectiousness. This first tier is called *standard precautions.*

The second-tier condenses the disease-specific approach to isolation into transmission categories: airborne, droplet, and contact precautions. These precautions are designed to be used in the care of patients with a specific type of confirmed or suspected infection (Box 9.8 and Figs. 9.5 to 9.7).

The type of isolation techniques followed for a given patient depends on how transmissible the pathogen in question is. The patient care technician should follow

---

PROCEDURE 9.4
Donning a Mask

Perform the following steps when donning a mask:
1. Remove mask from container.
2. Don mask when ready to begin patient care by covering your nose, mouth, and eyes (or glasses) with the device. Wear a mask with a protective eye shield when there is risk of splashing. Secure mask in place with elastic band or by tying the strings behind your head.

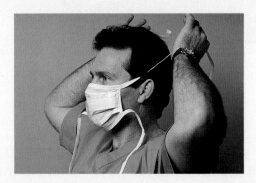

3. Wear mask until it becomes moist, but no longer than 20 to 30 minutes.

4. Remove mask by untying the strings or moving the elastic. Be certain not to touch contaminated area.

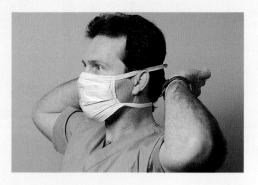

5. Dispose of soiled mask in appropriate container.
6. Wash hands thoroughly.
7. Record use of mask during patient care (some agencies require documentation of specific barriers used).
8. If contamination occurs, it is necessary to reassess technique.

(Figures from Potter PA, Perry AG: Fundamentals of nursing: concepts, process, and practice, ed 9, St. Louis, 2017, Mosby.)

Box 9.8 Types of Precautions and Patients Who Require Those Precautions

Standard Precautions (Tier 1)

Use standard precautions for the care of all patients. This general mandate is necessary because whether the patient is colonized or infected with certain pathogenic microorganisms is sometimes not known. Barrier precautions reduce the need to handle sharps.

Transmission Precautions (Tier 2)

Airborne Precautions

In addition to standard precautions, use airborne precautions for patients known or suspected to have serious illnesses transmitted by airborne droplet nuclei. Examples of such illnesses include the following:

- Measles
- Varicella zoster virus (including disseminated zoster), responsible for chickenpox and shingles
- Tuberculosis (TB)

Droplet Precautions

In addition to standard precautions, use droplet precautions for patients known or suspected to have serious illness transmitted by large particle droplets. Examples of such illnesses include the following:

- Invasive *Haemophilus influenzae,* including meningitis, pneumonia, epiglottitis, and sepsis
- Invasive *Neisseria meningitidis* disease, including meningitis, pneumonia, and sepsis

  Examples of other serious bacterial respiratory infections spread by droplet transmission include the following:
- Diphtheria (pharyngeal)
- Mycoplasma pneumonia
- Pertussis
- Pneumonic plague
- Streptococcal pharyngitis, pneumonia, and scarlet fever in infants and young children

  Examples of serious viral infections spread by droplet transmission include the following:
- Adenovirus
- Influenza
- Mumps
- Parvovirus B19
- Rubella
- TB caused by *Mycobacterium tuberculosis*

Tuberculosis Isolation

- TB isolation should be practiced for all patients with known or suspected TB. (Suspected TB is defined by agency policy and generally means any patient with a positive acid-fast bacillus [AFB] smear, a cavitated lesion seen on a chest x-ray, or identification as high risk with a screening tool.)
- Isolation is mandatory in a single-patient room designated as negative-pressure airflow and having at least 6 to 12 air exchanges per hour. It is necessary to vent room air to the outside and to ensure that the door is closed (before and after entering the room) to maintain negative pressure.
- It is mandatory that healthcare workers wear an N-95 or higher particulate respirator mask or a powered air

purifying respirator (PAPR) when entering an AFB isolation room (check agency's policy for type of mask).

- It is mandatory for healthcare workers to undergo a fit-test* before using a respirator for the first time. This ensures that the type and the size of the respirator are appropriate for the individual.
- It is mandatory for healthcare workers to fit-check[†] the respirator's fit before each use.
- Respirators are permitted to be reused and stored according to manufacturer's recommendations and agency policy.

Contact Precautions

In addition to standard precautions, use contact precautions for patients known or suspected to have serious illnesses easily transmitted by direct patient contact or by contact with items in the patient's environment. Examples of such illnesses include the following:

- Gastrointestinal, respiratory, skin, or wound infections or colonization with multidrug-resistant bacteria judged by the infection prevention and control committee, and current state, regional, and national recommendations, to be of special clinical and epidemiologic significance
- Enteric infections with a low infectious dose or prolonged environmental survival, including the following:
  a. Clostridium difficile
  b. Diapered or incontinent patients with the following:
  1. *Escherichia coli* O157:H7
  2. Shigella
  3. Hepatitis A
  4. Rotavirus
- Respiratory syncytial virus, parainfluenza virus, and enteroviral infections in infants and young children
- Skin infections that are highly contagious or that tend to occur on dry skin, including the following:
  a. Diphtheria (cutaneous)
  b. Herpes simplex virus (neonatal or mucocutaneous)
  c. Impetigo
  d. Major (noncontaminated) abscesses, cellulitis, or decubitus ulcers
  e. Pediculosis
  f. Scabies
  g. Staphylococcal furunculosis in infants and young children
  h. Methicillin-resistant *Staphylococcus aureus* (MRSA)
  i. Vancomycin-resistant enterococci (VRE)
  j. Extended-spectrum beta-lactamase (ESBL); this enzyme attaches to the cell wall of *E. coli* and some *Klebsiella* organisms, which in turn makes the organisms multidrug resistant
  k. Varicella zoster virus (disseminated or in the immunocompromised host)
  l. Viral or hemorrhagic conjunctivitis
  m. Viral hemorrhagic infections (Ebola, Lassa, or Marburg)

Patients With Immunocompromise

Patients with immunocompromised conditions vary in their susceptibility to healthcare-associated infections depending

Continued

Box 9.8   Types of Precautions and Patients Who Require Those Precautions—cont'd

on the severity and the duration of immunosuppression. They are generally at increased risk for bacterial, fungal, parasitic, and viral infections from both endogenous and exogenous sources. In general, the use of standard precautions for all patients and transmission-based isolation precautions for specified patients reduces the acquisition by these patients of institutionally acquired organisms from other patients and environments. Patients with leukopenia sometimes require additional protective measures other than standard precautions. In such

instances, the physician or infection control nurse instructs nursing staff about the necessary protective measures (e.g., masks, private room). They place an isolation sign on the door, which lists the additional protective measures that staff and visitors are required to follow for the safety of the patient.

Monitoring of Isolation
Transmission-based isolation practices are monitored on an ongoing basis by the infection control nurse.

*Fit-test: Procedure to determine adequate fit of respirator, usually with qualitative measure (wearers are exposed to a concentrated saccharin solution and asked if they can detect taste while wearing respirator).
†Fit-check: Procedure in which worker uses negative pressure to see if mask is properly sealed to face.

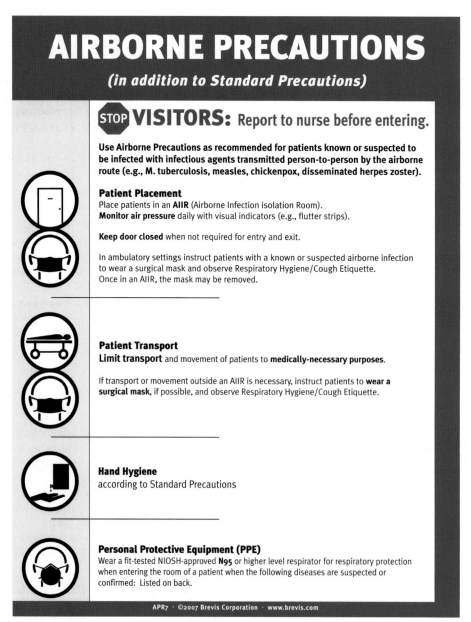

FIGURE 9.5 Airborne precautions. (Copyright 1997–2007 by Brevis Corporation. Courtesy Brevis Corporation, Salt Lake City, Utah.)

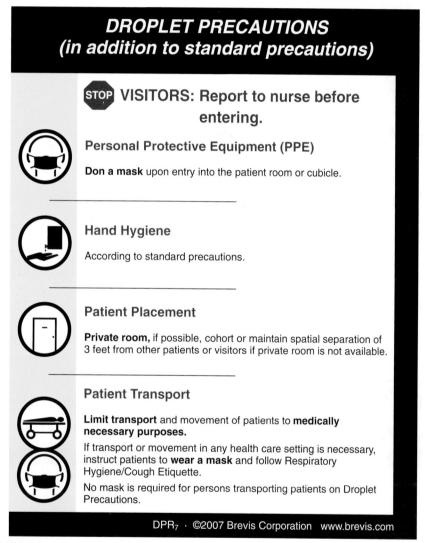

FIGURE 9.6 Droplet precautions. (Copyright 1997–2007 by Brevis Corporation. Courtesy Brevis Corporation, Salt Lake City, Utah.)

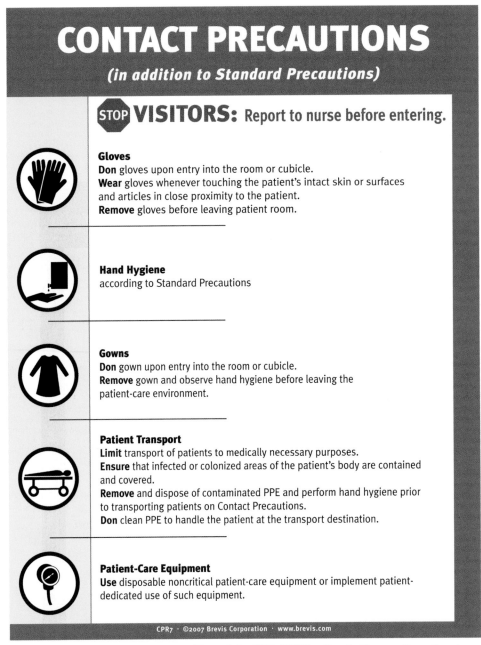

FIGURE 9.7 Contact precautions. (Copyright 1997–2007 by Brevis Corporation. Courtesy Brevis Corporation, Salt Lake City, Utah.)

some basic principles regardless of which technique is used:

- The patient care technician should perform thorough hand hygiene before and after caring for a patient.
- The patient care technician should have an adequate understanding of the method of transmission of the infectious microorganism to help determine which protective barriers to use.
- The patient care technician should dispose of contaminated equipment and articles in a safe and

effective manner to prevent transmission of pathogens to other individuals.
- If the patient is to be transported to other areas in the agency (away from the isolation room), the patient care technician should take necessary measures to protect those who will potentially be exposed. The patient should be transported in accordance with hospital protocol.

Environmental barriers keep pathogens in a confined area. Examples of such barriers are placing a patient in a private or isolation room, closing the patient's door, and wearing personal protective equipment (such as a gown, mask, goggles, and gloves).

The patient with an infectious disease should be placed in a private or isolation room equipped with the appropriate hand hygiene and toilet facilities. Private rooms used for airborne illness isolation have negative-pressure airflow that prevents infectious particulates from flowing out of the closed environment. Special rooms with positive-pressure airflow are also used for patients with immunocompromised conditions, such as patients who are receiving an organ transplant or patients who are receiving certain kinds of chemotherapy treatment for cancer. In this case, a reduced number of microorganisms can enter the room. All articles that come into contact with the patient are contaminated, and these items should be handled appropriately to help reduce the transmission of microorganisms. Only necessary equipment for assessment of vital signs remains in the room if possible. Otherwise it is mandatory for the healthcare worker to disinfect the equipment when it must be removed from the room to use on another patient.

The increased incidence of tuberculosis (TB) has led to a heightened stress, along with these precautions, on wearing the particulate respirator mask to protect against airborne pathogens

Pulmonary Tuberculosis Precautions

Pulmonary TB infections continue to concern healthcare workers. Some strains of the bacteria that cause TB are multidrug resistant, which makes treatment of the infection very difficult. The best way to prevent the transmission of pulmonary TB is to quickly identify, isolate, and treat patients. Isolation for patients with known or suspected TB includes the use of a negative-pressure isolation room. Such rooms have negative pressure in relation to surrounding areas in the facility so that room air is exhausted directly to the outside or through special high-efficiency particulate air (HEPA) filters if recirculation is unavoidable. High-risk procedures on patients with suspected or confirmed infectious TB must be performed in negative-pressure rooms.

The Occupational Safety and Health Administration (OSHA) and CDC guidelines require healthcare workers who care for patients with known or suspected TB to wear HEPA respirators (Jensen et al., 2005; U.S. Department of Labor, 2009). The respirators have the capacity to filter particles smaller than 5 μm in size with a filter efficiency of 95% or higher. The healthcare employees who work with TB cases must undergo a mask fit-test to obtain a face-seal leakage of 10% or less. To ensure correct fit and efficiency, workers who experience a significant weight loss or weight gain should repeat the fitting process. Under National Institute for Occupational Safety and Health (NIOSH) criteria, the minimally acceptable level of respiratory protection for TB is the N-95 respirator (Procedure 9.5). Training on how to wear and store the respirator is required for hospital staff. Other requirements include annual TB skin testing for healthcare workers and appropriate follow-up when a previously negative skin test becomes positive.

Another option for healthcare workers who work around patients with known or suspected airborne infections such as TB is called a powered air purifying respirator (PAPR). A PAPR may be selected instead of an N-95 respirator if an N-95 respirator does not fit adequately. Facial hair and facial deformities may interfere with the face seal of an N-95. A PAPR may also be worn if an N-95 respirator is unavailable.

SURGICAL ASEPSIS

Surgical asepsis, or sterile technique, requires that the patient care technician use different precautions from

---

PROCEDURE 9.5

Isolation Precautions

1. Follow agency policy for specific type of transmission-based precautions used.
2. Ensure that the environment has the equipment and supplies for the type of isolation:
   a. Private or isolation room with anteroom
   b. Adequate hand hygiene facilities
   c. Containers for trash, soiled linen, and sharp instruments (such as needles)
3. Provide explanation of isolation precautions to patient, family, and visitors.
4. Post sign on door of patient's room or wall outside room stating the type of protective measures in use for patient care.

5. Be certain to supply the room with lined containers designated for soiled linens and for trash.
6. Assess vital signs with designated equipment if possible, administer medications, administer hygiene, and collect specimens.
7. Report any changes in patient's health status to nurse.
8. Record assessments and performance of transmission-based precautions. Document per agency policy.
9. Additional techniques for acid-fast bacillus (AFB) isolation (airborne precautions) are as follows:
   a. Before entering room, don N-95 respirator mask that you have undergone a fit-test for.
   b. Record assessments and performance of patient care.

those of medical asepsis. *Surgical asepsis* is the complete removal of all microorganisms, including spores, from an object. The patient care technician must understand that the slightest break in technique, when working with a sterile field or with sterile equipment, results in contamination. The patient care technician must practice surgical asepsis during certain periods of care to keep microorganisms away from the area.

Although surgical asepsis is most often practiced in the operating room, the labor and delivery area, and major diagnostic or procedure areas, the patient care technician also sometimes uses surgical aseptic techniques at the patient's bedside. This includes, for example, when the patient care technician inserts urinary catheters or applies sterile dressings. When the patient care technician is changing a dressing at a patient's bedside, hand hygiene is performed, sterile gloves are donned, and sterile area is maintained during the procedure.

Because surgical asepsis requires exact techniques, the patient care technician needs the patient's cooperation. For this reason, the patient care technician should prepare the patient before any procedure. Some patients may fear moving or touching objects during a sterile procedure, whereas other patients may try to assist. The patient care technician should explain how a procedure is to be performed and instruct the patient how to avoid contaminating sterile items, including the following measures:

- The patient should try not to make sudden movements of body parts covered by sterile drapes.
- The patient should refrain from touching sterile supplies, drapes, and the patient care technician's gloves and gown.
- The patient should avoid coughing, sneezing, or talking over a sterile area.

Principles of Sterile Technique

When beginning a surgically aseptic procedure, the patient care technician should follow the principles listed in Box 9.9 to ensure maintenance of surgical asepsis. Failure to follow each principle conscientiously endangers patients by placing them at risk for infection.

Assemble all the equipment necessary for a sterile procedure before the procedure begins. By doing so, the patient care technician avoids the need to leave a sterile area unattended to locate missing equipment or supplies. Always have a few extra supplies available in case something accidentally becomes contaminated. If an object becomes contaminated during the procedure, it should be discarded immediately per facility policy.

Using Alcohol-Based Hand Rub

Use of an alcohol-based surgical hand rub is acceptable means of sanitizing hands as long it has met U.S. Food and Drug Administration requirements to be used for that purpose. Procedure 9.6 addresses the technique of using the alcohol-based hand rub. Fingernails should be short, clean, and natural. The patient care technician must not wear artificial nails. Artificial nails harbor microorganisms and fungus. The patient care technician should remove all rings, watches, and bracelets before the alcohol-based hand rub is applied. Alcohol-based hand rubs are not suitable if the hands are soiled with any kind of matter. Regular handwashing is the preferred method when the hands are soiled.

PROCEDURE 9.6

Using an Alcohol-Based Waterless Antiseptic for Routine Hand Hygiene

The Centers for Disease Control and Prevention recommends the use of alcohol-based waterless antiseptics to improve hand hygiene practices, protect healthcare workers' hands, and reduce transmission of pathogens to patients and personnel in healthcare settings. Alcohols have excellent germicidal activity and are more effective than either plain soap or antimicrobial soap and water. Emollients are added to alcohol-based antiseptics to prevent drying of the skin.

If hands are not visibly soiled, use an alcohol-based waterless antiseptic for routine decontamination of hands in most clinical situations.

1. Apply an ample amount of product to palm of one hand.
2. Rub hands together, covering all surfaces of hands and fingers with antiseptic.
3. Rub hands together for several seconds until alcohol is dry. Allow hands to dry before applying gloves. If an adequate volume is used, 15 to 25 seconds are needed for hands to dry.
4. If hands are dry or chapped, a small amount of facility-approved lotion or barrier cream can be applied.

Alcohol-based waterless antiseptics are not recommended if caring for a patient with *Clostridium difficile* diarrhea or *Candida* species infections. The spores are unaffected by the alcohol in the hand sanitizer.
(Data from Boyce JM, Pittet D: HICPAC/SHEA/APIC/IDSA Hand Hygiene Task Force and the CDC Healthcare Control Practices Advisory Committee draft guidelines for hand hygiene in healthcare settings. Infect Control Hosp Epidemiol 23[12 Suppl]:S3-S40, 2002.)

Box 9.9 Principles of Sterile Technique

1. *A sterile object remains sterile only when touched exclusively by other sterile objects.* (This principle guides your placement of sterile objects and how you handle them.)
   a. Sterile touching sterile remains sterile; for example, wear sterile gloves and use sterile forceps to handle objects on a sterile field.
   b. Sterile touching clean becomes contaminated; for example, if the tip of a syringe or other sterile object touches the surface of a clean disposable glove, the object is contaminated.
   c. Sterile touching contaminated becomes contaminated; for example, when you touch a sterile object with an ungloved hand, the object is contaminated.
   d. Sterile touching questionable is contaminated; for example, when you find a tear or break in the covering of a sterile object, discard the object regardless of whether it appears untouched or not.
2. *Place only sterile objects on a sterile field.* Properly sterilize all items before use. It is essential to keep the package or container holding a sterile object intact and dry. A package that is torn, punctured, wet, or open is unsterile.
3. *A sterile field out of the range of vision or an object held below a person's waist is contaminated.* Never turn your back on a sterile field or leave it unattended. Contamination can occur accidentally from a dangling piece of clothing, falling hair, or an unknowing patient touching a sterile object. Consider any object below waist level contaminated because you are not able to keep it in constant view. Keep sterile objects in front of you with your hands as close together as possible.
4. *A sterile object or field becomes contaminated by prolonged exposure to air.* Avoid activities that potentially create air currents, such as excessive movements or rearranging linen after a sterile object or field becomes exposed. When opening sterile packages, keep to a minimum the number of people walking into the area. Microorganisms also travel by droplets through the air. Be sure no one talks, laughs, sneezes, or coughs over a sterile field or when gathering and using sterile equipment. Never perform sterile procedures if you have a cold or other respiratory ailment unless you are wearing a specialized mask. Microorganisms have the potential to travel through the air and fall on sterile items or fields if you reach over the work area. When opening sterile packages, hold the item or piece of equipment as close as possible to the sterile field

without touching the sterile surface. Do not continue to rearrange the sterile items on the sterile field to help reduce the contamination that can occur by microorganisms traveling through the air.
5. *When a sterile surface comes in contact with a wet, contaminated surface, the sterile object or field becomes contaminated.* Moisture seeping through a sterile package's protective covering permits microorganisms to travel to the sterile object. When stored sterile packages become wet, discard the objects immediately or send the equipment for resterilization. When working with a sterile field or tray, you sometimes have to pour sterile solutions. Any spill is a possible source of contamination unless the object or field rests on a sterile surface impervious to moisture. For example, urinary catheterization trays contain sterile supplies that rest in a sterile, plastic container. Any sterile solution spilled within the container does not contaminate the catheter or other objects. In contrast, if you place a piece of sterile gauze in its wrapper on a patient's bedside table and the table surface is wet, consider the gauze to be contaminated.
6. *Fluid flows in the direction of gravity.* A sterile object becomes contaminated if gravity causes a contaminated liquid to flow over the object's surface. To prevent contamination during a surgical hand scrub, raise and hold your hands above your elbows. This allows water to flow downward without contaminating your hands and fingers. The principle of water flow by gravity is also the reason for drying in a sequence from fingers to elbows, with hands held up, after the scrub.
7. *Consider the edges of a sterile field or container to be contaminated.* Frequently, you place sterile objects on a sterile towel or drape. Because the edge of the drape touches an unsterile surface, such as a table or bed linen, a 1-inch (2.5-cm) border around the drape must be considered to be contaminated. The edges of sterile containers become exposed to air after they are open and are thus contaminated. After you remove a sterile needle from its protective cap or after removing a forceps from a container, do not allow the objects to touch the container's edge. The lip of an opened bottle of solution also becomes contaminated after it is exposed to air. When pouring a sterile liquid, first pour a small amount of solution and discard it. The solution thus washes away microorganisms on the bottle lip. Then pour a second time on the same side to fill a container with the desired amount of solution.

Managing Sterile Packages

Sterile items such as syringes, gauze dressings, and catheters are packaged in paper or plastic containers that are impervious to (unable to be penetrated by) microorganisms as long as the items remain dry and intact. Paper packages are permeable to steam and other suitable methods of sterilization and thus allow for the contents to be sterilized. A disadvantage of paper wrappers is that they tear or puncture relatively easily. Sterile items should be placed in clean, enclosed storage cabinets and never kept in the same room as dirty equipment.

Sterile supplies may have dated labels or chemical tapes that indicate the date when the sterilization expires. The tapes change color during the sterilization process. Failure of the tapes to change color means that the item is not sterile. Never use or allow use of a sterile item or piece of equipment after the expiration date. Some agencies use the "event-related" contamination rule. If the integrity of the sterile package is questionable (i.e., wet, torn, discolored), the item is discarded or sterilized per policy. If the patient care technician finds moisture present after a sterile tray is opened, the item is either discarded or returned to the institution's supply area for sterilization.

Before a sterile item is opened, thorough hand hygiene is performed. The supplies are assembled at the work area, such as the bedside table or in the treatment room, before packages are opened. A bedside table or countertop provides a large, clean working area for opening of items. Patient care technicians should ensure that the work area is above their waist level. Sterile supplies should not be opened in a space where a dirty object may fall on or come into contact with them.

Sterile packaged items can be opened without contamination of the contents even when the patient care technician is not wearing sterile gloves. Commercially packaged items are usually designed so that you only have to tear away or separate the paper or plastic cover from the rest of the tray or kit. Hold the item in one hand while pulling the wrapper with the other (Fig. 9.8). Be careful after opening to keep the inner contents sterile before use. When opening items packed in linen and some commercially prepackaged items, use the steps described in Box 9.10 and illustrated in Fig. 9.8 and Fig. 9.9.

Preparing a Sterile Field

When performing sterile procedures, the patient care technician needs a sterile work area that provides room for handling and placing sterile items. A sterile field is an area that is free of microorganisms and has been prepared to receive sterile items. Prepare the field by using the inner surface of a sterile wrapper as the work surface or by using a sterile drape (Procedure 9.7).

Sometimes the patient care technician chooses to wear sterile gloves while preparing items on the field. The patient care technician may then be able to touch

Box 9.10	Opening Sterile Packages

1. Perform hand hygiene.
2. Place the item flat in the center of the work surface.
3. Remove the tape or seal that indicates the sterilization date.
4. Grasp the outer surface of the tip of the outermost flap.
5. Open the outer flap away from your body, keeping your arm outstretched and away from the sterile field.
6. Grasp the outside surface of the first side flap.
7. Open the side flap, allowing it to lie flat on the table surface. Keep your arm to the side and not over the sterile surface. Do not allow flaps to spring back over the sterile contents.
8. Grasp the outside surface of the second side flap and allow it to lie flat on the table surface.
9. Grasp the outer surface of the last and innermost flap.
10. Stand away from the sterile package and pull the flap back, allowing it to fall flat on the surface.
11. Use the inner surface of the package cover (except for the 1-inch border around the edges) as a sterile field to handle this or additional sterile items. Grasp the 1-inch border to maneuver the entire field on the table surface.
12. When opening a small sterile item, hold it in your hand so that you can pass it to a person wearing sterile gloves or transfer it to a sterile field. Hold the package in your nondominant hand while you open the top flap and pull it away from you. With your dominant hand, carefully open the side and top flaps away from the enclosed sterile item in the same order in the previous steps.

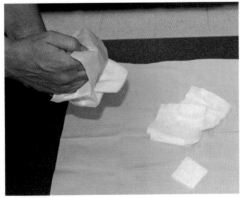

FIGURE 9.8 When opening a commercially packaged sterile item, tear the wrapper away from your body. (From Cooper K, Gosnell K: *Foundations of nursing*, ed 7, St. Louis, 2015, Mosby.)

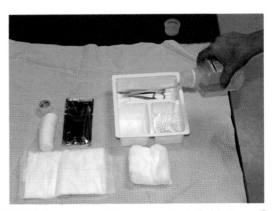

FIGURE 9.9 Placement of items on a sterile field. (From Cooper K, Gosnell K: *Foundations of nursing*, ed 7, St. Louis, 2015, Mosby.)

PROCEDURE 9.7
Preparing a Sterile Field

1. Prepare sterile field just before planned procedure. Be sure to use supplies immediately.
2. Select clean work surface that is above waist level.
3. Assemble necessary equipment.
4. Check dates, labels, and condition of package for sterility of equipment.
5. Wash hands thoroughly.
6. Place package containing sterile drape on work surface and open.
7. With fingertips of one hand, pick up folded top edge of sterile drape.
8. Gently lift drape up from its outer cover and let it unfold by itself without touching any object. Discard outer cover with your other hand.
9. With other hand, grasp adjacent corner of drape and hold the entire edge straight up and away from your body. Now, properly place drape while using two hands and being sure to keep the drape away from unsterile surfaces.
   a. Holding drape, first position the bottom half over intended work surface.
   b. Allow top half of drape to be placed over work surface last.
10. Perform procedure using sterile technique.

---

the entire drape, but an assistant has to open and pass sterile items to him or her unless the patient care technician applies new sterile gloves to prevent contamination of the sterile items. The patient care technician should not allow the gloves to touch the outside wrappers of the package that contains the sterile items.

Donning Sterile Gloves

Sterile gloves are an additional barrier used to prevent the transmission of microorganisms. The two methods of donning gloves are open (Procedure 9.8) and closed (Fig. 9.11). Those who work on general medical-surgical floors use open gloving before procedures such as dressing changes or urinary catheter insertions. The patient care technician should select the proper glove size. The glove must be snug enough to be able to pick up things easily and yet not so tightly stretched that it tears easily.

Opening and Pouring Sterile Solutions

The patient care technician may be required to pour sterile solutions into sterile containers. A bottle that contains a sterile solution is sterile on the inside and contaminated on the outside. The bottle's neck is also contaminated, but the inside of the bottle cap is sterile. After opening a cap or lid, the patient care technician can hold it in the hand or place it, sterile side (inside) up, on a clean surface. Thus the patient care technician can see the inside of the lid as it rests on the table surface. The patient care technician can never allow a bottle's cap or lid to rest sterile side down on a sterile surface because the cap's outer edge is unsterile and will contaminate the surface. Likewise, placement of a sterile cap down on an unsterile surface increases the chances of the inside of the cap becoming contaminated.

Always hold the bottle with its label in the palm of the hand to prevent the solution from wetting the label. If the solution is allowed to wet the label, it may cause it to fade and reduce its legibility. Keep the edge of the bottle from touching the edge or the inside of the receiving container, which is unsterile. The solution should be poured slowly to avoid splashing the underlying drape or field. The bottle should never be held so high above the recipient container that even slow pouring causes splashing. The bottle should be held over the outside of the edge of the sterile field (Fig. 9.10). See Procedure 9.9.

CLEANING, DISINFECTION, AND STERILIZATION

Microorganisms are present on items in the home and public areas, including healthcare agencies. By following basic clean or aseptic techniques, the patient care technician can help interrupt the spread of infection. Antiseptics are a means to inhibit the growth of microorganisms, although killing them this way is not possible. Antiseptics are also referred to as *bacteriostatic* solutions. *Bacterio* means "microorganism," and *static* means "referring to that which cannot move or grow." Use of antiseptics (like alcohol or chlorhexidine gluconate) on human tissue is acceptable and is often performed before sterile procedures like surgery and during wound care. Antiseptics can be used for mouth care and when performing hand hygiene.

Cleaning

Cleaning is the removal of foreign materials, such as soil and organic material, from objects. Generally, cleaning involves use of water and mechanical action with or without detergents.

PROCEDURE 9.8

Performing Open Sterile Gloving

1. Have package of properly sized sterile gloves at treatment area.
2. Perform thorough hand hygiene.
3. Remove outer glove package wrapper by carefully separating and peeling apart sides.

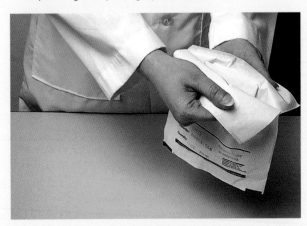

4. Grasping inner side of package, lay package on clean flat surface just above waist level. Open package, keeping gloves on wrapper's inside surface.

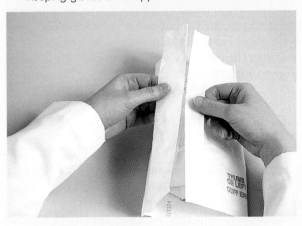

5. Identify right and left gloves. Each glove has a cuff approximately 2 inches (5 cm) deep.
6. Glove dominant hand first. With thumb and first two fingers of nondominant hand, grasp edge of cuff of glove for dominant hand. Touch only glove's inside surface.

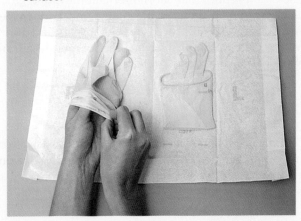

7. Carefully pull glove over dominant hand, leaving cuff; be sure that cuff does not roll up wrist. Be sure that thumb and fingers are in proper spaces.

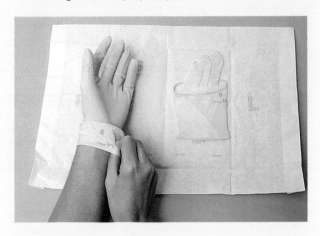

8. With gloved dominant hand, slip fingers underneath second glove's cuff in such fashion that the cuff will protect the gloved fingers.

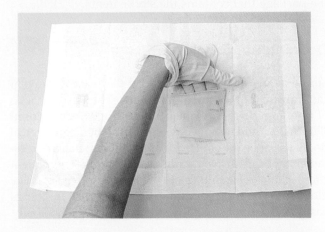

9. Carefully pull second glove over nondominant hand. Do not allow fingers and thumb of gloved dominant hand to touch any part of exposed nondominant hand. Keep thumb of dominant hand abducted back.

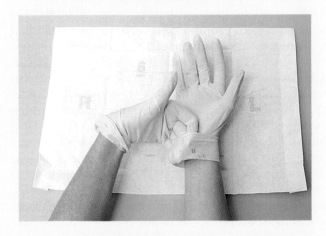

PROCEDURE 9.8

Performing Open Sterile Gloving—cont'd

10. After second glove is on, interlock hands. *Be sure to touch only sterile sides.* The cuffs usually fall down after application.

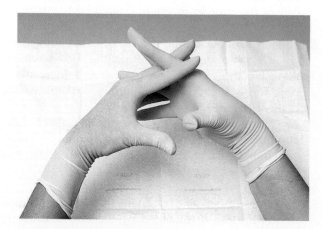

Glove Removal and Disposal

11. Grasp outside of one cuff with other gloved hand; avoid touching wrist.

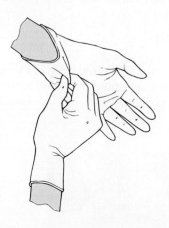

12. Pull glove off, turning it inside out. Discard in receptacle.

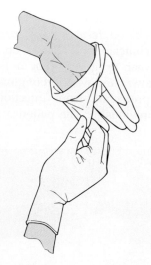

13. Take fingers of bare hand and tuck inside remaining glove cuff. Peel glove off, inside out. Discard in receptacle.

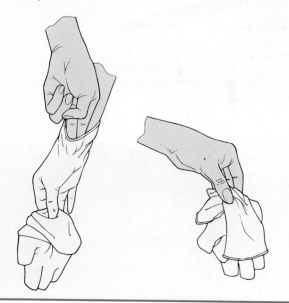

(Steps 3, 4, and 6 to 9 figures from Elkin MK, Perry AG, Potter PA: Nursing interventions and clinical skills, ed 3, St. Louis, 2004, Mosby. Step 10 figure from Potter PA, Perry AG: Fundamentals of nursing: concepts, process, and practice, ed 7, St. Louis, 2009, Mosby.) (Photos from Cooper K, Gosnell K: Foundations of nursing, ed 7, St. Louis, 2015, Mosby.)

PROCEDURE 9.9

Opening and Pouring a Sterile Solution

1. Verify the expiration date of the sterile solution before opening.
2. Open the cap or lid of the bottle, taking great care to not touch the inside of the bottle cap or the inside of the bottle.
3. After removing the cap or lid, either hold it in your hand or place it sterile side up (inside up), on a clean surface.
4. Hold the bottle with the label in the palm of the hand to prevent the solution from wetting the label.
5. Keep the edge of the bottle from touching the edge of the receiving container.
6. Pour the solution slowly to avoid splashing the underlying drape or sterile field.
7. Hold the bottle over the outside edge of the sterile field.

When an object comes in contact with potentially infectious material, the object is contaminated. If the object is disposable, it is discarded per facility policy. Reusable objects must be thoroughly cleaned and then either disinfected or sterilized before reuse, per facility policy.

When cleaning equipment that is soiled by organic material such as blood, fecal matter, mucus, or pus, the patient care technician should put on a mask and protective eyewear or goggles (or a face shield), a fluid-resistant gown, and waterproof gloves. These barriers provide protection from infectious organisms (as discussed previously). The patient care technician

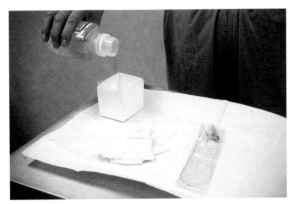

FIGURE 9.10 Place receptacle into which you pour fluids near edge of sterile table to prevent the need for reaching over the sterile field to pour. (From Elkin MK, Perry AG, Potter PA: *Nursing interventions and clinical skills,* ed 4, St. Louis, 2008, Mosby.)

needs a stiff-bristled brush and detergent or soap for cleaning.

Perform the following steps when cleaning equipment:

1. Rinse a contaminated object or article with cold running water to remove organic material. Hot water causes the protein in organic material to coagulate and stick to objects, making removal difficult.
2. After rinsing, wash the object with soap and warm water. Soap or detergent reduces the surface tension of water and emulsifies dirt and remaining material. Rinse the object thoroughly to remove the emulsified dirt.
3. Use a brush to remove dirt or material present in the equipment's grooves or seams. Friction dislodges contaminated material for easy removal. Open any hinged items for cleaning.
4. Rinse the object in warm water.
5. Dry the object and prepare it for disinfection or sterilization if indicated by the intended use of the item.
6. The brush, the gloves, and the sink in which the equipment is cleaned are considered contaminated and must be cleaned and dried per facility policy.

Disinfection

Disinfection is used to destroy microorganisms. However, it does not destroy spores. The solutions used during disinfection are called *disinfectants,* or possibly *bactericidal*

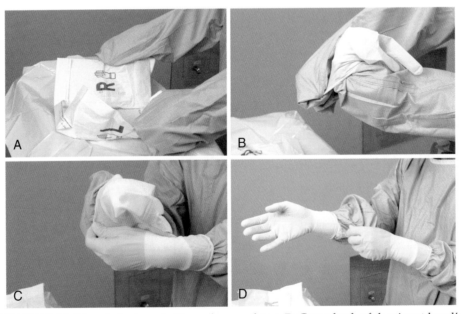

FIGURE 9.11 Closed gloving. **A,** Open glove package. **B,** Grasp back of dominant hand's glove cuff with nondominant hand and stretch over end of dominant hand's sleeve. **C,** Glove nondominant hand in same manner. **D,** Use gloved dominant hand to pull on glove, keeping nondominant hand inside sleeve until it emerges into glove. (From Potter PA, Perry GA: *Fundamentals of nursing,* ed 9, St. Louis, 2017, Mosby.)

solutions (the suffix *cidal* is derived from a Latin word meaning "to kill"). These solutions are too strong to use on human skin and are appropriate to use on inanimate objects. If a disinfectant solution comes in contact with human tissue, the tissue may feel "slippery." This is the first step of tissue breakdown. When using a disinfectant, the patient care technician should use clean gloves to protect the skin.

Sterilization

Sterilization refers to methods used to kill all microorganisms, including spores. The two types of sterilization methods are physical and chemical (Box 9.11).

Box 9.11   Methods of Disinfection and Sterilization

Physical Method
1. Steam under pressure, or moist heat, is the most practical and dependable method for destruction of all microorganisms. This process is called sterilization. Examples of sterilization equipment are the autoclave, which is used in hospitals and other agencies, and the pressure cooker, which is used in a home environment.
2. Boiling water is the best method for home use and is the least expensive. However, this technique does not destroy bacterial spores and some viruses. The article must be boiled for a minimum of 15 to 20 minutes for disinfection.
3. Radiation is used to sterilize pharmaceutical goods, foods, and heat-sensitive items. It is extremely effective on articles that are difficult to sterilize with other methods.
4. Dry heat is a method used for disinfecting articles that are destroyed by moisture. Health agencies seldom use this method, but in the home, an article can be disinfected by being placed in the oven for 2 hours at 320° F or for 45 minutes at 350° F.

Chemical Process
1. Gas (ethylene oxide) is used for sterilization. It destroys spores formed by bacteria.
2. Chemical solutions are often used to disinfect instruments because they are effective in destroying microorganisms. One way to store clinical thermometers is in a chemical solution, and some articles are soaked in a solution to prepare them for another, more definitive method of disinfection or sterilization.

Most health agencies have a central supply department that disinfects and sterilizes reusable equipment and supplies. Although most supplies used today for patient care are disposable, some supplies and equipment still require the use of disinfection and sterilization. The patient and family members should be taught the principles of cleansing and disinfecting for use in the home environment.

There are two accepted methods of disinfection and sterilization (see Box 9.11). One is a physical process that uses heat or radiation; the second process uses chemicals. Both methods destroy microorganisms. The method used depends on the following factors: (1) the type of microorganisms present (spore-forming bacteria are resistant to destruction); (2) how many microorganisms may be present (it takes longer to kill a large number); and (3) the type of item that needs to be disinfected and sterilized (some materials are so sensitive that heat or certain chemicals destroy them). Other determinants of the sterilization method used are (1) the intended use of the article (e.g., surgery requires that all organisms be destroyed, whereas medical asepsis consists of techniques that inhibit the growth and transmission of pathogenic microorganisms), and (2) the methods of sterilization available.

Liquid and gaseous chemicals are used to sterilize and disinfect equipment. Examples may include iodine, alcohol, dialdehyde, and chlorine bleach compounds. Chlorine bleach is useful for household disinfection and disinfection of water, but it must never be mixed with ammonia because of the resulting emission of toxic fumes. Chlorine bleach has a tendency to corrode some metals. Iodine is a good bactericidal agent (i.e., it kills bacteria but not spores). Iodine leaves behind stains and is not used as widely as it was previously.

Injury & Illness Prevention Box 9.2

- The basic principles of hygiene are bathing; not sharing personal articles such as combs, toothbrushes, razors, and washcloths; and covering one's mouth when coughing and sneezing.
- These practices are important to help prevent the spread of infection in the home setting.

CHAPTER SUMMARY

The mucous membranes of the respiratory, gastrointestinal, and genitourinary tracts, and intact skin provide primary defense against pathogenic microorganisms. An infection has potential to develop as long as the six elements that compose the infectious chain are uninterrupted. A microorganism's virulence (the degree to which a microorganism produces disease) depends on its ability to resist attack by the body's normal defenses. Age, poor nutrition, stress, inherited conditions, chronic disease, and treatments or conditions that compromise the immune system increase susceptibility to infection. The signs of local inflammation and infection are similar, but the inflammatory response can occur in the absence of an infectious process.

The CDC recommends that healthcare workers consider all patients as infectious and to use standard precautions to reduce the risk of exposure to blood and body fluids. Following aseptic principles is the key to a patient care technician's success in preventing patients from acquiring infection.

Isolation transmission–based precautions are used to prevent personnel and patients from acquiring infections and prevent transmission of microorganisms to other people. Wearing gloves, gowns, and masks in combination with eye protection devices such as goggles or glasses with solid side shields is mandatory when contact with blood or potentially infectious material is possible or whenever splashing or spraying of blood or potentially infectious material is possible.

Standard precautions are used to prevent the spread of organisms present in blood, all other body fluids, nonintact skin, and mucous membranes. Standard precautions are used with all patients because it is often unknown which patients have an infection. This includes the use of barrier protection when appropriate.

Case Scenario

You have nasopharyngitis, otherwise known as the common cold. You do not have a fever, but you do have clear drainage coming from your nose. Should you come to work today? Why or why not? If you do come to work, what precautions should you take to limit the transmission of your microorganism to the patients you will be caring for?

REVIEW QUESTIONS

1. A 24-year-old is admitted to a medical unit with the diagnosis of hepatitis A and placed in contact precautions. What is the reason for placing this person on contact precautions?
   a. To prevent transmission of infectious microorganisms
   b. To control the environment of the patient
   c. To protect the patient from infectious microorganisms
   d. To protect only the family

2. The patient care technician is working in a medical area with 15 patient rooms. Each patient has a different illness. When planning care, the patient care technician recognizes which of the following as the most important action to provide protection to each patient from healthcare-associated infections?
   a. Wearing a gown
   b. Placing each patient in isolation
   c. Hand hygiene
   d. Wearing gloves

3. The student is reviewing sterile technique. When using the technique, the student is reminded to hold sterile objects in which location?
   a. Close to shoulder level
   b. Just below waist level
   c. Anywhere as long as they are handled with sterile gloves
   d. Above waist level

4. The patient care technician is preparing to don sterile gloves. What action indicates understanding of the needed procedure?
   a. Touch only the inside surface of the first glove while pulling it onto the hand.
   b. Place the fingers of the dominant hand into the outside cuff of the first glove.
   c. Let the cuff of the glove roll up over the hand as it is being pulled onto the hand.
   d. Begin the procedure by pulling the first glove upward and over the nondominant hand.

5. The patient care technician has completed a sterile procedure and is preparing to remove the soiled gloves. To remove the gloves, what action is required?
   a. Pull each finger from each of the gloves first, and then roll the glove back over the hand.
   b. Remove the glove from the nondominant hand by reaching inside the glove and pulling it off.
   c. Remove one glove, and then use the bare fingers to push the remaining glove off from inside the cuff.
   d. Hold both gloved hands under running water and roll the gloves down to keep microorganisms contained.

6. The student patient care technician (PCT) is preparing to open the outer sterile wrap of an indwelling catheter tray. Which flap of the wrap (in which direction) should be opened first?
   a. The flap that opens away from the PCT
   b. The flap that opens to the left
   c. The flap that opens to the right
   d. The flap that opens toward the PCT

Workplace Safety and Body Mechanics

1. Discuss safety concerns in a healthcare environment.
2. List the steps to be followed in the event of a fire.
3. Discuss terrorism and how it relates to workplace safety.
4. Discuss fire safety issues in a healthcare environment.
5. Discuss critical elements of an emergency plan for response to a natural disaster or other emergency.
6. Identify emergency preparedness plans in the community.
7. Discuss potential roles of the patient care technician in emergency preparedness.
8. Identify principles of body mechanics and ergonomics.
9. Explain the rationale for use of appropriate body mechanics.

alignment The relationship of various body parts to each other.

base of support A stance with feet shoulder-width apart.

bioterrorism The use of biologic agents to create fear and threat. Healthcare facilities must be prepared to treat mass casualties from such an attack.

Centers for Disease Control and Prevention (CDC) A federal agency that provides facilities and services for the investigation, identification, prevention, and control of disease.

codes A system of notification to be transmitted rapidly.

disaster manual Sometimes called the emergency response plan or emergency management plan.

disaster situation An uncontrollable, unexpected, psychologically shocking event that is unique and likely to have a significant impact on a variety of healthcare facilities.

ergonomics The science of matching workplace conditions and job demands to the capabilities of workers, especially in regard to musculoskeletal disorders and their prevention.

Occupational Safety and Health Administration (OSHA) A federal organization that provides guidelines to help reduce safety hazards in the workplace.

PASS The mnemonic (Pull the pin, Aim low, Squeeze handle, Sweep the unit) that will help the patient care technician remember how to operate the fire extinguisher.

poison Any substance that is harmful to your body when ingested (eaten), inhaled, injected, or absorbed through the skin.

RACE Rescue patients, sound the Alarm, Confine the fire, and Extinguish or Evacuate.

terrorism A violent or dangerous act used to intimidate or coerce a person or government to further a political or social agenda.

WORKPLACE SAFETY

The hospital environment is a source of potential safety hazards to healthcare workers (HCWs) and the clients and families they serve. Of significant impact is the threat of workplace violence (Box 10.1). In addition, various biologic, chemical, radiologic, and physical hazards are present.

Hospital workers are also exposed to blood and body fluids, contaminated needles, radiation, and vaccine-preventable diseases. Immunization programs help protect hospital personnel and, in turn, patients at risk

---

Box 10.1   Workplace Violence

Violence does not always involve physical injury, especially in relation to workplace violence. The term *workplace violence* refers to any intense extreme behavior used to frighten, intimidate, threaten, or injure a person or damage or destroy property. The behavior is sometimes physical, sometimes verbal, and sometimes even nonverbal, such as a gesture. Legally, if by either threat or gesture someone causes a person to fear being struck, an assault has occurred. Any unwelcomed physical contact from another person is battery. In other words, one does not have to be physically "hurt" to get protection under the law. As of 2010, more than 4500 fatal injuries occurred in the workplace in the United States, with just over 500 of those being workplace homicides (U.S. Department of Labor, n.d.).

According to information from the Bureau of Labor Statistics, in 2010 more than 11,300 assaults occurred against healthcare and social assistance workers, with nearly 19% occurring in nursing and residential care facilities. Most workplace violence, including in the healthcare setting, results in nonfatal injuries.

Unfortunately, these statistics do not provide the full picture because many workplace violence incidents are not reported. Sometimes healthcare workers do not report a violent incident because they are unsure what constitutes violence, do not know of the requirement to report the incident, or do not know who to inform; sometimes they do not file a report because the injuries do not require emergency treatment or time off from work.

Risk factors for work-related assaults in healthcare agencies include the following:
- On-site presence of patients, families, friends, and coworkers in the possession of handguns
- Patients who are hospitalized and under police custody at the same time (people arrested or convicted of crimes)
- On-site presence of acutely disturbed and violent people seeking healthcare
- On-site presence of mentally ill people who do not take medicine, do not receive follow-up care, and are not hospitalized unless they are an immediate threat to themselves or others
- On-site presence of upset, agitated, and disturbed family members and visitors
- Long emergency department waits that increase a person's agitation and frustration
- On-site agency pharmacies that are a source of drugs and therefore a target for robberies
- Gang members and substance abusers having access to agencies as patients or visitors

- Staff being alone with patients during care or transport to other agency areas during examination or treatment
- Low staffing levels during meals, during emergencies, and at night
- Poorly lighted parking areas or distant parking areas
- Lack of staff training in recognizing and managing potentially violent situations

OSHA provides guidelines for violence identification and prevention programs with a goal of eliminating or reducing employee exposure to situations that have potential to cause death or injury. These guidelines can be found at the OSHA Workplace Violence Safety and Health Topics page. The worksite is analyzed for hazards. Prevention strategies are developed and implemented. Also, employees are required to receive safety and health training per facility protocol. Your responsibilities in violence prevention programs include the following:
- Understand and follow the workplace violence prevention program.
- Understand and follow safety and security measures.
- Voice safety and security concerns.
- Report violent incidents promptly and accurately.
- Serve on health and safety committees that review incidents of workplace violence.
- Take part in training programs that focus on recognizing and managing agitation, assaultive behavior, and criminal intent.

Practice the following safety measures when dealing with agitated or aggressive people:
- Stand away from the person. Judge the length of the person's arms and legs. Stand far enough away that the person will not be able to hit or kick you.
- Position yourself close to the door. Do not allow yourself to become trapped in the room.
- Note the location of panic buttons, call bells, alarms, closed-circuit monitors, and other security devices.
- If you wear your identification badge around your neck, be sure it will break away if pulled.
- Keep your hands free.
- Stay calm. Talk to the person in a calm manner. Do not raise your voice or argue, scold, or interrupt the person.
- Do not touch the person.
- Tell the person that you will get the supervisor to speak to the person.
- Leave the room as soon as you are able. Be sure that the person is safe.
- Notify the supervisor or security officer of the situation.
- Complete an incident report according to agency policy.

(From Occupational Safety and Health Administration (OSHA): Workplace violence. Retrieved from https://www.osha.gov/SLTC/workplaceviolence; National Institute for Safety and Health (NIOSH) Bureau of Labor Statistics (BLS): Occupational violence. Retrieved from www.cdc.gov/niosh/topics/violence/traumaviol_research.html.)

of being infected by hospital personnel (see Injury & Illness Prevention Box 10.1). The Centers for Disease Control and Prevention (CDC, 2016) has published healthcare personnel vaccination recommendations (Box 10.2). These recommendations also apply to student nurses because they are fulfilling clinical requirements in healthcare facilities.

The National Institute for Occupational Safety and Health (NIOSH) focuses on safety and issues related to health. Identifying risks associated with the preparation of certain drugs and looking at ways to control exposure during preparation and administration is just one example of how this group works to ensure a safe healthcare environment for HCWs. The **Hazard Communication Act** of the Occupational Safety and Health Administration (OSHA) (a federal organization that provides guidelines to help reduce safety hazards in the workplace) requires healthcare facilities to inform employees about the presence of or potential for harmful exposures and how to reduce the risk of exposure. The Centers for Disease Control and Prevention (CDC) (a federal agency that provides facilities and services for the investigation, identification, prevention, and control of disease) also provides guidelines for working with infectious patients. Referring to the information on standard precautions (see Chapter 9) and following recommended guidelines for reducing exposure to the

---

Injury & Illness Prevention Box 10.1

- As an HCW, you are more susceptible to illnesses such as influenza. To protect yourself and your family, it is recommended that you take an influenza vaccination each year.
- Immunizations recommended by your healthcare institution are typically provided to you at no cost.

---

variety of hazards present in the healthcare environment is the responsibility of the patient care technician.

Needle Sticks and Pathogen Exposure

Needle sticks are another source of potential injury to healthcare personnel. Intravenous tubing and accessories that do not require needles are available, thus reducing the risk of needle sticks. Needle sticks can be further reduced by never recapping needles and following proper disposal of needles into sharps containers after use. A stray needle lying in bed linens or carelessly thrown into a wastebasket is a prime source of exposure to blood-borne pathogens. Many facilities use safety devices that prevent the need to recap needles (Fig. 10.1). Blood-borne diseases that can be transmitted through accidental needle sticks include hepatitis B and C and human immunodeficiency virus (HIV). Current guidelines and recommendations by the CDC and OSHA related to safety needle devices have dramatically reduced the number of HCW needle stick injuries. Studies by the CDC indicate a 95% reduction in HCWs infected with hepatitis B (HBV) from needle sticks from 1983 to 2001; 400 HCWs were infected in 2001 compared with 17,000 in 1983. The CDC reports the number of hepatitis C (HCV)–related HCW needle stick infections is unknown. They do report that the prevalence rate of HCV in HCWs is similar to the general population (1% to 2%) and that the risk of an HCW becoming infected with HCV from a needle stick is 1.8%. Also, the chance of an HCW becoming infected with HIV from a sharps injury is 0.03%. There were 58 documented cases and 150

Box 10.2 CDC Healthcare Personnel Vaccination Recommendations

Hepatitis B: Give 3-dose series (dose 1 now; dose 2 in 1 month; dose 3 approximately 5 months after dose 2). Give intramuscularly (IM). Obtain anti-HBVs serologic testing 1 to 2 months after dose 3.

Influenza: Give 1 dose of influenza vaccine annually. Give inactivated injectable influenza vaccine intramuscularly or live attenuated influenza vaccine (LAIV) intranasally.

Measles, mumps, and rubella (MMR): For healthcare personnel (HCP) born in 1957 or later without serologic evidence of immunity or prior vaccination, give 2 doses of MMR, 4 weeks apart. For HCP born before 1957, see below. Give subcutaneously (SC).

Varicella: For HCP who have no serologic proof of immunity, prior vaccination, or history of varicella disease (*chickenpox*), give 2 doses of varicella vaccine, 4 weeks apart. Give SC.

Tetanus, diphtheria, Pertussis: Give a one-time dose of Tdap as soon as feasible to all HCP who have not received Tdap previously. Give Td boosters every 10 years thereafter. Give IM.

Meningococcal: Give 1 dose to microbiologists who are routinely exposed to isolates of *Neisseria meningitidis*. Give IM or SC.

Hepatitis A, typhoid, and polio vaccines are not routinely recommended for HCP. http://www.cdc.gov/vaccines/adults/rec-vac/hcw.html

---

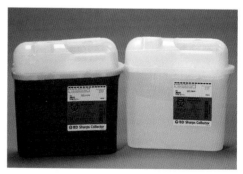

FIGURE 10.1 Needle disposal systems reduce the risk of accidental injury while removing the needle. (From Bonewit-West K: *Clinical procedures for medical assistants*, ed 7, St. Louis, 2008, Saunders.)

possible cases of HIV among HCWs from sharps injury (puncture or cut) between 1981 and 2013 (CDC, 2016).

Fire Safety

Between the years of 2006 and 2010, more than 6000 healthcare facility fires required fire department intervention. Almost half were in long-term care facilities, and one quarter were in hospitals. Of these fires, 6 deaths and 171 injuries occurred, with cooking equipment being the primary cause of fires. Fortunately, only 4% of fires spread from the room where the fire originated (Ahrens, 2012).

An established fire safety program is mandatory for all healthcare facilities (Box 10.3). Most facilities have a safety committee that is actively involved in establishing and monitoring prevention and fire education programs. Fire prevention includes good housekeeping, maintenance, and employee discipline (Box 10.4).

Housekeeping responsibilities include eliminating all unnecessary combustible material, and maintenance responsibilities include ensuring the proper functioning of fire protection devices, such as alarms, extinguishers, and sprinklers. It is mandatory to identify, light, and unlock exits. Cooking and laundry equipment, filters, and air ducts are to be kept free of lint and grease. It is required that a facility must inspect and maintain all mechanical and electrical equipment and outlets regularly to keep fire hazards to a minimum.

All employees need to know the telephone number or procedure for reporting a fire, and the location of the nearest alarms and firefighting equipment. In addition,

---

Box 10.3   Fire Safety Interventions and Safe Evacuation of Patients

Action (Rationale)

I. Follow facility fire plan in the event of a fire. *(Fire plan outlines procedures to follow.)*
   A. If you can, determine patient's age, sensory impairments, level of mobility, ability to comprehend instructions, and overall need for protection.
   B. Receive from the nurse the type of evacuation assistance needed.
   C. Provide clear explanations to patients and visitors in a calm manner.
   D. Assist with evacuations if needed:
      1. Usually patients are moved horizontally (e.g., out of rooms, across halls, and through the next set of fire doors). *(The fire and its potential for spreading often necessitate movement to a safer area. Some agencies have fire doors that are normally held open by magnets and close automatically when a fire alarm sounds. It is important to keep equipment away from these doors.)*
      2. If smoke or fire prevents you from moving patients across the hall, proceed vertically down to a lower level. **Never use elevators as an exit route. A fire spreads very quickly up through the elevator shaft.**
      3. If a patient cannot walk or be moved by bed, stretcher, or wheelchair from the fire area, the patient must often be carried. *(Use the carrying method that is safe for both you and the patient; fire department personnel will help with the evacuation.)*

4. Infant and child removal
   a. Place a blanket or sheet on floor.
   b. Place two infants in each bassinet, using diapers or small blankets for padding.
   c. Place the bassinet in the middle of the blanket.
   d. Use the baby vest if available or fold the blanket over one end, fold the corners in, and then roll the sides in to form a pocket.
   e. Grasp the folded corners of the blanket and pull the infants to safety. Two people (or, if necessary, one person) are able to drag eight babies to the prescribed area.
   f. Alternatively, place as many children as possible in one crib and pull the crib to the prescribed area.
5. Universal carry: The universal carry is a method of removing a patient from a bed to the floor. It is a quick and effective method for removing a patient who is in immediate danger. This carry can be used by anyone, regardless of patient size.
   a. Spread a blanket, sheet, or bedspread on the floor alongside the bed, placing one third of it under the bed and leaving about 8 inches to extend beyond the patient's head.
   b. Grasp the patient's ankles, and move the patient's legs until they fall at the knee over the edge of the bed.
   c. Grasp each shoulder, slowing pulling the patient to a sitting position.

Box 10.3	Fire Safety Interventions and Safe Evacuation of Patients—cont'd

d. From the back, encircle the patient with your arms, place your arms under the patient's armpits, and lock your hands over the patient's chest.

e. Slide the patient slowly to the edge of the bed, and lower the patient to the blanket. If the bed is high, instruct the patient to slide down one of your legs.

f. Taking care to protect the patient's head, gently lower the head and upper torso to the blanket and wrap the blanket around the patient.

g. At the patient's head, grip the blanket with both hands, one above each shoulder, holding the patient's head firmly in the 8 inches of blanket. Do not let the patient's head snap back.

h. Lift the patient to a half-sitting position, and pull the blanketed patient to safety.

6. Blanket drag

7. If vertical or downward evacuation by an interior stairway is necessary, in many cases one person can handle a helpless patient by using the blanket drag.

a. Double a blanket lengthwise, and place it on the floor parallel and next to the bed, leaving 8 inches to extend above the patient's head.

b. Using cradle drop, kneel drop, universal carry, or other suitable means, remove the patient from the bed to the folded blanket on the floor alongside the bed.

c. Grasp the blanket above the patient's head and pull to the stairway; start down the stairs with patient coming headfirst onto the stairway.

d. Position yourself one, two, or three steps lower than the patient, depending on your height and the patient's height. The patient's lower body inclines upward.

e. Place your arms under the patient's arms, and clasp your hands over the patient's chest.

f. Back slowly down the stairs, constantly maintaining close contact with the patient, keeping one leg against the patient's back.

8. When considering the two-person swing, and all evacuation methods, take into consideration the patient's size and weight (see Fig. 10.3).

a. Two staff members grasp each other's forearms to form a seat for the patient to sit in.

b. Other personnel lift the patient into the seat formed and patient is removed from area.

II. Follow-up

A. Listen to the "All clear" announcement after a drill or follow specific instructions from the fire department or supervisor regarding the return of patients. ("This area is safe for patients and staff.")

B. Reduce the potential for fire-related injuries by doing the following:

1. Follow and enforce the smoking policy. Most facilities have adopted a *No Smoking* policy to promote a smoke-free environment for patients and employees.

2. Know the location of fire alarm boxes and type of fire extinguishers available.

3. Know the location of the fire exits.

4. Be familiar with the hospital fire safety program and protocols for evacuation.

5. Keep hallways free of unnecessary supplies, furniture, and other obstacles.

6. Check to see that electrical equipment is operating safely. *(Planning saves valuable time and improves overall performance.)*

C. Participate, when possible, in fire drills. Fire safety education programs are necessary to meet the requirements of accrediting agencies, such as The Joint Commission.

III. Evaluation

A. The immediate environment of the patient is safe from potential fire hazards.

B. In the event of a fire, established procedures are followed.

HCWs must know their roles in the overall hospital evacuation plan. Checking for fire hazards on an ongoing basis is a must and should be a part of the facility's ongoing quality improvement plan.

An important element in any fire safety program is an understanding of what type of fire extinguisher to use on different types of fires. Use the appropriate fire extinguisher for each type of fire:

- Paper, wood, and cloth fires require a type A fire extinguisher.
- Flammable liquid fires, such as those caused by grease and anesthetics, require a type B fire extinguisher.
- Electrical fires require a type C fire extinguisher.
- Fire extinguishers marked ABC are acceptable for use on any type of fire.

Knowledge of which type of extinguisher is on the unit before a fire occurs is vital. Most fire safety programs afford HCWs the opportunity to handle the different types of fire extinguishers.

Certain areas of the healthcare facility require additional fire safety programs and precautions. Fire and smoke inhalation are potential problems associated with the use of lasers in surgery and with oxygen therapy. Other common ignition sources in the operating area are electric cautery equipment and high-intensity light cords. In the event of a fire, patients receiving life-support systems may need manual respiratory support with an Ambu bag.

By remembering the formula RACE (Rescue patients, sound the Alarm, Confine the fire, and Extinguish or Evacuate), the patient care technician is prepared when safety is threatened by fire. In the event of fire, rescue patients in *immediate* danger, and then follow the facility's procedure for activating the fire alarm and reporting the location and extent of the fire. Measures are then taken to contain or extinguish the fire if no immediate threat to safety exists. These measures include closing doors and windows, turning off oxygen and electrical equipment, and using the appropriate fire extinguisher (Fig. 10.2). The mnemonic PASS (Pull the pin, Aim low, Squeeze handle, Sweep the unit) will help the patient care technician remember how to operate the fire extinguisher (see Box 10.4).

Enforcement of the facility's smoking policy and monitoring for potential electrical hazards help prevent fires. Frayed or broken electrical cords or a faulty piece of equipment should never be used. Notify the maintenance department of any defects in the equipment, and report any shocks felt while using equipment. The HCW must enforce no smoking policies. If you find that a patient or family member is smoking in the patient's room, report it directly and immediately to the nurse. The safety of patients and caregivers depends on the staff's knowledge of fire prevention guidelines and fire procedures (see Box 10.3).

Laser Beam Safety

The increased use of lasers in the healthcare setting requires specific safety precautions because a laser has

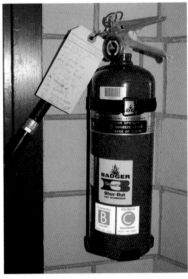

FIGURE 10.2 Fire extinguisher. (From VanMeter KC, VanMeter WG, Huber RJ: *Microbiology for the healthcare professional*, ed 2, St. Louis, 2016, Mosby.)

Box 10.4	Fire Prevention Guidelines for Patient Care Technicians

- Keep the phone number for reporting fires visible on the telephone at all times.
- Know the agency's fire drill and evacuation plan.
- Know the location of all fire alarms, exits, and fire extinguishers.
- Use the mnemonic *RACE* to set priorities in case of fire:
  - **R** Rescue and remove all patients in immediate danger.
  - **A** Activate the alarm. Always do this before attempting to extinguish even a minor fire.
  - **C** Confine the fire by closing doors and windows and turning off all oxygen and electrical equipment.
  - **E** Extinguish the fire using an extinguisher.
- Memorize the mnemonic *PASS* to operate the fire extinguisher:
  - **P** Pull the pin to unlock the handle.
  - **A** Aim low at the base of the fire.
  - **S** Squeeze the handle.
  - **S** Sweep the unit from side to side.

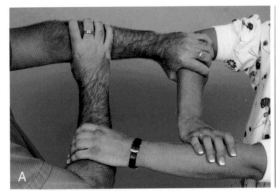
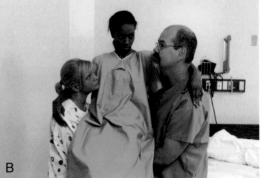

FIGURE 10.3 The two-person evacuation carry. A, Hands positioned to form two-person evacuation swing. B, Patient is seated firmly on swing and holds healthcare workers by shoulders for emergency evacuation. (From Cooper K, Gosnell K: *Foundations of nursing*, ed 7, St. Louis, 2015, Mosby.)

the potential to cause skin and eye injury and start a fire if used incorrectly. Therefore eye protection is necessary for the patient and the staff working with the laser. Personnel involved with laser-based procedures wear specially designed eyewear. Because a laser beam gives out an enormous amount of energy, dry substances that are combustible, meaning that they are able to start a fire, can accidentally ignite, posing a threat to the patient and staff. Ensure that water and a halon fire extinguisher are readily available. For prevention of injury to patients, staff, and equipment, sufficient and appropriate fire extinguishers must be located in magnetic resonance imaging (MRI) areas.

Accidental Poisoning

The CDC defines a poison as "any substance that is harmful to your body when ingested (eaten), inhaled, injected, or absorbed through the skin. Any substance can be poisonous if too much is taken." Poisoning (refers to the condition or physical state produced by the ingestion, injection, inhalation, or exposure of a poisonous [toxic] substance) continues to be an issue in the United States. According to the CDC (2016), in 2011, unintentional poisoning took over the first place for being the leading cause of unintentional injury deaths in all age groups, with motor vehicle fatalities coming in as second. Eighty-two percent of all unintentional poisonings are related to drugs (both over-the-counter and prescription drugs). Although legislation passed in the early 1970s required the use of child safety packaging for certain substances, a significant number of accidental poisonings continue to occur. Companies are now producing bottles that are easier to open, for those who suffer from arthritis and may not have a strong grip. This makes it easier for the child to access, whereas in the past the safety lids made it more difficult for the bottle to be opened. Emergency department visits for medication poisoning are twice as common as household substance poisonings among children. One of every 180 visits to the emergency department by 2-year-olds is for medication poisoning (CDC, 2014). Specific poisoning-reversal substances such as activated charcoal and some medications such as Mucomyst or Narcan are antidotes and are available for certain types of poisons. Note that syrup of ipecac is no longer recommended for use (see Injury & Illness Prevention Box 10.2 on the nonuse of ipecac).

The older adult is also at risk. Changes that occur with aging interfere with the individual's ability to absorb and excrete drugs. Some older adults share medications with friends or limit their medications because of the cost associated with buying them. Changes in vision sometimes lead to an accidental ingestion. If elderly patients have any memory impairment, they are likely to forget when they last took either prescribed or over-the-counter medication.

Injury & Illness Prevention Box 10.2

The Nonuse of Ipecac at Home

The National Capital Poison Center states the following:
- The American Academy of Pediatrics and the American Association of Poison Control Centers recommend that ipecac syrup not be kept in homes for available use.
- The U.S. Food and Drug Administration (FDA) is considering making ipecac syrup available to the public by prescription only.
- Most pharmacies no longer carry ipecac syrup.
- The first action recommended in the event of ingestion of a poison is to call the poison control center at 1-800-222-1222.

(Data from National Capital Poison Control Center: Ipecac syrup. *Retrieved from www.poison.org/prepared/ipecac.asp.)*

Hospitalized patients and those in other types of healthcare facilities are at risk for accidental poisoning because of poisonous substances in the environment. Cleaning solutions and disinfectants must be properly labeled and stored. To prevent poisoning, toxic agents are removed from areas where accidental poisoning is possible. Do not remove toxic or poisonous substances from their original containers because incorrect labeling is one of the likely results, and never use substances from unmarked containers.

DISASTER PLANNING

Disaster planning, or emergency preparedness, enables rescuers to respond effectively and efficiently when confronted with a disaster situation. A disaster situation is an uncontrollable, unexpected, psychologically shocking event that is unique and likely to have a significant impact on a variety of healthcare facilities. Examples of natural threats to safety are earthquakes, hurricanes, floods, and tornados. Bombings, arson, riots, shootings, and hostage-taking represent acts of violence carried out by people always affect a facility's day-to-day operations.

Factors that affect disaster response include the time of the day; the scope and duration of the triggering event; readiness of the healthcare facility, personnel, and equipment; preparations for appropriate procedures; and the degree to which the various community agencies and institutions work together with one another. Healthcare facilities are expected to receive victims and survivors and to assist rescuers.

Disasters are referred to as either external or internal. The external disaster originates outside the healthcare facility and results in an increased number of patients being brought to the facility (e.g., an explosion in a chemical plant, a tornado, a train accident). The emergency department is the main focus of activity. Typically, no immediate safety threat to staff, patients, or hospital property exists.

The internal disaster represents an extraordinary situation that is brought about by events within the healthcare facility, such as a fire. In many cases, the organization's ability to function normally is threatened. An internal disaster has the ability to threaten the safety of patients, visitors, staff, and facility property.

Disaster planning consists of putting appropriate measures into place to ensure that healthcare facilities and personnel have the capacity to manage a disaster effectively (Box 10.5 and Box 10.6). Most state and federal regulators require disaster drills to be conducted routinely to prepare healthcare facilities and personnel to be able to respond to such a disaster in an organized way. All staff must be familiar with the location and the contents of the facility's disaster manual (sometimes called the emergency response plan or emergency management plan). This manual specifies chain of command (who makes the decisions), callback procedures, assignment procedures, departmental responsibilities, patient evacuation procedure and routes, procedures for the receipt and management of casualties (how to count and keep record of which patients have come in, living or nonliving), and policies related to the overall management of supplies and equipment. Supplies and equipment can become exhausted in a short time during a disaster, so it is important to have a plan in place for extra resources should one hospital run out. An example is ventilators, also known as a breathing machine. A

Box 10.5   Disaster Planning Interventions

1. **Planning**
   a. Review facility disaster plan frequently to update knowledge. The development of the disaster preparedness plan is an evolving and ongoing process. The purpose of disaster preparedness planning is to prepare the facility and healthcare workers for both external and internal disasters.
   b. Know your own particular responsibilities in a disaster emergency.
   c. Participate, when possible, in disaster drills. Learning experiences are provided through disaster drills and formal critiques of the responses. Disaster drills may be initiated on a particular nursing unit, facility wide, community wide, or even state wide.
   d. Participation in a crisis support group is desirable if directly involved in a disaster or a disaster response. Individuals often experience some level of emotional or critical incident stress.
2. **Follow facility disaster plan in the event of a disaster.**
   a. Identify the type of disaster emergency by recognizing the code that is used to announce it.

   b. Identify each patient's age, sensory impairments, level of mobility, ability to comprehend instructions, and overall need for protection. Your nurse can provide this information to you if you do not know it.
   c. Provide clear explanations to patients and visitors in a calm manner if directed to do so by the nurse.
   d. If a disaster occurs when you are off duty, follow your facility protocols for reporting in (i.e., some facilities require you to report for duty at your regularly scheduled times, whereas others require you to contact your manager for instruction). Community agencies and resources are incorporated into the overall plan.
   e. If an internal disaster occurs, assist with planned evacuations as needed.
   f. Listen for the "All clear" announcement after a disaster drill. This indicates that the drill is over.
3. **Evaluation.** The healthcare team will typically have an evaluation of how the team did with carrying out the plan. This is where you will identify what worked well and what did not work, and how changes can be made in preparation for the next disaster.

Box 10.6   Variations for Disaster Planning: Nursing Home

Nursing home residents also sometimes need evacuation and relocation in the case of an internal disaster. The successful nursing home disaster preparedness plan, like those for hospitals, outlines the sequence of events to be followed:

- Residents need some type of identification (picture identification or identification bracelet, such as those used in the memory support unit for patients found to have Alzheimer's disease).
- At the designated triage site, nurses decide where residents will go.

- Residents sometimes need admission to a hospital or other building, such as a school or church, for temporary shelter and care.
- The disaster plan must include instructions and guidelines for what is to be done after the relocation is completed.
- Notification of families and physicians is critical.
- A log is kept to document events. List the name of the patient, who transported the patient and how, and where the patient was sent so that family and physicians are aware of the patient's location and transfers as they occur.

hospital typically has an inventory of only a certain quantity. If there is a large disaster that involved an alteration in breathing, and many required ventilators to live, the facility could quickly run out of their stock. It is necessary to know this information ahead of time so that there is planning for where additional pieces of equipment such as ventilators could be located.

Various codes (a system of notification to be delivered rapidly) are used by healthcare facilities to alert personnel to the various emergencies affecting the facility. All personnel in a healthcare facility must be knowledgeable of the code system and how to act in response to codes. This may include providing your contact phone numbers so that you can be reached in the case of an emergency situation such as a disaster. Some facilities require all levels of care, including the patient care technician, to respond to a disaster by coming back to work, regardless of whether it is your scheduled day or not. Responding to a disaster often requires the help of the entire healthcare team in order to provide care to the increased numbers of those injured or sick.

TERRORISM

Terrorism, or the possibility of a terrorist attack, is viewed as an environmental health threat. Terrorism is a violent or dangerous act used to intimidate or coerce a person or government to further a political or social agenda. Before 1990 and the Gulf War, the possibility of the United States coming under attack from terrorist groups using biological, chemical, or nuclear weapons seemed remote. After the terrorist attacks on the World Trade Center in New York City and the Pentagon on September 11, 2001, the government implemented the Homeland Security Act of 2002. Its purpose was to have a single agency to oversee the development of a comprehensive approach to a large domestic incident. The Department of Homeland Security is primarily concerned with preventing and managing potential attacks by an individual or small group on one of our cities, a large sporting event, a school, or a unit of our military forces.

Bioterrorism

Bioterrorism is the use of biologic agents to create fear and threat. Healthcare facilities must be prepared to treat mass casualties from such an attack. A facility's emergency management plan provides details on how to respond to a terrorist attack: for example, determining the agent used, determining the time and location of the attack and the affected population, obtaining and delivering supplies, and providing treatment. Education and training is required to prepare all staff to respond to an attack by taking the necessary steps to initiate an agency's emergency management plan.

Terrorism by Nuclear Exposure

One example of how the threat of nuclear terrorism will possibly manifest is an attack on a domestic nuclear weapon facility. Another is the use of a so-called "dirty bomb," which is a radiation-dispersal device that joins nuclear waste with a conventional bomb.

A patient is contaminated by radiation from a source on the body or the clothing, from ingesting it, or by absorbing it through a skin opening. The effects on the patient are determined by the amount of radiation absorbed (absorbed radiation is measured in grays [Gy]; 1 Gy = 100 rads). When less than 0.75 Gy is absorbed, patients usually do not have any symptoms. Patients who absorb 8 Gy usually die, and an absorption of 30 Gy is always fatal.

Death typically occurs from infection or other complications related to the exposure. OSHA requires that hospitals have an emergency plan for treating patients contaminated with radioactive substances. A decontamination unit is set up near the emergency department.

Active Shooters

The U.S. Department of Homeland Security has issued guidelines to follow if and when there is an active shooter in a healthcare facility. Your facility may have specific policies and procedures, so be sure to review that information when you begin working. It does no good to look for the information once you are in the middle of an active shooter situation. It pays to be informed, and can save lives.

The RUN-HIDE-FIGHT initiative was developed by the U.S. Department of Homeland Security and focuses on how to remove yourself from the situation if possible. The following information is taken from www.dhs.gov. If you find yourself in an active shooter situation, the first thing you want to do is to remain calm. Avoid screaming or yelling if possible. Follow these guidelines:

RUN: Have an escape route and plan in mind. Leave your belongings behind. Keep your hands visible. If you are in an office or patient room, stay there and close the door. Lock it if possible.

HIDE: Hide in an area out of the shooter's view. Block entry to your hiding place and lock the doors. Silence your cell phone and/or pager.

FIGHT: Only as a last resort and when your life is in imminent danger will you fight. Act with physical aggression and throw items at the shooter. Call 911 when it is safe to do so.

BODY MECHANICS

Healthcare personnel must learn and practice proper principles of body mechanics to prevent injury to themselves and injury to their patients. When assisting patients with mobility, patient care technicians must be constantly aware of their own body mechanics. According to the Bureau of Labor Statistics (www.bls.gov), nursing personnel (which includes unlicensed assistive personnel [UAP], such as certified nurse assistants [CNAs], patient care technicians, and orderlies, rank second in the number of occupational injuries requiring days away from work. Nurses fall just below the top five occupations that require days away from work because of injuries. The vast majority of these injuries are classified as **musculoskeletal disorders (MSDs),** with back injuries prominent among healthcare personnel.

Most injuries occur when nursing personnel perform tasks that require repetitive movement, uncomfortable posture, and exertion to assist patients in activities such as feeding, dressing, bathing, toileting, repositioning, and ambulation. Awareness of proper ergonomic principles (ergonomics is the science of matching workplace conditions and job demands to the capabilities of workers, especially in regard to MSDs and their prevention) and good body mechanics help prevent injury.

Mechanical lifting devices (sling and standing lifts) and assistive patient-handling equipment, such as roller boards, sliders, friction-reduction pads, transfer chairs, and gait belts, work by taking on the energy and force that otherwise are imposed on the patient care technician's body during the lifting, transferring, or repositioning of a patient. Regular use of lifts and other assistive devices reduces the risk of injury.

Safe patient transfer requires adequate staffing, the right mix of personnel, and appropriate, readily available, well-maintained patient-lifting equipment. The patient care technician is responsible for being competent in the appropriate and safe use of equipment and proper use of assistive devices.

Use of Appropriate Body Mechanics

Understanding **body mechanics** (the area of physiology for the study of muscle action and how muscles function in maintaining the posture of the body and prevention of injury during activity) includes knowledge of how certain muscle groups are used. The patient care technician uses body mechanics daily while making beds, assisting the patient to walk, carrying supplies and equipment, lifting, providing patient care, and carrying out other procedures.

To prevent an injury to the patient care technician and the patient, principles of body mechanics for HCWs (Table 10.1) should be followed by all healthcare professionals and personnel. The appropriate use of body mechanics should consistently be practiced in the workplace and in one's personal life so that MSDs do not occur. Maintenance of appropriate body alignment is the key factor in proper body mechanics. The term alignment refers to the relationship of various body parts to each other. Alignment assists with balance and helps coordinate movements smoothly and effectively.

Maintenance of a wide base of support (a stance with feet shoulder-width apart) when standing is one of the basic concepts of good body mechanics and alignment that should be followed because it helps in providing better stability (Fig. 10.4). Better stability prevents the patient care technician from losing proper balance while carrying out patient care, which could result in strain or injury to muscles.

The skeletal muscles and the nervous system maintain equilibrium, or balance, which facilitates appropriate

Table 10.1	Body Mechanics for Healthcare Workers

Action	Rationale
When planning to move a patient, arrange for adequate help. Use mechanical aids if help is unavailable.	Two workers lifting together divide the workload by 50%.
Encourage patient to assist as much as possible.	This promotes patient's abilities and strength while keeping workload to a minimum.
Keep back, neck, pelvis, and feet aligned. Avoid twisting.	Twisting increases risk of injury.
Flex knees; keep feet shoulder length apart.	A broad base of support increases stability.
Position yourself close to patient (or object being lifted).	This minimizes strain and undue stress on the lifter. Holding an object or patient away from the body increases the workload.
Use arms and legs (not back).	The leg muscles are stronger larger muscles capable of greater work without injury.
Slide patient toward yourself using a pull sheet.	Sliding requires less effort than lifting. Pull sheet keeps to a minimum any shearing forces, which can damage patient's skin.
Set (tighten) abdominal and gluteal muscles in preparation for move.	Preparing muscles for the load limits strain to the least possible level.
Person with the heaviest load coordinates efforts of team involved by counting to 3.	Simultaneous lifting keeps the load for any one lifter to a minimum.

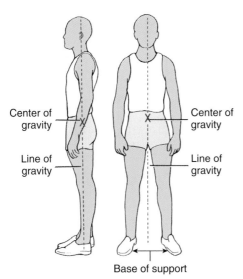

FIGURE 10.4 Good position for body mechanics: chin is high and parallel to the floor, abdomen is tightened (internal girdle) in and up with gluteal muscles tucked in, and feet are spread apart for a broad base of support. (From Potter PA, Perry AG, Stocket PA, et al.: *Fundamentals of nursing: concepts, process, and practice*, ed 9, St. Louis, 2017, Mosby.)

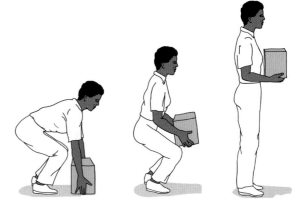

FIGURE 10.5 Picking up a box with use of good body mechanics. Box is carried close to the person's body and base of support. (From Sorrentino SA, Remmert LN: *Mosby's essentials for nursing assistants*, ed 5, St. Louis, 2014, Mosby.)

body alignment when lifting, bending, moving, and performing other activities. Bending one's knees and hips before attempting these activities protects the back from the stress and potential injury inherent in the physical work of nursing. When stooping, the hips and knees should be flexed or bent and appropriate body alignment maintained (i.e., the back kept straight). Bending from the waist should be avoided because this will, in time, strain the lower back (Fig. 10.5). The patient care technician should work at a height or level that is comfortable to help prevent undue stress and strain on the back muscles. This can be easily accomplished by adjusting the height of the bed to a level appropriate for the patient care technician's height.

Use of large muscle groups (such as arm and shoulder muscles, hips, and thigh muscles) helps in performing a bigger workload more safely. The more muscle groups used, the more evenly the workload is distributed. If the base of support is widened in the direction of movement, less effort is needed to carry out an activity. To avoid twisting the spine, the patient care technician should stand directly in front of the person or object being worked with.

Patient care technicians have numerous other ways to protect themselves and the patient from injury. Carrying objects close to the midline of the body (see Fig. 10.5), avoiding reaching too far, avoiding lifting when other means of movement are available (such as sliding, rolling, pushing, or pulling), using devices instead of or in combination with lifting, and using alternating periods of rest and activity are just a few of the ways to prevent injury. Knowing the maximum weight that is safe to carry is also important. Many facilities suggest a 50-lb weight limit on lifting for their staff. If you have a need to lift an item that is heavier than the 50-lb weight limit, it is appropriate for you to seek help from a peer. It is important that each member of the healthcare team maintain proper body mechanics throughout the lifting to avoid injury.

Patient care technicians should assess their own abilities and limitations and those of the person helping when working in pairs. Correct use of body mechanics is required to provide good care while preventing injury (Table 10.1).

CHAPTER SUMMARY

Discuss safety measures for coping with violence in the workplace. Prevention of falls, electrical injuries, fires, burns, and accidental poisoning is key to maintaining a safe environment. Electrical accidents are often prevented by reporting frayed or broken electrical cords or any shocks felt when using equipment. Fire-related injuries can be reduced by knowing the location of exits, fire alarm boxes, and fire extinguishers. By remembering the formula RACE (**R**escue patients, sound the **A**larm, **C**onfine the fire, and **E**xtinguish or **E**vacuate), you will be prepared when safety is threatened by a fire. Participation in fire and disaster drills helps staff become familiar with established protocols.

A terrorist attack is a potential environmental health threat. Follow the RUN-HIDE-FIGHT plan if ever in an active shooter situation. Bioterrorism, or the use of biologic agents to create fear and threat, is the most likely form a terrorist attack will take.

Protection of the musculoskeletal system is essential to prevent injury to both patient and patient care technician. Less effort is needed to carry out an activity if the base of support is widened in the direction of movement. Appropriate body mechanics should be practiced consistently. Maintenance of correct body alignment is the key to proper body mechanics. Correct body alignment promotes balance and helps coordinate movements. Permanent disability can occur from inappropriate positioning.

Case Scenario

The patient care technician enters the patient's room to answer the call bell and sees the patient frantically pointing to the trashcan next to the bed. The patient care technician sees a burning cigarette in the trashcan that has now created small flames. What should the first action of the patient care technician be? Describe in order the steps that should be taken next. How can this be prevented in the future?

REVIEW QUESTIONS

1. The patient care technician discovers smoke in a soiled utility room across the hall from a patient's room. What should the patient care technician's initial action be?
   a. Sound the fire alarm
   b. Disconnect the oxygen supply
   c. Use any extinguisher on the fire
   d. Remove the patient from the area

2. A type C fire extinguisher is required for which type of fire?
   a. Paper
   b. Cloth
   c. Grease
   d. Electrical

3. During the 7 AM to 3 PM shift on the adult surgical unit, the code is announced for an external disaster emergency. Which event best represents this type of situation?
   a. A school bus accident
   b. A bomb threat in the mail room
   c. A hostage-taking event in the emergency department
   d. An electrical fire in the maintenance department

4. The patient accidentally knocks the emesis basin to the floor. When picking up the emesis basin, which movement demonstrates proper body mechanics by the patient care technician (PCT)?
   a. The PCT lowers the body by flexing the knees and bending the hips.
   b. The PCT bends from the waist and hips.
   c. The PCT flexes the knees and bends at the waist.
   d. The PCT keeps the legs straight and flexes the waist.

5. A 72-year-old patient with a stroke has slid to the foot of the bed. With use of appropriate body mechanics, the patient care technician maintains a wide base of support and faces the patient in the direction of movement. What do these actions allow the patient care technician to do?
   a. Use the back muscles
   b. Use the large muscles across the scapula
   c. Exert less physical effort
   d. Use the gluteal muscles

6. The student nurse demonstrated principles of good body mechanics with which activity?
   a. Keeping the knees in a locked position
   b. Maintaining a wide base of support and bending at the knees
   c. Bending at the waist to maintain one's balance
   d. Holding objects away from the body for improved leverage

Patient Safety

LEARNING OBJECTIVES

1. Identify safety precautions that help to prevent falls.
2. Relate specific safety considerations to the developmental age and needs of individuals across the life span.
3. Identify tasks that are appropriate for individuals across the life span to ensure a safe environment.
4. Describe safe and appropriate methods for the application of safety reminder devices when caring for patients.
5. Discuss how the patient care technician can promote a restraint-free environment.
6. Discuss safety concerns in the healthcare environment.

KEY TERMS

fear of retribution Having a fear of being punished.
safety reminder device (SRD) Formerly referred to as restraints.
sentinel event Any unexpected occurrence involving death or serious physical or psychological injury, or the risk thereof.

Safety of the patient is a primary concern of the health-care team. Ensuring a safe physical environment and helping patients feel safe in their environment are goals for patient care technicians (PCTs) practicing within a healthcare facility. Numerous factors can endanger the patient's physical and psychological safety. This chapter looks at potential threats to a patient's safety in various environments and how the PCT can meet the safety needs of the patient.

SAFETY IN THE HOSPITAL OR HEALTHCARE ENVIRONMENT

Traditionally, the patient's overall safety in the hospital or other healthcare environment has been a primary concern of nursing. Today, the focus on a safe environment has expanded to include all the individuals that come in contact with patients, as we have come to recognize and identify potential hazards and threats faced by hospital personnel, patients, and visitors (Box 11.1).

Box 11.1 Precautions to Promote Safety

- Orient patient to the environment to provide familiarity.
- Place bedside table and overbed table within reach. Ensure that frequently used items, such as the telephone, eyeglasses, or other personal belongings, are easily accessible.
- Assist patients when they get out of bed if they have had surgery, received narcotics for analgesia, have an unsteady gait, or have been in bed for an extended period.
- Keep environment free of clutter because such items as books, magazines, and shoes sometimes cause the patient to trip and fall.
- Follow facility policies regarding the use of side rails.
- Keep adjustable beds in the low position except when giving care.
- If bed is equipped with an alarm, turn on for the restless, disoriented patient.
- Lock wheels on beds, wheelchairs, and gurneys.
- Encourage patients to wear nonslip slippers or shoes when ambulating.
- Wipe or mop up spilled liquids promptly. Personnel and patients all need to be alert to signs warning of wet or slippery floors.
- Encourage the use of hand rails in the bathrooms and halls.
- Provide adequate lighting.
- Demonstrate the proper use of emergency call buttons or cords.
- Instruct patient to use the call bell for assistance.
- Some institutions have adopted "fall precaution" policies in which every patient is evaluated on admission to determine the degree of likelihood for a potential fall (see Box 11.2).

A safe environment implies freedom from injury with focus on helping to prevent falls, electrical injuries, fires, burns, and poisoning. The PCT must be alert to potential safety problems and must know how to report and respond when safety is threatened.

Providing and maintaining a safe environment involves the patient, visitors, and members of the healthcare team. Protection and education are primary responsibilities of the healthcare team. It is up to each member to do his or her part in protecting the patient from harm. Checking to see that the call light or signal system is working and accessible is an example of how the PCT helps maintain a safe environment.

Each year, The Joint Commission releases and evaluates national patient safety goals for healthcare facilities. These goals are developed from a review of various national databases and assist facilities in identifying keys elements for maintaining patient safety. A component of these goals includes the identification of sentinel events. The Joint Commission defines a sentinel event as "any unexpected occurrence involving death or serious physical or psychological injury, or the risk thereof" (The Joint Commission, n.d.). The reporting of certain sentinel events to The Joint Commission is required, and includes a thorough review of the event (root causes) and the plan for improvements that will prevent the event from occurring again. Examples of sentinel events include medication errors and errors in procedures and treatments that led to the death of an individual and inappropriate application of safety reminder devices (SRDs; formerly referred to as restraints).

Delegation and Documentation Box 11.1

- Always document accurately, even when an error occurs.
- Healthcare institutions should not make you feel scared to admit to making a mistake; this is known as fear of retribution.
- Anytime you make an error, report it to the nurse as soon as possible.

Falls

Falls are a common problem in healthcare facilities, requiring the PCT to be alert to patients who are at an increased risk for falls. A fall risk assessment will be completed by the nurse when the person is admitted to the unit and whenever a significant change in the patient's condition has occurred. A fall risk assessment is necessary on admission to a facility or if a significant change in the patient's condition has occurred. Box 11.2 is a sample list of questions found on a fall risk assessment tool. Note that the nurse will ask these questions to the patient. Facilities require fall precautions if the

Box 11.2	Sample Questions Found on a Fall Risk Assessment Tool

Yes   No

1. Is there a history of a fall(s) in the past year?
2. Does the patient have an unsteady gait or difficulty ambulating?
3. Is the patient receiving any high-risk medications?
4. Does the patient require equipment to assist in ambulating?
5. Does the patient have an altered mental status?
6. Is the patient experiencing blood pressure problems, dizziness, or vertigo?
7. Is the patient age 70 years or above?
8. Does the patient experience bowel or bladder incontinence?
9. Does the patient have an intravenous (IV), chest tube, or oxygen line or attachment to any other tubing?
10. Does the patient have any vision or other sensory problems?

answer is "yes" to a specified number of questions on a fall risk assessment tool. This information will help you to know which patients are at risk for falls. The nurse will also be able to tell the PCT which patients are at risk for falls. Patient falls are a major safety consideration for *all* institutions. The very young and older adults are not the only individuals at risk in the healthcare environment. Individuals who become sick or who are injured are also at risk. Being placed in a strange environment and the various feelings and complaints patients often experience when they are sick may put them more at risk for falls. The use of certain drugs such as anesthesia (drugs that numb you or put you to sleep), sedatives (drugs that relax you), or narcotics (painkillers) increases the risk of falling, as well as being unstable when patients walk or if they have a problem with balance.

Safety Considerations for Infants and Children

Ensuring the safety of infants and children means protecting the child and educating the parents to do so as well. Accidents involving children are largely preventable, so parents and caregivers need to be aware of specific dangers at each stage of growth and development. As the child grows larger and becomes older, the risk for injury changes. Growth and the learning of new motor skills place the child at great risk for injury.

The PCT can assist with educating families about the safety in the home. Many dangers exist in a child's

environment. All household cleaning items are potentially poisonous when swallowed and must be kept out of children's reach. Children cannot read or understand labels on cleaning materials or medication containers. Infants in the oral stage of development put almost anything into their mouths, and as infants learn to crawl, electrical sockets and cords also become a danger. Toddlers and young children can be protected from burns by turning pot handles on a stove away from the child's reach. Bath water can be another potential hazard for children because of the temperature of the water or from leaving children unattended for any length of time. Pool safety should also be emphasized to parents and caregivers. Protecting infants and toddlers from falling out of bed while in the healthcare facility is a concern. Keeping side rails up or using a pediatric crib are safety measures to prevent falls. When giving care, placing the hand on the infant or toddler when turning to obtain supplies prevents the infant or child from falling off a bed or examination table.

Older Adults

Changes associated with aging may significantly affect the ability of older adults to protect themselves from injury (see Injury & Illness Prevention Box 11.1). Unsteady gait, age-related vision changes, and medication side effects (such as vertigo) pose a threat to the older adult's safety. Ensuring that older adults wear their eyeglasses and hearing aids and use assistive devices for ambulating when necessary are important nursing interventions to promote patient safety.

Assisting weak or disoriented older patients when drinking hot liquids such as soups, coffee, or tea can prevent burns. People in this age group are more vulnerable to burns from spilled hot liquids and from heating pads and electric blankets.

Safety Reminder Devices

A safety reminder device (SRD) is defined as any of the numerous devices used to immobilize a patient or part of the patient's body, such as arms or hands. Many facilities have adopted a restraint-free environment, thus eliminating the use of any type of SRD. This is especially true in long-term care facilities. The long-term care setting is the permanent home for many residents, so maintaining a safe environment while protecting the individual's dignity is a priority.

The use of SRDs tends to cause increased restlessness, disorientation, agitation, anxiety, and a feeling of powerlessness. These devices may contribute to a patient's inability to walk and increase associated problems with immobility such as dehydration, healthcare-associated infection, and incontinence. Patients often

Injury & Illness Prevention Box 11.1

Physiologic changes in aging increase the need for safety precautions:

- Changes in vision, including altered depth perception, increased sensitivity to glare, and decreased visual acuity in dim light, increase the risk of falls because of misperception of visual cues.
- Changes in hearing, including varying degrees of deafness and tinnitus (ringing in the ears), increase the risk of injury from hazards in the environment because certain warnings that are commonly detected with auditory cues, such as motor vehicle horns, alarms, or even spoken warnings, go unheard.
- Prevent sensory overload (too much stimulation to the senses) in older adults because both reflexes and the ability to respond to multiple stimuli slow with aging.
- Changes in muscle strength and joint function that result in slowed reaction time, altered gait, and altered sense of balance make it more likely that stumbling will result in a fall.
- Changes in the peripheral vascular system sometimes result in loss of sensitivity to heat, cold, or foreign objects, which increases the risk of tissue damage from burns, frostbite, and pressure.

- Older adults take many medications that increase the need for safety precautions. Some of these drugs affect reaction time and increase the risk of injury. Antihypertensives, diuretics, and antihistamines increase the risk of orthostatic hypotension (a drop of 25 mm Hg in systolic pressure and 10 mm Hg in diastolic pressure), which increases the risk of falls.
- Keep to a minimum the use of SRDs with older adults and, when necessary, the amount of any restraint used. SRDs reduce mobility and result in a loss of strength that can increase the risk of falls or injury.
- Accidental poisoning is a significant problem in older adults. Visual changes raise the potential for misreading of labels on medication or other package labels and lead to overdose or other errors in administration. Medication organizers or dispensers help reduce the risk of medication errors in the home. In addition, many older adults do not consider over-the-counter medications to be "real" medicine, so they take them freely and fail to mention them when questioned by the nurse or physician regarding drug use. Many over-the-counter medications increase the risk of injury to the older adult by potentiating or interfering with the effects of prescription drugs.

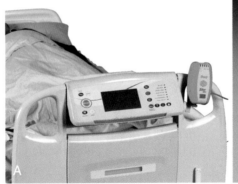 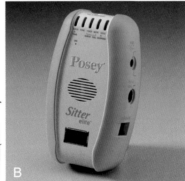

FIGURE 11.1 A, Weight-sensitive alarm. B, Chair alarm. (Courtesy of Posey Company, Arcadia, California.)

pull against the SRDs, causing skin and circulation problems.

SRDs may be used for various reasons and are primarily for considerations of patient safety. Certain groups of patients, such as the disoriented patient, are more likely to need SRDs. This prevents the disoriented patient from wandering and prevents or decreases the risk of the patient falling from a bed, chair, or wheelchair (Fig. 11.1). The patient who is aggressive because of mental health or drug-related issues may also need an SRD. The SRD may be necessary for this type of patient to protect other patients and staff from harm.

An SRD may serve to safeguard the continuity and safety for providing treatment (e.g., the wrist SRD keeps patients from removing intravenous lines, feeding tubes, drainage tubes, or an endotracheal tube when on a ventilator).

When dealing with issues related to the use of SRDs, the focus of patient care is on attempting alternative strategies before turning to the use of these devices (Box 11.3). By determining individual patient needs and looking at what's going on in their environment, the PCT often is able to reduce or eliminate the need for SRDs. Most healthcare facilities have specific policies

---

Box 11.3   Designing a Restraint-Free Environment

Care of the patient who may be prone to threats to safety and security requires a creative, systematic, and attentive approach. A wide variety of electronic devices have been developed to alert staff to a patient's need for assistance. A weight-sensitive alarm can be placed under a patient in bed or in a chair. When the patient tries to get up, an alarm sounds (see Fig. 11.1A). A chair alarm may be used to remind the patient or alert the staff when a patient who requires assistance when standing or ambulating tries to get up without assistance (see Fig. 11.1B).

To design a restraint-free environment:
- Orient patient and family to surroundings; explain all procedures and treatments.
- Encourage family and friends to stay, or use sitters for patients who need supervision.

- Assign confused or disoriented patients to rooms near the nurses' station. Observe these patients frequently.
- Provide appropriate visual and auditory stimuli (e.g., family pictures, clocks, radio).
- Eliminate bothersome treatments as soon as possible. For example, discontinue tube feedings and begin oral feedings as quickly as the patient's condition allows.
- Use relaxation techniques (e.g., massage).
- Institute exercise and ambulation schedules as the patient's condition allows.
- Encourage participation in diversional activities (e.g., long-term care facilities typically have daily activities planned for the residents, such as games, movies, and entertainment).
- Maintain toileting routines.

Box 11.4   Long-Term Care Variations for Safety Reminder Devices

Legislation has greatly affected the use of safety reminder devices (SRDs) in the long-term care facility. Under the Omnibus Budget Reconciliation Act (OBRA) of 1987, residents' rights are specifically addressed in terms of SRDs. This act, effective October 1, 1990, mandates specific guidelines and prohibits routine use of SRDs in long-term care facilities. The act regulates the use of extremity SRDs, hand mitts, safety vests, and wheelchair safety bars. SRDs may be used only to ensure the physical safety of the resident or other residents. A written order by the physician must detail the duration and circumstances under which the SRDs are to be used.

OBRA states the following as acceptable reasons for the use of physical restraints:
- All other interventions have been attempted before the use of restraints.

- Other disciplines have been consulted for their assistance.
- Supporting documentation has been completed.

Essentials of SRD Documentation
- Reason for the physical restraint
- Explanation given to patient and family
- Date and time of the patient's response to treatment
- Duration
- Frequency of observation and patient's response
- Safety
- Release the physical restraint at least every 2 hours
- Routine exercise of extremities, including range-of-motion exercises
- Assessment for circulation and skin integrity
- Assessment for continued need for the physical restraint
- Patient outcome

---

and procedures related to the use of SRDs (Box 11.4), and most require a specific order from a healthcare provider. Some facilities require a healthcare provider order for SRDs be renewed every 24 hours. The nurse will explain to the patient the need for the devices even if the patient does not seem to understand the explanation. Also, the nurse must inform family members about the need for SRDs.

Hourly Rounding

Studies have shown that hourly rounding has decreased the rate at which patients fall. Many falls occur when patients try to ambulate to the bathroom. By asking the patients on an hourly basis whether they have toileting needs, patients are less likely to attempt to get up on their own and perhaps risk falling. The PCT is often responsible for completing the hourly rounding. Many facilities use checklists for the PCT to document that the patient has been rounded on each hour. This checklist may be hand-written and on a clipboard, or may be part of the electronic health record.

The Patient Care Technician as Sitter

There are times when the PCT will serve the role as a sitter during the assigned shift. This may be for an older adult patient who continues to try to get up out of the bed and is not allowed to do so, or this could be for a patient who has exhibited suicidal behaviors. Sometimes the patient who is suicidal will try and convince the person to leave the room, stating that he or she is okay. Under no circumstances is the sitter to leave the patient in the room alone. It is very important that the PCT stay with the patient throughout the shift, only leaving when someone else arrives to cover for the absence.

Delegation and Documentation Box 11.2

Although preventing falls is the responsibility of all caregivers, including unlicensed assistive personnel (UAP) such as the PCT, ultimately, assessment for risk of fall or injury requires the nurse and is not delegated. You need to know the following information from the nurse for those who are at risk for falls.

* The patient's limitations to walking and any specific ways to minimize risks
* Environmental safety precautions (e.g., bed locked and in low position, call bell and personal items within reach, clear pathway in room, nonskid footwear)
* What to do when a patient starts to fall while being assisted with ambulation (i.e., ease patient into a sitting position in a chair or on the floor and alert the nurse)

Monitoring patient behavior for risk of injury and promoting a safe environment is acceptable to delegate as a responsibility of the PCT and of nursing staff. Assessment of a patient's behaviors and decisions about using less restrictive interventions require the critical thinking and knowledge application unique to the nurse. PCTs do not make the decision as to which SRDs should be in place to decrease the patient's risk for falls.

Although the application of SRDs is acceptable to delegate to UAP, assessment of when SRDs are needed and the appropriate type to use requires the nurse and is not delegated. The PCT should have the following information before assisting with any SRDs:
* Correct placement of the SRD
* Observation for constriction of circulation, skin integrity, and adequate breathing
* When and how to change position and provide range-of-motion exercises, skin care, toileting, and opportunities for socialization

---

Radiological and Therapeutic Radiation

Radiation presents a health hazard, if used incorrectly, in healthcare settings and the community. Radiation and radioactive materials are used in the diagnosis and treatment of patients. Hospitals have strict guidelines on the care of patients who are receiving radiation and on the handling of radioactive materials. To reduce the amount of exposure to radiation, the PCT must limit time spent near the source, keep as great a distance from the source as possible, and use shielding devices such as lead aprons. Staff members who work near radiation routinely are required to wear devices that record their cumulative, or total, exposure to radiation. This is usually a type of clip-on plastic device that is attached to the person's shirt or pants. After collection and processing of these devices, those staff members whose radiation exposure readings fall above a set limit are frequently assigned to an alternative work area away from radiation exposure. Follow-up medical attention is often mandated for them as well.

The community is put at risk for radiation exposure if radioactive waste products are disposed of or transported incorrectly. Community health agencies, the Environmental Protection Agency (EPA), the Nuclear Regulatory Commission (NRC), the Department of Energy (DOE), and the Department of Transportation (DOT) have established specific, strict guidelines for the disposal of radioactive waste (EPA, 2012). If a radioactive leak occurs, these agencies institute measures to prevent exposure of surrounding neighborhoods, to clean up radioactive leaks as quickly as possible, and to ensure that anyone injured receives prompt medical care.

Care of the patient receiving internal radiation therapy is acceptable to delegate to UAP. Care measures that the PCT should know about before caring for someone receiving internal radiation therapy are as follows:

* Patient's activity limitations
* Safety regulations (e.g., time and distance limits)
* Use of protective equipment (shields, gloves)
* Visitor restrictions (no one younger than 18 years of age or who is or may be pregnant)
* Care and handling of patient care–related items and substances (e.g., linen, trash, dietary tray, specimens, urine, feces)

Mercury Spill

The PCT must know whom to contact when exposure to a hazardous chemical such as mercury occurs in the healthcare setting. Exposures in a healthcare facility include broken thermometers or sphygmomanometers (blood pressure device), although these devices are seldom used or allowed in most healthcare facilities. These may continue to be used in long-term care settings. Mercury enters the body through inhalation and absorption through the skin. Exposures that occur in a healthcare facility setting are usually brief but still have the potential to affect the brain or kidney. Full recovery is likely to occur once the body cleans itself of the contamination. Box 11.5 summarizes steps to take in the event of a mercury spill. Although a mercury spill is not likely to occur in the healthcare setting, it is important to be aware of the facility's policy for proper cleanup of a mercury spill. Mercury-containing equipment may be used in factory settings, so the occupational health nurse should be aware of mercury spill safety in the event that an employee comes into contact with mercury while on the job.

Box 11.5   Mercury Spill Cleanup Procedure

In the event of a mercury spill, follow these steps while waiting for trained personnel to arrive:

1. Evacuate the room except for a housekeeping crew (if available).
2. Ventilate the area. Close interior doors and open any outside windows.
3. DO NOT VACUUM THE SPILL.

After the mercury has been recovered:

4. Mop the floor with a mercury-specific cleanser (see agency policy).
5. Dispose of collected mercury according to local environmental safety regulations.

CHAPTER SUMMARY

Prevention of falls, electrical injuries, fires, burns, and accidental poisoning is key to maintaining a safe environment. Infants, young children, older adults, and the ill or injured patients are at risk of falling. Proper patient orientation includes information about the use of the call light and bed controls. Be sure that patients know how their bed controls and call light work. Place frequently used items within reach of patients. Always keep adjustable beds in the low position except when care is given to decrease the risk of falls.

Gait belts are an added safety feature to use when assisting patients to ambulate. Discuss with the nurse any patients who are at risk for falls before beginning the shift. Attempt to design a safe environment for the patient. This may include keeping equipment out of the walkway of the patient, using nonskid socks with grips on the bottoms, and keeping cords neatly tucked away.

Case Scenario

The PCT walking down the hall hears a patient calling out for help. The PCT comes into the room and realizes that the patient does not remember how to use the call light. The patient is sitting in the bed pushing various buttons on the call light and the television is turning on and off. What factors possibly contribute to the patient's inability to remember, and what should the PCT do? What are some strategies to use that would assist patients in remembering how to use their call light?

REVIEW QUESTIONS

1. The nurse is observing the PCT who is assisting a resident in a long-term care facility ambulate with a gait belt. Which action by the PCT indicates to the nurse that further instruction is necessary? *(Select all that apply.)*
   a. The PCT loosely fastens the gait belt around the patient's waist.
   b. The PCT places the gait belt on the resident before assisting the resident to a standing position.
   c. The PCT grasps the gait belt while assisting the resident out of bed.
   d. The PCT fastens the belt around the arm of the chair to prevent the resident from slipping out of the chair.
   e. The PCT explains to the resident that the gait belt is used to prevent injury to the resident and the PCT when assisting with ambulation.

2. The home health nurse is assessing a child for the risk of injury. Which factor places a child at greatest risk for specific types of injuries?
   a. Gender of the child
   b. Overall health
   c. Educational level
   d. Developmental level

3. The PCT is reviewing the patient list for the shift. Which information is of most concern to the PCT that this patient is at high risk of falling?
   a. The patient has diabetes.
   b. The patient had a stroke 3 years ago with no complications.
   c. The patient becomes disoriented in the evening hours.
   d. The patient wears eyeglasses and a hearing aid.

4. The PCT learns of a mercury spill that occurred in the doctor's office in which she is employed. Which action by the PCT is correct?
   a. The PCT cleans the mercury spill with alcohol and ordinary cleaning cloths.
   b. The PCT closes all windows and doors to prevent the mercury spill from spreading out of the area.
   c. The PCT instructs the housekeeping staff to vacuum up the spill.
   d. The PCT evacuates the area and contacts trained personnel to clean up the spill.

5. It is the responsibility of the PCT to apply safety reminder devices to the patient who is at risk for falls.
   a. True
   b. False

Moving, Positioning, and Preventing Falls

LEARNING OBJECTIVES

1. Discuss considerations related to mobility for older adults.
2. Discuss the complications of immobility.
3. Demonstrate the use of assistive devices for proper positioning.
4. Demonstrate placement of patient in various positions, such as Fowler's, supine (dorsal), Sims's, side-lying, prone, dorsal recumbent, and lithotomy positions.
5. Describe and demonstrate range-of-motion exercises and explain their purpose.
6. Identify complications caused by inactivity.
7. Describe safe and appropriate methods for the application of safety reminder devices when caring for patients.
8. Discuss strategies that promote a restraint-free environment.

KEY TERMS

abduction The movement of a limb or other part away from the midline of the body, or from another part.

adduction Movement toward the midline of the body; also applies to movements inward and across the body.

alignment The process of adjusting body parts so that they are in proper relative position.

contracture When muscles, ligaments, and tendons are not shortened and lengthened with movement, a permanent shortening of these structures may occur.

disuse syndrome Inactivity that can lead to deterioration of many body functions.

dorsal (supine) Lying flat on the back.

dorsal recumbent Supine position with patient lying on back, head, and shoulder with extremities moderately flexed; legs are sometimes extended.

dorsiflexion To bend or flex backward.

extension Movement of certain joints that decreases angle between two adjoining bones.

flexion The action of bending or the condition of being bent, especially the bending of a limb or join.

Fowler's Posture assumed by patient when head of bed is raised 45 to 60 degrees.

genupectoral Also known as knee-chest; patient kneels so that weight of the body is supported by knees and chest, with abdomen raised, head turned to one side, and arms flexed.

hyperextension Extreme or abnormal extension.

immobility The inability to move around freely.

lithotomy Patient lies supine with hips and knees flexed and thighs abducted and rotated externally.

mobility A person's ability to move around freely in his or her environment.

orthopneic A posture assumed by the patient sitting up in bed at 90-degree angle, or sometimes resting in forward tilt while supported by pillow on overbed table.

palpitations A pounding or racing of the heart; may or may not indicate a serious heart disorder.

pronation Rotation of the hand or forearm so that the surface of the palm is facing downward or toward the back.

prone Lying facedown in horizontal position.
range-of-motion (ROM) The full movement potential of a joint.
semi-Fowler's Posture assumed by patient when head of bed is raised approximately
    30 degrees.
Sims's Position in which patient lies on side with knee and thigh drawn upward toward chest.
supination The kind of rotation that allows the hand to turn up.
Trendelenburg's Position in which patient's head is low and the body and legs are on
    inclined plane.

Safely moving and positioning a patient can have a great effect on the reduction of patient falls. Mechanical lifting devices (sling and standing lifts) and assistive patient-handling equipment, such as roller boards, sliders, friction-reduction pads, transfer chairs, and gait belts, work by taking on the energy and force that otherwise are applied on the patient care technician (PCT) during the lifting, transferring, or repositioning of a patient. Regular use of lifts and other assistive devices reduces the risk of injury.

Safe patient transfer requires having enough staff, the right mix of personnel, and appropriate, readily available, well-maintained patient-lifting equipment. The PCT is responsible for being competent in the proper and safe use of equipment and assistive devices.

FALLS

Falls are a common problem in healthcare facilities, requiring the patient care technician to be alert to patients who are at an increased risk for falls. A fall risk assessment is usually performed by the admitting nurse on admission to the unit and whenever a significant change in the patient's condition has occurred. Patient falls are a major safety consideration for *all* institutions. The very young and older adults are not the only ones at risk for falls in the healthcare environment. Those who become ill or who are injured are also at risk. An unfamiliar environment and the various symptoms and signs associated with the patient's diagnosis often place an individual at risk. The use of anesthesia, sedatives, or narcotics increases the risk of falling, as does an unstable gait or a problem with balance.

Gait belts are another way to help patients ambulate safely. A gait belt is a canvas (or other very strong material) belt that encircles the patient's waist (some belts have handles attached for the staff to grasp) while the patient ambulates. Correct technique in the use of the gait belt is as follows:

1. Apply gait belt securely around the patient's waist.
2. Walk to the side of patient, grasping the gait belt toward the patient's back. The other hand may either support the patient's arm or grasp the gait belt towards the patient's side. Unless the patient has a tendency to lean toward one particular side, walk on the patient's weaker side so that you are able to give assistance if the patient starts to fall.
3. Have patient support self by leaning on or holding your arm.
4. Walk slightly behind the patient for better support.
5. Walk with your knees and hips flexed.
6. After ambulation, loosen or remove the gait belt.
7. Document procedure.

Infants and Children

Ensuring the safety of the environment of infants and children requires protecting the child and educating the parents to do so as well. The nurse is responsible for anticipating potential injuries and individualizing patient care and teaching, but the patient care technician can support the nurse by reminding the patients how to prevent injuries such as falls. Accidents involving children are largely preventable, but parents and caregivers need to be aware of specific dangers at each stage of growth and development. Growth and the learning new motor skills place the child at great risk for injury.

Many dangers are present in a child's environment. All household cleaning items are potentially poisonous when ingested and must be kept out of children's reach. Remind parents that most younger children are not able to read or understand labels on cleaning materials or medication containers. The nurse will educate parents that infants in the oral stage of development put almost anything into their mouths and that as infants learn to crawl, electrical sockets and cords also become a danger. Toddlers and young children can be protected from burns by turning pot handles on a stove away from the child's reach. Bath water can be another potential hazard for children because of the temperature of the water or from leaving children unattended for any length of time. Pool safety should also be emphasized to parents and caregivers. Protecting infants and toddlers from falling out of bed while in the healthcare facility is a concern. Keeping side rails up or using a pediatric crib are safety measures to prevent falls. When giving care, placing the hand on the infant or toddler when turning to obtain supplies prevents the infant or child from falling off a bed or examination table.

Older Adults

Changes associated with aging significantly affect the ability of older adults to protect themselves from injury. Unsteady gait, age-related vision changes, and medication side effects (such as vertigo) pose a threat to the older adult's safety. Ensuring that older adults wear their eyeglasses and hearing aids and use assistive devices for ambulating when necessary are important nursing interventions to promote patient safety.

POSITIONING OF PATIENTS

Positioning of patients is a common task performed by PCTs. Many positions can be used to prevent patients from development of complications (Procedure 12.1). Inappropriate positioning poses the risk of causing permanent disability.

Mobility Versus Immobility

Mobility is a person's ability to move around freely in his or her environment. Moving about serves many purposes, including exercising, expressing emotion, attaining basic needs, performing recreational activities, and completing activities of daily living (those activities of physical self-care such as bathing, dressing, and eating). In addition, mobility is fundamental to maintaining the body's normal physiologic activities. For normal physical mobility, the body's nervous, muscular,

---

PROCEDURE 12.1
Positioning Patients

1. Assemble equipment and supplies.
   - Pillows
   - Footboard
   - Trochanter roll
   - Splinting devices
   - Hand rolls
   - Safety reminder devices
   - Side rails
2. Request assistance as needed.
3. Introduce self.
4. Identify patient.
5. Explain procedure.
6. Perform hand hygiene. Wear gloves as necessary according to agency policy and guidelines from the Centers for Disease Control and Prevention (CDC) and Occupational Safety and Health Administration (OSHA).
7. Prepare patient.
8. Close door or pull curtain.
9. Raise level of bed to comfortable working height.
10. Remove pillows and devices used in previous position.
11. Put bed in flat position, or as low as patient can tolerate, and lower side rail closest to you.
12. Position patient.
    a. **Dorsal (supine)** position (lying flat on the back) (see illustration).
       (1) Place patient on back with head of bed flat.
       (2) Place small rolled towel under lumbar area of back.
       (3) Place pillow under upper shoulder, neck, and head.
       (4) Place trochanter rolls parallel to lateral surface of thighs.
       (5) Place small pillow or roll under ankle to elevate heels.
       (6) Support feet in dorsiflexion with firm pillow, footboard, or high-top sneakers.

(7) Place pillows under pronated forearms, keeping upper arms parallel to patient's body (see illustration).
(8) Place hand rolls in patient's hands.

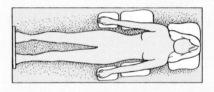
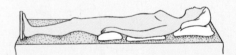

    b. **Dorsal recumbent** position (supine position with patient lying on back, head, and shoulder with extremities moderately flexed; legs are sometimes extended).
       (1) Move patient and mattress to head of bed.
       (2) Turn patient onto back.
       (3) Assist patient to raise legs, bend knees, and allow legs to relax.
       (4) Replace pillow. Patient sometimes needs a small lumbar pillow.
    c. **Fowler's** position (posture assumed by patient when head of bed is raised 45 to 60 degrees) (see illustration).
       (1) Move patient and mattress to head of bed.
       (2) Raise head of bed to 45 to 60 degrees.
       (3) Replace pillow.
       (4) Use footboard or firm pillow.
       (5) Use pillows to support arms and hands.
       (6) Place small pillow or roll under ankles.

Continued

PROCEDURE 12.1

Positioning Patients—cont'd

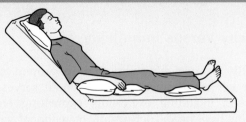

d. **Semi-Fowler's** position (posture assumed by patient when head of bed is raised approximately 30 degrees).
   (1) Move patient and mattress to head of bed.
   (2) Raise head of bed to about 30 degrees.
   (3) Replace pillow. See Step 9c for positioning of pillows.
e. **Orthopneic** position (posture assumed by the patient sitting up in bed at 90-degree angle, or sometimes resting in forward tilt while supported by pillow on overbed table) (see illustration). Often used for the patient with a cardiac or respiratory condition.
   (1) Elevate head of bed to 90 degrees. Patient sometimes sits on side of bed with legs dangling or propped on a chair.
   (2) Place pillow between patient's back and mattress.
   (3) Place pillow on overbed table and assist patient to lean over, placing head on pillow.

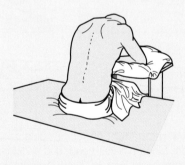

f. **Sims's** position (position in which patient lies on side with knee and thigh drawn upward toward chest) (see illustration). The left Sims's position is appropriate for the enema procedure and administration of a rectal suppository.
   (1) Place patient in supine position.
   (2) Position patient in lateral position, lying partially on the abdomen.
   (3) Draw knee and thigh up near abdomen and support with pillows.
   (4) Place patient's lower arm along the back.
   (5) Bring upper arm up, flex elbow, and support with pillow.
   (6) Allow patient to lean forward to rest on chest.

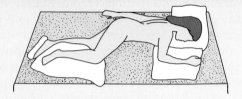

g. **Prone** position (lying face down in horizontal position) (see illustration).
   (1) Assist patient onto abdomen with face to one side.
   (2) Flex arms toward the head.
   (3) Position pillows for comfort. Place a pillow under lower leg to release any "pull" on the lower back, or place a pillow under the head as shown (or both).

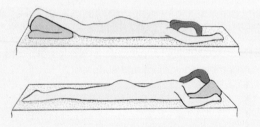

h. **Knee-chest (genupectoral)** position (patient kneels so that weight of body is supported by knees and chest, with abdomen raised, head turned to one side, and arms flexed) (see illustration).
   (1) Turn patient onto abdomen.
   (2) Assist patient into kneeling position; arms and head rest on pillow while upper chest rests on bed.

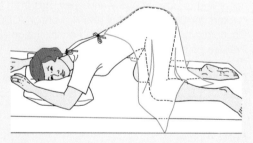

i. **Lithotomy** position (patient lies supine with hips and knees flexed and thighs abducted and rotated externally [sometimes feet are positioned in stirrups]) (see illustration).
   (1) Position patient to lie supine (lying on the back).
   (2) Request patient to slide buttocks to edge of examining table.
   (3) Lift both legs; have patient bend knees and place feet in stirrups.
   (4) Drape patient.
   (5) Provide small lumbar pillow if desired.

PROCEDURE 12.1

Positioning Patients—cont'd

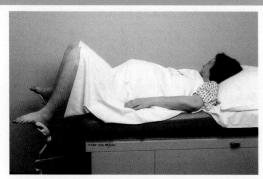

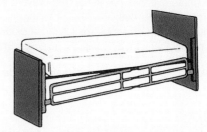

j. **Trendelenburg's** position (patient's head is low and the body and legs are on inclined plane) (see illustration).

(1) Place patient's head lower than body, with body and legs elevated and on an incline. Foot of bed is sometimes elevated on blocks. (Not used if patient has a head or chest injury.) Trendelenburg's position was used to treat shock but now is used less often because it causes pressure on the diaphragm by organs in the abdomen and shunts more blood to the brain rather than all of the vital organs. This position is sometimes used to assist in venous distention during central line placement.

13. Ensure that the patient is in proper body alignment.
14. Provide comfort by performing a back massage after turning from one position to another.
15. Reposition debilitated, unconscious, or paralyzed patients at least every 2 hours.
16. Perform hand hygiene.
17. Document.

(Step 12a and 12h figures from Potter PA, Perry AG: Basic nursing: essentials for practice, ed 7, St. Louis, 2011, Mosby. Step 12g adapted from Potter PA, Perry AG: Basic nursing: essentials for practice, ed 7, St. Louis, 2011, Mosby. Step 12f figure from Elkin MK, Perry AG, Potter PA: Nursing interventions and clinical skills, ed 4, St. Louis, 2008, Mosby. Step 12i figure from Ball J, Dains J, Flynn J, et al: Seidel's guide to physical examination, ed 8, St. Louis, 2015, Mosby.)

Injury & Illness Prevention Box 12.1

Older Adults and Mobility

- The skin of older adults is more fragile and susceptible to injury. When moving or transferring older adults, avoid pulling them across bed linens because this has the potential to cause shearing or tearing of the skin (See Box 12.2).
- Always support older adults under the joints when moving them in bed. Lifting in any other manner increases the stress on the joint and causes increased pain, particularly if some degenerative joint disease exists. Explain each step in simple language, and avoid jerky sudden movements.
- Aging tends to result in loss of flexibility and joint mobility, which often interferes with normal transfer techniques and necessitates modifications to protect patient and PCT.
- Weakness and low blood pressure are common signs and symptoms noted in an older adult on bed rest. Proceed slowly and cautiously when helping a patient ambulate for the first time after they have been immobile for an extended amount of time. While facilitating independence and proper utilization of patient's body mechanics, use assistive devices such as canes, walkers, and trapeze bars. Provide adequate help to ensure patient safety when moving a patient from a lying to a sitting position and from a sitting to a standing position.
- Older adults who have many diseases or have undergone prolonged bed rest have greater risk for low blood pressure with postural change (orthostatic hypotension).
- Patients who use medications to reduce blood pressure are at greater risk for orthostatic hypotension.
- Older adults, particularly those with altered sensory perception, sometimes become fearful when hydraulic lifts are used for transfers. Provide eyeglasses and basic instructions.
- Limited positioning alternatives are available for the older adult who has arthritis, neuropathies, or other restrictive conditions.
- Discourage older adult patients from sitting for prolonged periods without stretching and moving. Lack of movement presents a risk for contractures of joints.
- Ensuring good body **alignment** when the patient is sitting is a way to prevent joint and muscle stress.

Continued

and skeletal systems must be intact, functioning, and used regularly. Although a person may welcome a rare day to lie in bed and rest, the person who is *immobile* (experiencing immobility, the inability to move around freely) is predisposed to a wide variety of complications (Box 12.1).

Many types of health problems potentially lead to a decline in a patient's mobility. Patients with certain illnesses, injuries, or surgeries sometimes experience a period of immobilization as a result of changes in medical and physical status. In some cases, immobilization is also used therapeutically to limit the movement of the whole body or a body part, and some patients are under ambulation restrictions. Interventions to prevent complications of immobility are varied, and many do not require a physician's order (see Box 12.1). See Box 12.2 for mobility considerations for those in long-term care settings.

Various assistive devices help maintain correct body positioning and prevent complications that commonly arise when a patient needs prolonged bed rest (Table 12.1). Several of the devices are especially useful in the care of patients who have a loss of sensation, mobility, or consciousness (Figs. 12.1 to 12.3). When a patient is required to remain in the bed for an extended amount of time, range-of-motion (ROM) exercises may need to be performed. These exercises help to prevent loss of muscle mass and joint contracture. The patient care technician may be asked to perform range-of-motion exercises (see Procedure 12.2).

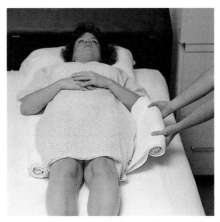

FIGURE 12.1 Trochanter roll. (From Potter PA, Perry AG, Stocket PA, et al: *Basic nursing: essentials for practice*, ed 7, St. Louis, 2011, Mosby.)

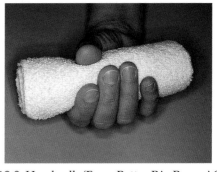

FIGURE 12.2 Hand roll. (From Potter PA, Perry AG, Stocket PA, et al: *Basic nursing: essentials for practice*, ed 7, St. Louis, 2011, Mosby.)

Moving the Patient

A common task for PCTs is assisting patients with movement. Patients may need assistance in various ways, for example, moving the patient up in bed, out of bed, or from a chair or wheelchair; turning the patient; and assisting the patient in and out of the bed for ambulation (see Procedure 12.3). In some situations, the PCT uses mechanical equipment for lifting patients, such as the hydraulic lift, roller board, and gurney lift. The PCT

should first plan and mentally think through the lift in an effort to be prepared for lifting the patient and then physically perform the lift.

Use of the Lift for Moving Patients

Mechanical devices, such as the patient lift with a sling (Fig. 12.4), are useful for moving patients safely and protecting the PCT's back and for full-weight lifting of

Box 12.1　Complications of Immobility and Preventive Measures

Complications

- *Muscle atrophy and asthenia* (muscle weakness): Muscles decrease in size and strength when not continually used.
- *Contractures:* When muscles, ligaments, and tendons are not shortened and lengthened with movement, a permanent shortening of these structures may occur.
- *Disuse osteoporosis:* Lack of weight bearing on bones causes bone demineralization, allowing fractures to occur more easily.
- *Pressure ulcer:* Tissue ischemia (lack of blood flow to an area) from unrelieved pressure results in skin breakdown.
- *Constipation:* Immobility slows peristalsis, resulting in stool remaining in the colon longer and muscle atrophy in the abdominal muscles that aid in expulsion of stool.
- *Urinary tract infection:* Urinary stasis causes changes in pH and allows bacterial growth.
- *Renal calculi* (kidney stones): Urinary stasis from immobility leads to slowed calcium metabolism, thus leading to stone formation.
- *Hypostatic pneumonia:* Decreased aeration and accumulation of secretions lead to inflammation and infection in the lungs.
- *Orthostatic hypotension* (drop in systolic blood pressure of 20 mm Hg or a decrease of 10 mm Hg in diastolic blood pressure within 3 minutes of standing when moving from lying or sitting to standing position): Immobility can lead to a decrease in venous return or decreased cardiac output in response to postural change.
- *Anorexia* (decreased appetite): Lack of mobility slows the digestive process and slows the metabolic rate, causing decreased appetite.
- *Insomnia:* Decreased stimuli, depression, and frequent napping during the day as a result of immobility may cause difficulty sleeping at night.

- *Disorientation:* Lack of stimulation, decreased endorphin production, decreased need for thought processes, and decreased socialization may lead to disorientation.
- *Thrombophlebitis and deep vein thrombosis (DVT;* blood clot with accompanying inflammation of the involved vein, usually of the lower extremity): Decrease in venous circulation allows blood to pool in lower extremities, leading to inflammation of vessels and clot formation.
- *Pulmonary embolism* (blood clot that has traveled to the lungs): DVT that has broken loose from vessel and has traveled to the lungs, causing a blockage in a pulmonary vessel.

Interventions to Prevent Complications of Immobility

- Reposition at least every 2 hours
- Ensure adequate intake; encourage fluids
- Encourage a well-balanced diet
- Prevent deformities (e.g., footboard or other measures to prevent foot drop)
- Handle and transfer patients carefully; maintain proper body alignment
- Position lower extremities properly (a pillow or wedge between the legs, never under knees)
- Early ambulation
- Antiembolism measures if directed by the nurse (thromboembolic deterrent [TED] hose or decompression boots)
- Progressive ambulation
- Roll up head of bed
- Dangle over side of bed
- Stand
- Take a few steps
- Sit in the chair
- Up to bathroom
- Up and about the room
- Up and out in the hallway
- Up as desired

Table 12.1　Assistive Devices for Proper Positioning

Device	Reason for Use
Pillow	Provides support to body or extremity; elevates body part; splints incisional area to reduce postoperative pain during activity or coughing and deep breathing
Foot boots or foot boards	Maintain feet in dorsiflexion, which prevents plantar flexion (foot drop)
Trochanter roll (see Fig. 12.1)	Prevents external rotation of legs when patient is in supine position; possible to make with a bath blanket
Sandbag	Provides support and shape to body contours; immobilizes extremity; maintains specific body alignment
Hand roll (see Fig. 12.2)	Maintains thumb slightly adducted and in opposition to fingers; maintains fingers in slightly flexed position
Hand-wrist splint	Individually molded for patient to maintain proper alignment of thumb; slightly adducted in opposition to fingers; maintains wrist in slight dorsiflexion
Trapeze bar (see Fig. 12.3)	Enables patient to raise trunk from bed; enables patient to transfer from bed to wheelchair; allows patient to perform exercises that strengthen upper arms
Side rail	Helps weak patient to roll from side to side or to sit up in bed
Bed board	Provides additional support to mattress and improves vertebral alignment
Wedge pillow	Also called *abductor pillow* (triangular pillow made of heavy foam); used to maintain the legs in abduction after total hip replacement surgery

(Modified from Potter PA, Perry AG, Stocket PA, et al: Basic nursing: essentials for practice, ed 7, St. Louis, 2012, Mosby.)

patients who cannot assist. Follow agency policy for use of the lift (Procedure 12.4).

The National Institute for Occupational Safety and Health's (NIOSH) Division of Safety Research recommends that healthcare personnel should never attempt to lift more than 35 pounds of a patient's body weight (Howard, 2010). For the safety of the staff and the patient, additional assistance should always be secured when the transferability of a patient is in doubt.

Many special problems are to be considered in transfer. Patients who have been immobile for several days or longer may be weak or have vertigo (dizziness) and sometimes have orthostatic hypotension (a drop in blood pressure) when transferred. A patient with neurologic deficits perhaps has paresis (muscle weakness) or paralysis unilaterally or bilaterally, which complicates

safe transfer. A flaccid arm can easily sustain injury during transfer if unsupported. Be creative when necessary in the transfer of trauma patients, always discussing the plan for such transfer with the nurse. As a general rule, a gait (transfer) belt should be used and assistance obtained for mobilization of such patients.

Safety Reminder Devices

A **safety reminder device (SRD)** is defined as any of the numerous devices used to immobilize a patient or part of the patient's body, such as arms or hands. An SRD is also known as a restraint in some facilities. Many facilities have adopted a restraint-free environment, thus

Text continued on p. 223

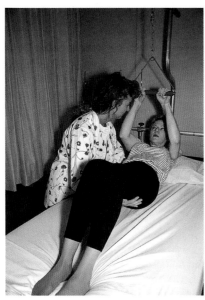

FIGURE 12.3 Patient using a trapeze bar. (From Potter PA, Perry AG, Stocket PA, et al: *Basic nursing: essentials for practice,* ed 7, St. Louis, 2011, Mosby.)

Box 12.2	Long-Term Care Considerations for Mobility

- Patients who have maintained bed rest for a long time sometimes revert back to a favorite position. Frequently assess these patients, and turn them more often as needed.
- Use a lift (draw) sheet as often as possible to prevent shearing force on fragile skin.
- Allow the patient to assist with moving and positioning whenever possible to promote independence.
- Perform safety and maintenance checks of ambulation devices on a routine basis.
- Perform periodic assessments to ensure that the patient is using ambulation device properly.
- Consult the physical therapist for additional assistance or exercises and to ascertain the patient's response to the exercise program.
- Group activities (e.g., simple games, walking, tossing a ball in a large circle) are useful in maintaining range-of-motion.

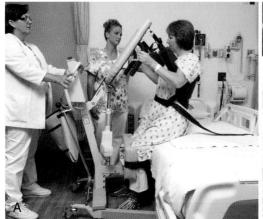
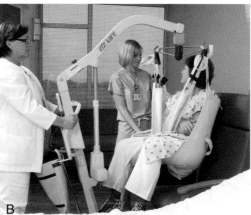

FIGURE 12.4 A, Motorized lift. B, Use of a mechanical lift to lower patient into chair. (From Potter PA, Perry AG, Stocket PA, et al: *Basic nursing: essentials for practice,* ed 7, St. Louis, 2011, Mosby.)

PROCEDURE 12.2

Performing Range-of-Motion Exercises

1. Refer to medical record or care plan for special interventions.
2. Assemble equipment.
   - Clean gloves, if necessary (see step 6).
3. Introduce self.
4. Identify patient.
5. Explain procedure.
6. Perform hand hygiene and don clean gloves according to agency policy and guidelines from CDC and OSHA.
7. Prepare patient for exercises:
   a. Close door to room or pull curtain.
   b. Drape for procedure if appropriate.
   c. Raise bed to comfortable working level.
   d. Assist patient to a comfortable position, either sitting or lying down.
8. Support the body part above (proximal to) and below (distal to) the joint by cradling the extremity or by using cupped hand to support the joint being exercised.

9. Begin by doing exercises in normal sequence (see Table 12.2). Repeat each full sequence 5 times during the exercise period. Discontinue exercise if patient reports pain or if resistance or muscle spasm occurs.
10. Assist patient by putting each joint through full range of motion (see Table 12.2).
11. Position patient for comfort. To prevent **contracture** (an abnormal shortening of a muscle), do not allow patients with joint pain to remain continuously in position of comfort; joints must be exercised routinely. Periodically provide back massage.
12. Adjust bed linen.
13. Remove and dispose of gloves and wash hands.
14. Document the following:
    - Joints exercised
    - Presence of edema or pressure areas
    - Any discomfort resulting from the exercises
    - Any limitations of range-of-motion
    - Patient's tolerance of the exercises

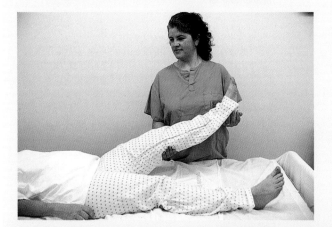

(Step 8 figure from Perry AG, Potter PA: Nursing interventions and clinical skills, ed 6, St. Louis, 2016, Elsevier.)

PROCEDURE 12.3

Moving the Patient

1. Refer to the medical record or care plan for special interventions.
2. Assemble equipment.
   - Hospital bed
   - Chair
   - Side rails
   - Patient's slippers
   - Cotton blanket
   - Pillows
   - Extra personnel
   - Lifting devices (see Procedure 12.4)
3. Introduce self.
4. Identify patient.
5. Explain procedure.
6. Perform hand hygiene.
7. Prepare patient for procedure.
   a. Close door or pull curtain.
   b. Adjust bed level for safe working height.

8. Arrange for assistance as necessary.
9. Lift and move patient up in bed (sometimes requires one staff member and sometimes more):
   a. Place patient supine with head flat.
   b. Face the patient and establish base of support.
   c. Use a lift (draw) sheet to assist patient up in bed.
      (1) Roll patient first to one side and then the other, placing lift sheet underneath patient from shoulders to thighs.
      (2) Flex knees and face body in the direction of the move. The foot farthest away from the bed faces forward for broader base of support.
      (3) With one nurse on each side of patient, grasp lift sheet firmly with hands near patient's upper arms and hips, rolling the sheet material until hands are close to the patient.

Continued

(4) Instruct patient to rest arms over body and to lift head on the count of 3; at the same time, pull the sheet to move the patient up to head of bed.

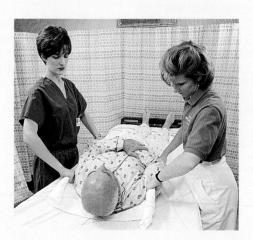

10. Turning the patient:
    a. Stand with feet slightly apart and flex knees.
    b. If the patient is unable to assist in turning, two people should use the lift sheet to turn the patient.
    c. Move patient's body to one side of the bed.
    d. If patient is assisting in turning, turn the patient on side facing raised side rail, toward the patient care technician. If patient is not assisting, then use the lift sheet to turn the patient.
    e. Flex one of patient's legs over the other. Place pad or pillow between legs.
    f. Align patient's shoulders; place pillow under head.
    g. Support patient's back with pillows as necessary. A "tuck back" pillow is made by folding pillow lengthwise. Tuck smooth area slightly under patient's back.
11. Dangling patient:
    a. Assess pulse and respirations.
    b. Move patient to side of bed toward the patient care technician.
    c. Lower bed to lowest position.
    d. Raise head of bed.
    e. Support patient's shoulders and help to swing legs around and off bed; do this all in one motion by simply pivoting patient. Ensure patient's feet touch floor.

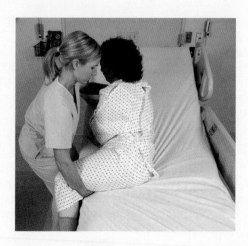

    f. Another way to accomplish this is by rolling the patient onto his or her side before sitting the patient up. The patient care technician then stoops and, when standing, brings the patient along with the patient care technician.
    g. Help patient place slippers on; cover legs. For safety, have patient place slippers on while in bed.
    h. Assess patient's pulse and respirations.
12. Log-rolling the patient (back, neck, or head conditions sometimes necessitate log-rolling after injury or surgery):
    a. Enlist the help of at least one additional person.
    b. Lower the head of the bed as much as the patient can tolerate.
    c. Place a pillow between the patient's legs. Use of a pull sheet placed between shoulders and knees facilitates turning (see Step 9c[1]).
    d. Extend the patient's arm over the patient's head unless shoulder movement is restricted. If shoulder movement is restricted, keep the arm in extension next to the body.
    e. With two assistive staff on the same side of the bed, one of the staff places one hand on the patient's shoulder and the other on the hip, while the other staff places one hand to support the patient's back and the other behind the knee. If a lift sheet is used, space hands in such a way to provide even support for the length of the rolled sheet and to distribute weight evenly.

PROCEDURE 12.3
Moving the Patient—cont'd

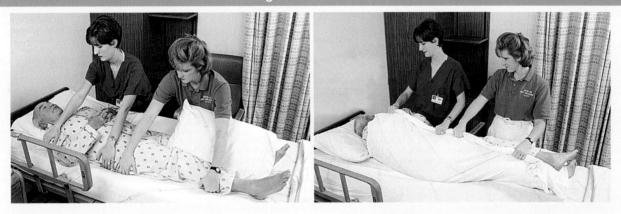

f. On a count of 3, turn the patient with a continuous, smooth, and coordinated effort.
g. Support the patient with pillows as previously discussed (see step 10g).
13. Transferring the patient from bed to straight chair or wheelchair:
    a. Lower bed to lowest position.
    b. Raise head of bed.
    c. Support patient's shoulders and help swing legs around and off bed; perform all in one motion.

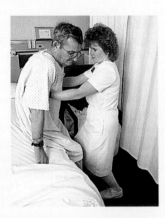

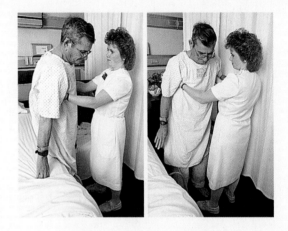

g. Assist patient to stand and swing around with back toward seat of chair. Keep the strong side toward the chair.
h. Help patient to sit down as the nurse bends his or her knees to assist process.

d. Help patient don robe and slippers (or do this before beginning procedure).
e. Have chair positioned beside bed with seat facing foot of bed.
    (1) Place wheelchair at right angle to bed and lock wheels after bed is lowered.
    (2) Place straight chair against wall or have another staff member hold the chair.
f. Stand in front of patient and place hands at patient's waist level or below; allow patient to use his or her arms and shoulder muscles to push down on the mattress to facilitate the move.

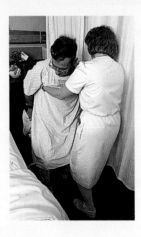

Continued

PROCEDURE 12.3

Moving the Patient—cont'd

i. Apply blanket to legs.

j. If transfer belt is used, apply after patient is sitting on side of bed and follow these guidelines:

 (1) Stand in front of the patient.

 (2) Have the patient hold on to the mattress, or ask the patient to place his or her fists on the bed by the thighs.

 (3) Be sure that the patient's feet are flat on the floor.

 (4) Have the patient lean forward.

 (5) Instruct the patient to place his or her hands on the patient care technician's shoulders, not around the patient care technician's neck or at the side as shown.

 (6) Grasp the transfer belt at each side.

 (7) Brace knees against the patient's knees. Block the patient's feet with the patient care technician's feet.

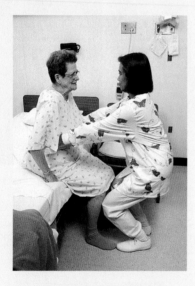

 (8) Ask the patient to push down on the mattress and to stand on the count of 3. Pull the patient into a standing position as you straighten your knees.

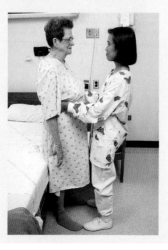

 (9) Pivot the patient so that he or she is able to grasp the far arm of the chair. Back of the legs will be touching the chair.

(10) Continue to turn the patient until the other arm rest is grasped.

(11) Gradually lower the patient into the chair as you bend your hips and knees. The patient assists if able by leaning forward and bending his or her elbows and knees.

(12) Ensure that buttocks are to the back of the chair.

(13) Cover patient's lap and legs.

(14) Transferring from bed to stretcher then back to bed:

 a. Position bed flat and raise to the same height as stretcher or gurney. Lower side rails.

 b. Cover patient with top sheet or blanket and remove linens without exposing patient.

 c. Assess for IV line, Foley catheter, tubes, or surgical drains, and position them to avoid tension during the transfer.

 d. Position the stretcher as close to the bed as possible, and lock the wheels of the bed and stretcher (with side rails lowered).

 e. When patient is able to assist, stand near side of stretcher and instruct patient to move feet, then buttocks, and finally upper body to the stretcher, bringing blanket along. Be certain that patient's body is centered on the stretcher.

 f. When patient is unable to assist, place a folded sheet or bath blanket under the patient so that it supports patient's head and extends to midthighs. Roll the sheet or bath blanket close to the patient's body. Assist patient to cross arms over chest. Two assistive staff reach over the bed to patient, and two more stand as close to the stretcher as possible. A fifth person stands at the foot to transfer the feet. Using a coordinating count of 3, all five staff lift the patient to the edge of the bed. With another effort, lift the patient from edge of bed to gurney. Roller devices are available in some facilities to facilitate this transfer.

PROCEDURE 12.3

Moving the Patient—cont'd

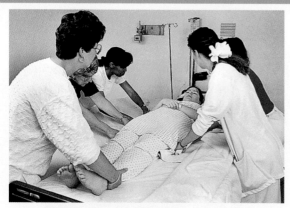

14. Transferring patient from a wheelchair to a bed:
    a. Adjust the height of the bed to the level of the seat of the wheelchair if possible.
    b. Position the wheelchair at a 45-degree angle next to the bed.
    c. Face the wheelchair toward the foot of the bed midway between the head and foot of the bed.
    d. Lock the wheelchair. Locks are located above the rims of the wheels. Push handle forward to lock.
    e. Raise the footplates, and place the transfer belt on patient (if not already in place).
    f. Assist patient to move to the front of the wheelchair.
    g. Position yourself slightly in front of patient to guard and protect patient throughout the transfer.
    h. Coordinate transfer to the bed by having patient stand and then pivot to the side of the bed. Then have patient sit on the side of the mattress.
    i. With patient sitting on side of the bed, place your arm near the head of the bed under the person's shoulders while supporting the head and neck. Take your other arm and place it under the person's knees. Bend your knees and keep your back straight.
    j. Tell patient to help lift the legs when you begin to move. On a count of three, standing with a wide base of support, raise patient's legs as you pivot his or her body and lower the shoulders onto the bed. Remember to keep your back straight.
15. Perform hand hygiene.
16. Assess patient for appropriate body alignment after move. When repositioning, always assess previously dependent skin surfaces (pressure areas). Position pillows for comfort. Do not overtire patient during ambulation. As in all transfers, be certain call device is in easy reach.
17. Document procedure.

(Step 9c(4), 12e, 13j(7), and 13j(8) figures from Sorrentino SA: Assisting with patient care, ed 1, St. Louis, 1998, Mosby. Step 11e figure from Perry AG, Potter PA: Clinical nursing skills and techniques, ed 8, St. Louis, 2014, Mosby. Step 13c, 13f, and 13h figures from Potter PA, Perry AG: Basic nursing: essentials for practice, ed 6, St. Louis, 2006, Mosby. Step 13j, 14f figure from Elkin MK, Perry AG, Potter PA: Nursing interventions and clinical skills, ed 4, St. Louis, 2008, Mosby. Step 15 taken from Perry AG, Potter PA: Nursing interventions and clinical skills, ed 6, St. Louis, 2016, Elsevier.)

PROCEDURE 12.4

Using Lifts for Moving Patients

1. Refer to medical record or care plan for special interventions. Read manual for direction.
2. Assemble equipment:
   - Mechanical lift frame (see Fig. 12.4)
   - Seat sling attachment (may be one piece or two) or a standing frame
   - Two cotton bath blankets
3. Introduce self.
4. Identify patient.
5. Explain procedure.
6. Perform hand hygiene.
7. Prepare patient for interventions.
   a. Close door or pull curtains.
   b. Adjust bed level to working height (even with level of arm of chair [of lift] if chair is not removable or level with seat if chair is removable.)
   c. Place cotton bath blanket over chair for patient's comfort.
   d. Cover patient with remaining bath blanket.
8. Secure adequate number of personnel.
9. Place chair near bed.
10. Appropriately place canvas seat under patient; support head and neck.
11. Slide horseshoe-shaped bar under bed on one side.
12. Lower horizontal bar to level of sling.
13. Fasten hooks on chain to openings in sling.
14. Raise head of bed.
15. Fold patient's arms over chest.

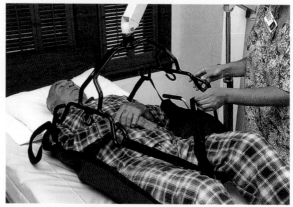

Continued

PROCEDURE 12.4

Using Lifts for Moving Patients—cont'd

16. Pump lift handle until patient is raised off bed.

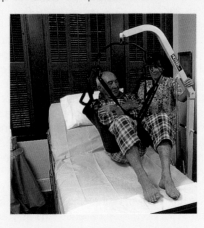

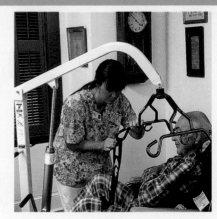

17. With steering handle, pull lift off bed and down to chair.
18. Release valve slowly to lift and lower patient toward chair.
19. Close off valve and release straps.
20. Remove straps and lift.

21. Perform hand hygiene.
22. Document procedure.
    - Evaluate body alignment to help prevent skin impairment.
    - Evaluate patient's response to movement to help determine patient's mobility potential.

Steps 15, 16, and 20 figures from Birchenall J, Streight E, Mosby's Textbook for the Home Care Aide, ed. 3, 2013, Elsevier

---

Table 12.2	Joint Range-of-Motion Exercises

Body Part	Type of Joint	Type of Movement
Neck and cervical spine	Pivotal	*Flexion*[a]: Bring chin to rest on chest. *Extension*[b]: Return head to erect position. *Hyperextension*[c]: Bend head back as far as possible. Use caution with older adults.
		Lateral flexion: Tilt head as far as possible toward each shoulder.
		Rotation: Turn head as far as possible to right and left.
Shoulder	Ball and socket 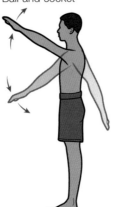	*Flexion:* Raise arm from side position forward to position above head. *Extension:* Return arm to position at side of body. *Hyperextension:* Move arm behind body, keeping elbow straight.

Table 12.2   Joint Range-of-Motion Exercises—cont'd

Body Part	Type of Joint	Type of Movement
	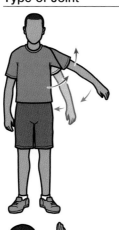	*Abduction*[d]: Raise arm to side to position above head with palm away from head. *Adduction*[e]: Lower arm sideways and across body as far as possible.
	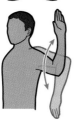	*Internal rotation:* With elbow flexed, rotate shoulder by moving arm until thumb is turned inward and toward back. *External rotation:* With elbow flexed, move arm until thumb is upward and lateral to head.
	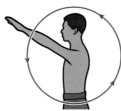	*Circumduction:* Move arm in full circle. (Circumduction is combination of all movements of ball-and-socket joint.)
Elbow	Hinge	*Flexion:* Bend elbow so that lower arm moves toward its shoulder joint and hand is level with shoulder. *Extension:* Straighten elbow by lowering hand. *Hyperextension:* Bend lower arm back as far as possible.
Forearm	Pivotal	*Supination*[f]: Turn lower arm and hand so that palm is up. *Pronation*[g]: Turn lower arm so that palm is down.
	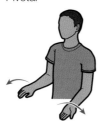	
Wrist	Condyloid	*Flexion:* Move palm toward inner aspect of forearm. *Extension:* Move fingers so that fingers, hands, and forearm are in same plane, in a straight line. *Hyperextension:* Bring dorsal surface of hand back as far as possible.
	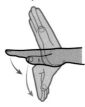	
		*Radial flexion:* Bend wrist medially toward thumb. *Ulnar flexion:* Bend wrist laterally toward fifth finger.

Continued

Table 12.2	Joint Range-of-Motion Exercises—cont'd	

Body Part	Type of Joint	Type of Movement
Fingers	Condyloid hinge	*Flexion:* Make fist. *Extension:* Straighten fingers. *Hyperextension:* Bend fingers back as far as possible. *Abduction:* Spread fingers apart. *Adduction:* Bring fingers together.
Thumb	Saddle	*Flexion:* Move thumb across palmar surface of hand. *Extension:* Move thumb straight away from hand. *Abduction:* Extend thumb laterally (usually done when placing fingers in abduction and adduction). *Adduction:* Move thumb back toward hand. *Opposition:* Touch thumb to each finger of same hand.
Hip	Ball and socket	*Flexion:* Move leg forward and up with knee in extension. *Extension:* Move leg back beside other leg while knee joint remains in extension. *Hyperextension:* Move leg behind body. *Abduction:* Move leg laterally away from body. *Adduction:* Move leg back toward medial position and beyond if possible. *Internal rotation:* Turn foot and leg toward other leg. *External rotation:* Turn foot and leg away from other leg.

Table 12.2	Joint Range-of-Motion Exercises—cont'd	

Body Part	Type of Joint	Type of Movement
		Circumduction: Move leg in circle.
Knee	Hinge	*Flexion:* Bring heel back toward back of thigh. *Extension:* Return heel to floor.
Ankle	Hinge	*Dorsiflexion*[h]: Move foot so that toes are pointed upward. *Plantar flexion:* Move foot so that toes are pointed downward.
Foot	Gliding	*Inversion:* Turn sole of foot medially. *Eversion:* Turn sole of foot laterally.
Toes	Condyloid hinge	*Flexion:* Curl toes downward. *Extension:* Straighten toes.
		Abduction: Spread toes apart. *Adduction:* Bring toes together.

(Figures from Potter PA, Perry AG: Fundamentals of nursing: concepts, process, and practice, ed 6, St. Louis, 2006, Mosby.)
[a]**Flexion:** Movement of certain joints that decreases angle between two adjoining bones.
[b]**Extension:** Movement of certain joints that increases angle between two adjoining bones.
[c]**Hyperextension:** Extreme or abnormal extension.
[d]**Abduction:** Movement of limb away from body.
[e]**Adduction:** Movement of limb toward axis of body.
[f]**Supination:** Kind of rotation that allows palm of hand to turn up.
[g]**Pronation:** Palm of hand turned down.
[h]**Dorsiflexion:** To bend or flex backward.
(Modified from Potter PA, Perry AG, Stocket PA, et al: Basic nursing: essentials for practice, ed 7, St. Louis, 2012, Mosby.)

eliminating the use of any type of SRD. This is especially true in long-term care facilities. The long-term care setting is the permanent home for many residents, so maintaining a safe environment while protecting the individual's dignity is a priority.

The use of SRDs also tends to result in increased restlessness, disorientation, agitation, anxiety, and a feeling of powerlessness by the patient. These devices may also contribute to patient immobility and associated problems with immobility such as dehydration, healthcare-associated infection, and incontinence. The resulting disuse of body parts has the potential to increase disability and lead to further patient weakness and unsteadiness. This is known as disuse syndrome. Patients often pull against the SRDs, causing skin and circulation problems.

SRDs may be used for various reasons but are primarily used to keep patients safe. An SRD may serve to support the ongoing treatment the patient is receiving (e.g., the wrist SRD prevents patients from removing IV lines, feeding tubes, drainage tubes, or an endotracheal tube when on a ventilator). Certain patient populations, such as those who are disoriented or confused, are more likely to need SRDs. The use of SRDs prevents the disoriented patient from wandering and prevents or reduces the risk of the patient falling from a bed, chair, or wheelchair. The patient who is aggressive because of mental health or drug-related issues may also need an SRD. The SRD may be necessary to protect other patients and staff from harm.

Attempting alternative strategies before turning to the use of SRDs (Box 12.3) is always the first consideration. By assessing individual patient needs, characteristics of the environment, and organizational change, the PCT often is able to use strategies that reduce or eliminate the need for SRDs. Patient safety and the safety of others is the only reason an SRD is used. Most healthcare facilities have specific policies and procedures related to the use of SRDs (Box 12.4 and Procedure 12.5), and most require a specific order from a healthcare provider. Some facilities require that a healthcare provider order for SRDs be renewed every 24 hours. Explain to the patient the need for the devices even if the patient does not seem to understand the explanation. Also, inform family members about the need for SRDs. Include information about the specific device used and the approximate period for use.

Box 12.3   Designing a Restraint-Free Environment

Care of the patient who may be prone to threats to safety and security requires a creative, systematic, and attentive approach. A wide variety of electronic devices have been developed to alert staff to a patient's need for assistance. A weight-sensitive alarm can be placed under a patient in bed or in a chair. When the patient tries to get up, an alarm sounds. A chair alarm may be used to remind the patient or alert the staff when a patient who requires assistance when standing or ambulating tries to get up without assistance.

To design a restraint-free environment:
- Orient patient and family to surroundings; explain all procedures and treatments.
- Encourage family and friends to stay, or use sitters for patients who need supervision.

- Assign confused or disoriented patients to rooms near the nurses' station. Observe these patients frequently.
- Provide appropriate visual and auditory stimuli (e.g., family pictures, clocks, radio).
- Eliminate bothersome treatments as soon as possible. For example, discontinue tube feedings and begin oral feedings as quickly as the patient's condition allows.
- Use relaxation techniques (e.g., massage).
- Institute exercise and ambulation schedules as the patient's condition allows.
- Encourage participation in diversional activities (e.g., long-term care facilities typically have daily activities planned for the residents, such as games, movies, and entertainment).
- Maintain toileting routines.

Box 12.4   Long-Term Care Variations for Safety Reminder Devices

Legislation has greatly affected the use of safety reminder devices (SRDs) in the long-term care facility. Under the Omnibus Budget Reconciliation Act (OBRA) of 1987, residents' rights are specifically addressed in terms of SRDs. This act, effective October 1, 1990, mandates specific guidelines and prohibits routine use of SRDs in long-term care facilities. The act regulates the use of extremity SRDs, hand mitts, safety vests, and wheelchair safety bars. SRDs may be used only to ensure the physical safety of the resident or other residents. A written order by the physician must detail the duration and circumstances under which the SRDs are to be used.

OBRA states the following as acceptable reasons for the use of physical restraints:
- All other interventions have been attempted before the use of restraints.

- Other disciplines have been consulted for their assistance.
- Supporting documentation has been completed.

Essentials of SRD Documentation
- Reason for the physical restraint
- Explanation given to patient and family
- Date and time of the patient's response to treatment
- Duration
- Frequency of observation and patient's response
- Safety
- Release the physical restraint at least every 2 hours
- Routine exercise of extremities, including range-of-motion
- Assessment for circulation and skin integrity
- Assessment for continued need for the physical restraint
- Patient outcome

PROCEDURE 12.5

Applying Safety Reminder Devices

1. Refer to medical record, care plan, and Kardex. Review agency policy. (*A physician's order is required before safety reminder devices [SRDs] are applied.*)
2. Perform hand hygiene.
3. Introduce self.
4. Identify patient.
5. Procedure:
   1. Explain procedure.
   2. Prepare for procedure by providing privacy and assembling necessary supplies.
   3. Receive instructions for application of an SRD from the nurse (a comprehensive nursing assessment of the patient's potential for injury and treatment in relation to the need for an SRD is crucial before applying SRD).
6. Apply appropriate type of SRD:
   1. **Wrist or ankle (extremity) SRD designed to immobilize one or more extremities**
      1. If using Kerlix gauze, make a clove hitch by forming a figure of 8 and picking up the loops. (*The clove hitch does not tighten when pulled.*)
      2. Place gauze or padding around the extremity.
      3. Slip the wrist(s) or ankle(s) through loops directly over the padding; if using a commercially made SRD, wrap the padded portion of the device around affected extremity, thread tie through slit in device, and fasten to second tie with a secure knot.

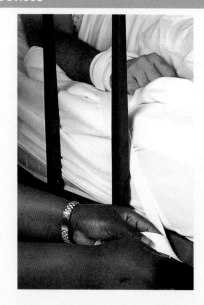

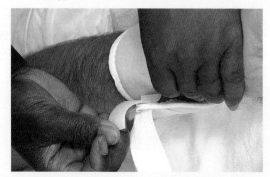

   4. Secure ends of ties to the movable portion of the bed frame that moves with the patient when the bed is adjusted, **not to side rails.**

   5. Leave as much slack as possible (1 to 2 inches).
   6. Palpate pulses below the SRD.
   2. **Elbow SRD**
      1. Place SRD (a piece of fabric with slots for the insertion of tongue blades to keep the elbow straight) over the elbow or elbows. (*Elbow SRDs are often used with children to prevent elbow flexion so that they cannot disturb tubes, catheters, and dressings.*)

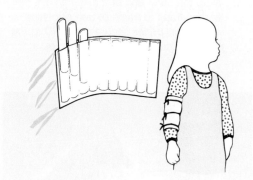

Continued

PROCEDURE 12.5

Applying Safety Reminder Devices—cont'd

2. Wrap SRDs snugly, tying them at the top. For small infants, tie or pin SRDs to their shirts.
3. **Vest (sometimes referred to as a wrap jacket or chest SRD)**
   1. Apply device over the patient's gown.
   2. Put vest on patient with V-shaped opening in the front.

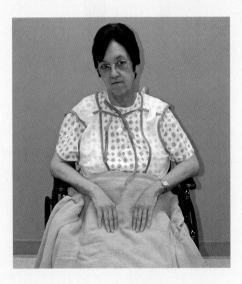

3. Pull tie at end of vest flap across the chest and slip tie through slit on opposite side of vest.
4. Wrap the other end of the flap across patient and tie the straps to frame of bed or behind wheelchair. *(Helps secure vest SRD to the patient.)* Use the quick-release knot.

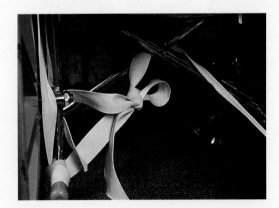

5. With a proper fit, there is room for a fist in the space between the vest and the patient.

4. **Gait or safety reminder belts**
   1. Apply belt over the patient's gown.

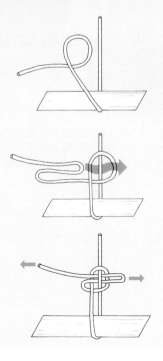

2. If patient is ambulating, place belt around the patient's waist. The belt usually has a buckle to secure the belt in place.
3. If the belt does not have a buckle, use a slip knot.
4. Use a quick-release knot rather than a regular knot to secure the safety reminder device to bed frame.

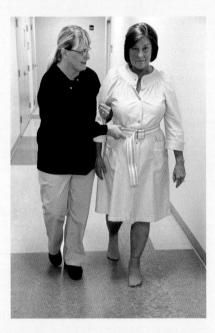

PROCEDURE 12.5

Applying Safety Reminder Devices—cont'd

5. Secure SRDs so that the patient cannot untie them.
6. Apply SRD with gentleness and compassion.
7. Perform hand hygiene.
8. Document procedure.
   - Reason(s) SRD needed
   - If appropriate, the notification of the physician and time order obtained
   - The time and type of SRD applied
   - The ongoing assessment and monitoring of the patient's skin, extremity circulation, and mental status
   - The response(s) of the patient
   - The periodic removal of the SRD and any skin care performed
   - If SRD removed, note time and follow-up assessments
   - If reapplication is needed, note reasons, time, and patient assessment
   - A flow sheet is an excellent tool for this documentation (see Fig. 11.1)

7. Follow-up
   1. Monitor for skin impairment.
   2. With the use of extremity SRD, assess extremity distal to SRD every 30 minutes or more often according to agency policy.
   3. Remove SRD on one extremity at a time at least every 2 hours (know agency policy) for 5 minutes.
   4. Monitor position of SRD, circulation, skin condition, and mental status frequently. Remove SRD when no longer needed.
   5. With the use of vest SRD, monitor respiratory status.
   6. Do NOT leave the patient unattended during temporary removal of SRD. Do take advantage of removal to change patient's position and inspect skin.
   7. Gently massage the skin beneath SRD; apply lotion or powder if desired.
   8. Change SRD when soiled or wet.
   9. Assess frequently for tangled ties or pressure points from knots; adjust SRD device(s) as needed.

8. Evaluation
   1. The SRD is adequate and appropriate for the individual patient's condition.
   2. SRDs are correctly applied. *(Correct application prevents injury to the patient or to others.)*

3. Quick-release knots are easily released.
4. Related problems (e.g., of the skin or of the musculoskeletal system) are identified.

9. Pediatric considerations
   - When a child must be restrained for a procedure, it is best that the person applying the restraint not be the child's parent or guardian.
   - A mummy restraint is a safe, efficient, short-term method to restrain a small child or infant for examination or treatment.
     1. Open a blanket, and fold one corner toward the center. Place the infant on the blanket with shoulders at the fold and feet toward the opposite corner.

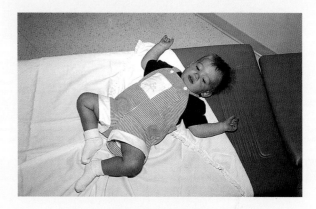

   2. With infant's right arm straight down against body, pull the right side of the blanket firmly across the right shoulder and chest, and secure beneath the left side of body.

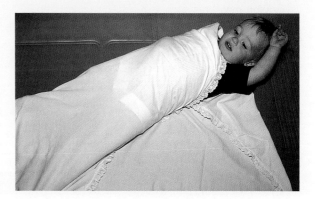

Continued

PROCEDURE 12.5

Applying Safety Reminder Devices—cont'd

3. Place the left arm straight against the body, bring the left side of the blanket across the shoulder and chest, and lock beneath the infant's body on the right side.

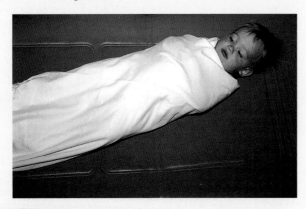

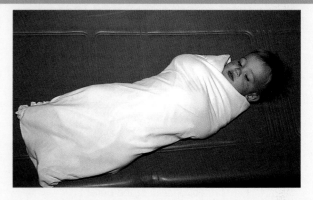

- Remain with the infant during restraint, and remove the restraint immediately after treatment is complete. If restraint is required for an extended period, remove it at least every 2 hours and perform range-of-motion exercises on all extremities.

4. Align the infant's legs, pull the corner of the blanket near the feet up toward the body, and tuck snugly in place or fasten securely with safety pins.

(Step 6a(3), 6b(3), 6d(1), 6d(4) figures from Cooper K, Gosnell K: Foundations of nursing, ed 7, St. Louis, 2015, Mosby. Step 6a(4), 6b(1), and 6c(4) figures from Potter PA, Perry AG: Fundamentals of nursing: concepts, process, and practice, ed 7, St. Louis, 2009, Mosby. Step 9(1) through 9(4) figures from Elkin MK, Perry AG, Potter PA: Nursing interventions and clinical skills, ed 3, St. Louis, 2004, Mosby.)

Injury & Illness Prevention Box 12.2

Patient Safety Promotion

- Explain to the patient and members of the family why SRDs are necessary.
- The nurse should provide information about the type of SRD to be used and the approximate time frame for use.
- Inform patient and family that the patient will still receive comfort measures such as repositioning and limb exercises.
- Instruct family to keep bedside tables and overbed tables close to the patient.
- Encourage family to mount grab bars around toilets and showers; instruct the patient how to use them.
- Recommend that rugs and carpets be securely attached to floors and stairs.

- Recommend that bath mats and nonskid strips be attached to bathtubs and the floors of shower stalls.
- Recommend that electrical cords be secured against baseboards so that the patient will not trip over them easily.
- Ensure that the call bell is within easy reach of the hospitalized patient, and show patient the location of emergency call bells in bathrooms. (The PCT must respond to call lights quickly, especially for patients who need assistance to the bathroom.)
- See that wheelchairs remain locked when transporting a patient from bed to wheelchair or back to bed.
- Instruct caregivers to check that side rails are up and safety straps secured around the patient who is on a stretcher.

Delegation and Documentation Box 12.1

Moving the patient is a task delegated to the PCT by the nurse. The following steps should be followed when moving the patient:
- Have the patient wear shoes with a nonslip surface during transfer or ambulation.
- Make slow, gradual position changes.
- Help the patient sit in a chair or return to bed if the patient has symptoms of orthostatic hypotension.

- When assisting with ambulation, the following steps should be followed:
  - Do not try to hold patients if they become dizzy or faint. Ease them into a sitting position in a chair or onto the floor (See Procedure 12.6).
  - Use assistive devices such as walkers, crutches, gait belt, or cane when appropriate.
  - Be sure that the area is free of clutter, wet areas, and rugs that may slide.

Delegation and Documentation Box 12.2

It is acceptable to have the skills of safe and effective transfer from bed to chair delegated to you as the PCT.

- Have the patient wear shoes with a nonskid surface during ambulation.
- Be sure that the area is free of clutter, wet areas, and rugs that may slide or buckle.
- Use an intravenous (IV) pole to assist in ambulation for patients with continuous IV therapy.

- Be sure that the patient uses the correct gait and weight bearing during ambulation.
- Ease patients to a sitting position in a chair or on the floor if they become dizzy or faint.
- Alert the nurse if a patient becomes dizzy or lightheaded or suffers a fall.

PROCEDURE 12.6

Assisting With Falls During Ambulation

1. Observe the patient closely.
2. Encourage the patient to do the following:
   - Take slow, deep breaths
   - Keep eyes open and look straight ahead
   - Keep head up
3. If the patient starts to fall, do not attempt to prevent the fall. Ease the patient to the floor. This allows you to break the fall, control its direction, and also protect the patient's head. Follow these steps when assisting a patient's fall:
   - Stand with your feet apart. Keep your back straight.
   - Bring the patient close to your body as quickly as possible. Use the gait belt if one is worn. If not, wrap your arms around the patient's waist. Move your leg so that the patient's buttocks rest on it. Move the leg near the patient (see illustration).

- Lower the patient to the floor by letting the patient slide down your leg. Bend at your hips and knees as you lower the patient (see illustration). *(The gravitational pull enables the patient to be lowered to the floor with a minimal amount of strain to your musculoskeletal system.)*
- Call for assistance.
- Assist patient to return to bed.
- Report and document the following:
  - How the fall occurred
  - How far the patient walked
  - How activity was tolerated before the fall
  - Any report of symptoms before the fall
  - The amount of assistance needed by the patient while walking
- Complete an incident report, if required.

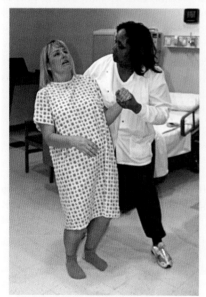

May support the falling patient under the arms as shown.

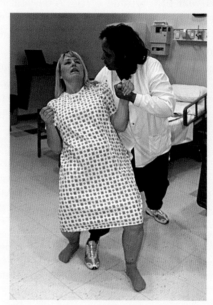

The patient's buttocks rest on your leg.

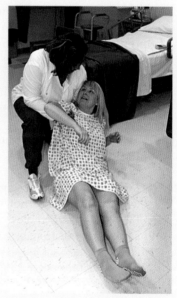

Slide the patient down your leg to the floor.

(From Cooper K: Foundations of nursing, ed 7, St. Louis, 2015, Mosby.)

CHAPTER SUMMARY

The PCT has an important role in the positioning of patients. Failure to position them correctly can result in permanent disability. Proper positioning permits activity, enhances comfort, and prepares patients for procedures.

Immobility sometimes results from illness or trauma, and sometimes it is prescribed for therapeutic reasons. Whatever the reason, immobility poses the risk of serious complications. Interventions to avoid these complications are possible.

When turning, moving, lifting, or carrying a patient, the PCT should secure adequate assistance to reduce strain and prevent injury to both the PCT and the patient. Perform procedures safely and properly, facilitating the patient's independence. Mechanical devices such as a hydraulic lift, roller board, and gurney lift are used for moving patients safely.

Documentation related to the need for the SRDs, the type of device used, and the patient's response is crucial. Be sure to communicate with the nurse regularly when a patient has an SRD.

Case Scenario

The PCT is in the process of transferring Mr. D from his bed to a chair with use of a mechanical lift. The PCT has prepared the chair and placed it near the bed. The PCT turns Mr. D to his side, places the sling under Mr. D to ensure adequate support of his head, returns Mr. D to his back, and slowly begins to lift him from his bed. What has the PCT forgotten to do, and why is it important? The patient has a trapeze bar across the bed, trochanter rolls, and a footboard. Explain the rationale for use of each of these devices to maintain proper body alignment.

REVIEW QUESTIONS

1. The PCT helps ambulate an 84-year-old female patient. The patient becomes very weak, reports feeling faint, and begins to fall. What is the most appropriate action to prevent injury to the patient?
   a. Support her while she is falling and allow her to sit on the floor.
   b. Carefully attempt to return her to her room.
   c. Tell her to hold onto the wall and that you will get more assistance.
   d. Ask her to take deep breaths and look straight ahead.

2. It is the patient's first night after an abdominal hysterectomy. She has not voided for 9 hours, and the PCT is to insert a Foley catheter into her bladder. What patient position best allows insertion of the catheter?
   a. Dorsal recumbent
   b. Lithotomy
   c. Sims's
   d. Prone

3. A 64-year-old patient has difficulty breathing and is unable to rest in a supine position. The patient's head of the bed is elevated to 90 degrees, a pillow is placed on the overbed table, and the nurse encourages the patient to lean forward, placing his head on the pillow. What position would this patient be considered as being in?
   a. Semi-Fowler's
   b. Dorsal
   c. Sims's
   d. Orthopneic

4. Which assistive device allows patients to pull with the upper extremities to raise their trunk off the bed, to assist in transfer from bed to wheelchair, and to perform upper arm exercises?
   a. Trapeze bar
   b. Trochanter roll
   c. Hand rolls
   d. Footboard

5. In which position is the patient lying face down or chest down?
   a. Supine
   b. Lateral
   c. Prone
   d. Fowler's

6. When using a lift sheet to assist in moving a patient up in bed, what should the PCT ask the patient to do?
   a. Bend the knees to assist in moving
   b. Keep the hands at sides
   c. Raise the arms above the head
   d. Maintain a straight body position

Basic Emergency Care

LEARNING OBJECTIVES

1. Describe the patient care technician's role in emergency response.
2. Summarize the typical emergency supplies and equipment.
3. Demonstrate the use of an automated external defibrillator.
4. Summarize the general rules for managing emergencies.
5. Recognize and respond to life-threatening emergencies in the ambulatory care setting.
6. Perform professional-level cardiopulmonary resuscitation (CPR).
7. Identify and assist a patient with an obstructed airway.
8. Assist and monitor a patient who has fainted.
9. Control a hemorrhagic wound.
10. Discuss the legal and ethics concerns arising from medical emergencies.

KEY TERMS

cyanosis A blue coloration of the mucous membranes and body extremities caused by lack of oxygen.

fibrillation Rapid, random, ineffective contractions of the heart.

idiopathic Pertaining to a condition or a disease that has no known cause.

myocardium The muscular lining of the heart.

rapid response team A team of medical personnel who respond to a patient whose condition may be rapidly getting worse.

ASSISTING WITH MEDICAL EMERGENCIES

First aid is defined as the immediate care given to a person who has been injured or has suddenly taken ill. Knowledge of first aid and related skills often can mean the difference between life and death, temporary and permanent disability, or rapid recovery and long-term hospitalization. The patient care technician may be responsible for initiating first aid in the healthcare facility and continuing to administer first aid until the physician or the trained medical team arrives. Every patient care technician should successfully complete a course for the healthcare personnel in cardiopulmonary resuscitation (CPR) and should continue to hold a current CPR card as long as he or she is employed.

Basic knowledge of CPR and life support skills needs to be updated regularly, because procedures change as new techniques are developed. For example, both the American Red Cross and the American Heart Association (AHA) now recommend the inclusion of training on automated external defibrillators (AEDs) for all healthcare workers.

Patient care technicians need up-to-date training in current emergency practices. They should try to attend a renewal course before their certification expires for first aid and CPR. Being prepared for both types of emergencies is important. The facility's employees must be ready to respond both to emergencies on site and to natural disasters or other emergencies that affect the community.

Patient care technicians are not responsible for diagnosing emergencies, but they are expected to make decisions about emergency situations on the basis of their medical knowledge and training. If any doubt exists about how to manage a particular situation, the patient care technician should not hesitate to consult the nurse or some other more experienced member of the healthcare team.

Rapid Response Team

Many healthcare facilities have created a specialized team of healthcare providers whose main job is to respond to potential patient emergencies inside the building before they become actual emergencies. The term rapid response describes how fast the team typically responds to the patient. The goal of this team is to respond when a patient is rapidly declining so that they may be able to prevent the patient from getting worse than he or she already is, or even dying. Members of this team usually include nurses from critical care units, a physician, and a respiratory therapist. Most facilities who use a rapid response team will allow any staff who are at the patient's bedside and note that the patient is getting significantly worse to call. Additionally, some

Table 13.1	Typical Rapid Response System Calling Criteria

- Heart rate more than 140/min or less than 40/min
- Respiratory rate more than 28/min or less than 8/min
- Systolic blood pressure greater than 180 mm Hg or less than 90 mm Hg
- Oxygen saturation less than 90% despite oxygen supplementation
- Acute or sudden change in mental status
- Urine output less than 50 ml/4 hours
- Staff member has a significant concern about the patient's condition

Additional criteria used at some facilities:
- Chest pain unrelieved by medication
- An airway that is threatened to be blocked
- Seizure
- Uncontrolled pain

Refer to your facility's policy and procedure for activating the rapid response team.

(Taken from: https://psnet.ahrq.gov/primers/primer/4/ rapid-response-systems.)

facilities allow the patient's family members to call the rapid response team if they feel that their loved one is getting suddenly worse. Typically, facilities will have certain criteria that may be met in order to call the rapid response team (Table 13.1).

Injury & Illness Prevention Box 13.1

- Perform only the emergency procedures for which you have been trained.
- If an emergency occurs in the facility, notify the nurse.
- If a nurse cannot be located, immediately contact the rapid response team.

Emergency Supplies

Emergency supplies consist of a properly equipped "crash cart" or box of items needed for a variety of emergencies (Fig. 13.1). The supplies vary to some degree, depending on what types of patients a particular unit cares for (Box 13.1). For example, a labor and delivery unit will have drugs that are specific to the pregnant patient and newborn baby, whereas an emergency department (ED) will have supplies that include treatment of poisoning. Emergency supplies should be kept in an easily accessible place that is known to everyone who works on the unit, and the supplies should be inventoried regularly. Expiration dates of medications and sterile supplies must be checked weekly or monthly, along with the status of available oxygen tanks and related supplies, and the cart should be replenished with fresh supplies after every use. This is a job that is often required of the patient care technician. Careful attention to the expiration dates can prevent not having

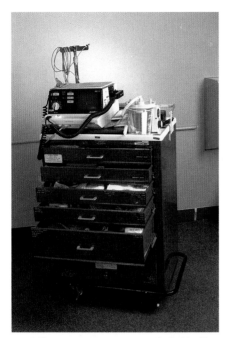

FIGURE 13.1 Office emergency cart with defibrillator. Drawers are marked for easy retrieval of emergency supplies. (From Proctor DB, Adams AP: *Kinn's The medical assistant: An applied learning approach,* ed 12, St. Louis, 2012, Saunders.)

the medication when it is needed. It is never a good idea to check expiration dates during an emergency. Use downtime, or slow times on the unit, to double-check expiration dates of medications and supplies.

Chain of Survival

The American Heart Association CPR course includes instruction on the *Chain of Survival*, which includes five links of a chain that identify the proper steps to take in caring for someone with cardiac arrest. Care is provided as soon as possible, as any delay can decrease the patient's chance of survival. (See AHA's website at http://www.heart.org/HEARTORG/CPRAndECC/WhatisCPR/EC-CIntro/Chain-of-Survival_UCM_307516_Article.jsp#.VqXD7Mc4 now for further details.)

Chain of Survival actions in the hospital include the following:

1. Surveillance and prevention
2. Recognizing cardiac arrest and activating the emergency medical services (EMS) system
3. Immediate, high-quality CPR
4. Rapid defibrillation
5. Advanced life support and postarrest care

Defibrillators

The patient care technician may be required to assist the healthcare team with defibrillation of emergency

| Box 13.1 | Basic Emergency Supplies |

Equipment

- Adhesive tape in 1- and 2-inch widths
- Airways—variety of types and sizes
- Alcohol wipes
- Ambu bag with assorted sizes of facial masks
- Antimicrobial skin ointment
- Bandage scissors
- Cotton balls and cotton swabs
- CPR masks—both adult and pediatric
- Defibrillator (with defibrillator daily checklist)
- Elastic bandages in 2- and 3-inch widths
- Filter needles
- Flashlight with batteries
- Gauze pads (2×2- and 4×4-inch widths) and roller bandage (both sterile and nonsterile)
- Gloves, sterile and nonsterile, in multiple sizes
- Hot and cold packs (instant type)
- Intravenous catheters, tubing, solutions (variety of types, including D_5W and Ringer's lactate), and tourniquet
- Laryngoscope with blades
- Lubricant
- Personal protective equipment (PPE), including impervious gowns, splash guards or goggles, and booties
- Portable oxygen tank with regulator, mask, and nasal cannula
- Roller gauze (Ace bandages and gauze dressing) in various sizes
- Sharps container
- Sphygmomanometer—both pediatric and adult regular and large sizes
- Splints—various sizes
- Sterile dressings—miscellaneous sizes, including two abdominal pads
- Steri-Strips or suturing material
- Suction machine and catheters
- Syringes and needles in assorted sizes and gauges
- Tongue blades
- Tubex cartridge system
- Venipuncture supplies and butterfly units

Certain medications will be included as well. It is not the patient care technician's responsibility to know all of the medications; however, it is the patient care technician's responsibility to ensure that all medications are within their respective expiration date and stocked according to the guidelines.

patients. Defibrillation is indicated when a patient is in ventricular fibrillation (VF). VF is a severe cardiac arrhythmia that is caused by uncoordinated, rapid firing of the electrical system of the heart, which makes it impossible for the ventricles to empty. In the absence of ventricular emptying, the patient has no pulse, blood pressure drops to zero, and the patient could die within 4 minutes unless help is given immediately.

Defibrillators are devices that send an electrical current through the myocardium by means of handheld paddles (in a healthcare facility) or self-adhesive pads applied to the chest. This electrical shock causes momentary asystole, giving the heart's natural pacemaker an opportunity to resume the heart rate at a normal rhythm.

An AED has a computerized system that analyzes a cardiac rhythm and delivers voice-prompt instructions on how to operate the device (Fig. 13.2 and Procedure 13.1). AEDs use self-adhesive pads that record and monitor the cardiac rhythm, and the device instructs the rescuer when to deliver the electrical charge. The apex-anterior position is the most commonly used paddle position, with the anterior (sternum) pad placed to the right of the upper sternum, and the apex pad placed under the patient's left nipple at the left middle axillary line. To defibrillate a female patient, the apex pad is placed next to or underneath the left breast.

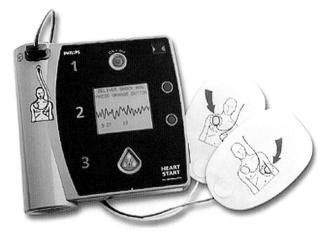

FIGURE 13.2 Fully automated external defibrillator. (Images provided courtesy of Philips Medical Systems IN Aehlert B: *Mosby's comprehensive pediatric emergency care*, St. Louis, 2005, Mosby.)

PROCEDURE 13.1

Maintain Provider/Professional-Level CPR Certification: Use an Automated External Defibrillator

These steps are to be performed only on an approved mannequin unless providing emergency care to a real patient who requires use of the AED.

If the healthcare worker witnesses a cardiac arrest, an automated external defibrillator (AED) should be used as soon as possible. If cardiopulmonary resuscitation (CPR) has already been started, continue performing CPR until the AED machine is turned on, pads are applied, and the machine is ready.

1. Place the AED near the victim's left ear. Turn on the AED.
2. Attach electrode pads to the victim's bare dry chest as pictured on the AED. Place the electrodes at the sternum and apex of the heart. Ensure that the pads are in complete contact with the victim's chest and that they do not overlap (see Figure 13.3).
3. All rescuers must clear away from the victim. Press the ANALYZE button. The AED analyzes the victim's coronary status, announces whether the victim is going to be shocked, and automatically charges the electrodes.

4. All rescuers must clear away from the victim. Press the SHOCK button if the machine is not automated. You may repeat 3 analyze-shock cycles.
5. Deliver one shock, leaving the AED attached, and immediately perform CPR, starting with chest compressions.
6. After 2 minutes of CPR, repeat the AED analysis and deliver another shock, if indicated. If a nonshockable rhythm is detected, the AED should instruct the rescuer to resume CPR immediately, beginning with chest compressions.
7. If the machine gives the "No Shock Indicated" signal, assess the victim. Check the carotid pulse and breathing status and keep the AED attached until EMS arrives. (Continue to monitor breathing and circulation, because these can stop at any time. Keep the AED pads in place to diagnose ventricular fibrillation quickly if it occurs.)

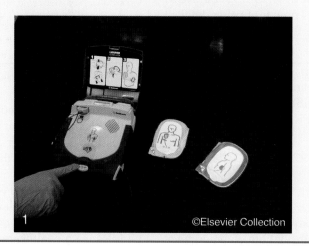

©Elsevier Collection

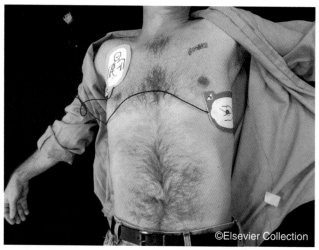

FIGURE 13.3 Connect the adhesive pads to the automated external defibrillator (AED) cables; apply the pads to the patient's chest at the upper right sternal border and at the lower left ribs over the cardiac apex.

Precautions for Automated External Defibrillators

- Neither the patient nor the caregiver should be in contact with any metal during defibrillation. Do not place the AED pad over jewelry, and remove the patient's glasses to prevent injuries.
- When available, a pediatric-dose AED system should be used for children 1 to 8 years of age (it should not be used on infants younger than 1 year). These systems deliver a reduced shock dose for victims up to about 8 years old or weighing 55 pounds.
- All clothing (including bras) must be removed; pads must be applied directly to the skin. If the individual has a great deal of hair on the chest, try to push the hair aside before applying the pads, or apply the pads and quickly remove them to remove hair from the area, then reapply new pads. The machine will prompt you by stating "Check electrode" if the connection is poor.
- To prevent burns, ensure that the patient is lying on a dry surface and the chest is dry before applying the pads.
- If the patient has an implanted defibrillator or pacemaker, it will be obvious from the bulged area under the surface of the skin on the chest. Apply the AED pads at least 1 inch away from implants to prevent interference.

GENERAL RULES FOR EMERGENCIES

Regardless of what type of facility you work in, consider the following general rules when faced with an emergency:

- It is most important to stay calm. Reassure the patient and make him or her as comfortable as possible.
- Assess the situation to determine the nature of the emergency. Decide whether the need is immediate. This decision requires calm judgment and medical knowledge.
- Obtain as much information as possible to determine the appropriate action.
- Immediately refer any concerns to the nurse.

Telephone Screening

Each time the phone rings in a healthcare facility, a person with a possible life-or-death situation may be on the other end of the line. One of the most important tasks performed by patient care technicians may be answering the phones and managing patients' needs efficiently and appropriately. Emergency action principles serve as a guide for managing emergency phone calls:

- If the patient's situation is life-threatening, tell the patient to activate EMS by calling 911.
- *Never put a caller with a life-threatening emergency on hold, and always be the last to hang up.*
- Remain on the line until help arrives and you have talked to EMS personnel.
- Immediately record the names of the caller and the patient, the location, and the phone number in case the connection is lost.
- If you are unsure how to manage the emergency situation, contact the nurse while you remain on the phone.
- Gather as much information as possible about what is wrong with the patient and when the problem started. Obtain details about the patient's condition, including the following:
  - What is the patient's level of consciousness? Alert, responsive, lethargic, or confused? Did the patient lose consciousness at any time? If so, for how long?
  - What is the character of the patient's respirations (and pulse if the caller is able to determine this): normal, rapid, shallow, or difficult?
  - Is there bleeding? If so, how much and from where?
  - Is there a suspected head or neck injury? If so, has the patient been moved?
  - Is there a suspected fracture? Where?
  - Does the patient have a history of this problem?
  - Are there other symptoms, such as fever, vomiting, diarrhea, or pain?
  - Details about what has been done for the patient.
  - Medication: What, when? Dose, effectiveness? Current allergies?
- Thoroughly document the information gathered and any actions taken, including notification of EMS, whether the patient was sent to the ED or an appointment was scheduled, all home care recommendations, and whether the physician was notified and when.

Management of On-Site Emergencies

An emergency can occur at any time to anyone. Always follow standard precautions when at risk for coming into contact with blood or body fluids. When an emergency occurs, it is impossible to determine the level of infection. All body fluids must be considered infectious, and appropriate precautions must be taken to prevent cross-contamination. It is important to document all details of the incident in the patient's medical record.

Fainting (Syncope)

Fainting, or *syncope*, is a common emergency. It usually is caused by a transient loss of blood flow to the brain (e.g., a sudden drop in blood pressure), which results in a temporary loss of consciousness. It can occur without warning, or the patient may appear pale; may feel cold, weak, dizzy, or nauseated; and may have numbness of the extremities before the incident. The greatest danger to the patient is an injury from falling during the attack. Therefore if a patient or family member has syncopal symptoms, immediately place the individual in a supine position. Loosen all tight clothing and maintain an open airway. Apply a cold washcloth to the forehead. Measure and record the patient's pulse, respiratory rate, and blood pressure, and report the findings to the physician. Keep the patient in a supine position for at least 10 minutes after the person regains consciousness. A complete patient history can help determine the possible causes of the attack (e.g., a history of heart disease or diabetes). Document the details of the episode and how long it took the patient to recover completely (Procedure 13.2).

If the patient does not recover quickly, a physician member of the healthcare team may activate the rapid response team. Syncope might be a brief episode in the development of a serious underlying illness, such as an abnormal heart rhythm, that could lead to sudden cardiac death.

Unresponsive Patient

If a patient is able to talk to you, he or she has an open airway. If the patient does not respond to a simple question (e.g., "Are you OK?"), gently shake the person's shoulder to check responsiveness. If the patient does not respond, you must assume that the patient is unconscious. Immediately call for help and activate EMS if that is the healthcare facility's policy.

To care for an unresponsive patient, first assess the patient's respirations to determine whether the person is breathing. When the patient collapsed, the tongue may have gone limp and occluded the airway. Just by changing the individual's position and opening the

---

---

airway, you may provide all the assistance the patient needs to breathe independently.

If the patient is face down, roll the victim onto his or her back while supporting the head, neck, and back. Apply the head tilt–chin lift movement to open the airway. The tongue is attached to the lower jaw, so moving the jaw forward automatically opens the patient's airway. If a head or neck injury is suspected, the neck should be manipulated as little as possible. If a neck injury is suspected, the airway should be open with the jaw-thrust maneuver. Both of these actions relieve possible obstruction of the trachea by the tongue.

Check for breathing no longer than 10 seconds by looking for a rise in the chest and by listening or feeling for air exchange (Fig. 13.4). Breathing may stop suddenly for a variety of reasons, including shock, disease, and trauma. If no breaths are detected, artificial ventilation must be started immediately, because death can occur within 4 to 6 minutes. Barrier devices should be kept on hand for artificial respiration (Fig. 13.5), and these should be used if rescue breaths are required (Procedure 13.3).

After giving the patient two slow breaths, check for signs of normal breathing or movement. If no signs of responsiveness are evident, check for cardiac circulation at the carotid pulse (in an adult or a child) or at the brachial pulse (in an infant) (Fig. 13.6). Gently feel for the pulse while continuing to assess the patient for possible signs of recovery for 5 to 10 seconds. If a pulse is present, continue ventilating the lungs with slow breaths every 4 to 5 seconds (adult) or every 3 seconds (child or infant). If the pulse is absent, begin cycles of 30 chest compressions at a rate of about 100 per minute followed by two slow breaths.

When both breathing and pulse stop, the victim has suffered sudden death. Sudden death has many causes,

PROCEDURE 13.2

Perform First Aid Procedures: Care for a Patient Who Has Fainted

1. If warning is given that the patient feels faint, have the patient lower the head to the knees to increase the blood supply to the brain.

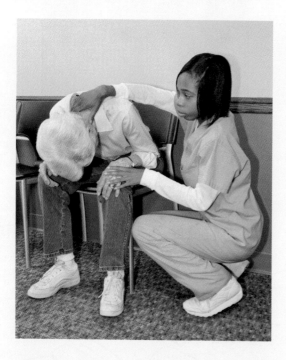

If this does not stop the episode, have the patient lie down on the examination table or lower the patient to the floor. If the patient collapses to the floor when fainting, treat with caution because of possible head or neck injuries.

2. Immediately notify the physician of the patient's condition and assess the patient for life-threatening emergencies, such as respiratory or cardiac arrest. If the patient is breathing and has a pulse, monitor the patient's vital signs.

3. Loosen any tight clothing and keep the patient warm, applying a blanket if needed.

4. If a head or neck injury is not a factor, elevate the patient's legs above the level of the heart using the footstool with pillow support if available.

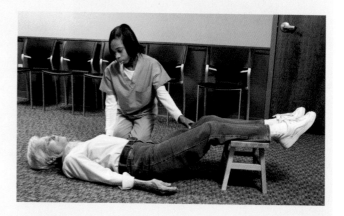

(Elevating the legs assists with venous blood return to the heart. This may relieve symptoms of fainting by elevating the blood pressure and increasing blood flow to vital organs.)

5. Continue to monitor vital signs and apply oxygen by nasal cannula if ordered by the physician.

6. If vital signs are unstable or the patient does not respond quickly, activate emergency medical services (EMS).

7. If the patient vomits, roll the patient onto his or her side to prevent aspiration of vomitus into the lungs.

8. Once the patient has completely recovered, assist the patient into a sitting position. Do not leave the patient unattended on the examination table.

Document the incident, including a description of the episode, the patient's symptoms and vital signs, the duration of the episode, and any complaints.

including heart disease, choking, drowning, poisoning, suffocation, electrocution, and smoke inhalation. CPR must be started immediately to attempt to revive the patient and to prevent permanent damage to body organs, especially the brain. Continue CPR until the victim begins to move, an AED is available and ready to use, professional help arrives, or you are too exhausted to continue. If the patient has a pulse but is not breathing, continue rescue breathing and occasionally monitor the pulse until help arrives.

Refer to the *Standard First Aid Manual* of the American Red Cross or the *American Heart Association CPR Manual*, or the organizations' websites, for specific procedures and precautions in the management of respiratory and cardiac emergencies. As stated earlier, all healthcare workers should have a current certification for the healthcare worker in CPR.

Choking

Choking is usually caused by a foreign object, often a ball or bolus of food, lodged in the upper airway. The victim may grab his or her neck between the thumb and the index finger (Fig. 13.7); this universal distress signal should be viewed as a sign that the victim needs help.

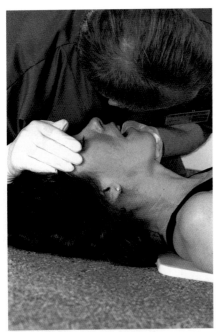

FIGURE 13.4 Checking for breathing in an unconscious patient. (From Proctor DB, Adams AP: *Kinn's The medical assistant: An applied learning approach,* ed 12, St. Louis, 2012, Saunders.)

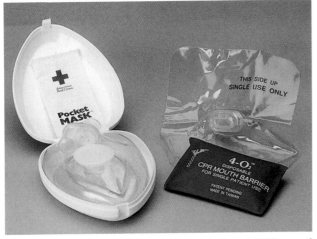

FIGURE 13.5 Cardiopulmonary resuscitation (CPR) mouth barriers. (From Proctor DB, Adams AP: *Kinn's The medical assistant: An applied learning approach,* ed 12, St. Louis, 2012, Saunders.)

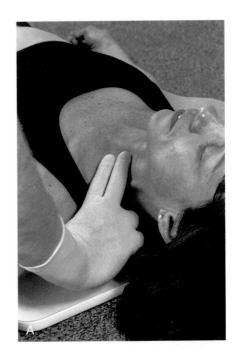

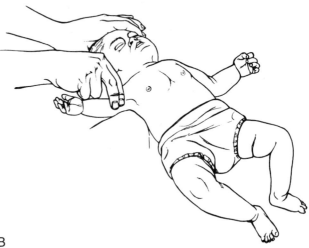

FIGURE 13.6 **A,** In an adult, check for a carotid pulse. **B,** In an infant, check for a brachial pulse. (From Proctor DB, Adams AP: *Kinn's The medical assistant: An applied learning approach,* ed 12, St. Louis, 2012, Saunders.)

If the victim has good air exchange or only partial airway obstruction and can speak, cough, or breathe, do not interfere, but encourage the patient to continue coughing until the object is expelled. Monitor the patient for signs of respiratory distress, such as pallor and cyanosis. If the patient has a pronounced wheeze (whistling sound in their airway) or a very weak cough, he or she has a partial airway obstruction with poor air exchange and may need help. If the patient is unable to

speak, breathe, or cough, a complete airway obstruction exists, and quick action must be taken to clear the airway. With complete obstruction, the patient eventually loses consciousness from lack of oxygen to the brain. This condition may lead to respiratory and cardiac arrest. If the object is not removed, the victim may die within 4 to 6 minutes. Procedure 13.4 presents the steps involved in clearing an obstructed airway in an adult. The procedure for removal of a foreign airway obstruction is exactly the same for a child older than 1 year of age.

To dislodge a foreign object from the airway of an infant up to 1 year of age, place the baby face down over

PROCEDURE 13.3

Maintain Provider/Professional-Level CPR Certification: Perform Adult Rescue Breathing, One-Rescuer and Two-Rescuer CPR; Perform Pediatric and Infant CPR

These steps are to be performed only on approved mannequins.

To Perform One-Rescuer CPR on an Adult Victim

1. Establish unresponsiveness. Tap the victim and ask, "Are you OK?" Wait for the victim to respond.
2. Activate the emergency response system. Get the AED. Use your personal cell phone if nearby to avoid leaving the patient. Put on gloves and get a ventilator mask. (As soon as it is determined that an adult victim requires emergency care, activate emergency medical services [EMS]. Most adults with sudden, nontraumatic cardiac arrest are in ventricular fibrillation. The time from collapse to defibrillation is the single most important predictor of survival.)
3. Tilt the victim's head by placing one hand on the forehead and applying enough pressure to push the head back; with the fingers of the other hand under the chin, lift up and pull the jaw forward. Look, listen, and feel for signs of breathing. Place your ear over the mouth and listen for breathing. Watch the rising and falling of the chest for evidence of breathing.

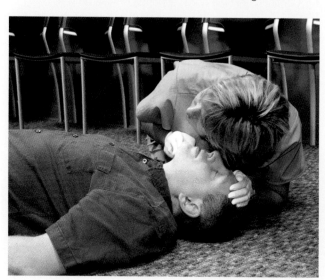

4. At the same time you are checking for breathing, check the patient's pulse (at the carotid artery for an adult or older child; at the brachial artery for an infant). If a pulse is present, continue rescue breathing (1 breath every 4 to 5 seconds—about 10 to 12 breaths per minute for an adult; 1 breath every 3 seconds—about 12 to 20 breaths per minute for an infant or child). If no signs of circulation are present, begin cycles of chest compressions at a rate of 100 to 120 compressions per minute for an adult followed by 2 slow breaths.
5. To deliver chest compressions, kneel at the victim's side a couple of inches away from the chest. Hand placement is over the sternum, between the nipples but above the xiphoid process.
6. Place the heel of your hand on the chest over the lower part of the sternum.

7. Place your other hand on top of the first and interlace or lift your fingers upward off the chest.

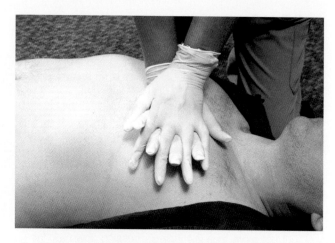

8. Bring your shoulders directly over the victim's sternum as you compress downward, keeping your elbows locked.

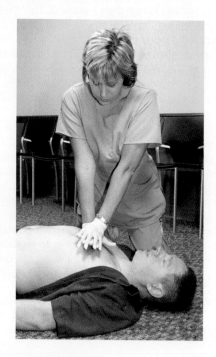

9. Depress the sternum at least 2 inches in an adult victim. Avoid pressing down more than 2.4 inches; injury can occur. Relax the pressure on the sternum after each compression but do not remove your hands from the sternum.
10. After performing 30 compressions (at a rate of 100 to 120 compressions per minute), perform the head tilt–chin lift maneuver to open the airway, and give 2 rescue breaths. Each breath should take only 1 second.
11. Continue the cycle of 30 compressions to 2 breaths until help arrives, or an AED arrives. If the patient starts

Continued

PROCEDURE 13.3

Maintain Provider/Professional-Level CPR Certification: Perform Adult Rescue Breathing, One-Rescuer and Two-Rescuer CPR; Perform Pediatric and Infant CPR—cont'd

to respond with movement as well as a pulse and respiratory rate, move the patient to a recovery position.

Adult Two-Rescuer CPR

1. Rescuer 1 should check for a response from the person by asking them, "Are you OK?"
2. Rescuer 1 should check for breathing and a pulse for not more than 10 seconds. If there is no breathing or a pulse within the 10 seconds, CPR is begun.
3. Expose the person's chest and ensure that they are in a supine position.
4. If the victim does not have a pulse, then the compressor begins to give chest compressions at a rate of 100 to 120 per minute. Count out loud so that you can establish a regular rhythm. Allow the chest to recoil between each compression. Give 30 compressions.
5. Press down with each compression at least 2 inches but not more than 2.4 inches. Pressing down too far can cause injury to the patient.
6. Open the person's airway using the head tilt–chin lift method and give two rescue breaths. Each breath should not last longer than 1 second. The chest should rise and fall with each breath.
7. Continue the cycle of 30 compressions to 2 breaths minimizing interruptions to no longer than 10 seconds.
8. Rescuer 2 obtains the AED, opens the case, and turns it on (see Procedure 13.1). Once the AED has performed an analysis, the AED will indicate whether or not a shock will be given.
9. Once the AED has given a shock, CPR will be resumed by Rescuers 1 and 2. One rescuer will give 30 chest compressions; the other will give 2 rescue breaths.
10. When the AED signals for a rhythm check, pause and change positions.
11. Resume CPR after the rhythm check by giving 30 chest compressions and 2 rescue breaths. Continue with this pattern until the person begins to move or until a code team or rapid response team arrives to provide advanced cardiac life support. If the person begins to move, position him or her in the recovery position.

To Perform CPR on a Child

The procedure for giving CPR to a child aged 1 to 8 years is essentially the same as that for an adult. The differences are as follows:
- Start CPR if the child's heart rate is less than 60 beats per minute.
  - Perform five cycles of compressions and breaths on the child (30:2 ratio, about 2 minutes) before calling 911 or the local emergency number or using an AED. If another person is available, have that person activate EMS while you care for the child. (It is important to provide immediate circulation of

oxygenated blood to a child to prevent brain damage. Most pediatric cardiac arrests occur because of a secondary problem, such as airway occlusion, rather than a cardiac problem. If you know that there is an airway obstruction, clear the obstruction and then proceed with CPR.)
- Use only one hand to perform chest compressions. (The pediatric sternum requires less force to achieve the needed depression.)
- Breathe more gently.
- When two rescuers are present, change the compression-to-breath ratio to 15 compressions to 2 breaths. For one rescuer, the same ratio for adults is used for children, 30 compressions followed by 2 breaths per cycle; after 2 breaths, immediately begin the next cycle of compressions and breaths.
  - Give only enough air to make the chest rise.
  - Chest compressions should compress about 1/3 of the depth, or 2 inches.
- After five cycles (about 2 minutes) of CPR without response, use a pediatric AED if available.
- Continue until the child responds or help arrives.

Infant CPR

Infant cardiac arrest typically is caused by lack of oxygen from drowning or choking. If you know that the infant has an airway obstruction, clear the obstruction; if you do not know why the infant is unresponsive, perform CPR for 2 minutes (about five cycles) before calling 911 or the local emergency number. If another person is available, have that person call for help immediately while you attend to the baby.

Rescue Breathing for an Infant

Use an infant ventilator mask or cover the baby's mouth and nose with your mouth.
- Give two rescue breaths by gently puffing out the cheeks and slowly breathing into the infant's mouth, taking about 1 second for each breath.

To Perform CPR on an Infant

- For single-rescuer CPR, draw an imaginary line between the infant's nipples. Place two fingers on the sternum just below this intermammary line.
  - For two-rescuer CPR, use the two-thumb encircling hands method.
- Gently compress the chest.
- Compression rate should be 100 to 120 per minute.
- Administer 2 breaths after every 30 compressions.
- After about five 30:2 cycles, activate EMS.
- Continue CPR until the child responds or help arrives.
  - Remove your gloves and the ventilator mask valve and discard them in the biohazard container. Disinfect the ventilator mask per the manufacturer's recommendations. Sanitize your hands.
  - Document the procedure and the patient's condition.

your forearm and across your thigh. The head should be lower than the trunk, and you should support the baby's head and neck with one hand. Using the heel of your other hand, deliver five blows to the back, between the infant's shoulder blades (Fig. 13.8A). Holding the baby between your arms, turn the infant face up, keeping the head lower than the trunk. Using two fingers, deliver five thrusts to the midsternal area at the infant's nipple line (Fig. 13.8B). Examine the infant's mouth, and if the object is visible, pluck it out with your fingertips. *Never perform a finger sweep on an infant.* A baby's oral cavity is too small for a finger sweep, and such an action may only push the obstruction farther into the airway. If the obstruction is not visible, administer two rescue breaths by covering the baby's nose and mouth with your mouth, or use a pediatric ventilator mask if available. Repeat the sequence until the foreign body is expelled or help arrives.

If a choking victim is in the late stages of pregnancy, chest compressions should be delivered to prevent possible trauma to the infant. If the patient is obese and you are unable to wrap your arms around the abdomen, perform chest compressions as you would for a pregnant woman.

The abdominal thrust maneuver also can be performed on yourself if you are choking and no one is nearby to help you. Press your fist into your upper abdomen with quick, upward thrusts, or lean forward and press the abdomen quickly against a firm object, such as the back of a chair.

Seizures

Seizures may be idiopathic, meaning that we do not know why they occur, or they may result from trauma, injury, or metabolic alterations, such as hypoglycemia

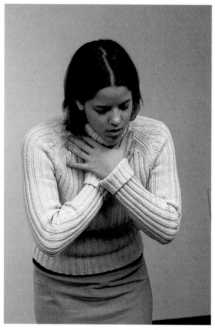

FIGURE 13.7 Universal sign of choking. (From Proctor DB, Adams AP: *Kinn's The medical assistant: An applied learning approach,* ed 12, St. Louis, 2012, Saunders.)

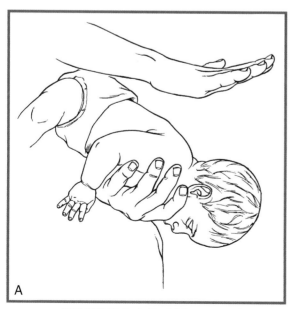 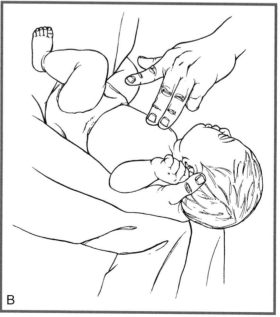

FIGURE 13.8 A, Back blows are administered to an infant supported on the arm and thigh. B, Chest thrusts are administered in the same position as for cardiac compressions. (From Henry MC, Stapleton ER: *EMT prehospital care,* ed 3, Philadelphia, 2004, Saunders.)

PROCEDURE 13.4

Perform First Aid Procedures: Respond to an Airway Obstruction or Choking in an Adult

The technique for an unresponsive victim is to be performed only on an approved mannequin.

1. Ask, "Are you choking?" If the victim indicates yes, ask, "Can you speak?" If the victim is unable to speak, tell the victim that you are going to help. (If the victim is unable to speak, is coughing weakly, and/or is wheezing, he or she has an obstructed airway with poor air exchange, and the obstruction must be removed before respiratory arrest occurs.)
2. Stand behind the victim with your feet slightly apart. (With an obstructed airway, the victim may lose consciousness at any time. The rescuer must be prepared to lower the unconscious victim to the floor safely.)
3. Reach around the victim's abdomen and place an index finger into the victim's navel or at the level of the belt buckle. Make a fist of the opposite hand (do not tuck the thumb into the fist) and place the thumb side of the fist against the victim's abdomen above the navel. If the victim is pregnant, place the fist above the enlarged uterus. If the victim is obese, it may be necessary to place the fist higher in the abdomen. It may be necessary to perform chest thrusts on a victim who is pregnant or obese. (The fist should be placed in the soft tissue of the abdomen to avoid injury to the sternum or rib cage.)
4. Place the opposite hand over the fist and give abdominal thrusts in a quick inward and upward movement.

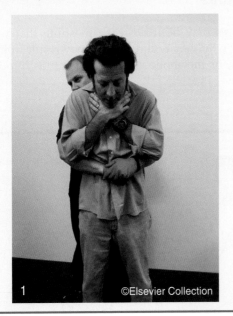

1   ©Elsevier Collection

Repeat the abdominal thrusts until the object is expelled or the victim becomes unresponsive.

Unresponsive Adult Victim

1. Carefully lower the patient to the ground, activate the emergency response system, and put on disposable gloves.
2. Immediately begin cardiopulmonary resuscitation (CPR) with 30 compressions and 2 breath cycles using the ventilator mask. (Higher airway pressures are maintained with chest compressions than with abdominal thrusts.)
3. Each time the airway is opened to deliver a rescue breath during CPR, look for an object in the victim's mouth and remove it if visible. If no object is found, immediately return to the cycle of 30 chest compressions.
4. A finger sweep should be used only if the rescuer can see the obstruction.
5. Continue cycles of 30 compressions to 2 rescue breaths until the obstruction is removed or emergency medical services (EMS) arrives.
6. If the obstruction is removed, assess the victim for breathing and circulation. If a pulse is present but the patient is not breathing, begin rescue breathing.
7. Once the patient has been stabilized or EMS has taken over care, remove your gloves and the ventilator mask valve and discard them in the biohazard container. Disinfect the ventilator mask per the manufacturer's recommendations. Sanitize your hands.
8. Document the procedure and the patient's condition.

or hypocalcemia. A *febrile* seizure is transient and occurs with a rapid rise in body temperature above 101.8°F (38.8°C). Febrile seizures typically occur in children between 6 months and 5 years of age. Many different types of seizures occur, but all are caused by a disruption in the electrical activity of the brain.

If a patient suffers a grand mal seizure, which involves uncontrolled muscular contractions, the most important point is to protect the patient from possible injury. Clear everything away from the patient that could cause accidental injury, and observe him or her until the seizure ends. Do not place anything into the person's mouth because it may damage the teeth or tongue and force the tongue back over the trachea. Do not hold the patient down because this may result in muscle injuries or fractures. If unconsciousness persists after the seizure has subsided, place the patient in the recovery position to maintain an open airway and allow drainage of

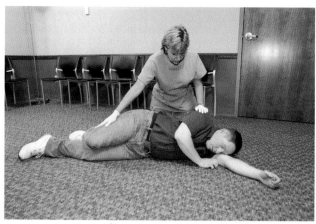

FIGURE 13.9 Recovery position. (From Proctor DB, Adams AP: *Kinn's The medical assistant: An applied learning approach,* ed 12, St. Louis, 2012, Saunders.)

excess saliva. After the seizure is over, let the patient rest or sleep, but never leave the person alone. Notify the nurse at once, or call the rapid response team.

To prevent choking, position the head so that any secretions drain from the side of the mouth. If the patient is lying on the floor, did not fall, and shows no indications of a head or neck injury, he or she can be placed in the recovery position as follows (Fig. 13.9):

1. Place the patient's arm that is farthest from you alongside and above the head; place the other arm across the chest.
2. Bend the leg that is closest to you, and after placing one arm under the patient's head and shoulder and the other hand on the flexed knee, roll the patient away from you while you stabilize the head and neck. The patient's head should be resting on the extended arm.

The recovery position uses gravity to drain fluids from the mouth and keep the trachea clear. Keep the patient in this position until the person is alert or help arrives. Do not give the patient anything to eat or drink. Vital signs should be measured at regular intervals and recorded for the physician.

Bleeding

Patients may report any of several different types of wounds. A *contusion* is a closed wound with no evidence of injury to the skin; it typically is caused by blunt trauma, appears swollen and discolored, and is painful. A contusion results in a painful bruise, but the skin remains intact. A scrape on the surface of the skin (e.g., a skinned knee, rug burn) is called an *abrasion*. A deeper, more jagged wound is called a *laceration*. Additional tissue damage may occur around a laceration, and, depending on its depth, the wound may need to be repaired surgically. A *puncture* wound occurs when an object is forced into the body (e.g., stepping on a nail). If an object is lodged in body tissues, the best course is to leave it there, stabilize it as much as possible with rolled-up material, and transport the individual to a clinic or ED. The puncture may have severed blood vessels, and if the object is removed, considerable bleeding may occur. An injury in which tissue is torn away (e.g., complete or partial removal of a finger) is known as an *avulsion*.

Lacerations are common presentations in a primary care physician's office. A lacerated wound shows jagged or irregular tearing of the tissues. The severity depends on the cause of the laceration, the site and extent of the injury, and whether the area is contaminated. The injury that caused the laceration also may have damaged blood vessels, nerves, bones, joints, and organs in the body cavities.

When the patient arrives at the facility, put on gloves, have the patient lie down, and cover the injured area with a sterile dressing; use a dressing that is thick enough to absorb the bleeding (Procedure 13.5). Reassure the patient and explain your actions as much as possible.

Wounds that are not bleeding severely and that do not involve deep tissue damage should be cleaned with antimicrobial soap and water to remove bacteria and other foreign matter. If the laceration is extremely dirty, the physician may want the area irrigated with sterile normal saline solution.

A butterfly closure strip may be used over small lacerations to hold the edges together. If the wound is superficial and has straight edges, it may be closed with a microporous tape (e.g., Steri-Strips) (Fig. 13.10), which eliminates the discomfort of suturing and suture removal. Another wound closure option is a tissue adhesive product such as Dermabond™ fluid or Liquiband™, which forms a strong, flexible closure similar in strength to nylon suture material. Tissue adhesive products are very useful for closing simple lacerations in children while providing an antimicrobial and waterproof coating to the wound site that lasts several days, even with repeated washing.

After the clinician closes the wound, the patient care technician typically applies a sterile dressing to the site. The size and thickness of the dressing depend on the type of wound.

Nosebleeds (Epistaxis)

A nosebleed, or *epistaxis*, is a hemorrhage that usually results from the rupture of small vessels in the nose. Nosebleeds can be caused by injury, disease, hypertension, strenuous activity, high altitudes, exposure to cold,

PROCEDURE 13.5

Perform First Aid Procedures: Control Bleeding

1. Sanitize your hands and put on appropriate personal protective equipment.
2. Assemble equipment and supplies.
3. Apply several layers of sterile dressing material directly to the wound and exert pressure.
4. Wrap the wound with bandage material. Add more dressing and bandaging material if the bleeding continues.
5. If bleeding persists and the wound is on an extremity, elevate the extremity above the level of the heart. Notify the physician immediately if the bleeding cannot be controlled.
6. If the bleeding still continues, maintain direct pressure and elevation; also apply pressure to the appropriate artery. If the bleeding is in the arm, apply pressure to the brachial artery by squeezing the inner aspect of the middle upper arm. If the bleeding is in the leg, apply pressure to the femoral artery on the affected side by pushing with the heel of the hand into the femoral crease at the groin. If the bleeding cannot be controlled, emergency medical services (EMS) may need to be activated.
7. Once the bleeding has been brought under control and the patient has been stabilized, discard contaminated materials in an appropriate biohazard waste container.
8. Disinfect the area, then remove your gloves and discard them in a biohazard waste container.
9. Sanitize your hands.
10. Document the incident, including details of the wound, when and how it occurred, the patient's symptoms and vital signs, treatment provided by the physician, and the patient's current condition.

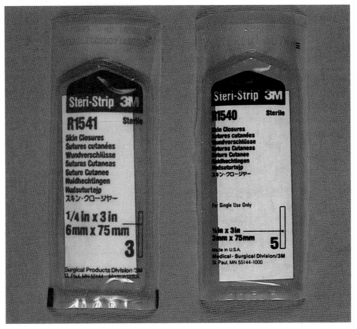

FIGURE 13.10 Steri-Strips. (From Proctor DB, Adams AP: *Kinn's The medical assistant: An applied learning approach,* ed 12, St. Louis, 2012, Saunders.)

overuse of anticoagulant medications (e.g., aspirin), and nasal recreational drug use. Bleeding from the anterior nostril area usually is venous, whereas bleeding from the posterior region usually is arterial and is more difficult to stop. Treatment of epistaxis varies according to the amount of bleeding and the presence of other conditions, as well as the use of anticoagulant medications.

If the bleeding is mild to moderate and from one side of the nose, the patient should sit up, lean slightly forward, and apply direct pressure to the affected nostril by pinching the nose. Continue constant pressure for 10 to 15 minutes to allow clotting to take place. Repeat if the bleeding cannot be controlled, insert a clean gauze pad into the nostril, and notify the nurse.

Legal and Ethical Issues

The patient care technician works in the healthcare environment and reports to the nurse or physician. Although you are responsible for your own actions, the nurse or physician is legally responsible for the care you administer to patients while working in the healthcare facility. You are responsible for knowing the limitations placed on patient care technicians in your state and for adhering strictly to your employer's emergency care policies and procedures. Patient care technicians are not qualified to diagnose a patient problem but are responsible for acting appropriately in a medical emergency. In addition to legal responsibilities, you have an ethical responsibility to your patients to provide the highest standard of care. Always act in the best interest of the patient, and never hesitate to ask the nurse for immediate assistance when faced with a medical emergency.

Most states have enacted *Good Samaritan* laws to encourage healthcare professionals to provide medical assistance at the scene of an accident without fear of being sued for negligence. These statutes vary greatly, but all have the intent of protecting the caregiver. A physician or other healthcare professional is not legally obligated to provide emergency care at the site of an accident, regardless of the ethical and moral considerations. Legal liability is limited to gross neglect of the victim or willfully causing further injury to the victim. As a caregiver, you are required to act as a reasonable person and cannot be held liable for personal injury resulting from an act of omission, or not doing something to help. Good Samaritan statutes provide for evaluation of the caregiver's judgment but are in effect only at the site of an emergency, not at your place of employment.

If you have not been trained in CPR, you cannot be expected to perform the procedure at the emergency site. However, in many states, a healthcare provider with CPR training and skills who is present at the scene can be declared negligent if cardiac arrest occurs and he or she does not administer CPR to the victim.

If the victim is conscious, or if a member of his or her immediate family is present, obtain verbal consent to perform emergency care. Consent is implied if the patient is unconscious and no family member is present.

Patient care technicians also can play a key role in community response to natural or human-made disasters. The patient care technician is cross-trained to perform multiple clinical duties that would prove very useful in an emergency. These include interacting professionally with patients, performing diagnostic tests, performing phlebotomy, assisting with procedures, and administering first aid and CPR as needed. Because of this wide range of skills, patient care technicians serve as useful volunteers on local emergency response teams. Investigate agencies and organizations that are committed to emergency preparedness in your community, and see how a patient care technician could help these organizations if an emergency arises.

CHAPTER SUMMARY

The patient care technician must be constantly on guard to protect patients from possible injury. Methods for achieving this goal include communicating openly about patient safety issues, following standard procedures when delivering patient care, and working as part of a team to secure patients' safety. Patient care technicians can be of considerable help in a community emergency. They can provide therapeutic communication to gather patient data, monitor injured victims, perform first aid and monitor vital signs, and help with any medically related service.

Each healthcare unit must have a centrally located crash cart or emergency bag stocked with all emergency supplies, equipment, and medication. This material must be inventoried consistently and maintained.

Management of emergencies requires a calm, efficient approach. Life-threatening emergencies require immediate assessment, and notification to the nurse. While waiting for assistance from the nurse or the rapid response team, the patient care technician should check for breathing and circulation. Rescue breaths or CPR is administered if indicated. Depending on the patient's signs and symptoms, the patient should be monitored for signs of a heart attack; the Heimlich maneuver is performed for an airway obstruction. The patient care technician should ask for help when indicated and should perform appropriate procedures based on the patient's presenting condition.

Infants with an obstructed airway should receive alternating back blows and chest thrusts with attempted rescue breaths until the item is dislodged or help arrives. The patient care technician should always follow standard precautions when caring for a patient with a medical emergency. Documentation of emergency treatment should include information about the patient; vital signs; allergies, current medications, and pertinent health history; the patient's chief complaint; the sequence of events, including any changes in the patient's condition since the incident; and any physician's orders and procedures performed.

Good Samaritan laws, which vary from state to state, are designed to protect any individual from liability, whether a healthcare professional or a layperson, if he or she provides assistance at the site of an emergency. The law does not require a medically trained person to act, but if emergency care is given in a reasonable and responsible manner, the healthcare worker is protected from being sued for negligence. This protection, however, does not extend to the workplace.

Case Scenario

Cheryl Skurka, PCT, has been working for Dr. Peter Bendt in the urgent care for approximately 6 months. During that time, a number of patient emergencies have presented. Cheryl is concerned that she is not prepared to assist with emergencies in the ambulatory care setting. She decides to ask Dr. Bendt for assistance, and he suggests that she work with the experienced screening staff to learn how to manage emergencies.

- Is it important for Cheryl to be able to recognize life-threatening emergencies and to be prepared to respond to them? Why or why not?

- What are some of the typical patient emergencies that occur in a healthcare facility?
- How should Cheryl instruct a patient to control bleeding from a hemorrhaging wound?
- What legal factors should Cheryl keep in mind when handling emergencies?

REVIEW QUESTIONS

1. Which members of the healthcare team typically make up a rapid response team?
   a. Critical care nurse
   b. Patient care technician
   c. Housekeeping
   d. Unit secretary

2. What is the primary goal of the rapid response team?
   a. Respond to the patient's complaints
   b. Provide the patient with a quicker response time to requests for the dietary tray
   c. Improve the patient outcomes by responding to a decline in his or her condition in a quick manner
   d. Improve the patient's satisfaction with care

3. CPR provided to adults is the same procedure as with infants.
   a. True
   b. False

4. A patient care technician who is certified in CPR could be found negligent if someone needed CPR and he or she chose not to assist.
   a. True
   b. False

5. Which of the following guidelines are true with use of an automated external defibrillator (AED)?
   a. Fingernail polish must be removed from the patient's fingernails.
   b. Excessive chest hair may need to be removed.
   c. The patient care technician is not allowed to assist in the use of the AED.
   d. Use of the AED requires at least two people.

Patient Assessment

Assisting With the Physical Examination

1. Outline the patient care technician's role in preparing for the physical examination.
2. Summarize the instruments and equipment the physician typically uses during a physical examination.
3. Describe the six methods of examination and give an example of each.
4. Outline the basic principles of properly gowning and draping a patient for examination.
5. Position and drape a patient in six different examining positions while remaining mindful of the patient's privacy and comfort.
6. Outline the sequence of a routine physical examination.
7. Prepare for and assist in the physical examination of a patient, correctly completing each step of the procedure in the proper sequence.
8. Summarize the role of the patient care technician in the physical examination process.
9. Discuss the legal and ethical implications of the physical examination.

auscultation The act of listening to body sounds, typically with a stethoscope, to assess various organs throughout the body.

bruit An abnormal sound or murmur heard on auscultation of an organ, vessel (such as a carotid artery), or gland.

clubbing Abnormal enlargement of the distal phalanges (fingers and toes) associated with cyanotic heart disease or advanced chronic pulmonary disease.

colonoscopy Procedure in which a fiberoptic scope is used to examine the large intestine.

electrocardiogram A graphic record of electrical conduction through the heart.

emphysema Pathologic accumulation of air in the alveoli, which results in alveolar destruction and overall oxygen deprivation; in the lungs, the bronchioles become plugged with mucus and lose elasticity.

gait Manner or style of walking.

hospitalist A physician, nurse practitioner, or physician's assistant who provides care to patients who are hospitalized.

manipulation Movement or exercising of a body part by means of an externally applied force.

murmur Abnormal sound heard during auscultation of the heart that may or may not have a pathologic origin; it is associated with valve disease or a congenital heart defect.

nodules Small lumps, lesions, or swellings that are felt when the skin is palpated.

palpation The use of touch during the physical examination to assess the size, consistency, and location of certain body parts.

primary care physician A physician who treats patients, typically in an outpatient setting, for a broad range of diseases across all age ranges.

sclera The white part of the eye that forms the orbit.

transillumination Inspection of a cavity or organ by passing light through its walls.

trauma Physical injury or a wound caused by an external force or violence.

In an effort to promote health maintenance, healthcare professionals must understand the anatomy and physiology of the body, the role each body part plays, how each component functions, and what happens to the body when disease occurs in body systems.

PRIMARY CARE PHYSICIAN/HOSPITALIST

Primary care physicians (PCPs) treat patients of all ages for a broad range of diseases and complaints. A PCP is qualified to provide healthcare for the entire family from birth to old age. Most health insurance programs have converted to the *primary care referral system.* This often means that most patients are required to have a PCP as the gatekeeper for personal healthcare-related issues. Therefore the PCP must be contacted first, before the patient can be referred to specialty physicians for care.

The hospitalist is a physician, nurse practitioner, or physician assistant who is employed by the hospital to provide care to patients who present in a hospital setting. The hospitalist is not from a particular office; rather, the physician's place of employment is the hospital. More hospitals are choosing to hire hospitalists in an effort to provide around-the-clock care, which improves continuity in care, increases quality, and decreases patient wait times for physical examinations and treatment. In hospitals where hospitalists are employed, care is available 24 hours a day, 7 days a week, including holidays. This allows PCPs and other providers who have their own practice to maintain that practice without having to travel to the hospital to round on their patients and make admission and discharge decisions. The hospitalist makes those decisions in collaboration with the PCP, and is a person who is always present within the hospital building. Typically, hospitalists will take shift rotations, such as 8-hour, 12-hour, or 24-hour rotations.

The PCP evaluates the patient's total healthcare needs, provides personal medical care within one or more fields of medicine, and refers the patient to a specialist when an advanced or serious condition warrants additional expertise. The patient care technician's clinical responsibilities in a primary care office include assisting with patients who may have problems in any of the body systems and with procedures in all age groups. With such a diversified scope of practice, the physician and patient care technician must work as a team to use their time efficiently and still provide quality, patient-centered healthcare. This is also true as well in the hospital setting. The team may be patient care technician and hospitalists. In the emergency department, hospitalists will perform physical examinations and will depend on the patient care technician to set up the room for a physical examination, as well as prepare the patient for the physical examination. This chapter will cover the physical examination, what is required to complete one, and your role in the examination as the patient care technician.

PHYSICAL EXAMINATION

The purpose of a physical examination is to determine the patient's overall state of well-being. All major organs and body systems are checked during a physical examination. As the physician examines the entire body, he or she interprets the findings, and by the time the examination has been completed, the physician has formed an initial diagnosis of the patient's condition. Often laboratory and other diagnostic tests are ordered to supplement the physician's initial diagnosis. The results of these tests are used to refine the patient's diagnosis, to help the physician plan or revise treatment for the patient, to evaluate and maintain current drug therapy, and/or to determine the patient's progress.

Preparing for the Physical Examination

Role of the Patient Care Technician in the Physical Examination

Before the examination, the patient care technician has the opportunity to ensure that the patient feels comfortable during the examination process and that all the necessary medical information has been obtained. As part of patient preparation, the patient care technician should verify the patient's name and date of birth and ask about any allergies. These are known as acceptable patient identifiers to ensure that you have the correct patient. At least two patient identifiers must be used when performing a procedure or obtaining a specimen. The patient's room number and physical location are not acceptable patient identifiers. The patient care technician's duties include preparing and maintaining the examination room and equipment, preparing the patient, and assisting the physician during the physical examination.

Room Preparation

The patient care technician is responsible for ensuring that the examination room is ready for any procedure that might be performed during the physical examination. The area should be as comfortable as possible for the patient and free of any potential dangers. The examination room is prepared as follows:

- The area should be checked at the beginning of each shift and between patients to ensure that it is completely stocked with equipment and supplies and that all equipment is functioning properly and the room properly cleaned. The patient care technician must understand how to take care of and operate all equipment and instruments and should refer to operation manuals supplied by manufacturers as needed.

- Expiration dates must be checked regularly on all packages and supplies, and expired materials should be discarded.
- The room should be private, well lit, and at a comfortable temperature for the patient during the physical examination. Warm blankets should be available for the patient who may get chilled during the examination.
- The area should be cleaned and disinfected daily and between patients as needed to prevent the spread of infection and to ensure patients' comfort. All potentially contaminated surfaces, including the examination table, are disinfected between patients, with an appropriate disinfectant prescribed by the facility's policy and procedure. After cleaning the table, change the examination paper by unrolling a new piece. In the hospital setting, this cleaning may be completed by another service such as housekeeping; however, it is the entire healthcare team's responsibility to ensure that cleaning has been completed; never assume that it has been done without checking first.
- Drapes, gowns, and all other patient supplies are arranged before the patient enters the room so that they are ready for use.
- To save time, the instruments and equipment needed for the examination are prepared and arranged for easy access before the physician or practitioner enters the room.
- The examination room should contain all materials required for observing standard precautions, including disposable gloves, a sink with an antibacterial hand-washing agent, paper towels, biohazard waste containers, sharps containers, and impervious gowns and face guards. Sharps containers are replaced when they are two-thirds full, as indicated by standard precautions.

Patient Preparation

Getting the patient ready for the examination includes taking care of paperwork before the patient enters the examination room and performing related clinical skills.

- Ensure that the medical record is available and that any needed consent forms have been signed; as the patient care technician, you are not responsible for obtaining any signatures on consents. This is the role of the nurse and physician. You can, however, check to be sure that the forms are on the medical record.
- Introduce yourself and address the patient by his or her preferred name, ensuring to maintain respect at all times. Pay close attention to the patient's nonverbal language to make sure that the patient understands what to expect.
- Obtain specimens (e.g., urine, blood) if they have been preordered by the physician, or if this practice is part of the department policy. Your nurse may delegate this to you. For example, some emergency departments obtain a urine sample on all female patients. This should not be assumed; always check with your nurse before obtaining any specimens.
- Measure and record the patient's height, weight, body mass index (BMI), and vital signs.
- Explain the examination procedure to the patient. Be prepared to answer the patient's questions and allay any fears.
- Ask the patient whether he or she needs to empty the bladder before the examination, because a full bladder may interfere with the examination and may be uncomfortable for the patient.
- Help the patient physically prepare for the examination. Explain to the patient which clothing should be removed and in which direction to put on the gown (open to the front or to the back, depending on the type of examination), and provide a drape to ensure the patient's privacy. Offer assistance as needed.
- Assist the patient into and out of various examination positions as needed.
- Throughout this entire sequence of events, explain what is happening, and consistently maintain the patient's privacy and confidentiality.
- Document patient data in the medical record, completing all forms required.
- Place the patient's medical record in the designated area for the physician, perhaps at the main nurse's station of the unit or the front desk of an office; ensure that no identifiable patient information is visible, in accordance with regulations established by the Health Insurance Portability and Accountability Act (HIPAA).
- Help the patient with dressing as needed after the examination.

Delegation and Documentation Box 14.1

- Obtaining informed consent before a procedure or examination is the role of the physician.
- As the patient care technician, you may serve as the witness to the patient's signature of informed consent.
- If the patient has questions about the procedure, notify the nurse at once.

Assisting the Physician

The patient care technician should be prepared to help the physician complete the physical examination as comprehensively and efficiently as possible. You have already prepared the room, so all equipment and supplies are available and in good working order; you also have prepared the patient by gathering the needed information and measuring and recording vital signs. During the examination, the physician may expect the patient care technician to do the following:

- Hand him or her instruments and equipment as requested and provide supplies as needed.
- Alter the position of a lamp to better illuminate the area being examined and turn lights off and on during specific phases of the examination.
- Position and drape the patient during different phases of the examination.
- Assist in collecting and properly labeling specimens such as urine, Pap smear specimens, and throat cultures.
- Conduct follow-up diagnostic procedures as ordered, including an electrocardiogram (ECG), eye or ear screening, urinalysis, and phlebotomy.
- Schedule postexamination diagnostic procedures such as mammography, x-ray examination, or colonoscopy.

Supplies and Instruments Needed for the Physical Examination

The instruments typically used during the physical examination are shown in Fig. 14.1. They enable the physician or practitioner to see, feel, inspect, and listen to parts of the body. All equipment must be in good working order, properly disinfected, and readily available for the physician's use during the examination. The instruments most frequently used for a physical examination are described in the following paragraphs. Physical examinations typically are performed from the head to the feet; the instruments are listed in the order in which the physician typically would request them.

Ophthalmoscope

An ophthalmoscope is used to inspect the inner structures of the eye. It consists of a stainless-steel handle containing batteries and an attached head, which has a light, magnifying lenses, and an opening through which the eye is viewed. Examination rooms usually are equipped with wall-mounted electrical units for the ophthalmoscope and otoscope, a dispenser for disposable speculums, and a wall-mounted sphygmomanometer.

Otoscope

An otoscope is used to examine the external auditory canal and tympanic membrane. It has a stainless-steel handle containing batteries or is part of a wall-mounted electrical unit. The head of the otoscope has a light that is focused through a magnifying lens and should be covered with a disposable ear speculum. The light also may be used to illuminate the nasal passages and throat.

Nasal Speculum

A nasal speculum is a stainless-steel instrument used to inspect the lining of the nose, nasal membranes, and internal septum (Fig. 14.2). When the handles of the nasal speculum are squeezed, the tips spread apart to

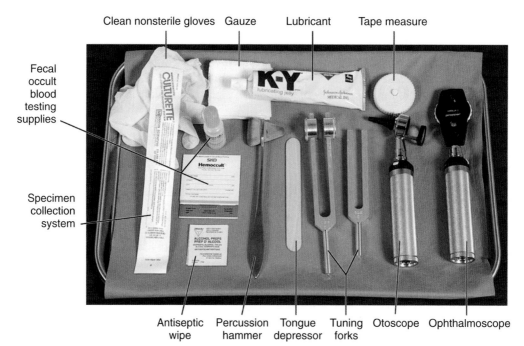

FIGURE 14.1 Instruments for the physical examination. (From Bonewit-West K: *Clinical procedures for medical assistants*, ed 9, St. Louis, 2015, Saunders.)

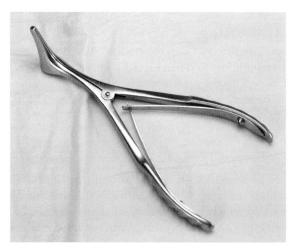

FIGURE 14.2 Nasal speculum. (From Proctor D, Adams A: *Kinn's the patient care technician*, ed 12, St. Louis, 2014, Saunders.)

dilate the nostrils, allowing the physician to visualize the internal aspects. An otoscope with a special attachment may also be used for nasal visualization.

Tuning Fork

Tuning forks are aluminum fork-shaped instruments that consist of a handle and two prongs (Fig. 14.3A). The prongs produce a humming sound when the physician strikes them against his or her hand. Tuning forks are available in different sizes, and each size produces a different pitch level. A tuning fork is used to check the patient's auditory acuity (Fig. 14.3B) and to test bone vibration (Fig. 14.3C). This aluminum instrument consists of a handle and two prongs that produce a humming sound when the physician strikes the prongs against his or her hand.

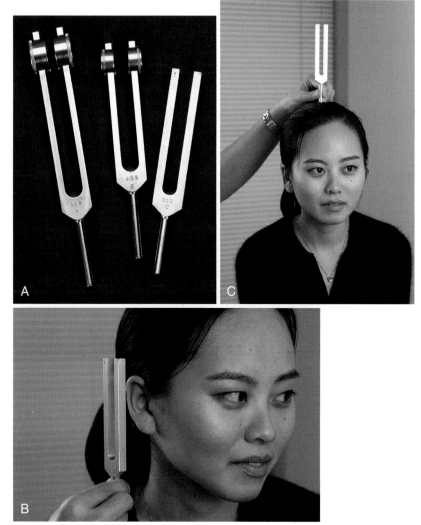

FIGURE 14.3 A, Tuning forks. B, Sound vibration test. C, Bone vibration test. (From Proctor D, Adams A: *Kinn's the patient care technician*, ed 12, St. Louis, 2014, Saunders.)

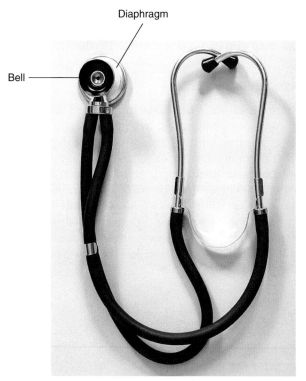

FIGURE 14.4 Stethoscope. (From Ball J, Dains J, Flynn J, et al: *Seidel's guide to physical examination*, ed 8, St. Louis, 2015, Mosby.)

Stethoscope

A stethoscope is a listening device used when certain areas of the body are auscultated, particularly the heart and lungs. This instrument is available in many shapes and sizes. All have two earpieces that are connected to flexible rubber or vinyl tubing (Fig. 14.4). At the distal end of the tubing is a diaphragm or bell (many have both), which, when placed securely on the patient's skin, enables the physician to hear internal body sounds.

Reflex Hammer

A reflex hammer is sometimes called a *percussion hammer.* This stainless-steel instrument has a hard rubber head that is used to strike the tendons of the knee and elbow to test the neurologic reflexes.

Gloves

Disposable examination gloves protect the healthcare worker and the patient from microorganisms. According to standard precautions, gloves must be worn whenever the potential exists for contact with any body fluid, broken skin or wounds, or contaminated items.

Tongue Depressor

A tongue depressor is a flat wooden blade used to hold down the tongue when the throat is examined.

Tape Measure

A tape measure is a flexible ribbon ruler that is usually printed in inches and feet on one side and in centimeters and meters on the opposite side. Measurements may be used to assess length and head circumference in infants, wound size, and so on.

Additional Supplies

Gauze squares, cotton balls, cotton-tipped applicators, specimen containers, hemoccult packets (occult blood tests), Pap smear supplies for female patients, lubricating jelly for vaginal and rectal examinations, and laboratory request forms should be easily accessible during the examination.

Assisting With the Physical Examination

Methods of Examination

Examinations are performed as both a routine confirmation of the absence of illness and a means of diagnosing disease. Healthcare providers use six methods to examine the human body. All six are part of a complete physical examination.

Inspection

During inspection, the examiner uses observation to detect significant physical features or objective data. This method of examination ranges from focusing on the patient's general appearance (general state of health, including posture, mannerisms, and grooming) to more detailed observations, including body contour, gait, symmetry, visible injuries and deformities, tremors, rashes, and color changes.

Palpation

In palpation, the examiner uses the sense of touch (Fig. 14.5A). A part of the body is felt with the hand to determine its condition or the condition of an underlying organ. Palpation may involve touching the skin or performing a firmer exploration of the abdomen for underlying masses. This technique involves a wide range of perceptions, including temperature, vibration, consistency, form, size, rigidity, elasticity, moisture, texture, position, and contour. Palpation is performed with one hand, both hands (bimanual), one finger (digital), the fingertips, or the palmar aspect of the hand. A pelvic examination is done bimanually, whereas an anal examination is performed digitally. Do not confuse palpation with *palpitation*, which is a throbbing pulsation felt in the chest.

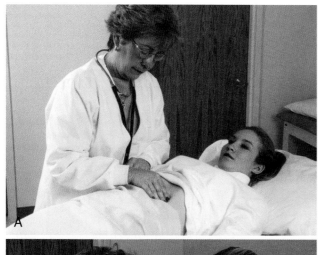
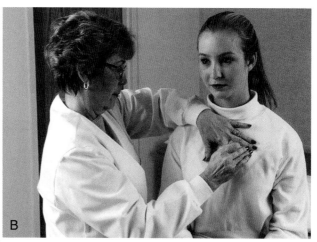
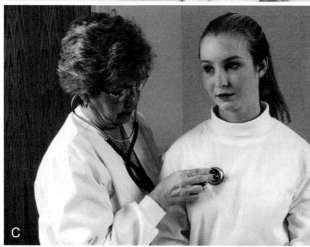

FIGURE 14.5 A, Demonstration of palpation. B, Demonstration of percussion. C, Demonstration of auscultation. (From Zakus SM: *Mosby's clinical skills for medical assistants*, ed 4, St. Louis, 2001, Mosby.)

Percussion

Percussion involves tapping or striking the body, usually with the fingers or a small hammer, to elicit sounds or vibratory sensations. Percussion aids determination of the position, size, and density of an underlying organ or cavity. The effect of percussion is both heard and felt by the examiner; it is helpful in determining the amount of air or solid matter in an underlying organ or cavity. The two basic methods of percussion are *direct percussion* and *indirect percussion.* Direct (immediate) percussion is performed by striking the body with a finger. With indirect (mediate) percussion, which is used more frequently, the physician places his or her hand on the area and then strikes the placed hand with a finger of the other hand (Fig. 14.5B). Both a sound and a sense of vibration are evident. The examiner quantifies the sound in terms of pitch, quality, duration, and resonance.

Auscultation

During auscultation, the physician uses a stethoscope to listen to sounds arising from the within the body (not the sound produced by the physician, as in percussion, but sounds that originate within the patient's body).

Auscultation is a difficult method of examination, because the physician must distinguish between a normal sound and an abnormal sound (Fig. 14.5C). It is particularly useful for evaluating sounds originating in the lungs, heart, and abdomen, such as a murmur, a bruit, and bowel sounds.

Mensuration

Mensuration is the process of measuring. Measurements that are recorded include the patient's height and weight, the length and diameter of an extremity, the extent of flexion or extension of an extremity, the size of the uterus during pregnancy, the size and depth of a wound, and the pressure of a grip. Measurements are taken with a flexible tape measure, a circular wound measurement device (Fig. 14.6), or a specialized piece of equipment (e.g., a goniometer, which is used to measure joint angles) and usually are recorded in centimeters.

Manipulation

Manipulation is the passive movement of a joint to determine the range of extension or flexion of a part of

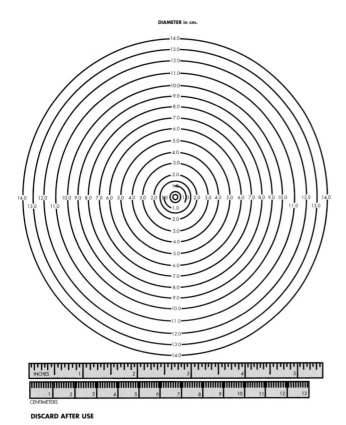

FIGURE 14.6 Circular wound measurement device. (From Perry AG, Potter P: *Clinical nursing skills and techniques,* ed 7, St. Louis, 2010, Mosby.)

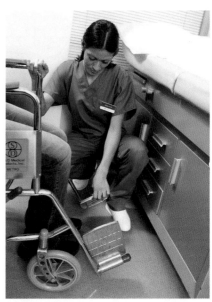

FIGURE 14.7 Wheels locked and foot rests elevated. (From Proctor D, Adams A: *Kinn's the patient care technician,* ed 12, St. Louis, 2014, Saunders.)

the body. Manipulation may or may not be grouped with palpation. It usually is considered separate from the four standard methods of examination (inspection, palpation, percussion, and auscultation) and is grouped with mensuration, especially by an orthopedist or a neurologist. Insurance and industrial reports often request this information in detail. For example, a patient involved in a work-related accident that caused joint damage may have to perform assisted range-of-motion (ROM) exercises to the joint, with subsequent measurements of joint flexion and extension.

Positioning and Draping the Patient for the Physical Examination

Various patient positions are used to facilitate a physical examination. The patient care technician instructs the patient about and assists the patient into these positions, ensuring as much ease and modesty as possible, and helps the patient maintain the position during the examination with as little discomfort as possible. Do not place a patient into a position that is uncomfortable or that compromises the patient's privacy until it is necessary to complete that part of the examination. Never leave the patient's side if he or she is in a position that could result in a fall.

Draping the patient with an examination sheet protects the individual from embarrassment and keeps the patient warm. However, the sheet must be positioned so that it allows complete visibility for the examiner and does not interfere with the examination. During the general examination, each part of the body is exposed one portion at a time. For gynecologic and rectal examinations, the sheet is positioned on the diagonal across the patient, or in a diamond shape, to provide maximum comfort for the patient while allowing the physician to perform the examination.

A number of positions are used for medical examinations. Review positions from Chapter 12: Fowler's, semi-Fowler's, supine, dorsal recumbent, lithotomy, Sims's, prone, knee-chest, and Trendelenburg. The nurse can assist you with determining which position the physician will want the patient placed in.

Transferring a Patient

Frequently, patients need assistance with moving from a chair to the examination table or back again. Patients can be transferred in multiple ways, but all transfers should focus on correct body mechanics by the patient care technician. If the patient is in a wheelchair, move the chair close to the examination table, lock the wheels, and lift the foot rests of the wheelchair out of the way (Fig. 14.7). Explain the procedure to the patient and ask for his or her assistance.

If one side of the patient is stronger than the other, always provide support on the strong side. Place a step stool in front of the wheelchair next to the side of the examination table. Support the patient close to your

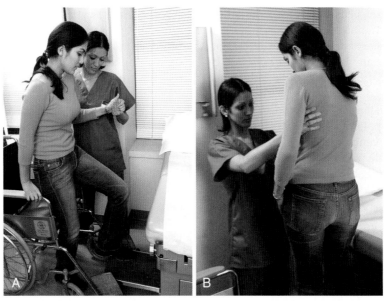

FIGURE 14.8 A, Strong side support. B, Pivot with support. (From Proctor D, Adams A: *Kinn's the patient care technician*, ed 12, St. Louis, 2014, Saunders.)

body on the strong side, with one hand under the axillary region and the other either grasping the patient's hand or holding the forearm. When bending, always bend at the knees and maintain the back's three natural curves, allowing the leg muscles to help in lifting. Give the patient a signal and lift as the patient assists. Anchor the step stool with one foot, and help the patient step up onto the stool with the strong leg, then pivot (Fig. 14.8). Ease the patient down onto the table, bending your knees while keeping your back aligned and avoid twisting your back at the hips. Ensure that the patient is comfortable and is safely positioned on the table (Fig. 14.9). You may need to remain with the patient until the examination has been completed to ensure the patient's safety. If the physician prefers the patient be in a supine position, place one arm across the patient's shoulders and the other under the knees, and smoothly lower the patient's upper body to the table while raising the legs. Use the same pivoting techniques with proper body mechanics to help transfer the patient from the examination table back to the locked wheelchair. If the patient must hold onto you, have the person hold your waist or shoulders, not your neck.

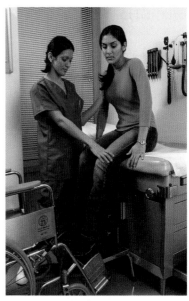

FIGURE 14.9 Sitting on a table with support. (From Proctor D, Adams A: *Kinn's the patient care technician*, ed 12, St. Louis, 2014, Saunders.)

Injury & Illness Prevention Box 14.1

- Always use good body mechanics when assisting patients to the examination table to prevent a musculoskeletal injury.
- Never assume that patients can lift themselves up onto the examination table; this could result in a patient fall.
- Always stay with the patient throughout the examination to provide comfort.

EXAMINATION SEQUENCE

The physical examination sequence is fairly standard; however, variations may occur depending on the physician's specialty, the medical necessity for the examination, and the physician's preference. Patients are more cooperative and less anxious if they understand what is expected of them; therefore you should start by giving the patient a brief explanation of the examination process. Assemble all supplies and instruments needed for the examination before the physician enters the room. As the physician proceeds with the examination, ensure that the patient remains unexposed by adjusting the drape and gown as needed. In every examination, the patient care technician assists the physician by handing him or her the correct instruments and needed supplies.

Having a female assistant in the room during the examination of a female patient is frequently a facility's policy and can help prevent potential lawsuits. If the physician is male, a female patient care technician must remain with a female patient throughout the examination unless the physician excuses the patient care technician from the room.

When the physician begins the examination, the patient care technician should keep conversation to a minimum and remain inconspicuous. The examination usually starts with the patient seated on the examining table in Fowler's position. If the physician uses reflected light, the light source should be behind the patient's right shoulder. If illuminated instruments are used, standard overhead lights are sufficient. Take care not to shine a light directly into the patient's eyes; this can be done by turning on lights while they are directed away from the patient and carefully moving the light toward the area.

Presenting Appearance (General Appearance)

The physician starts the physical examination by observing the patient's appearance. Either *presenting appearance* or *general appearance* may be used on the medical record. These terms note whether the patient appears well and in good health (e.g., the patient appears disoriented or in distress; well-nourished or undernourished; and answers questions with ease or confusion).

The patient's gait often provides important information. The patient may limp, walk with the feet wide apart, have a shuffle step, or have difficulty maintaining his or her balance. In addition to gait, all the patient's body movements are observed for possible muscle actions that the physician deems unusual. Posture also is checked for indications of pain, stiffness, or difficulty with limb movement. If the patient care technician notes any of these observations or the patient reports any complaints, these should be recorded in the patient's medical record along with the vital signs before the physician begins the examination.

Nutrition and Stature

If in an outpatient setting, the patient care technician measures the patient's height and weight before the examination begins, and these measurements are recorded in the patient record, along with the BMI. During the examination, the physician notes the body build and proportions. Any *gross* (immediately obvious) deformities are recorded. Sometimes abnormalities in height or body proportion may be caused by hormonal imbalances.

Speech

Speech may reveal a pathologic condition. Some basic speech defects include *aphonia*, the inability to speak because of loss of the voice, which is commonly seen with severe laryngitis or overuse of the voice; *aphasia*, the loss of expression by speech or writing because of an injury or disease of the brain; and *dysphasia*, lack of coordination and failure to arrange words in proper order, usually caused by a brain lesion. With *motor aphasia*, the patient knows what he or she wants to say but cannot use muscles properly to speak, perhaps seen as slurred or incoherent speech that might occur after a cerebrovascular accident (CVA). In *sensory aphasia*, the patient pronounces words easily but uses them inaccurately, as in jumbled speech.

Breath Odors

Breath odors may or may not be diagnostic, although they often are associated with poor oral hygiene or dental care. Acidosis produces a strong odor of acetone, which is sweet and fruity, and may result from diabetes mellitus, starvation, or renal disease. A musty odor usually is associated with liver disease, and the odor of ammonia may be noted in cases of uremia.

Skin

The condition of the skin can be a good reflection of the patient's nutritional status and hydration level. If dehydration is suspected, skin *turgor* is checked by pinching the skin on the posterior surface of the hands. The tissue is observed to see how quickly it returns to the normal location. A delay indicates a decrease in tissue fluid, confirming the diagnosis of dehydration. Extreme dryness, scaling, extended time for wound healing, or frequent breaks in the skin may indicate systemic disease.

Fingernails and toenails often give some indication of a person's health. Brittle, grooved, or lined nails may indicate local infection or systemic disease. Clubbing of the fingertips is associated with some congenital heart or lung diseases. *Spooning* of the nail is seen in some patients with severe iron-deficiency anemia. *Beau's lines* appear after an acute illness but grow out and disappear. The physician may refer a patient with skin disorders to a dermatologist for diagnosis and treatment.

Head

Once the physician makes the overall observations of the patient's general condition, physical examination typically begins with the head and face and moves downward to the feet. The face reflects the patient's state and tells the physician a great deal about how the patient handles stress and illness. The skull, scalp, and face are palpated for size, shape, and symmetry. The distribution or lack of hair and the hair texture may indicate hormonal changes. Excessive hair, especially facial hair in female patients, indicates a hormonal imbalance. As the head is palpated, the physician assesses possible nodules, masses, or signs of trauma.

Eyes

The pupils are checked for reaction by shining a light into one eye at a time. If both pupils constrict equally and smoothly to a light stimulus, the physician documents "PERRLA" (which means the pupils are equal, round, respond to light, and adjust and focus on objects). The sclera is checked for color, which ranges from white to pale yellow. If the eye is inflamed, it will be evident in the sclera. A sclera with a yellow tone indicates liver disease. Movements of the eyes are tested by having the patient follow the physician's finger. If eye movement is within average range, the note "extraocular movement (EOM) intact" is written. The physician uses the ophthalmoscope to examine the interior of the eye, including the retina and the intraocular vessels. Some diseases, such as diabetes mellitus or hypertension, damage the blood vessels of the retina.

Ears

The ears are examined with an otoscope. The external ear is checked first for inflammation of the external auditory canal or for earwax (cerumen). The tympanic membrane (eardrum) is examined and should appear pearly gray. Scars on the eardrum frequently are the result of earlier, chronic ear infections or perforations. The color of the eardrum is important to the diagnosis because it may indicate fluids such as blood or pus behind the eardrum in the middle ear. The patient may be asked to swallow several times to allow observation of movement of the tympanic membrane, which occurs because of pressure changes in the eustachian tube. The eustachian tube equalizes air pressure between the middle ear and the throat. The ability of the tympanic membrane to move is crucial to the hearing process.

Nose and Sinuses

The mucosa of the nasal cavity is examined for color and texture. The sinuses cannot be seen, but the frontal and maxillary sinuses may be examined by firm palpation over the area and by transillumination. When disorders of the eyes, ears, nose, and throat are observed, and the physician believes that the condition warrants the attention of a specialist, the patient is referred to an ophthalmologist or an otorhinolaryngologist (ear, nose, and throat specialist).

Mouth and Throat

The mouth, or oral cavity, usually is thought of in terms of oral hygiene and dental care. Dental hygiene includes the condition of the teeth, how the patient cares for the teeth and gums, and whether the teeth of the upper and lower jaws meet properly (occlude) for chewing. Healthy gums are pale pink, glossy, and smooth and do not bleed when pressure from a tongue depressor is applied. The palatine tonsils usually are visible. The physician may use a tongue depressor and a piece of gauze to grasp the tongue to examine it carefully. The floor of the mouth is examined by both inspection and palpation for enlarged lymph nodes, salivary gland function, and ulcerations. The insides of the cheeks and the gumline are also examined for any abnormal marks or color.

Neck

The neck is examined for range of motion by having the patient move the head in various directions. The thyroid gland is given special attention for symmetry, size, and texture. The physician manually palpates the thyroid area, and the patient is asked to swallow several times. The carotid artery is palpated and auscultated for possible bruits. The lymph nodes are palpated. *Lymphadenopathy* (enlargement of the lymph nodes) occurs if the patient has an infection of the face, head, or neck.

Reflexes

The patient's reflexes are checked with the patient in high Fowler's and supine positions. While the patient is sitting, the biceps are checked with the patient's arm flexed and supported by the examiner. The knee jerk (patellar reflex) and the ankle jerk (Achilles reflex) are checked using *tapotement* (a tapping or percussing movement) with either the fingers or the reflex hammer. The plantar reflexes (Babinski and Chaddock reflexes) are tested with the patient in an upright or supine position.

Chest

While the patient is still in the sitting position, the chest, heart, and lungs are examined. The chest is examined for symmetric expansion. A tape measure may be used, especially if variation exists between the upper and lower chest expansion. A patient with a history of emphysema may have a barrel-shaped chest. The physician may use percussion to determine the density of lung tissues.

With the stethoscope to the patient's back, the examiner auscultates lung sounds. The patient is asked to take deep, regular breaths. This may produce slight dizziness, but the patient should be assured that it is only the result of the deep respirations and will rapidly pass. The physician notes the types of respirations and the presence of lung sounds in all lobes.

Because considerable concentration is required to interpret heart sounds, the physician must have complete silence in the examination room when listening to the patient's heart. The heart is examined with a stethoscope from both anterior and posterior approaches to the patient. Further examination may include auscultation on the left lateral side. In patients with heart disease, the physician may spend an extended time listening to heart sounds. If chest or heart abnormalities are found, the physician typically orders further diagnostic tests, including blood analysis, x-ray evaluation, and an ECG. Once the results of these studies have been analyzed, the physician may refer the patient to a cardiologist for treatment of a heart condition, or a pulmonologist or a respiratory care specialist for treatment of a breathing disorder.

Abdomen

For the abdominal part of the examination, the patient is lowered to the dorsal recumbent position and the drape is lowered to the pubic hair line. The gown is raised to just under the breasts. The physician stands to the patient's right side if at all possible. The patient's arms may be placed at the side, or the hands may be crossed over the chest or under the head. Relaxation of the abdominal muscles is absolutely essential for the abdominal examination. To assist in this and to promote patient comfort, a small pillow can be placed under the head and knees. The physician auscultates the abdomen in all quadrants to confirm the presence of complete bowel sounds and palpates the abdomen for any abnormalities. The physician also may use percussion to determine the density, position, and size of underlying abdominal organs.

Breast and Testicles

Careful breast examination is part of the physical examination for every female patient, regardless of whether she is symptomatic. The breasts are examined both visually and by palpation with the patient in high Fowler's position and then again in the supine position. Breast cancer is the most common malignancy in women, and early detection is the key to successful treatment. This is a good opportunity to discuss and reinforce the consistent use of monthly self-breast examination (SBE).

For male patients who have reached puberty or are 15 years of age or older, the physician will perform a testicular examination. This is an important self-examination for all males to perform each month, because testicular carcinoma is a major health risk.

Rectum

The rectal examination usually follows the abdominal examination or may be part of the examination of the male or female genitalia. Preserving the patient's comfort and dignity is vital. For this part of the examination, the physician needs examination gloves and lubricating jelly. The examination light should be directed at the perineal area during the examination.

Hemoccult test specimens, which are stool specimens to determine if blood is present, often are collected at the time of the digital rectal examination. If this is a procedure the physician performs, be sure to include the necessary collection folder with the examination equipment. Patients found to have gastrointestinal (GI) disorders may be referred to a gastroenterologist.

ROLE OF THE PATIENT CARE TECHNICIAN

The physical examination establishes a baseline from which a patient's healthcare needs are determined. The examination should never be considered routine. Each patient's needs are special, and the patient care technician must be prepared to assist when needed. Throughout the procedure, the patient care technician must treat the patient with respect and guard the individual's privacy as much as possible.

The primary role of the patient care technician is to have the room, equipment, and supplies stocked and ready; the patient prepared, with vital signs, height, weight, and BMI measured and recorded; documentation completed regarding the patient's chief complaint or reported data; and the patient properly gowned and in position for the examination. During the examination, the patient care technician should be prepared to hand the physician needed equipment or to assist in any other way necessary. After the examination has been completed, the patient care technician should assist the patient as needed; complete any diagnostic procedures ordered by the physician; assist in the patient's discharge or transfer back to their patient room; answer the patient's questions; and disinfect and restock the room in preparation for the next patient.

Legal and Ethical Issues

The patient care technician must recognize that a legal and ethical contract exists between the patient and the healthcare facility. As the healthcare facility's employee, the patient care technician is part of that contract. Information gained during the physical examination is confidential and must remain that way. The patient care technician must uphold ethical responsibilities to render service, respect confidential information, and uphold the honor and high principles of the profession.

HIPAA Applications

- Remember that conversations in the healthcare facility may be overheard. Guard patient confidentiality when gathering information about the chief complaint, scheduling diagnostic tests, or processing samples. If the main desk has a privacy glass, make sure that it remains closed; turn away from the waiting room when talking on the phone; and avoid any conversations about the patient that may be overheard.
- Place medical records on the desk with identifying information facing down to prevent those passing by from recognizing the patient's name. If electronic medical records (EMRs) are used, safeguard patient information by closing patient files and locking computers when you will be out of the room.
- Maintain patient confidentiality during the admissions procedure in the facility.

CHAPTER SUMMARY

Before the examination, the patient care technician has the opportunity to interact with the patient to ensure that he or she feels comfortable during the examination process, and that all necessary medical information has been obtained. The patient care technician's duties include preparing and maintaining the examination room and equipment; preparing the patient by conducting the initial interview and measuring vital signs; assisting the physician with positioning and draping; and providing instruments and supplies as needed during the physical examination.

Instruments and supplies typically used in a physical examination include nasal speculum, ophthalmoscope, otoscope, tongue depressor, reflex hammer, various tuning forks, stethoscope, sphygmomanometer, thermometer, examination gloves, tape measure, scale, examination light, disposable gloves, biohazard container, specimen bottles, laboratory requisitions, hemoccult test supplies, patient gown, drapes, and lubricating gel.

The examiner uses *inspection* to detect significant physical features, such as the patient's general appearance. With *palpation*, the sense of touch is used to feel the brachial pulse before a blood pressure reading is taken. *Percussion* involves tapping or striking the body to elicit sounds or vibratory sensations, as in percussion of the chest to detect fluid in the lungs. A stethoscope is used to *auscultate* or listen to the lungs and heart. *Mensuration* is the process of measuring the patient's height and weight. *Manipulation* is the passive, assisted movement of a joint to determine the range of extension or flexion.

The patient should be instructed on whether to wear the gown open in the front or open in the back, depending on the type of examination to be done. Draping requires constant attention to maintaining the patient's privacy throughout the examination while assisting the physician with exposure of the area being examined. The general rule is to cover all exposed body parts until the point in the examination when the physician must evaluate that particular area.

Good body mechanics principles include maintaining balanced posture, bending the knees while maintaining the back's three natural curves, and using leg muscles to help lift. Move the wheelchair close to the examination table, lock the wheels, and lift the foot rests of the wheelchair out of the way. Provide patient support close to your body on the patient's strong side. Place a step stool in front of the wheelchair next to the side of the examination table, and with one hand under the axillary region and the other grasping the patient, anchor the step stool with one foot and help the patient step up onto the stool with the strong leg; then help the patient pivot into a sitting position on the table.

The examination sequence depends on the type of examination and the physician's preference. The physician typically begins the examination by noting the patient's general health appearance, nutrition status, speech, breath odor, skin condition, and reflexes. The physician then begins the physical examination, starting at the head and working down through the body to the rectum. Any abnormalities are noted and may be further investigated with diagnostic tools after the examination has been completed.

Prepare the examination room and the patient; complete the initial patient interview and measure and record vital signs; gather the needed equipment and place it in the order of use; gown and drape the patient as needed; provide patient instruction and check for understanding throughout the process; assist during the examination by handing the physician instruments, managing changes in light, collecting samples as ordered, and conducting diagnostic procedures as ordered; assist the patient when the examination is done, including helping the patient dress, scheduling further diagnostic tests as ordered, and answering the patient's questions. Complete the documentation, disinfect the examination room and equipment, and restock supplies to ready the room for the next patient.

Case Scenario

Felicia Grand, a newly hired patient care technician, works for Dr. Anna Kosto, who is a hospitalist in a busy emergency care department. One of Felicia's chief responsibilities is to assist Dr. Kosto with physical examinations. Her duties include preparing and maintaining the examination room and equipment; getting the patient ready for specific physical examinations; and gowning, draping, and positioning the patient as needed. Because Felicia will be assisting with examinations, she must become familiar with the physical examination procedure and the order in which the physician needs various pieces of medical equipment. It also is important that Felicia protects herself from possible injury by using appropriate body mechanics throughout her day in the office.

- What equipment does Felicia need to gather before the physician enters the examination room to make sure that the examination goes smoothly and without interruption?
- With what examination and treatment positions should Felicia be familiar, and when should the various positions be used?
- What measures can Felicia take to protect herself from injury when lifting heavy items or assisting with the transfer of patients?

REVIEW QUESTIONS

1. Which member of the healthcare team is responsible for obtaining informed consent before conducting an examination or performing a diagnostic test?
   a. Physician
   b. Nurse
   c. Patient care technician
   d. Unit secretary

2. How often should the examination room be cleaned?
   a. Once per shift
   b. Once per day
   c. Whenever housekeeping cleans it
   d. Each time it is used

3. If the physician is male and the patient is female, which gender should be present during the physical examination?
   a. Male
   b. Female
   c. Either
   d. Both

4. As you are preparing the patient for the examination, the patient is nervous about the type of examination the physician has said he will perform and has further questions. What should the patient care technician do?
   a. Try to answer the patient's questions
   b. Notify the nurse at once
   c. Call the physician to the room
   d. Tell the patient to wait until the physician begins the examination to ask questions

5. How often should the examination room be checked for proper stocking of supplies?
   a. Daily
   b. Each shift
   c. After use by a patient
   d. Each shift and each time the room is used

Measuring and Recording Vital Signs

1. Recall the average body temperature, pulse rate, respiratory rate, and blood pressure for various age groups.
2. Describe emotional and physical factors that can cause the body temperature to rise or fall.
3. Convert temperature readings between the Fahrenheit and Celsius scales.
4. Obtain and record an accurate patient temperature using three different types of thermometers.
5. Describe pulse rate, rhythm, and volume.
6. Locate and record the pulse at multiple sites.
7. Demonstrate the best way to obtain an accurate respiratory count.
8. Specify physiologic factors that affect blood pressure.
9. Identify the different Korotkoff phases.
10. Accurately measure and document blood pressure.
11. Accurately measure and document height and weight for both infants and adults.
12. Convert kilograms to pounds and pounds to kilograms.
13. Obtain anthropometric measurements on infants and small children.
14. Determine the patient care technician's legal and ethical responsibilities in obtaining vital signs.

apnea Absence or cessation of breathing.

arrhythmia An abnormality or irregularity in the heart rhythm.

arteriosclerosis Thickening, decreased elasticity, and calcification of arterial walls.

bounding Term used to describe a pulse that feels full because of increased power of cardiac contraction or as a result of increased blood volume.

bradycardia A slow heartbeat; a pulse below 60 beats per minute.

bradypnea Respirations that are regular in rhythm but slower than normal in rate.

cerumen A waxy secretion in the ear canal; commonly called ear wax.

chronic obstructive pulmonary disease (COPD) A progressive, irreversible lung condition that results in diminished lung capacity.

dyspnea Difficult or painful breathing.

essential hypertension Elevated blood pressure of unknown cause that develops for no apparent reason; sometimes called primary hypertension.

febrile Pertaining to an elevated body temperature.

homeostasis Internal adaptation and change in response to environmental factors; multiple functions that attempt to keep the body's functions in balance.

hyperpnea An increase in the depth of breathing.

hypertension High blood pressure.

hyperventilation Abnormally prolonged and deep breathing, usually associated with acute anxiety or emotional tension.

hypotension Blood pressure that is below normal (systolic pressure below 90 mm Hg and diastolic pressure below 50 mm Hg).

intermittent pulse A pulse in which beats occasionally are skipped.

orthopnea Condition in which an individual must sit or stand to breathe comfortably.

orthostatic (postural) hypotension A temporary fall in blood pressure when a person rapidly changes from a recumbent position to a standing position.

otitis externa Inflammation or infection of the external auditory canal (swimmer's ear).

peripheral Term that refers to an area outside of or away from an organ or structure.

pulse deficit Condition in which the radial pulse is less than the apical pulse; may indicate a peripheral vascular abnormality.

pulse pressure The difference between systolic and diastolic blood pressures (30 to 50 mm Hg is considered normal).

pyrexia Febrile condition or fever.

rales Abnormal or crackling breath sounds during inspiration.

rhonchi Abnormal rumbling sounds on expiration that indicate airway obstruction by thick secretions or spasms.

secondary hypertension Elevated blood pressure resulting from another condition, typically kidney disease.

sinus arrhythmia Irregular heartbeat that originates in the sinoatrial node (pacemaker).

spirometer Instrument that measures the volume of air inhaled and exhaled.

stertorous Term that describes a strenuous respiratory effort marked by a snoring sound.

syncope Fainting; a brief lapse in consciousness.

tachycardia A rapid but regular heart rate; one that exceeds 100 beats per minute.

tachypnea Condition marked by rapid, shallow respirations.

thready Term that describes a pulse that is scarcely perceptible.

wheezing A high-pitched sound heard on expiration; indicates obstruction or narrowing of respiratory passages.

Measurement of vital signs is an important aspect of care for the patient being seen in a healthcare facility. These signs are the human body's indicators of internal homeostasis and the patient's general state of health. Because patient care technicians are the ones who most often obtain these measurements, it is important that they be done correctly and accurately each time. If you understand the principles of and the reasons for these measurements, you will have a better understanding of their benefit in the care of the patient.

Accuracy is essential. A change in one or more of the patient's vital signs may indicate a change in their health. These changes may suggest the presence or absence of a disease process and therefore may lead to a change in the treatment plan. Although the patient care technician obtains vital signs routinely, it is a task that requires consistent attention to accuracy and detail. These findings are extremely important in order to have a correct diagnosis, and vital signs should never be measured without you giving your full attention in obtaining them. In addition to performing accurate measurement, care must be taken when charting the findings on the patient's medical record. It can be easy to get confused when obtaining sets of vital signs on multiple patients. It is important to come up with a process to keep yourself from getting patients mixed up with other patients.

Delegation and Documentation Box 15.1

- It is important to keep patient vital signs organized to the specific patient and not confused with other patients.
- Instead of writing patient vital signs on scrap paper or a paper towel, use a spiral-bound small notebook in which each patient can have a section.
- If confidential information is included in this notebook, be sure to tear out the pages and shred or place in a confidential trash bin at the end of your shift.
- If an electronic medical record is used and you have the option of recording vital signs in the patient room, it is best to go ahead and enter them while you are beside the patient.
- If a clipboard is provided by the unit for you to record vital signs, be sure that you pay attention to the location you record them.
- Use two patient identifiers to ensure that you are taking vital signs on the correct patient.

Vital signs are the patient's temperature, pulse, respiration, and blood pressure. These four signs are abbreviated *TPR* and *BP* and may be referred to as *cardinal signs.* The patient care technician must understand the significance of the vital signs and must measure and record them accurately. *Anthropometric* measurements are not considered vital signs but usually are obtained at the same time as vital signs. These measurements include height, weight, recumbent length, body mass index (BMI), and other body measurements, such as fat composition and an infant's head circumference.

FACTORS THAT MAY INFLUENCE VITAL SIGNS

Vital signs are influenced by many factors, both physical and emotional. A patient may have had a hot or cold beverage just before the examination or may be angry or fearful about what the physician may find. For example, consider that a patient has been asked to return to have repeat labs drawn because the first set showed the presence of suspicious cells that might mean leukemia, or cancer of the blood. The patient care technician measures the patient's blood pressure and finds it significantly elevated compared with previous readings. The patient may be anxious and nervous about the test results, and the elevated blood pressure readings reflect his or her anxiety.

What temperature reading might be expected in a patient who could not find a parking place and had to walk four blocks to the hospital, knowing he or she would be late for his lab appointment? If you said that it would be elevated, you are right. Certainly, this patient's metabolism would increase because of the physical exercise, and as a result, patient's temperature would be elevated, along with pulse, respirations, and blood pressure.

For one reason or another, many patients are apprehensive during an office visit. These emotions may alter vital signs, and the patient care technician must help the patient relax before taking any readings. Measurements sometimes must be obtained a second time, after the patient is calmer or more comfortable. For a better picture of the patient's vital signs, the patient care technician may be asked to record the vital signs twice: at the initial time and 20 to 30 minutes later.

TEMPERATURE

Physiology

Body temperature is defined as the balance between heat lost and heat produced by the body. It is measured in degrees Fahrenheit (F) or degrees Celsius (C). The process of chemical and physical change in the body that produces heat is called *metabolism.* Body temperature is a result of this process. The core, or central, body temperature is maintained within a normal range by the thermoregulatory center in the hypothalamus, located in the brain. The average body temperature varies from person to person and is different in each person at different times throughout the day. In a healthy adult, this varies from 97.6°F to 99°F (36.4°C to 37.3°C); the average daily temperature is 98.6°F (36.8°C). Body temperature is lowest in the morning and highest in the late afternoon. Factors that may affect body temperature include the following:

- *Age:* The body temperature of infants and young children fluctuates more rapidly in response to external environmental temperatures. Teething may cause a slight elevation in temperature, but should not be the cause of a fever. Aging adults lose their ability to respond to temperature extremes, which makes them more susceptible to hypothermic or hyperthermic reactions.
- *Stress and physical activity:* Both exercise and emotional stress can increase the metabolic rate, causing an elevation in temperature.
- *Gender:* Hormone secretions result in fluctuations of the core body temperature in women throughout the menstrual cycle.
- *External factors:* Smoking, drinking hot fluids, and chewing gum can temporarily elevate an oral temperature.

When sick, a person's metabolic activity is increased; this causes an increase in internal heat production, which in turn raises the body temperature. The increase in body temperature is thought to be the body's defensive reaction because heat slows the growth of some bacteria and viruses. Some say a fever can be healing for a person.

When a fever is present, superficial blood vessels (those near the surface of the skin) constrict. The small papillary muscles at the base of hair follicles also constrict, creating goose bumps. Chills and shivering may follow, producing internal heat. As this process repeats itself, more heat is produced, and the body temperature becomes elevated or rises above the normal range. When more heat is lost than is produced, the opposite effect occurs, and body temperature drops below normal range.

Fever

Infection, either bacterial or viral, is the most common cause of fever in both children and adults.

Infants do not usually develop febrile illnesses during the first 3 months of life; if one is present, it usually is very serious. However, fever, or pyrexia, is very common in young children and accounts for an estimated 26% of office visits. Fevers are classified according to the 24-hour pattern they follow. See Box 15.1 for temperatures which are considered to be febrile. The three most common patterns of fevers are as follows:

- *Continuous fever*, which rises and falls only slightly during a 24-hour period. The temperature consistently remains above the patient's average normal temperature range and fluctuates less than 3 degrees.
- *Intermittent fever*, which comes and goes, alternating between elevated and normal levels.
- *Remittent fever*, which fluctuates considerably (i.e., by more than 3 degrees) and never returns to the normal range.

Variation from the patient's average body temperature range may be the first warning of an illness or a change in the patient's current condition. Patients with fever usually have loss of appetite *(anorexia)*, headache, thirst, flushed face, hot skin, and general malaise, or tiredness. Some patients experience an acute onset of chills and shivering followed by an increase in body temperature. A serious possible complication in young children with high fevers is a febrile seizure, which is a seizure brought on by a fever. Medication to reduce the fever, or *antipyretic* drugs (e.g., Tylenol), should be taken as instructed to prevent dangerous spikes in temperature. Age-related normal values for temperature readings are shown in Table 15.1.

Temperature Readings

A clinical thermometer is used to measure body temperature. It is calibrated in the Fahrenheit or the Celsius scale. The Fahrenheit scale is used most often in the United States, but hospitals and many ambulatory care settings use the Celsius scale. The formulas for conversion from one system to the other are as follows:

$$°C = (°F - 32) \times \frac{5}{9}$$

$$°F = \left(°C \times \frac{9}{5}\right) + 32$$

For example, if an infant's temperature is measured at 101°F, the Celsius conversion would be as follows:

$$°C = (101°F - 32) \times \frac{5}{9}$$

$$= 69 \times \frac{5}{9}$$

$$= 345 \div 9$$

$$= 38.3°C$$

If the ambulatory care setting where you work uses a Celsius thermometer, patients may ask you what the temperature is in Fahrenheit degrees because that is the scale they understand. If the facility does not have a conversion chart available, you will need to convert the temperature mathematically. For example, if an infant's temperature is 39°C, what is the Fahrenheit reading?

$$°F = \left(°C \times \frac{9}{5}\right) + 32$$

$$= \left(39°C \times \frac{9}{5}\right) + 32$$

$$= (351 \div 5) + 32$$

$$= 70.2 + 32$$

$$= 102.2°F$$

Several types of thermometers and several different methods can be used to take temperature readings. A digital thermometer is placed under the tongue, in the armpit, or rectally; a tympanic thermometer is inserted into the ear; and a temporal artery (TA) scanner is moved across the forehead. Average temperature values for adults at the four most common sites are shown in Table 15.2.

Axillary temperatures are approximately 1°F (0.6°C) lower than accurate oral readings because axillary readings are not taken in an enclosed body cavity. When taken correctly, the tympanic (ear) temperature is an

Box 15.1	Temperatures Considered Febrile

- Rectal, temporal, or aural (ear) temperature over 100.4°F (38°C)
- Oral temperature over 99.5°F (37.5°C)
- Axillary temperature over 98.6°F (37°C)
- Fever of unknown origin (FUO): a temperature over 100.9°F (38.3°C) that lasts 3 weeks in adults and 1 week in children without a known related diagnosis

Table 15.1	Age-Related Temperature Norms	
Age	Fahrenheit	Celsius
Newborn (axillary)	98.2°	36.8°
1 year	99.7°	37.6°
6 years to adult (oral)	98.6°	37°
Elderly aged above 70 years (oral)	96.8°	36°

Table 15.2	Average Adult Temperatures	
Site	Fahrenheit	Celsius
Oral	98.6°	37°
Axillary	97.6°	36.4°
Tympanic	98.6°	37°
Temporal artery	98.6°	37°

accurate measure because it records the temperature of the blood closest to the hypothalamus. However, recent research on the newest device for obtaining temperature, the TA thermometer, indicates that this method is more accurate than tympanic measurement for identifying elevated temperatures in infants. Pediatricians, therefore, may prefer TA temperatures in infants suspected of having a fever. The TA thermometer also records accurate temperature readings in all age groups of patients. The tympanic method still is considered a fast, accurate, and noninvasive way of recording temperatures for older children and adults. Noninvasive means that you do not have to place anything inside the body; children generally respond to this method better.

When obtaining an oral temperature, you do not have to indicate the site when documenting the reading in the patient's chart. However, you should write (T) for tympanic, (A) for axillary, or (TA) for temporal artery readings after recording the temperature to clarify that an alternative site was used. Oral temperature cannot be measured accurately in young children because the technique requires patients to hold the thermometer under the tongue and keep the mouth closed. To take an infant's temperature rectally, lubricate the probe tip, hold the baby securely with the legs elevated, and insert the probe approximately ½ inch; hold the probe carefully throughout the procedure to prevent rectal damage. Pediatricians may prefer that infants' temperatures be taken with a temporal thermometer because it is more comfortable for the baby, is less invasive, and eliminates the possible complication of a perforated rectum.

For patients older than 3 years and for those unable to hold a thermometer properly in their mouth during the procedure, a tympanic or temporal thermometer can be used; if not, a less accurate axillary temperature can be obtained.

Illness & Injury Prevention Box 15.1

- Do not place a glass thermometer in a child's mouth; they could bite down on the thermometer, which could result in the thermometer breaking inside the child's mouth.
- Teenagers or adults who are developmentally delayed may not be able to cooperate with an oral temperature reading, because they cannot hold a thermometer in their mouth with their mouths closed.
- Rectal thermometers are color-coded red; oral thermometers are usually blue. Be sure to pay attention to the type of thermometer you are selecting, using the route it is intended for.

Types of Thermometers and Their Uses

Digital Thermometer

Digital thermometers are battery operated and are available in both Fahrenheit and Celsius scales. Disposable covers fit snugly over the probes and are easily and quickly removed by pushing in the colored end of the probe (usually blue for oral; red for rectal). The instrument sounds a beep when the process is completed (10 to 60 seconds), and the reading appears on a light-emitting diode (LED) screen on the face of the instrument (Procedure 15.1). Because the only part of the instrument that comes in contact with the patient is the probe, which has a plastic covering over it, the risk of cross-infection is greatly reduced (Fig. 15.1). Another type of digital thermometer resembles the old mercury thermometers that the Occupational Safety and Health Administration (OSHA) no longer allows clinicians to use in healthcare facilities. These thermometers have a digital screen on which the temperature is read and should always be covered by a disposable sheath.

Temperature should not be taken orally if the patient recently has had something hot or cold to eat or drink or has just smoked, because these factors may artificially increase or decrease the patient's temperature. In addition, the patient must be able to hold the thermometer under the tongue with the lips tightly sealed around the probe to obtain an accurate oral reading.

Tympanic Thermometer

The tympanic membrane of the ear can be used for quick, accurate, and safe assessment of a patient's temperature. It shares the blood supply that reaches the

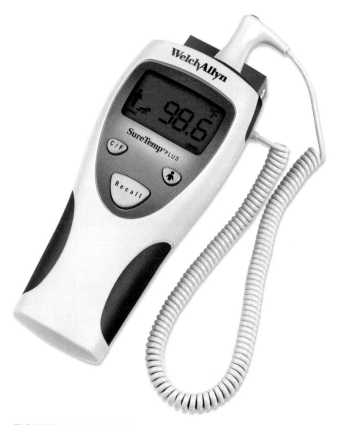

FIGURE 15.1 Digital thermometer. (Courtesy Welch Allyn.)

PROCEDURE 15.1

Obtain Vital Signs: Obtain an Oral Temperature Using a Digital Thermometer

1. Sanitize your hands.
2. Assemble the needed equipment and supplies.
3. Identify your patient and explain the procedure. Ensure that the patient has not eaten, consumed any hot or cold fluids, smoked, or exercised during the 30 minutes before the temperature is measured.
4. Prepare the probe for use as described in the package directions. Ensure that probe covers are always used.

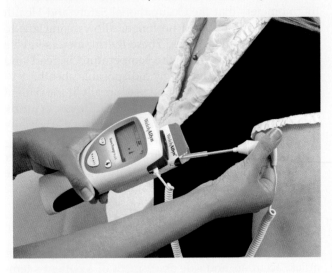

5. Place the probe under the patient's tongue and instruct the patient to close the mouth tightly without biting down

on the thermometer. Help the patient by holding the probe end.

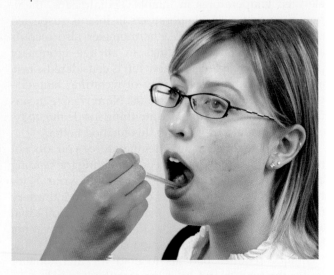

6. When a beep is heard, remove the probe from the patient's mouth and immediately eject the probe cover into an appropriate biohazard waste container. Note the reading in the LED window of the processing unit.
7. Record the reading in the patient's medical record (e.g., T = 97.7°F).
8. Sanitize your hands and disinfect the equipment as indicated.

---

hypothalamus, which is the brain's temperature regulator. The ear canal is a protected cavity, so aural temperature is not affected by factors such as an open mouth, hot or cold drinks, or even a stuffy nose, which would prevent a patient from keeping the mouth closed during the procedure. In addition, the covered probe is designed to bounce an infrared signal off the eardrum without touching it, so the risk of spreading communicable diseases during temperature measurement is greatly reduced. The tympanic measurement system consists of a handheld processor unit equipped with a tympanic probe, which is covered with a disposable speculum for use (Fig. 15.2).

When the probe is placed into the ear canal, it gently seals the external opening of the canal, and the infrared energy emitted by the tympanic membrane is gathered. This signal is digitized by the processor unit and is shown on the display screen. Accurate readings are obtained in less than 2 seconds (Procedure 15.2). Both the speed of the tympanic thermometer and the comfort it affords the patient have made it the more popular choice in healthcare facilities. However, this unit should not be used (1) if the patient has bilateral otitis externa (ear infection), because the procedure would be

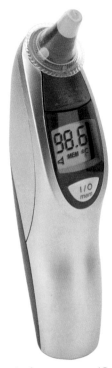

FIGURE 15.2 Tympanic thermometer. (Courtesy Welch Allyn.)

PROCEDURE 15.2

Obtain Vital Signs: Obtain an Aural Temperature Using the Tympanic Thermometer

1. Sanitize your hands.
2. Gather the necessary equipment and supplies.
3. Identify your patient and explain the procedure.
4. Place a disposable cover on the probe.

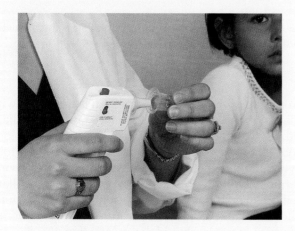

5. Follow the package directions to start the thermometer.
6. Insert the probe into the ear canal far enough to seal the opening. Do not apply pressure. For children younger than 3 years, gently pull the earlobe down and back; for patients older than 3 years, gently pull the top of the ear up and back.

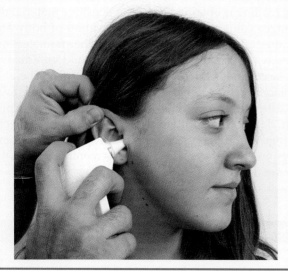

7. Press the button on the probe as directed. The temperature will appear on the display screen in 1 to 2 seconds.
8. Remove the probe, note the reading, and discard the probe cover into a biohazard container without touching it.

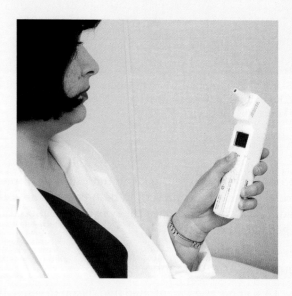

9. Sanitize your hands and disinfect the equipment if indicated.
10. Record the temperature results (e.g., T = 98.6° F [T]) in the patient's medical record.

(From Bonewit-West K: Clinical procedures for medical assistants, ed 7, St. Louis, 2008, Saunders.)

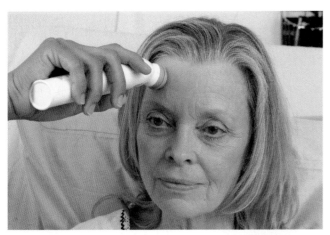

FIGURE 15.3 Temporal artery thermometer. (From Sorrentino SA, Remmert LN: *Mosby's Textbook for Nursing Assistants*, ed 9, St. Louis, 2017, Elsevier.)

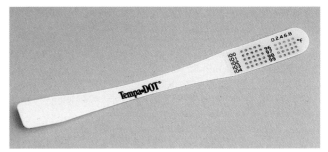

FIGURE 15.4 Tempa-Dot disposable oral strip thermometer. (Courtesy Medical Indicators, Inc., Hamilton, NJ.)

uncomfortable for the patient, and (2) if affected cerumen (earwax) is present in both ears, because the reading may be inaccurate. The wax could be too thick to get a good reading.

Temporal Artery Scanner

The TA scanner uses an infrared (red) beam to assess the temperature of the blood flowing through the TA of the side of the forehead, where the artery lies about 1 mm below the skin (Fig. 15.3). Because the artery is so close to the skin, it provides good surface heat conduction, allowing the thermometer to obtain a fast, accurate, and noninvasive measurement of the body temperature. This thermometer is easily used on children, and typically does not frighten them.

To perform the procedure, place the probe in the center of the forehead, halfway between the eyebrows and the hairline. Bangs should be pushed back off the forehead (this method cannot be used if bandages cover the area). Depress the button on the scanner and gently stroke the probe across the forehead toward the hairline (at the temples), keeping the probe flat on the patient's skin. As the scanner moves across the forehead, repeated temperature measurements are taken and the highest measurement is recorded; keeping the button depressed, lift the scanner from the temporal area and lightly place the probe behind the earlobe. Release the button and remove the probe. Recording an accurate temperature takes about 3 seconds (Procedure 15.3).

Axillary Thermometer

Studies indicate that axillary temperatures are accurate when performed correctly. Axillary temperatures take more time to register the correct body temperature, but the method is safe, simple, and easy to perform

(Procedure 15.4). Axillary temperatures are taken with a digital thermometer, which is placed into the axillary fold. If the digital thermometer has more than one probe, the oral (blue) probe with a disposable probe cover should be used. Because tympanic and temporal thermometers are relatively expensive, the axillary method may be a viable way for parents of young children to get accurate temperature readings at home. However, parents should be aware that the axillary temperature may be as much as 1 degree less than the child's actual core temperature.

Disposable Thermometer

Disposable thermometers (those that are used only once) are frequently used on small children in the home. The reading is obtained by a heat-sensitive material that changes color according to the elevation of body temperature. Two types of disposable thermometers frequently are used by parents of young children. One type is placed under the child's tongue (Fig. 15.4); the other is placed on the forehead. Although both types are fairly reliable, the temperature-sensing materials have expiration dates, which often are overlooked, and specific storage requirements may apply. Disposable thermometers are considered to be good screening devices but are not as accurate as other methods.

PROCEDURE 15.3

Obtain Vital Signs: Obtain a Temporal Artery Temperature

1. Sanitize your hands. Gather the necessary equipment and supplies.
2. Introduce yourself, identify your patient, and explain the procedure.
3. Remove the protective cap on the probe. The probe can be cleaned by lightly wiping the surface with an alcohol swab.
4. Push the patient's hair up off of the forehead to expose the site. Gently place the probe on the patient's forehead, halfway between the eyebrows and the hairline.
5. Depress and hold the SCAN button and lightly glide the probe sideways across the patient's forehead to the hairline just above the ear.

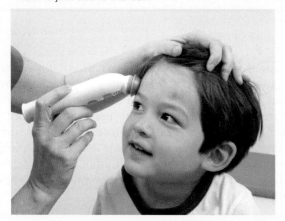

As you move the sensor across the forehead, you will hear a beep, and a red light will flash.

6. Keep the button depressed, lift the thermometer, and place the probe on the upper neck behind the ear lobe.

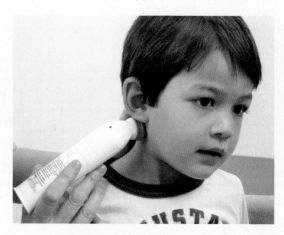

The thermometer may continue to beep, indicating that the temperature is rising.

7. When scanning is complete, release the button and lift the probe. Note the temperature recorded on the digital display. The scanner automatically turns off 15 to 30 seconds after release of the button.
8. Disinfect the thermometer if indicated and replace the protective cap.
9. Sanitize your hands.
10. Record the temperature results (e.g., T = 101.6° F [TA]) in the patient's medical record.

PROCEDURE 15.4

Obtain Vital Signs: Obtain an Axillary Temperature

1. Sanitize your hands.
2. Gather the needed equipment and supplies.
3. Introduce yourself, identify your patient, and explain the procedure.
4. Prepare the thermometer or digital unit in the same manner as for oral use.
5. Remove the patient's clothing and gown the patient as needed to access the axillary region.
6. Pat the patient's axillary area dry with tissues if needed.
7. Cover the thermometer or probe and place the tip into the center of the armpit, pointing the stem toward the upper chest, ensuring that the thermometer is touching only skin, not clothing.

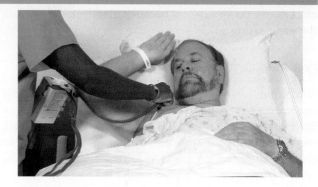

Continued

8. Instruct the patient to hold the arm snugly across the chest or abdomen until the thermometer beeps.

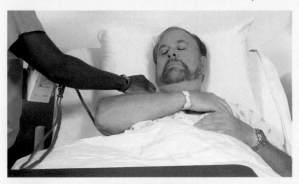

9. Remove the thermometer, note the digital reading, and dispose of the cover in the biohazard waste container.
10. Disinfect the thermometer if indicated.
11. Sanitize your hands.
12. Record the axillary temperature on the patient's medical record (e.g., T = 97.6° F [A]).

(Figures from Mosby's nursing assistant video skills 4.0, *St. Louis, 2015, Elsevier.)*

Cleaning Thermometers

Digital Thermometers

The digital unit or individual digital thermometers should be routinely cleaned with disinfectant. When ejecting the probe shield or removing the sheath, be careful not to contaminate the probe or the processing unit. If a chance exists that a patient's body fluids touched the unit, wipe it with disinfectant before returning it to the storage area.

Tympanic Thermometers

The same guidelines for a digital unit are followed in the cleaning of a tympanic thermometer. When using the device on a small child, be conscious of what the child touches. If the processing unit is touched, be sure to wipe it with disinfectant after use. However, be careful not to get the tip of the probe surface wet, and always use probe covers, because disinfectant can ruin the probe surface.

Disposable Thermometers

Sometimes disposable thermometers are used. These may be a cost-effective way with no use of batteries or maintenance required. Always discard a disposable thermometer in the appropriate waste container immediately after use to prevent contamination and the spread of pathogens to other patients.

PULSE

A patient's pulse rate reflects the palpable beat of the arteries throughout the body as they expand in response to contraction of the heart. With every beat, the heart pumps an amount of blood, known as the *stroke volume*, into the aorta. Arteries branch off the aorta as it travels down through the center of the abdomen, transferring the pulse beat throughout the body. To measure the pulse, an artery is used that is close to the body surface and can be pushed against a bone. Palpating a peripheral pulse gives the rate and rhythm of the heartbeat and local information about the condition of the artery used.

Pulse Sites

A pulse rate may be counted any place where an artery is near the surface of the body and the vessel can be pressed against a bone. The most common sites used to feel this rhythmic throbbing are the temporal, carotid, apical, brachial, radial, femoral, popliteal, and dorsalis pedis arteries (Fig. 15.5).

The *temporal* pulse is located in the temple area of the skull, parallel and lateral to the eyes (Fig. 15.6). It is seldom used as a pulse site but may be used as a pressure point to help control bleeding from a head injury.

The *carotid* artery is located between the larynx and the sternocleidomastoid muscle in the front and to the side of the neck (Fig. 15.7). It most frequently is used in emergencies and to check the pulse during cardiopulmonary resuscitation (CPR). It can be felt by pushing the muscle to the side and pressing against the larynx.

The *apical* heart rate, or the heartbeat at the apex of the heart, is heard with a stethoscope. It is used for infants and young children because the radial pulse is difficult to palpate in young patients or in adults if the radial pulse is difficult to feel or is irregular. An apical count may be requested if the patient is taking cardiac drugs or has bradycardia or tachycardia. To determine the presence of a pulse deficit, the physician may listen

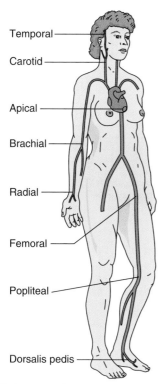

FIGURE 15.5 Pulse sites. (From Proctor D, Adams A: *Kinn's the patient care technician*, ed 12, St. Louis, 2014, Saunders.)

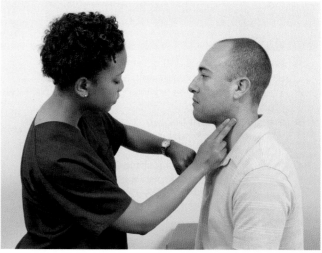

FIGURE 15.7 Carotid pulse. (From Proctor D, Adams A: *Kinn's the patient care technician*, ed 12, St. Louis, 2014, Saunders.)

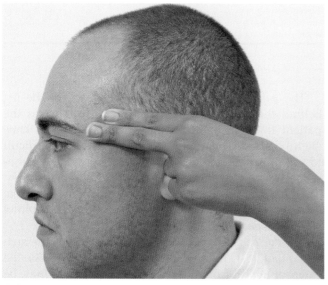

FIGURE 15.6 Temporal pulse. (From Proctor D, Adams A: *Kinn's the patient care technician*, ed 12, St. Louis, 2014, Saunders.)

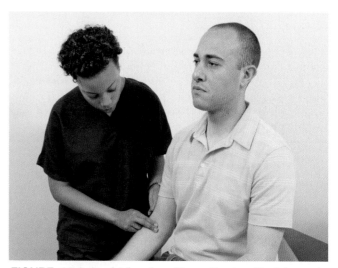

FIGURE 15.8 Brachial pulse. (From Proctor D, Adams A: *Kinn's the patient care technician*, ed 12, St. Louis, 2014, Saunders.)

to the apical beat while the patient care technician counts the pulse at another site. The apex of the heart is located in the left fifth intercostal space on the midclavicular line, that is, between the fifth and sixth ribs on a line with the midpoint of the left clavicle. The stethoscope is placed just below the left nipple between the fifth and sixth ribs. The pulse should be counted for 1 full minute and should be documented with (AP) beside the recorded count (Procedure 15.5).

The *brachial* pulse is felt at the inner *(antecubital)* aspect of the elbow. This is the artery that is felt and heard when blood pressure is measured (Fig. 15.8). It also can be felt in the groove between the biceps and triceps muscles on the inner surface of the middle upper arm. This is the pulse that is checked on infants and young children receiving CPR.

The *radial* artery is the most frequently used site for counting the pulse rate. It is best found on the thumb side of the wrist, 1 inch below the base of the thumb (Fig. 15.9).

The *femoral* pulse is located at the site where the femoral artery passes through the groin. The examiner must press deeply below the inguinal ligament to palpate this pulse.

PROCEDURE 15.5

Obtain Vital Signs: Obtain an Apical Pulse

1. Sanitize your hands and clean the stethoscope earpieces and diaphragm with alcohol swabs.
2. Introduce yourself, identify your patient, and explain the procedure.
3. If necessary, assist the patient in disrobing from the waist up and provide the patient with a gown that opens in the front.
4. Assist the patient into the sitting or supine position.
5. Hold the stethoscope's diaphragm against the palm of your hand for a few seconds.
6. Place the stethoscope just below the left nipple in the intercostal space between the fifth and sixth ribs over the apex of the heart.

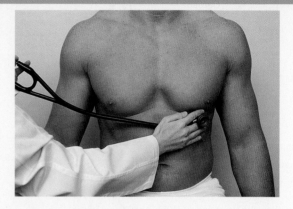

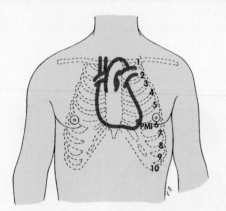

7. Listen carefully for the heartbeat.
8. Count the pulse for 1 full minute. Note any irregularities in rhythm and volume.
9. Help the patient sit up and dress.
10. Sanitize your hands.
11. Record the pulse in the patient's chart (e.g., AP = 96) and record any arrhythmias.

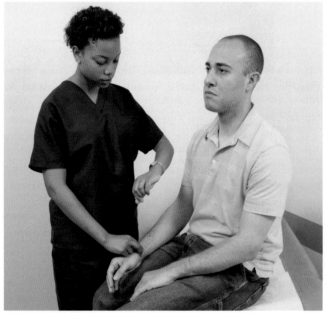

FIGURE 15.9 Radial pulse. (From Proctor D, Adams A: *Kinn's the patient care technician*, ed 12, St. Louis, 2014, Saunders.)

The *popliteal* pulse is found at the back of the leg behind the knee. Palpation of this pulse requires the patient to be in a recumbent position with the knee slightly flexed. The popliteal artery is deep and difficult to feel. It is palpated and also monitored with a stethoscope when a leg blood pressure reading is necessary. The physician checks blood flow through the popliteal artery if a circulatory system problem, such as a blood clot, is suspected in the lower leg.

The *dorsalis pedis* (pedal) artery is felt across the arch of the foot, just slightly lateral to the midline, beside the extensor tendon of the great toe. This pulse may be congenitally absent in some patients. Because a good pulse rate at this site is an indicator of normal lower limb circulation and arterial sufficiency, the physician checks the pedal pulses in patients with peripheral vascular problems (e.g., patients with diabetes mellitus).

Characteristics of a Pulse

When measuring a pulse, you must note three important characteristics: rate, rhythm, and volume. These characteristics vary with the size and elasticity of the artery and the strength and regularity of the heart's contractions. A patient's pulse may reveal valuable information about the cardiovascular system.

Rate

The pulse rate is a measure of the number of heartbeats felt from the movement of blood through an artery. When the heart contracts, pressure throughout the arteries is increased, and the arteries expand. When the heart relaxes, arterial pressure is decreased, and the arteries relax. Each contraction and relaxation of the heart muscle is a heartbeat, and each resulting expansion and relaxation of the arteries is the pulse rate. Normally, the heartbeat (rate) and the pulse rate are the same. The rate of the pulse is the number of heartbeats (pulsations) that occur in 1 minute. Because the body must balance heat loss by increasing circulation (a faster heart rate), the pulse rate is proportionate with the size of the heart. The smaller the body, the greater is the heat loss and the faster the heart must pump to compensate. Therefore infants and children normally have a faster pulse than adults; as the aging process progresses, the pulse rate declines.

Pulse rates normally vary as a result of a person's age, body size, gender, and health status. The rate is affected by an individual's activities and psychological state, and by certain medications. It usually is faster in women (70 to 80 beats per minute) than in men (60 to 70 beats per minute). Children tend to have more rapid pulse rates than adults. The rate is faster when sitting than when lying down, and it increases when an individual stands, walks, or runs. During sleep or rest, the pulse rate may drop to as low as 45 to 50 beats per minute. Well-conditioned athletes tend to have pulse rates of 50 to 60 beats per minute, because consistent aerobic exercise strengthens the heart muscle (the myocardium) so that each heart contraction ejects an increased volume of blood into the arterial system. Table 15.3 lists the normal pulse ranges for various age groups of patients.

Rhythm

The pulse rhythm is the time between pulse beats. A normal rhythm pattern has an even tempo, which indicates that the intervals between the beats are of equal duration. An abnormal rhythm, or arrhythmia, is described according to the rhythm pattern detected. An intermittent pulse may occur in healthy individuals during exercise or after drinking a beverage containing caffeine. A common irregularity found in children and young adults is sinus arrhythmia, in which the heart rate varies with the respiratory cycle, speeding up at the peak of inspiration and slowing to normal with expiration. If beats are frequently skipped or if the beats are markedly irregular, the physician should be advised, because this may indicate heart disease. If an irregular rhythm is detected, the apical pulse should be measured for a full minute to ensure accuracy, and the rate should be recorded for the physician's review. A note also should be made that the patient's pulse was irregular. For example: P-86 irregular.

Volume

The volume (pulse amplitude) reflects the strength of the heart when it contracts. Volume can be assessed by feeling the strength of the pulse as blood flows through the vessel. The force of each pulse beat is described as bounding, or full; strong, or normal; or thready, or weak (Box 15.2). The force of the heartbeat and the condition of the arterial wall, whether hard or soft, influence the volume. The pulse may vary only in intensity and otherwise may be perfectly regular. This condition also can indicate heart disease. The pulse force is recorded using a three-point scale.

Determining the Pulse Rate

Radial and Apical Pulse Rates

The patient should be in a comfortable position, with the artery to be used at the same level as or lower than the heart (Procedure 15.6). The limb should be well supported and relaxed. The patient may be lying down or sitting. As with all pulse readings, the pads of the first three fingers are placed over the artery. The thumb should never be used to determine the pulse rate, because the thumb has its own pulse, and the patient

Table 15.3	Approximate Age-Related Pulse Ranges	
Age	Range (Breaths per Minute)	Average (Breaths per Minute)
Newborn	120-160	140
1-2 years	80-140	120
3-6 years	75-120	100
7-11 years	75-110	95
Adolescence to adulthood	60-100	80

Box 15.2	Three-Point Scale for Measuring Pulse Volume	
3+	Full, bounding pulse	Pulsation is very strong and does not disappear with moderate pressure.
2+	Normal pulse	Pulsation is easily felt but disappears with moderate pressure.
1+	Weak, thready pulse	Pulsation is not easily felt and disappears with slight pressure.

PROCEDURE 15.6

Obtain Vital Signs: Assess the Patient's Radial Pulse

1. Sanitize your hands.
2. Introduce yourself, identify your patient, and explain the procedure.
3. Place the patient's arm in a relaxed position, palm downward, at or below the level of the heart.
4. Gently grasp the palm side of the patient's wrist with your first three fingertips approximately 1 inch below the base of the thumb.

5. Count the beats for 1 full minute using a watch with a second hand.
6. Sanitize your hands.
7. Record the count and any irregularities on the patient's medical record (e.g., P = 72). The pulse usually is recorded immediately after the temperature.

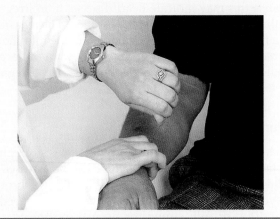

care technician's pulse rate may be confused with the patient's rate. Push the radial artery against the bone until the strongest pulsation is felt. The pulse should be counted for 1 full minute. The 15- or 30-second interval may be used once the patient care technician becomes proficient at performing the skill.

Variations from normal quality should be noted, such as an arrhythmia or a pulse that is thready or bounding. Some pulses are more difficult to feel than others, and finding the correct pressure to be used for each patient and site requires repeated practice and experience.

Both you and the patient should be in a relaxed position. The sensitivity in your counting fingers is greatly reduced if you are in an awkward position. Too much pressure obliterates the patient's pulse, and too little pressure prevents detection of irregularities or of all the beats. Record the number of beats in 1 minute. Assess the pulse, including rate, rhythm, and volume. If the pulse rate is counted at any site other than the radial artery, the rate should be recorded along with a notation of the site used. The apical pulse should always be auscultated for a full minute to detect any irregularities in rate and rhythm.

Femoral, Popliteal, and Pedal Pulses

Pulses in the lower extremities may be difficult to find and equally difficult to hear. A Doppler unit, which is

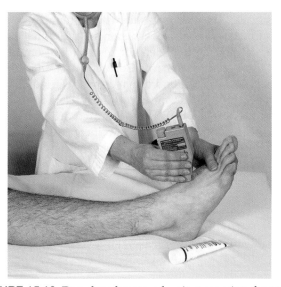

FIGURE 15.10 Doppler ultrasound unit measuring the pedal pulse. (From Jarvis C: *Physical examination and health assessment,* ed 5, St. Louis, 2008, W. B. Saunders.)

an ultrasound unit that magnifies the pulsation, may be used to locate and count these pulses accurately (Fig. 15.10). This unit is battery operated and can often be attached to a stethoscope so that only you hear the beat, or it can be set so that both you and your patient can hear the pulsations.

RESPIRATION

Physiology

The purpose of respiration is to provide for the exchange of oxygen and carbon dioxide among the atmosphere, the blood, and the body cells. Oxygen is taken into the body to be used for life-sustaining body processes, and carbon dioxide is released as a waste product.

One complete inspiration and expiration is called a *respiration*. During the inspiratory phase, the diaphragm contracts and drops down while the intercostal muscles pull the ribs up and outward, causing the lungs to expand and fill with air. During the expiratory phase, the diaphragm returns to its normal elevated position and the intercostal muscles relax, causing the lungs to expel the waste air back into the atmosphere.

Respiration is both internal and external. *External respiration* is the exchange of oxygen and carbon dioxide in the lungs. *Internal respiration* occurs at the cellular level, when oxygen in the bloodstream is transferred into the cells for energy, and carbon dioxide is released as a waste product and transported back to the lungs for exhalation.

The respiratory center in the medulla oblongata, located in the brain between the top of the spine and the brainstem, is sensitive to changes in blood oxygen and carbon dioxide levels. When blood carbon dioxide levels become elevated, the respiratory control center sends a message to the respiratory system that triggers breathing. Respiration, therefore, is controlled by the involuntary nervous system; this means that we breathe automatically. Because a person can control respiration to a certain extent, it also is a voluntary body function. However, breathing ultimately is under the control of the medulla oblongata, which is why we can hold our breath only for a given length of time. Once the blood's carbon dioxide level rises to the point where cells become oxygen starved, a stimulus is sent to the respiratory muscles (the diaphragm and intercostal muscles) and breathing begins involuntarily.

Characteristics of Respirations

Normally, a person's breathing is relaxed, automatic, and silent. When assessing a patient's respirations, you must note three important characteristics: rate, rhythm, and depth.

- *Rate:* The rate of respiration is the number of respirations per minute and is described as normal, rapid, or slow. Fig. 15.11 shows sample rate patterns recorded with a spirometer. Dyspnea occurs in patients with pneumonia, asthma, or chronic obstructive pulmonary disease (COPD). It also occurs after physical exertion or at very high altitudes. Other alterations in breathing are bradypnea, apnea, tachypnea, and hyperpnea. Hyperpnea

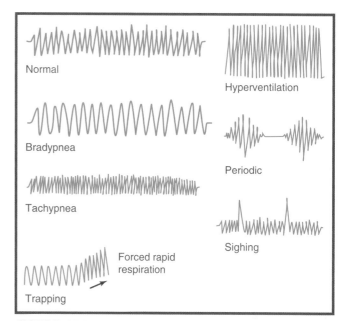

FIGURE 15.11 Respiratory rate patterns, called *spirograms*, are recorded using a spirometer. (From Proctor D, Adams A: *Kinn's the patient care technician*, ed 12, St. Louis, 2014, Saunders.)

Table 15.4	Approximate Age-Related Respiration Ranges	
Age	Range (Breaths per Minute)	Average (Breaths per Minute)
Newborn	30-50	40
1-3 years	20-30	25
4-6 years	18-26	22
7-11 years	16-22	19
Adolescence to adulthood	12-20	16

usually is accompanied by hyperventilation and often is found when the patient is extremely anxious or in pain. Orthopnea frequently occurs in patients with congestive heart failure (CHF) and COPD. Wheezing signals difficulty breathing in patients with asthma. Typically, a ratio of four pulse beats to one respiration is seen. As a rule, both the pulse and respiratory rates respond to exercise or emotional upset. Table 15.4 lists normal respiratory ranges for patients in various age groups.
- *Rhythm:* The term *rhythm* refers to the breathing pattern. A regular breathing pattern is normal in adults; however, the breathing pattern for infants varies. Automatic interruptions, such as sighing, are also considered normal.
- *Depth:* The *depth* of respiration is the amount of air inhaled and exhaled. When a patient is at rest, normal respirations have a consistent depth, which can be noted as you watch the rise and fall of the chest. Rapid, shallow breathing at rest occurs with some diseases, such as asthma and emphysema.

Normally, no noticeable breath sounds occur during the breathing process, except during snoring. Noticeable breath sounds are a sign of certain diseases, such as pneumonia, asthma, and pulmonary edema. After auscultating breath sounds with a stethoscope, the physician can describe the characteristics of breath sounds by using specific terminology (e.g., rales, rhonchi, stertorous breathing).

When an individual cannot inspire enough oxygen to supply all body cells with oxygenated blood, normal skin coloring, particularly around the mouth and the nail beds, changes to a bluish, dusky color. This coloration, which indicates an increased level of carbon dioxide in the blood, is called *cyanosis*. The patient also may have other signs and symptoms, such as vertigo, chest pain *(angina)*, and numbness in the fingers and toes.

Counting Respirations

Because most people are unaware of their breathing, do not mention that you will be counting their respirations (Procedure 15.7). The respiratory rate is easily controlled, and patients self-consciously alter their breathing rate when they know they are being watched. Therefore count the respirations while appearing to count the pulse. Keep your eyes alternately on the patient's chest and your watch while you count the pulse rate, and then, without removing your fingers from the pulse site, determine the respiratory rate. Counting respirations first may be easier, because that number is not as difficult to remember (Fig. 15.12). If the patient is supine, the arm may be crossed over the chest so that respirations can be felt with the rise and fall of the chest. Another way of observing respirations is to watch the movement of the patient's shoulders with each inspiration. Count the respirations for 30 seconds and multiply the number by 2. Do not use the 15-second interval, because this count can vary by a factor of +4 or −4, which is significant when one is dealing with such a small number. Note any variation or irregularity in the rate. Record the respiratory count on the medical record.

BLOOD PRESSURE

The blood pressure reading reflects the pressure of the blood against the walls of the arteries. Each time the ventricles contract, blood is pushed out of the heart and into the aorta, exerting pressure on the walls of the arteries. There are actually two blood pressure readings: the *systolic* pressure is the highest pressure level that occurs when the heart is contracting and the first pulse beat heard; the *diastolic* pressure is the lowest pressure level when the heart is relaxed and is the last sound heard. Systole (heart contraction) and diastole (heart relaxation) together make up the cardiac cycle. The difference between systolic and diastolic pressures is the pulse pressure.

Blood pressure is read in millimeters of mercury, abbreviated *mm Hg*. However, you need not include the abbreviation when documenting the reading on the patient's medical record. Blood pressure is recorded as a fraction, with the systolic reading the numerator (top) and the diastolic reading the denominator (bottom) (e.g., 130/80). Table 15.5 lists normal blood pressure ranges for patients of various age groups.

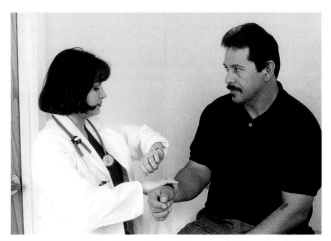

FIGURE 15.12 Hand position when counting respirations. The hands should be left in place as if still counting the patient's pulse. (From Proctor D, Adams A: *Kinn's the patient care technician*, ed 12, St. Louis, 2014, Saunders.)

PROCEDURE 15.7

Obtain Vital Signs: Determine the Respiratory Rate

1. Sanitize your hands.
2. Introduce yourself and identify the patient.
3. The patient's arm is in the same position used to count the pulse. If you have difficulty noticing the patient's breathing, place the arm across the chest to detect movement.
4. Note the rise and fall of the patient's chest.
5. Count the respirations for 30 seconds, using a watch with a second hand, and multiply by 2.
6. Release the patient's wrist.
7. Sanitize your hands.
8. Record the respirations on the patient's medical record after the pulse recording (e.g., R = 18).

Table 15.5	Approximate Age-Related Blood Pressure Ranges
Age	**Range (Systolic to Diastolic, mm Hg)**
Newborn	60-96 to 30-62
1-3 years	78-112 to 48-78
4-6 years	78-112 to 50-79
7-11 years	85-114 to 52-79
Adolescent	94-119 to 58-79
Adult	100-119 to 60-79

Table 15.6	Hypertension Categories		
Blood Pressure	**Normal**	**Prehypertension**	**Hypertension**
Systolic, mm Hg	Less than 120	120-139	140 or higher
Diastolic, mm Hg	Less than 80	80-89	90 or higher

Factors That Affect Blood Pressure

Physiologic factors that determine blood pressure include blood volume, peripheral resistance created by blood viscosity (the thickness of the blood), vessel elasticity, and the condition of the heart muscle and arterial walls.

Volume is the amount of blood in the arteries. An increased blood volume raises blood pressure, and a decreased blood volume lowers blood pressure. Therefore with extensive bleeding or hemorrhage, the blood volume drops, and so does the blood pressure.

The *peripheral resistance* of blood vessels refers to the relationship of the lumen (the diameter of the vessel) to the amount of blood flowing through it. The smaller the lumen, the greater is the resistance to blood flow. Blood pressure is higher with a small or reduced-size lumen and lower with a large lumen. Vessels affected by fatty cholesterol deposits called *atherosclerotic plaques* become narrower over time, resulting in smaller vessel lumens and therefore higher blood pressure.

Vessel elasticity is the ability of an artery to expand and contract to supply the body with a steady flow of blood. With advancing age, certain lifestyle factors, or the presence of arteriosclerosis, vessel elasticity may decrease, causing the arterial walls to become firm and resistant; as a result, the blood pressure is increased.

The condition of the myocardium (muscle layer of the heart) is a primary determinant of the volume of blood flowing through the body. A strong, forceful contraction empties the heart and tends to keep the blood pressure within normal limits. If the myocardium becomes weak, pressure in the vessels begins to increase in an attempt to maintain an adequate level of circulating blood to meet the oxygen and nutrient needs of the body.

Evaluating the Blood Pressure

When a patient's blood pressure is being tracked, frequent readings should be taken at about the same time of day and by the same person. Secondary hypertension is caused by another underlying pathologic condition, such as renal disease, complications of pregnancy,

endocrine imbalance, arteriosclerosis, atherosclerosis, and brain injury. Temporary hypertension may occur with stress, pain, exercise, and exhaustion. Many patients experience "white coat hypertension"; that is, their blood pressure becomes elevated in the medical environment, although it is normal when they are away from the healthcare facility. Essential hypertension is diagnosed in an adult (primary hypertension) if the systolic pressure is 140 mm Hg or higher and/or the diastolic pressure is 90 mm Hg or higher. Essential hypertension is the most common type of hypertension. It has no single identified cause but is associated with obesity, a high blood level of sodium, elevated cholesterol levels, and family history.

In 2013, the American Heart Association (AHA) published new guidelines for the diagnosis and management of hypertension. A new category of blood pressure, prehypertension, was identified, and normal blood pressure levels were lowered to less than 120/80. Table 15.6 identifies the categories of normal, prehypertensive, and hypertensive blood pressures.

The goal of the new recommendations is to reduce the number of people who die each year from hypertension-related illnesses such as coronary artery disease, heart attack, heart failure, kidney disease, and stroke. Hypertension can occur in children or adults, but individuals of African-American descent, middle-aged and elderly people, patients with diabetes mellitus, and those with kidney disease are at greatest risk. Hypertension has been called *the silent killer*, because it frequently has no symptoms, and individuals may go for long periods without knowing they have a problem. Hypertension often is discovered during medical treatment for another problem. Signs and symptoms may include blurred vision, angina, vertigo, dyspnea, fatigue, headache, flushing, nosebleeds (*epistaxis*), and palpitations.

The revised treatment guidelines for hypertension have four basic aspects:

1. Individuals with prehypertension should be diagnosed and encouraged to make lifestyle changes before they require medical treatment and/or move into the hypertensive category. The AHA recommends limiting intake of salt and eating a diet rich in potassium, calcium, magnesium, and protein

while reducing total fat intake, especially saturated fat and cholesterol. Prehypertensive individuals also should restrict their alcohol intake, engage in regular physical activity, and lose weight if necessary to maintain a healthy BMI range. Many times, just losing weight lowers blood pressure.

2. In people older than 50 years, the systolic reading is more important than the diastolic reading. Individuals aged above 50 years should be treated if they have a systolic pressure of 140 mm Hg or higher, regardless of their diastolic blood pressure. Medical treatment at this age can reduce the development of cardiac and kidney disease later in life.

3. Most patients with hypertension require two or more medications to achieve desired blood pressure levels. The goal of treatment is to maintain blood pressure below 140/90 mm Hg, or below 130/80 mm Hg in patients with diabetes or kidney disease. Patients should be treated with both a diuretic, which helps the body excrete excess amounts of fluid and sodium, and an antihypertensive medication.

4. A patient-centered treatment approach should be implemented to motivate patients and to maintain compliance with hypertension management. The patient care technician can play an active role in establishing a therapeutic relationship with patients by supporting them to ensure compliance with physician-recommended treatment such as making wise food choices when ordering their meal tray.

Hypotension is an abnormally low blood pressure, which may be caused by emotional or traumatic shock; hemorrhage; central nervous system disorders; and chronic wasting diseases. Persistent readings of 90/60 mm Hg or lower usually are considered hypotensive. Orthostatic (postural) hypotension can cause patients to experience vertigo or syncope. Some medications can cause orthostatic hypotension.

Measuring Blood Pressure

The instrument used to measure blood pressure is called the *sphygmomanometer*. The term *manometer* refers to an instrument used to measure the pressure of a liquid or a gas. *Sphygmo-* means pulse. Therefore *sphygmomanometer* means an instrument used to measure blood pressure in the arteries. The instrument consists of an inflatable cuff, an inflation bulb with a control valve, and a pressure gauge. The blood pressure mechanism consists of an aneroid dial attached to an inflatable cuff (Fig. 15.13A) or a blood pressure floor model (Fig. 15.13B).

Sphygmomanometers are delicately calibrated instruments that must be handled carefully. They should be recalibrated regularly and checked for accuracy, by you or by a medical supply dealer. The needle on the aneroid dial sphygmomanometer should rest within the small square or circle at the bottom of the dial. The dial can be calibrated by connecting it to a calibrated manometer. Pump both

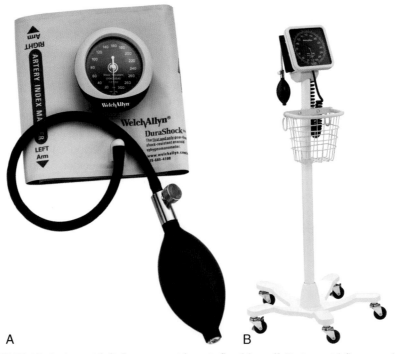

A   B

FIGURE 15.13 A, Aneroid dial system with an inflatable cuff. B, Aneroid floor model with a large, slanted face. (From Welch Allyn.)

manometers to 250 mm Hg and record readings on both machines at least four different times as the pressure is released. A correctly calibrated mechanism shows a difference of no more than 3 mm Hg between the two readings at any time during the deflation period. If the sphygmomanometer is not correctly calibrated, the patient's blood pressure reading will be inaccurate (Box 15.3).

The sphygmomanometer must be used with a stethoscope. The objective of the procedure is to use the inflatable cuff to obliterate (cause to disappear) circulation through an artery. The stethoscope is placed over the artery just below the cuff, and the cuff is slowly deflated to allow the blood to flow again. As blood flow resumes, cardiac cycle sounds are heard through the stethoscope, and gauge readings are taken when the first (systolic) and last (diastolic) sounds are heard (Procedure 15.8).

Blood pressure cuffs and stethoscopes are available in drug and retail stores for patients to use to measure their own blood pressure at home. These units can be aneroid, electronic, or computerized sphygmomanometers (Fig. 15.14).

Korotkoff Sounds

Two basic heart sounds are produced by the functioning of the heart during the cardiac cycle. The first sound, produced at systole (contraction), is dull, firm, and prolonged and is heard as a *lubb* sound. The second sound, produced at diastole (relaxation), is shorter and sharper and is heard as a *dupp* sound. Therefore *lubb-dupp* is the sound of one heartbeat.

Korotkoff sounds are the sounds heard during auscultation of blood pressure. These sounds are produced by vibrations of the arterial wall when the blood surges back into the vessel after it has been compressed by the blood pressure cuff. These sounds were first discovered and classified into five distinct phases by Russian neurologist Nikolai Sergeyevich Korotkoff.

Box 15.3	Common Causes of Error in Blood Pressure Readings

- The limb used for measurement is above the level of the heart.
- The rubber bladder in the cuff is not completely deflated before a reading is started or retaken.
- The pressure in the cuff is released too rapidly.
- The patient is nervous, uncomfortable, or anxious, which may cause a reading higher than the patient's actual blood pressure.
- The patient drank coffee or smoked cigarettes within 30 minutes of the blood pressure measurement.
- The cuff is applied improperly.
- The cuff is too large, too small, too loose, or too tight.
- The cuff is not placed around the arm smoothly.
- The bladder is not centered over the artery, or the bladder bulges out from the cover.
- The practitioner fails to wait 1 to 2 minutes between measurements.
- Instruments are defective:
  - Air leaks in the valve.
  - Air leaks in the bladder.
  - Aneroid needle is not calibrated to zero.

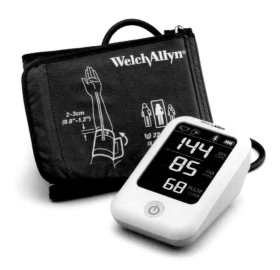

FIGURE 15.14 Personal blood pressure system, digital arm cuff. (From Welch Allyn.)

PROCEDURE 15.8

Obtain Vital Signs: Determine a Patient's Blood Pressure

1. Sanitize your hands.
2. Assemble the equipment and supplies needed. Clean the earpieces and diaphragm of the stethoscope with alcohol swabs.
3. Introduce yourself, identify the patient, and explain the procedure.
4. Select the appropriate arm for application of the cuff (no mastectomy on that side, without injury or disease). If the patient has had a bilateral mastectomy, the blood pressure should be taken using a large thigh cuff with the stethoscope over the popliteal artery.

Continued

PROCEDURE 15.8

Obtain Vital Signs: Determine a Patient's Blood Pressure—cont'd

5. Seat the patient in a comfortable position with the legs uncrossed and the arm resting, palm up, at heart level on the lap or a table.
6. Roll up the sleeve to about 5 inches above the elbow or have the patient remove the arm from the sleeve.
7. Determine the correct cuff size.
8. Palpate the brachial artery at the antecubital space in both arms. If one arm has a stronger pulse, use that arm. If the pulses are equal, select the right arm.

   CAUTION: If a female patient has had a mastectomy, the blood pressure should never be taken on the affected side. Compressing the arm may cause complications. If she has had a bilateral mastectomy, another site such as the popliteal artery must be used, which requires use of a thigh cuff.

9. Center the cuff bladder over the brachial artery with the connecting tube away from the patient's body and the tube to the bulb close to the body.

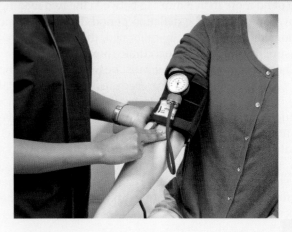

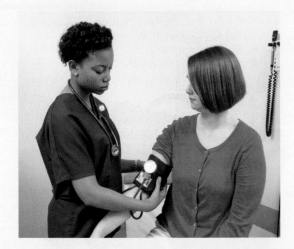

10. Place the lower edge of the cuff about 1 inch above the palpable brachial pulse, normally located in the natural crease of the inner elbow, and wrap it snugly and smoothly.
11. Position the gauge of the sphygmomanometer so that it is easily seen.
12. Palpate the brachial pulse, tighten the screw valve on the air pump, and inflate the cuff until the pulse can no longer be felt. Make a note at the point on the gauge where the pulse could no longer be felt. Mentally add 30 mm Hg to the reading. Deflate the cuff and wait 15 seconds.

13. Insert the earpieces of the stethoscope turned forward into the ear canals.
14. Place the stethoscope's diaphragm over the palpated brachial artery for an adult patient or the bell for a pediatric patient. Press firmly enough to obtain a seal but not so tightly that the artery is constricted.
15. Close the valve and squeeze the bulb to inflate the cuff, rapidly but smoothly, to 30 mm above the palpated pulse level, which was previously determined.

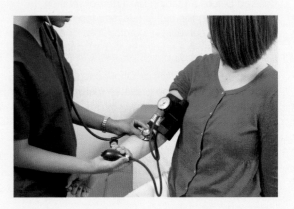

16. Open the valve slightly and deflate the cuff at a constant rate of 2 to 3 mm Hg per heartbeat.
17. Listen throughout the entire deflation; note the point on the gauge at which you hear the first sound (systolic) and the last sound (diastolic) until the sounds have stopped for at least 10 mm Hg. Read the pressure to the closest even number.

18. Do not reinflate the cuff once the air has been released. Wait 30 to 60 seconds to repeat the procedure if needed. (Not allowing the blood to refill in the brachial artery results in inaccurate readings.)
19. Remove the stethoscope from your ears and record the systolic and diastolic readings as BP systolic/diastolic (e.g., BP 120/80).
   NOTE: It is recommended that the blood pressure be checked and recorded in each arm during the initial assessment of the patient and then bilaterally periodically after that for patients with hypertension.
20. Remove the cuff from the patient's arm and return it to its proper storage area. Clean the earpieces of the stethoscope with alcohol and return it to storage.

21. Sanitize your hands.
   ADDENDUM: The physician may order the blood pressure with the patient be recorded in two different positions to determine whether orthostatic hypotension is a factor. For this, perform the following steps:
   1. Measure and record the patient's blood pressure (as detailed earlier) while the patient is either supine or sitting.
   2. Leave the cuff in place.
   3. Have the patient stand, and immediately measure the blood pressure again.
   4. Record the second blood pressure, as well as any patient symptoms, such as complaints of (c/o) vertigo or lightheadedness.

Phase I

Phase I is the first sound heard as the cuff deflates. The blood is resurging into the patient's artery and can be heard quite clearly as a sharp, tapping sound. Note the gauge reading when this first sound is heard. Record this as the systolic blood pressure.

Phase II

As the cuff deflates, even more blood flows through the artery. The movement of the blood makes a swishing sound. If you do not follow proper procedure in inflating the cuff, you may not hear these sounds because of their soft quality. Occasionally, blood pressure sounds completely disappear during this phase. Loss of the sounds followed by their reappearance later is called the *auscultatory gap*. The silence may continue as the needle falls another 30 mm Hg. Auscultatory gaps occur particularly in hypertension and certain types of heart disease, so if you notice such a gap, make sure to report it to the physician.

Phase III

In phase III, a great deal of blood is pushing down into the artery. The distinct, sharp tapping sounds return and continue rhythmically. If you do not inflate the cuff enough, you will miss the first two phases completely and you will incorrectly interpret the beginning of phase III as the systolic blood pressure (phase I).

Phase IV

At this point, the blood is flowing easily. The sound changes to a soft tapping, which becomes muffled and begins to grow fainter. Occasionally, these sounds continue to zero. This may occur in children, in patients of any age after exercise or with a fever, or in a pregnant patient with anemia. The AHA recommends that the beginning of phase IV be recorded as the diastolic reading for a child. Some physicians call the change at phase IV the *fading sound* and want it recorded between systolic and diastolic recordings (e.g., 120/84/70, with 84 representing the gauge reading when the sounds of phase III have ended and those of phase IV are beginning). Other physicians consider phase IV the true diastolic pressure.

Phase V

All sounds disappear in this phase. Note the gauge reading when the last sound is heard. Record this as the diastolic pressure.

Palpatory Method

The systolic pressure may be checked by feeling the radial pulse rather than hearing it with the stethoscope. Place the cuff in the usual position and palpate the radial pulse, noting rate and rhythm. Inflate the cuff until the pulse disappears, and then add 30 mm Hg more of inflation to get above the systolic pressure. Do not remove your fingers from the pulse or change the pressure of your fingers. Slowly release the pressure in the cuff and wait for the pulse to be felt again. Note the reading on the gauge, and record the first pulse felt as the systolic pressure. For example, if you first felt the radial pulse at 52 mm Hg, the palpated blood pressure is recorded as 52/P, with P indicating that the systolic reading was palpated. The diastolic and Korotkoff phases cannot be determined by this method. This method can be very useful in times of a medical emergency, such as shock, when the patient's blood pressure cannot be auscultated.

Pulse Oximetry

Pulse oximetry is the noninvasive measurement of arterial blood oxygen saturation, the percent to which hemoglobin is bound with oxygen. The assessment of oxygen saturation using pulse oximetry (SpO_2) is often included when obtaining vital signs (Procedure 15.9). A pulse oximeter is a probe with an LED connected by a cable to an oximeter. Normally, SpO_2 is greater than 95%. SpO_2 less than 90% is considered a clinical emergency (WHO, 2011).

The measurement of oxygen saturation is simple and painless and has few of the risks associated with more invasive measurements of oxygen saturation, such as arterial blood gas sampling. Conditions that decrease arterial blood flow, such as peripheral vascular disease, hypothermia, vasoconstrictors, hypotension, or peripheral edema, affect accurate measurement of oxygen saturation. Factors that affect light transmission, such as outside light sources, patient motion, or red-based nail polish, also affect the accurate measurement of oxygen saturation.

In adults, you can apply reusable and disposable oximeter probes to the earlobe, finger, bridge of the nose, or forehead. Oxygen saturation measurement using a forehead probe is quicker than finger probes (Yont et al., 2011) and more accurate in conditions that decrease arterial blood flow (Nesseler et al., 2012). Pulse oximetry is indicated in patients who have an unstable oxygen status or are at risk for impaired gas exchange.

In infants and small children, the oximeter probes are typically applied to the great toe. Often the biggest challenge is getting the probe to stay on with the movement that is typical of infants and children. In some cases, physicians will order continuous oxygen saturation monitoring. This means that there will be a monitor in the room of the patient that will typically have alarms set to notify staff of levels that are too low. Be sure to instruct the parents of the child to report if the probe falls off.

Delegation and Documentation Box 15.3

The skill of oxygen saturation measurement can be delegated to you as a patient care technician. Follow these guidelines when obtaining oxygen saturation:
- Consider the specific factors related to the patient that can falsely lower oxygen saturation.
- Obtain the appropriate frequency of oxygen saturation measurement.
- Apply the appropriate site and probe for measurement.
- Report any SpO_2 reading less than 95% to the nurse immediately.
- Refrain from using pulse oximetry as an assessment of heart rate because the oximeter will not detect an irregular pulse.

Delegation and Documentation Box 15.4

Vital signs are documented in this order: temperature (T), pulse (P), and respirations (R). Blood pressure is recorded after TPR. Correctly document the following vital signs:
1. Oral temperature 101.2°; apical pulse 90; respirations 22; and orthostatic blood pressure 138/88 supine and 110/70 standing
2. Tympanic temperature 36.8°; radial pulse 66; respirations 18; and bilateral blood pressure 128/76 in the left arm and 132/80 in the right arm
3. Temporal temperature 102.4°; apical pulse 102; and respirations 27
4. Axillary temperature 97.7°; carotid pulse 58; respirations 24; and palpated blood pressure 62

Illness & Injury Prevention Box 15.2

In order to prevent illness or injury to patients and yourself, be sure to follow these OSHA Guidelines for Measuring Vital Signs.
- Wash hands before and after each procedure.
- Always use protective disposable sheaths on all forms of thermometers.
- Immediately disinfect any equipment that has become contaminated during the procedure.
- Wear gloves if the potential exists for contacting any open areas or body fluids.
- When caring for a patient with a known respiratory infectious disorder, such as tuberculosis, use protective clothing, including a face shield or mask as indicated.
- Dispose of all contaminated material, including thermometer covers, gloves, and disinfectant swabs, in the proper biohazard waste containers.

ANTHROPOMETRIC MEASUREMENT

Anthropometry is the science that deals with measurement of the size, weight, and proportions of the human body. These measurements often are included in the initial recording of vital signs and before the physician performs a physical examination or a well-baby check. Because they are indicators of the patient's state of health and well-being, height and weight measurements and the associated BMI are discussed as aspects of the vital signs. Other measurements are discussed when pertinent in the specialty chapters.

Measuring Weight and Height

A patient's weight and height can be helpful in diagnosis, and the patient care technician must obtain these readings with accuracy and empathy (Procedure 15.10). In

PROCEDURE 15.9

Assessing Oxygen Saturation

1. Determine the need to measure patient's oxygen saturation from the nurse or patient medical record. (Examples may include acute or chronic respiratory problems, chest wall injury, monitoring during unconscious sedation, and recovery from sedation or anesthesia.)
2. Identify factors that influence measurement of SpO_2: oxygen therapy, respiratory therapy treatments such as postural drainage and percussion, hemoglobin level, hypotension, temperature, and medications such as bronchodilators.
3. Review patient's medical record for healthcare provider's order, or consult facility's procedure manual for oxygen saturation measurement standard of care.
4. Determine previous baseline SpO_2 (if available) from patient's record.
5. Determine most appropriate patient-specific site (e.g., finger, earlobe, bridge of nose, forehead) for sensor probe placement by measuring capillary refill. If capillary refill is greater than 2 seconds, select alternative site.
   a. Site must have adequate local circulation and be free of moisture.
   b. A finger free of polish or acrylic nail is preferred (Cicek et al., 2011).
   c. If patient has tremors or is likely to move, use earlobe or forehead.
   d. If patient is obese, clip-on probe may not fit properly; obtain a disposable (tape-on) probe.
6. Position patient comfortably. Instruct patient to breathe normally. If the finger is the monitoring site, support lower arm.
7. If using the finger, remove fingernail polish from digit with acetone or polish remover.
8. Attach the sensor to monitoring site. Instruct patient that the clip-on probe will feel like a clothespin on the finger but will not hurt.

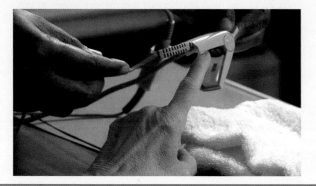

9. When the sensor is in place, turn on oximeter by activating power. Observe pulse waveform/intensity display and audible beep. Correlate oximeter pulse rate by taking patient's radial pulse.

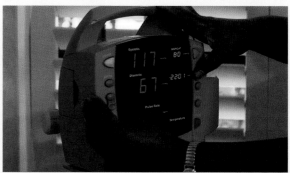

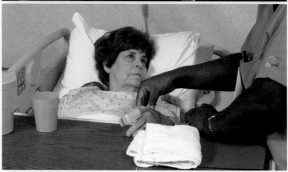

10. Leave the sensor in place until oximeter readout reaches a constant value and pulse display reaches full strength during each cardiac cycle. Inform patient that the oximeter alarm will sound if the sensor falls off or if patient moves the sensor. Read SpO_2 on digital display.
11. If you are told to monitor oxygen saturation continuously, verify that SpO_2 alarm limits are preset by the manufacturer at a low of 85% and a high of 100%. Determine limits for SpO_2 and pulse rate as indicated by patient's condition. Verify that alarms are on. Assess skin integrity under sensor probe every 2 hours; relocate sensor at least every 4 hours and more frequently if skin integrity is altered or tissue perfusion compromised.
12. If you plan on intermittent monitoring or spot-checking SpO_2, remove the probe and turn oximeter power off. Store the sensor in appropriate location.
13. Compare SpO_2 with patient's previous baseline and acceptable SpO_2 if indicated by the nurse. Note use of oxygen therapy, which can affect oxygen saturation.

(Figures from Mosby's nursing assistant video skills 4.0, *St. Louis, 2015, Elsevier.)*

PROCEDURE 15.10

Obtain Vital Signs: Measure a Patient's Weight and Height

NOTE: *Ensure that the scale is located in an area away from traffic to maintain the patient's privacy.*

1. Sanitize your hands.
2. Introduce yourself, identify your patient, and explain the procedure.
3. If the patient is to remove his or her shoes for weighing, place a paper towel on the scale platform. The patient may be given disposable slippers to wear.
4. Check to see that the balance bar pointer floats in the middle of the balance frame when all weights are at zero.
5. Help the patient onto the scale. Ensure that a female patient is not holding a purse and that a male or female patient has removed any heavy objects from pockets.
6. Move the large weight into the groove closest to the patient's estimated weight. The grooves are calibrated in 50-lb increments. If you choose a groove that is more than the patient's weight, the pointer will immediately tilt to the bottom of the balance frame. You then must move it back one groove.

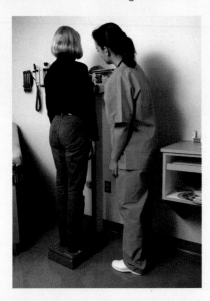

7. While the patient is standing still, slide the small upper weight to the right along the pound markers until the pointer balances in the middle of the balance frame. (The pointer floats between the bottom and the top of the frame when both lower and upper weights together balance the scale with the patient's weight.)

8. Leave the weights in place.
9. Ask the patient to stand up straight and to look straight ahead. On some scales, the patient may need to turn with the back to the scale.
10. Adjust the height bar so that it just touches the top of the patient's head.

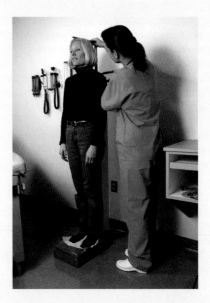

11. Leave the elevation bar set but fold down the horizontal bar (to maintain the height recording while protecting the patient from possible injury).
12. Assist the patient off the scale. Ensure that all items that were removed for weighing are given back to the patient.
13. Read the weight scale. Add the numbers at the markers of the large and small weights and record the total to the nearest $\frac{1}{4}$ lb on the patient's medical record (e.g., Wt: 136$\frac{1}{2}$ lb).
14. Record the height. Read the marker at the movable point of the ruler and record the measurement to the nearest $\frac{1}{4}$ inch on the patient's medical record (e.g., Ht: 64$\frac{1}{4}$ in).
15. Use the patient's weight and height to record the BMI if this is office procedure.
16. Return the weights and the measuring bar to zero.
17. Sanitize your hands.
18. Record the results on the patient's medical record.

---

many settings, weight and height are measured routinely as the patient is admitted to the hospital. Many physicians now use BMI to determine the risk for certain diseases, so the patient care technician may have to use accurately measured height and weight to determine the patient's BMI. BMI is a measurement of body fat based on height and weight. A person's BMI determines whether he or she is underweight, normal weight, overweight, or obese. The BMI values are as follows:

Underweight: <18.5
Normal weight: 18.5 to 24.9
Overweight: 25 to 29.9
Obesity: BMI of 30 or greater

| Box 15.4 | Weight Conversion Formulas |

To Convert Kilograms to Pounds
1 kg = 2.2 lb
   Multiply the number of kilograms by 2.2.
   Example
   A patient weighs 68 kg: 68 × 2.2 = 149.6 lb.

To Convert Pounds to Kilograms
1 lb = 0.45 kg
   Multiply the number of pounds by 0.45, or divide the number of pounds by 2.2 kg.
   Example
   A patient weighs 120 lb: 120 × 0.45 = 54 kg, or 120 ÷ 2.2 = 54.5 kg.

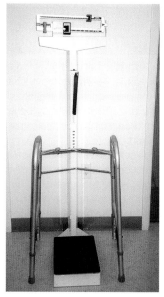

FIGURE 15.15 A walker is placed over the scale to aid the patient's balance. (From Proctor D, Adams A: *Kinn's the patient care technician*, ed 12, St. Louis, 2014, Saunders.)

BMI is a useful tool when planning a dietary and exercise plan for patients. It is one piece to the puzzle and certainly not the only indicator of health.

Certain medical specialties and specific medical problems may require continuous monitoring of weight. Hormone disorders (e.g., diabetes), growth patterns (seen in children), and eating disorders (e.g., obesity, bulimia) require accurate weight checks as part of every medical visit. In addition, maternity patients must have their weight monitored to ensure that they are gaining weight, but also as a precaution against too much weight gain, which may indicate fluid retention. Patients with cardiovascular disorders who tend to retain fluid should have their weight checked each time they are seen in the office. Some scales are calibrated in kilograms, and others in pounds. When weight must be converted from one to the other, use the formulas shown in Box 15.4.

Weight

Some patients are sensitive or secretive about their body weight, so the scale should be located in an area that provides privacy from staff and other patients. Your manner and approach are very important in keeping patients from feeling embarrassed or shy. Healthcare specialists are depending more on BMI than on traditional height and weight tables, but accurate measurements of height and weight are still required to accurately determine a patient's BMI. When patients are unstable, assist them onto the scale and help them balance themselves. A walker can be placed over the scale for the patient to use as hand support when getting on or off, or to maintain balance while on the scale (Fig. 15.15).

For infants who are unable to stand on a scale, a scale that allows them to lie down will be used (see Procedure 15.11).

Many times weights on infants and children are obtained in grams and kilograms. It is important that you know the conversion formula for kilograms to pounds.

Height

Height can be measured in inches or centimeters. Measurement is easily accomplished by moving the parallel bar attached to a wall ruler or on the scale. When an infant or child is not yet standing, the measurement of height is actually referred to as recumbent length (see Procedure 15.11).

Growth Charts

Growth charts that can be used to compare the child's individual growth pattern with national standards have been used since 1977, but in 2000 the Centers for Disease Control and Prevention (CDC) revised the charts to reflect cultural and racial diversity (samples are available at www.cdc.gov/growthcharts). The CDC charts take into account whether an infant was formula fed or breast-fed, because breast-fed infants may grow differently during the first year of life.

In addition, the CDC growth charts include information on the average BMI for infants and young adults 2 to 20 years of age, giving pediatricians another weapon in the fight against childhood obesity. BMI is a means of assessing the relationship between height and weight. BMI conversion charts typically are available, but the BMI can be calculated by dividing the child's weight in kilograms by the height in meters squared, or

$$BMI = \frac{Weight\,(kg)}{Height\,(m)^2}$$

PROCEDURE 15.11

Maintaining Growth Charts: Measuring an Infant's Length and Weight

Measuring an Infant's Length

1. Sanitize your hands, assemble the necessary equipment, and explain the procedure to the infant's caregiver.
2. Undress the infant. The diaper may be left on while the length is measured, but it must be removed before the infant is weighed.
3. Ask the caregiver to place the infant on his or her back on the examination table, which is covered with paper. If the table is a pediatric table with a headboard, ask the caregiver to hold the infant's head gently against the headboard while you straighten the infant's leg and note the location of the heel on the measurement area. If there is no headboard, ask the caregiver to gently hold the infant's head still while you draw a line on the paper at the back of the baby's head and at the heel after the leg is extended.

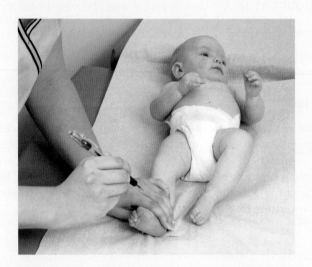

4. Measure the infant's length with the tape measure and record it.
5. Document the results in either inches or centimeters, depending on office policy, on the infant's growth chart, in the progress notes, and in the caregiver's record if requested. Complete the growth chart graph by connecting the dot from the last visit.

Weighing an Infant

1. Sanitize your hands, assemble the necessary equipment, and explain the procedure to the infant's caregiver.
2. Prepare the scale by sliding weights to the left; line the scale with disposable paper (reduces the risk of pathogen transmission).
3. Completely undress the infant, including removing the diaper. (Extra clothing or diapers will alter the weight, making it an inaccurate reading.)
4. Place the infant gently on the center of the scale, keeping your hand directly above the infant's trunk for safety.

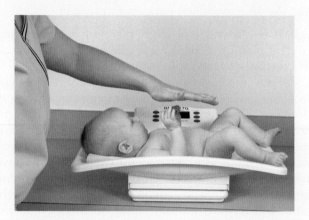

5. Slide the weights across the scale until balance is achieved. Attempt to read the infant's weight while he or she is still.
6. Return the weights to the far left of the scale and remove the baby. The caregiver can rediaper the baby while you discard the paper lining the scale. If the scale became contaminated during the procedure, follow Occupational Safety and Health Administration (OSHA) guidelines for use of gloves and disposal of contaminated waste. Disinfect the equipment according to the manufacturer's guidelines.
7. Sanitize your hands.
8. Document the results in either pounds or kilograms, depending on office policy, on the infant's growth chart, in the progress notes, and in the caregiver's record if requested. Complete the growth chart graph by connecting the dot from the last visit.

PROCEDURE 15.12

Maintain Growth Charts: Measure the Circumference of an Infant's Head

1. Sanitize your hands.
2. Identify the patient. If he or she is old enough, gain the child's cooperation through conversation.
3. Place an infant in the supine position, or the infant may be held by the parent. An older child may sit on the examination table.
4. Hold the tape measure with the zero mark against the infant's forehead, slightly above the eyebrows and the top of the ears. Ask the parent for assistance if necessary.
5. Bring the tape measure around the head, just above the ears, until it meets.

6. Read to the nearest 0.01 cm or ¼ inch.
7. Record the measurement on the growth chart and in the patient's medical record.
8. Dispose of the tape measure.
9. Sanitize your hands.

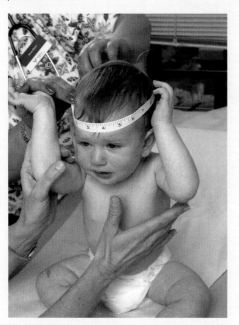

Examination of the child during routine well-child care includes measurement of the circumference of the infant's head to determine normal growth and development (Procedure 15.12). The size of the child's head reflects the growth of the brain. Brain growth is 50% complete by 1 year of age, 75% by age 3, and 90% by age 6. Routine head measurement is recommended in children until 36 months of age and in older children whose head size is not within norms. If the circumference of the head deviates greatly from normal measurements, be sure to notify the nurse at once. It is important to discover any congenital problem as early as possible so that appropriate treatment can be started.

The patient care technician should record the child's length or height, weight, and head circumference on growth charts so that the physician can compare the child's measurement statistics with national standards (Procedure 15.11). Growth charts consist of a series of percentile curves that illustrate the distribution of selected body measurements.

The current version of the CDC's growth records consists of 16 charts (8 for boys and 8 for girls) (Figs. 15.16 and 15.17). These charts represent revisions of the 14 previous charts and also the introduction of BMI-for-age charts for boys and for girls aged 2 to 20 years. As mentioned previously, the BMI is the recommended method of determining whether children or adults are overweight or obese. The BMI growth charts can be used beginning at 2 years of age, when height can be measured accurately.

Birth to 36 months: Boys
Length-for-age and Weight-for-age percentiles

NAME _____

RECORD # _____

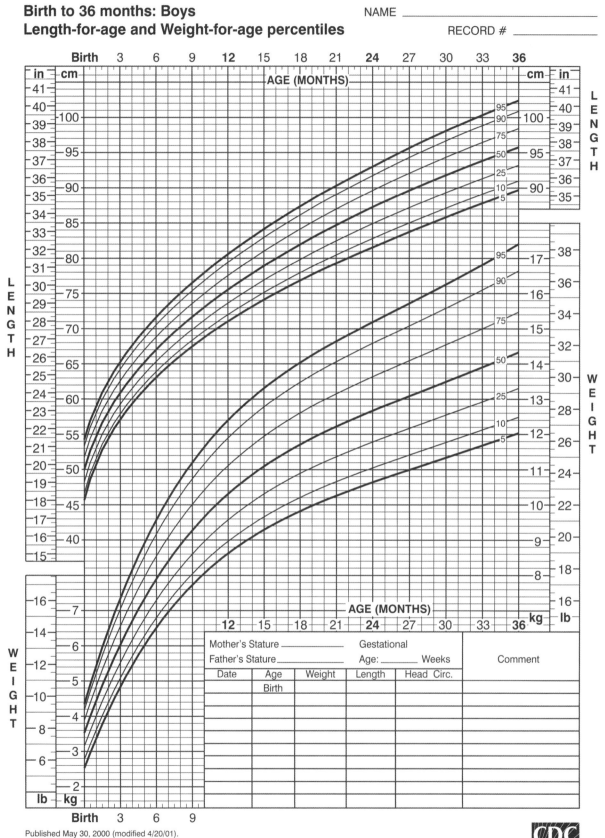

Published May 30, 2000 (modified 4/20/01).
SOURCE: Developed by the National Center for Health Statistics in collaboration with
the National Center for Chronic Disease Prevention and Health Promotion (2000).
http://www.cdc.gov/growthcharts

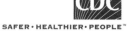

FIGURE 15.16 Growth chart: males. (From Proctor D, Adams A: *Kinn's the patient care technician*, ed 12, St. Louis, 2014, Saunders.)

2 to 20 years: Girls
Stature-for-age and Weight-for-age percentiles

NAME _____

RECORD # _____

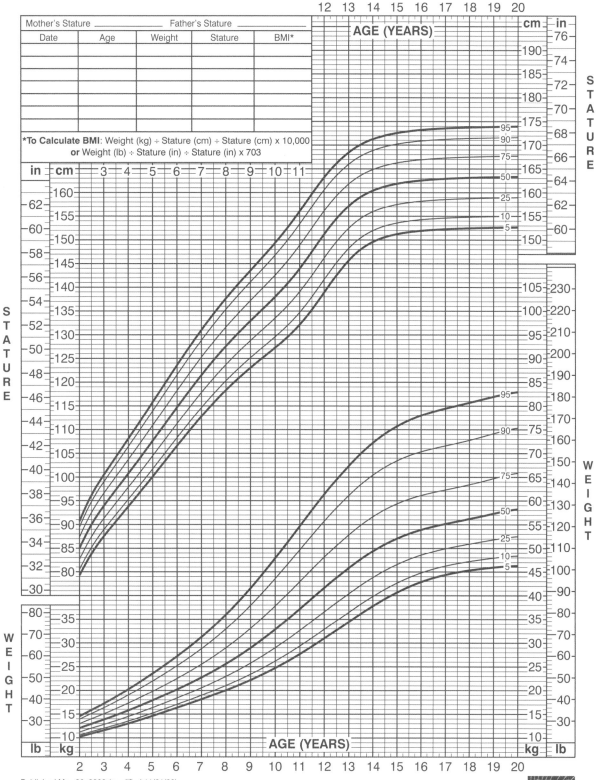

*To Calculate BMI: Weight (kg) ÷ Stature (cm) ÷ Stature (cm) x 10,000
or Weight (lb) ÷ Stature (in) ÷ Stature (in) x 703

Published May 30, 2000 (modified 11/21/00).
SOURCE: Developed by the National Center for Health Statistics in collaboration with
the National Center for Chronic Disease Prevention and Health Promotion (2000).
http://www.cdc.gov/growthcharts

SAFER • HEALTHIER • PEOPLE™

FIGURE 15.17 Growth chart: females (From Proctor D, Adams A: *Kinn's the patient care technician*, ed 12, St. Louis, 2014, Saunders.)

CHAPTER SUMMARY

Monitoring vital signs is a key responsibility of the patient care technician. It is crucial to measure and describe all facets of each vital sign correctly. The information must be accurately and clearly documented. The patient care technician should take advantage of all opportunities to answer questions and to help the patient understand the significance of healthy vital signs.

Patient privacy must be maintained throughout all procedures. The patient care technician should be sensitive to cultural and socioeconomic factors that may affect the patient's compliance with the physician's recommendations, such as diet, exercise, weight control, and the use of medication.

When obtaining vital signs, carefully select your response to a patient who asks about the results. Remember, patient care technicians are not qualified to diagnose a patient problem; that is, never evaluate or give an opinion of what the results may mean. For example, if a patient asks, "Is my blood pressure better?" you might reply, "The reading is 160/90 today." You have not said that it is worse, the same, or better, but you have informed the patient of the current blood pressure reading.

Always be accurate in transcribing results into the patient's medical record. If results are incorrectly recorded, the patient may be incorrectly diagnosed or treated. This can result in legal action that may implicate you. A careless attitude toward assessment of vital signs and documentation can lead to possible legal entanglement. Every procedure in this chapter is accompanied by a reminder to record the test results. If no entry has been made, the assumption is that the procedure was not done. Develop sensitivity toward proper conduct and performance so that you can protect yourself and your physician-employer.

Case Scenario

Dr. Susan Xu is a member of a multiphysician primary care practice. Each physician in the practice has a patient care technician who works directly with him or her. Carlos Ricci, CMA (AAMA), is Dr. Xu's assistant. Carlos graduated from a patient care technician program 3 years ago and feels he is able to see a variety of patients in Dr. Xu's practice. One of Carlos's primary responsibilities is to accurately measure and record each patient's vital signs before the patient is seen by Dr. Xu.

- What factors might alter a patient's vital signs?
- What methods can Carlos use to gather and record a patient's temperature, pulse, respirations, blood pressure, height, weight, and BMI to ensure that the readings are accurate?
- If Carlos obtains a reading that does not seem right, what should Carlos do?

REVIEW QUESTIONS

1. Using the correct formula, convert the following temperatures from one system to the other.

   99°F = _____ °C   102°F = _____ °C
   38°C = _____ °F   39.5°C = _____ °F

2. A 44-year-old patient is undergoing antibiotic therapy for pneumonia. His rectal temperature reading is 101.6°F. What is the expected oral temperature reading?
   a. 101.6°F (38.7°C)
   b. 100.6°F (38.1°C)
   c. 99.6°F (37.5°C)
   d. 97.6°F (36.4°C)

3. An adult patient is admitted to the emergency department with an exacerbation of asthma. Her respirations are 40 breaths per minute. After treatment, her rate returns to normal limits. What respiratory range is considered to be normal?
   a. 30 to 60
   b. 12 to 20
   c. 16 to 22
   d. 24 to 30

4. During a routine physical examination, a 48-year-old woman's blood pressure is noted at 180/90 mm Hg. She fears that she is hypertensive. A sustained elevation over what blood pressure reading must occur at two separate visits in order for a hypertensive diagnosis?
   a. 160/100 mm Hg
   b. 140/90 mm Hg
   c. 130/70 mm Hg
   d. 120/80 mm Hg

5. Which method of measuring temperature reveals core temperature?
   a. Skin
   b. Temporal
   c. Oral
   d. Axillary

6. The PCT begins to measure the blood pressure of an adult. The patient says that his doctor has instructed him to always use a large cuff. What is a reason for using a large cuff?
   a. A blood pressure cuff that is too small gives inaccurately high readings.
   b. A blood pressure cuff that is too small likely injures the brachial artery.
   c. Large cuffs are typically more accurate on adults than normal-size cuffs.
   d. Normal-size cuffs should be used for pediatric patients.

Obtaining and Monitoring an Electrocardiogram

1. Illustrate the electrical conduction system through the heart.
2. Explain the concepts of cardiac polarization, depolarization, and repolarization.
3. Identify the PQRST complex on an electrocardiographic tracing.
4. Summarize the properties of the electrocardiograph.
5. Describe the electrical views of the heart recorded by the 12-lead electrocardiograph.
6. Discuss the process of recording an electrocardiogram.
7. Perform an accurate recording of the electrical activity of the heart.
8. Compare and contrast electrocardiographic artifacts and the probable cause of each.
9. Identify a typical electrocardiograph tracing.
10. Describe common electrocardiographic arrhythmias.
11. Discuss the legal and ethical issues involved when performing ECGs.

atria The two upper chambers of the heart

atrioventricular (AV) node The part of the cardiac conduction system between the atria and the ventricles

bundle of His Specialized muscle fibers that conduct electrical impulses from the AV node to the ventricular myocardium

diastole The relaxation of the chambers of the heart during which blood enters the heart from the vascular system and the lungs

ectopic Originating outside the normal tissue

ischemia Decreased blood flow to a body part or organ, caused by constriction or blockage of the supplying artery

myocardial Pertaining to the heart muscle

sinoatrial (SA) node The pacemaker of the heart; it is located in the right atrium

systole The contraction of the heart; blood is pumped from the heart to the lungs and the rest of the body

ventricles The two lower chambers of the heart

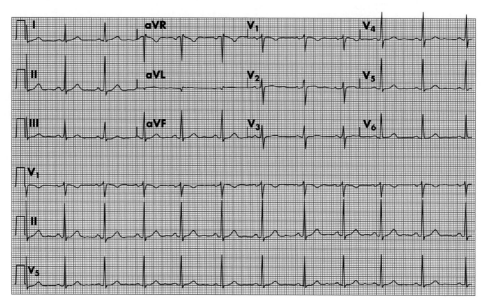

FIGURE 16.1 Example of a 12-lead ECG. (From Aehlert B: *ECGs made easy,* ed 3, St. Louis, 2006, Mosby.)

Electrocardiography is a painless, safe procedure and is the test often used for the diagnosis of heart disease. In electrocardiography, electrodes are attached to the patient's skin and connected to wires that go to the electrocardiograph. Electrocardiography amplifies the electrical impulses from the beating heart, and a pattern of these impulses is recorded and printed on electrocardiographic paper, or stored in the patient's electronic medical record. This record is called the *electrocardiogram* (ECG). The ECG is read and evaluated by the physician and becomes a part of the patient's medical record (Fig. 16.1). Some physician offices who use electronic medical records can record an ECG tracing directly into the patient's electronic record from their office.

It is very important that the ECG be performed as accurate as possible in order to capture exactly what is going on in the heart. Physicians often use the results of the ECG to make decisions for the patient's care. A patient care technician must have an understanding of both the normal cardiac function and the relationship of the ECG recordings to cardiac function. The patient care technician is responsible for ensuring that the patient is prepared mentally and physically for the test and that the equipment is set up properly. When performing electrocardiography, the patient care technician must be able to recognize problems with the recording and make appropriate corrections so that the physician has a clear record of the patient's cardiac activity. The goal is to obtain the most accurate ECG possible.

THE ELECTRICAL CONDUCTION SYSTEM OF THE HEART

The Cardiac Cycle

The cardiac cycle includes all the events that occur in the heart during one single heartbeat. Each chamber of the heart goes through two phases during the cardiac cycle: systole and diastole. During systole, both the atria and the ventricles contract and empty of blood. During diastole, the relaxation phase of the heart, the chambers refill with blood. Venous blood from the inferior and superior venae cavae empties into the right atrium during atrial diastole. As the right atrium fills, increased pressure in the chamber causes the tricuspid valve to open, and the right ventricle begins to fill. At the same time, blood returning from the lungs via the pulmonary veins fills the left atrium, causing the mitral valve to open, emptying blood into the left ventricle. Before systole occurs, the ventricles are already 70% filled. The cardiac cycle for a healthy adult lasts approximately 0.8 second. However, the amount of time it takes for the heart to empty and refill depends on many factors, including the condition of the myocardium, or muscle layer of the heart, and the heart's electrical system.

The electrocardiograph records both the intensity (strength) of the electrical impulses, and the actual time

---

History of Electrocardiography

Dutch physiologist Willem Einthoven developed techniques to record the electrical activity of the heart in the late 1800s. He called this recording an Electro Kardio Gramm, and hence the acronym EKG. Many physicians and other healthcare providers still call the recording an EKG, although the newer, preferred term for an electrocardiogram is *ECG*.

it takes for each part of the cardiac cycle to occur. It measures the electrical conductive impulses of the heart muscle, allowing the physician to see any abnormalities in normal heart activity. In addition to being recorded as an ECG, the cardiac cycle can appear as a continuously moving pattern on a monitor screen, accompanied by a sound for each beat. This pattern will display on a screen or print on the paper as you obtain the ECG.

The specialized electrical conduction system of the heart (Fig. 16.2) initiates each heartbeat. The main part of this system is the sinoatrial (SA) node, which is located in the upper back wall of the right atrium at the junction of the superior vena cava and the right atrium. The SA node controls the rate of heart contractions by initiating electrical impulses 60 to 100 times per minute. Each cardiac cycle, or heartbeat, starts with the SA node generating an electrical impulse that travels in a wave-like pattern across the cardiac muscle of the atria, causing them to contract almost simultaneously. This electrical impulse then stimulates the atrioventricular (AV) node, which is located in the posterior, superior portion of the right atrial septal wall, directly behind the tricuspid valve. A slight delay in conduction at this point allows the atria to empty completely. The electrical impulse then is transmitted to a special group of conduction fibers, the bundle of His, in the upper part of the interventricular septal wall. The bundle of His divides into two branches; the right bundle branch carries electrical impulses to the right ventricle, and the left bundle branch carries impulses to the left ventricle. The right and left bundle branches divide into smaller and smaller branches, ending in the Purkinje fibers, which spread across the apex of the heart and through the myocardium, stimulating ventricular contraction. The ventricles contract, forcing the blood out of the chambers and into the pulmonary artery emerging right ventricle and the aorta that emerges from the left ventricle.

Normal sinus rhythm (NSR) refers to a regular heart rate that falls within the average range of 60 to 80 beats per minute (beats/min). Sinus bradycardia is a heart rate below 60 beats/min; sinus tachycardia is a rate above 100 beats/min. In both of these conditions, the rhythm remains even, but the rate is pathologic, meaning that it could be caused by disease. An irregular cardiac rhythm is called an *arrhythmia*. Conditions that interrupt the conduction pathway, which can include the SA node to AV node, the bundle of His, or right and left bundle branches, all can cause arrhythmias.

Polarization, Depolarization, and Repolarization

Polarization is the resting state of the myocardial wall; no electrical activity occurs in the heart during this phase, which is recorded on the ECG strip as a flat line.

In this state the myocardial cells are ready for stimulation. When the electrical system of the heart stimulates a myocardial cell, depolarization occurs, resulting in the contraction of the stimulated heart muscle. After depolarization the heart muscle cells must return to a resting state before they can be electrically stimulated again. The process of reaching this resting state is called *repolarization.*

The electrocardiograph records a series of waves, or deflections, above or below a baseline on the ECG paper. Each deflection corresponds to a particular part of the cardiac cycle (Table 16.1). The normal ECG cycle consists of waveforms that are labeled the P wave, the Q wave, the R wave, the S wave, and the T wave. The Q, R, and S waves usually are grouped together; this is called the *QRS complex.* One entire cardiac cycle can be called the *PQRST complex.* In the next section, each part of the ECG is discussed in more detail.

PQRST Complex

The *P wave* occurs during the contraction of the atria and shows the beginning of cardiac depolarization. The P wave is the first deflection from the baseline; it typically is smooth and rounded and should occur before each QRS complex. Atrial repolarization is not recorded on the ECG strip, because its electrical impulse is small and is hidden in the QRS complex. The *PR segment* is the return to baseline after atrial contraction. The *PR interval* is the time from the beginning of atrial contraction to the beginning of ventricular contraction. It contains the P wave (depolarization of the atria) and the spread of the electrical impulse through the AV node, bundle of His, right and left bundle branches, and Purkinje fibers. As the heart rate increases, the PR interval typically shortens. The *QRS complex* shows the contraction of both ventricles and also reflects the completion of cardiac depolarization. Repolarization of the atria also occurs during this time, but it cannot be seen on the ECG because the recording of the much stronger QRS activity overshadows it. Depolarization of the ventricles results in the contraction of a much larger muscle mass than does depolarization of the atria. Therefore the QRS complex is recorded as a much more significant electrical activity than the P wave.

The *ST segment* reflects the time between the end of ventricular contraction and the beginning of ventricular recovery. The *T wave* represents ventricular recovery or repolarization of the ventricles. After the T wave comes a period of complete heart rest, also called *polarization*, which is indicated on the ECG as a straight line. The *QT interval* is the time between the beginning of the QRS complex through the T wave. During this time the ventricles contract and relax. A *U wave* occasionally can be seen as a small waveform just after the T wave in patients with a low serum potassium level or other

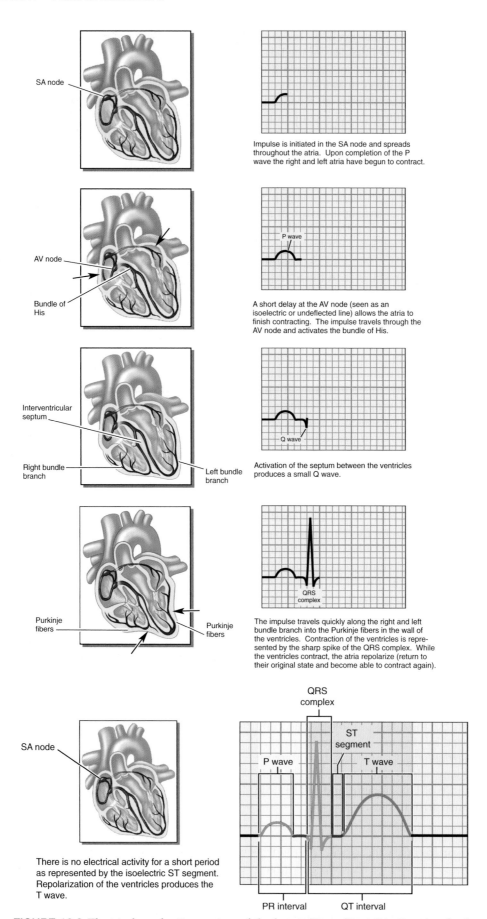

Impulse is initiated in the SA node and spreads throughout the atria. Upon completion of the P wave the right and left atria have begun to contract.

A short delay at the AV node (seen as an isoelectric or undeflected line) allows the atria to finish contracting. The impulse travels through the AV node and activates the bundle of His.

Activation of the septum between the ventricles produces a small Q wave.

The impulse travels quickly along the right and left bundle branch into the Purkinje fibers in the wall of the ventricles. Contraction of the ventricles is represented by the sharp spike of the QRS complex. While the ventricles contract, the atria repolarize (return to their original state and become able to contract again).

There is no electrical activity for a short period as represented by the isoelectric ST segment. Repolarization of the ventricles produces the T wave.

FIGURE 16.2 Electrical conduction system of the heart. (From Hunt SA: *Saunders fundamentals of medical assisting*, Philadelphia, 2002, WB Saunders.)

Table 16.1   The Cardiac Cycle

Stage	Heart Activity	Electrical Current
P wave*	Atrial contraction	Atrial depolarization
PR interval†	Contraction traversing the atrioventricular (AV) node	Depolarization traversing the AV node
QRS complex‡	Ventricular contraction	Ventricular depolarization
ST segment	Time interval between ventricular contraction and the beginning of ventricular recovery	Time interval between ventricular depolarization and ventricular repolarization
T wave	Ventricular contraction subsides	Ventricular repolarization (electric recovery)
U wave (not always present)	Associated with further ventricular relaxation	Associated with further ventricular repolarization
Baseline§	The heart at rest	Polarization
PR interval	Time interval between atrial contraction and ventricular contraction	Time interval between atrial depolarization and ventricular depolarization
QT interval	Time interval between the beginning of ventricular contraction and the subsiding of ventricular contraction	Time interval between the beginning of ventricular depolarization and ventricular repolarization (electric recovery)

*Wave: A uniformly advancing deflection (upward or downward) from a baseline on a recording.
†Interval: The lapse of time between two different electrocardiographic events; represents the time needed for an electrical current to move on.
‡Complex: The portion of the ECG tracing that represents the sum of three waves (contraction of the ventricles).
§Baseline: A neutral line against which waves are valued as they deflect upward (positive) or downward (negative) from the line.

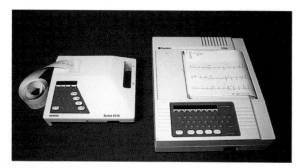

FIGURE 16.3 Many types of ECG machines are available, including single channel and multichannel models. (From Chester GA: *Modern medical assisting,* Philadelphia, 1999, WB Saunders.)

metabolic disorders. By measuring the actual configuration and location of each wave in relation to the other waves and to the baseline, in addition to the intervals between waves and segments, the physician is able to detect rhythmic disturbances of the heart and identify different types of cardiac disorders.

THE ELECTROCARDIOGRAPH

Electrocardiograph machines (Fig. 16.3) record 12 leads simultaneously and are also referred to as 6-channel ECG machines. Limb and chest electrodes must be placed on the patient at specific locations on the body before the recording starts. When the ECG is started, the machine records all 12 leads automatically and marks each lead with identifying letters. These multichannel ECG tracings take seconds to perform and can be placed in the patient's medical record without mounting or can be recorded directly into the patient's electronic medical record.

Electrocardiograph Paper

Electrocardiograph paper is heat and pressure sensitive, which means that either heat or pressure can cause a mark to appear. The stylus on an ECG machine makes the image on the ECG paper. When the machine is on, the stylus becomes hot and burns a marking on the paper as it moves side to side past the stylus. Because the paper is pressure sensitive, it must be handled carefully to prevent any additional markings that would blemish the tracing. Excessive fingerprints or smudges would interfere with the markings on the paper.

ECG paper is graph paper that has horizontal and vertical lines at 1-mm intervals. This is an agreed-on international standard that allows physicians anywhere in the world to interpret a patient's ECG in the same manner. A patient care technician needs to know both the size and the meaning of each square on the ECG paper to understand its significance.

The horizontal axis represents time, and the vertical axis represents amplitude. Each small square measures 1 mm on each side. Every fifth line, both vertically and horizontally, is darker than the other lines and creates a larger square measuring 5 mm on each side. When the electrocardiograph runs at normal speed, one small 1-mm square passes the stylus every 0.04 second, which means that one large 5-mm square passes the stylus every 0.2 second. Continuing this logic, in 1 second, five large squares pass the stylus. Therefore five sequential large squares show the record of what occurred in the heart during a time span of 1 second (5 large squares × 0.2 seconds = 1 second). Another way to say this is that at normal speed, the ECG paper travels past the stylus at a rate of 25 mm per second (Fig. 16.4).

The voltage, or strength, of the heartbeat also is recorded on the paper. Voltage can be displayed as

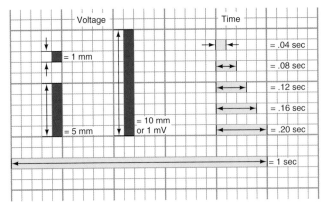

FIGURE 16.4 ECG paper. (From Chester GA: *Modern medical assisting,* Philadelphia, 1999, WB Saunders.)

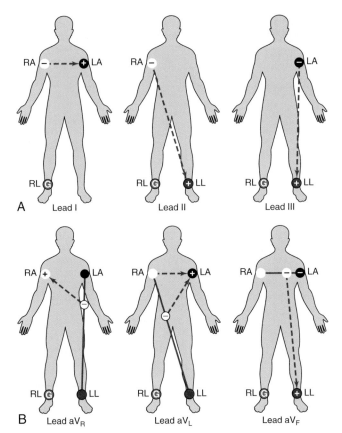

FIGURE 16.5 Standard (A) and augmented (B) limb leads. (From Chester GA: *Modern medical assisting,* Philadelphia, 1999, WB Saunders.)

either a positive or a negative deflection. One millivolt (mV) of electrical activity moves the stylus upward over 10 mm (two large squares). This is the standard normally used for obtaining an ECG, and it can be adjusted to match the strength of the electrical activity of the heart. The machine must be calibrated so that 1 mV of electrical activity produces a deflection that is 10 mm either above or below the baseline. When properly calibrated, the ECG records both the strength of the electrical activity of the heartbeat in millivolts and the speed of the heartbeat over time.

Electrodes and Leads

Ten sensors, called *electrodes,* are placed on the patient's arms (two), legs (two), and chest (six) to pick up the electrical activity of the heart. Electrodes must be applied to specific locations to record the heart's electrical activity from different angles and planes. Ten color-coded and labeled lead wires that end in a small metal clip are attached to the electrodes. The lead wires carry the signal of the heart's electrical activity to the ECG machine. Most machines require single-use, self-stick, disposable electrodes that are packaged with conductive jelly in the center.

The *leads* to the electrocardiograph carry the cardiac electrical impulses into the machine, where they are magnified by an amplifier. These amplified impulses are converted into mechanical action, which is recorded on the ECG paper by the stylus and/or shown on a monitor. A single lead records the electrical activity of the heart between two different electrodes, one positive and one negative. The placement of the positive electrode determines the particular view of the heart recorded. If depolarization occurs toward the positive electrode, the deflection is upright; if it moves toward the negative electrode, the waveform is deflected downward. Each lead records the average electrical flow at a specific time in a specific location of the heart. The ECG records views of the heart on both a frontal and a transverse plane. The frontal leads include leads I, II, III, aV_R, aV_L, and aV_F.

Horizontal plane leads include the six precordial, or chest, leads (V_1 to V_6).

Lead Recordings

The standard ECG consists of 12 separate leads, or recordings of the electrical activity of the heart, from different angles.

Standard Leads

The first three leads recorded are called the *standard* or *bipolar leads,* because each of them uses two limb electrodes to record the heart's electrical activity (Fig. 16.5A). The right arm electrode is the negative pole, and the left leg or left arm electrodes are the positive poles. Roman numerals I, II, and III are used to designate these leads.

- Lead I records tracings between the right arm and left arm, recording the electrical activity of the lateral part of the left ventricle.
- Lead II records tracings between the right arm and left leg, recording the electrical activity of the inferior surface of the left ventricle; this is the lead recorded on a cardiac monitor or on the rhythm strip at the bottom of the 12-lead ECG.

- Lead III records tracings between the left arm and left leg, which reflects the electrical activity of the inferior surface of the left ventricle.

Augmented Leads

The next three leads are the augmented, or combined, leads (Fig. 16.5B). These are designated augmented voltage right arm (aV_R), augmented voltage left arm (aV_L), and augmented voltage left leg (aV_F). Because the electrical activity recorded by these leads is relatively small, the ECG machine amplifies (or augments) the electrical potential when recorded. These are all unipolar leads with a single positive electrode that uses the right leg for grounding.

- aV_R records the electrical activity of the atria from the right shoulder; P waves and QRS complexes are deflected below the baseline.
- aV_L records the electrical activity of the lateral wall of the left ventricle from the left shoulder.
- aV_F records the electrical activity of the inferior surface of the left ventricle from the left leg.

Precordial Leads

The precordial, or chest, leads are unipolar and provide a transverse plane view of the heart. They are designated V_1, V_2, V_3, V_4, V_5, and V_6. The V means chest, and each of the numbers represents a specific location on the chest. The QRS complex shows as a negative deflection in V_1 and V_2, and views with each subsequent lead become more positive. Precordial leads measure the electrical activity among six specific points on the chest wall and a point within the heart (Fig. 16.6). It is important to avoid placing electrodes directly over a bony prominence.

- V_1—The electrode is placed in the fourth intercostal space, just to the right of the sternum.
- V_2—The electrode is placed in the fourth intercostal space, just to the left of the sternum.
- V_3—The electrode is placed midway between V_2 and V_4.
- V_4—The electrode is placed in the fifth intercostal space, at the left midclavicular line.
- V_5—The electrode is placed horizontal to V_4 in the left anterior axillary line.
- V_6—The electrode is placed horizontal to V_4 in the left mid-axillary line.

PERFORMING ELECTROCARDIOGRAPHY

Preparation of the Room and Patient

The room should be as quiet as possible when preparing for an ECG. Try to remain as far as possible from all

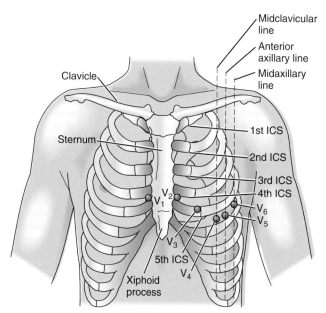

FIGURE 16.6 Chest leads. *ICS,* Intercostal space. (From Chester GA: *Modern medical assisting,* Philadelphia, 1999, WB Saunders.)

Injury & Illness Prevention Box 16.1

- When positioning the patient for an ECG, be sure to have the side rail of the bed up opposite of the side you are standing on.
- Always remember to lower the bed if you have raised it once you have completed the ECG to prevent falls.
- If the patient will be getting up after the ECG, be sure that you have removed the equipment and cords from the leads so that the patient does not trip and fall on them.

other electrical equipment, including x-ray machines, fans, refrigerators, and air conditioners. The room should be warm and should have adjustable lighting.

Position the patient so that you can work from the side of the patient that is most comfortable for you. You may need to raise the bed to a level that is comfortable to you. Electrocardiographers, or those who specialize in obtaining ECGs, most often work on the patient's left side, but as long as the electrodes are placed in the proper position, it really makes no difference which side you use.

Small pillows are helpful for helping the patient relax and providing maximum comfort during the procedure. Offer a pillow for the head and one for under the knees. If a head pillow is used, it should not elevate the patient's shoulders.

The patient with a patient gown on should have the opening in the front so that you can easily access the patient's chest and extremities. The patient who is coming into the office should disrobe to the waist and put on a patient gown with the opening in the front; easy access to the patient's extremities must be available. Pantyhose must be removed.

Place the patient in a supine position with the arms comfortably at the sides and the legs not touching one another. If the patient has difficulty breathing, a semi-Fowler's position should be used, or alternatively the patient can be seated on a wooden chair. However, ensure that you check with the physician before obtaining an ECG in an alternative position. If a seated position is used, the patient's feet must rest comfortably on the floor or on a footstool. Note any alternative position on the ECG recording. Positioning can make a difference in the reading of the ECG.

The patient should empty the bladder and then rest for at least 10 minutes before the ECG recording is made. Check to see whether the patient followed all the instructions provided in Fig. 16.7. Record the patient's vital signs and current medications on the patient's chart. This information can be programmed into some ECG machines and automatically printed on the ECG recording.

Explain to the patient the nature and purpose of the ECG. Attempt to answer all questions and make the patient as comfortable as possible during the procedure. Stress the importance of not moving during the entire procedure, and assure the patient that there is no danger of shock. Soften the lighting in the room to obtain maximum patient comfort. When you tell the patient to lie still, observe that he or she is breathing normally. Patients often hold their breath when asked to lie still.

Attaching Leads to the Patient

Disposable, single-use electrodes are placed on the patient's limbs and chest in very specific locations (Fig. 16.8). The lead wires from the machine then are connected to the electrodes. Making the proper connections is facilitated by specific lead markings or color coding on the end of each lead wire (Fig. 16.9).

- RA lead is attached to the electrode on the patient's right arm.
- LA lead is attached to the electrode on the patient's left arm.

INSTRUCTIONS FOR PATIENT BEFORE AN ELECTROCARDIOGRAM

Name: _____

Your cardiogram appointment is _____ , _____ at _____ AM
                                         Day   Date   Time   PM

These instructions are simple, but it is important that you follow them. Please call us if you are unable to follow these instructions or keep your appointment so we may make another appointment.

1. There is no discomfort or sensation in having an electrocardiogram. No electricity is put into the patient in any way. Small disposable electrodes are placed on the calf of each leg and on each arm and at different places on the chest. The minute impulse generated by your heart is simply picked up by these electrodes and recorded by the machine.

2. You will be asked to lie down on a comfortable table while the test is being performed by the technician.

3. For your convenience, it is best to wear loose clothing. You will be asked to disrobe to your waist to expose the chest. It will also be necessary to expose your lower legs from the knees down and the upper arms just below the shoulders.

4. The actual test only takes about 5 minutes, but you will be asked to rest for about one-half hour before the test. It is best you do not have a heavy meal for about 2 hours before the test. You should not consume any cold drinks or ice cream or smoke just before the test. It is also advisable to refrain from excessive exercise just before the test. Do not take any medications without the physician's usual instructions and knowledge.

5. During the test, you will be asked to lie absolutely still and relax, because the slightest movement interferes with an accurate tracing. Do not talk.

6. The skin on the legs, arms, and chest must be free from skin ointments, oils, and medications.

7. The technician taking the test is specially trained to perform the test but is unable to tell you the results of the test, because he or she is neither trained nor authorized to make any interpretations of the cardiogram. This is the task of the physician.

FIGURE 16.7 ECG patient instructions. (From Proctor DB, Adams AP: *Kinn's The medical assistant: An applied learning approach*, ed 12, St. Louis, 2012, Saunders.)

- RL lead is attached to the electrode on the patient's right leg.
- LL lead is attached to the electrode on the patient's left leg.
- The labeled lead wires then are placed on each precordial electrode.

Recording the Electrocardiogram

Procedure 16.1 explains how to record an ECG. It is important that you become familiar with the type of machine used in your institution. Machines vary according to the age and make of the model, but most electrocardiographs currently in use perform calibration functions and labeling automatically. You may have the option of entering specific information about the patient, such as age, gender, and prescriptions. Follow hospital or office protocol when performing the procedure. After the machine has been programmed, remind the patient to lie still and start the ECG procedure by pressing the appropriate key to run the ECG strip. Six-channel machines print and label all 12 leads, with a rhythm strip across the bottom of the paper in lead II, in a matter of seconds. Review the printout for clarity, and if it is acceptable, give the recording to the physician for review or save it in the patient's electronic medical record. Once approved, remove the leads and electrodes from the patient, assist him or her into a sitting position, and provide assistance in getting off the table and dressing if necessary.

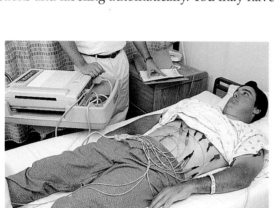

FIGURE 16.8 Chest lead locations. (From Cooper & Gosnell, *Foundations of nursing*, ed 7, 2015.)

The ECG Tracing and the Medical Record

ECG tracings usually are retained in medical records for many years to provide a history of patient cardiac activity. Paper clips and staples are never used, because they scratch and mark a tracing. Clear tape should not be used, because it can become sticky or yellow with age. Hospitals that still use the paper charting method will typically have lab sheets for attaching ECG strips using a peel-off strip that exposes double-sided tape. A single photocopy of the ECG can be made without damaging the original. If the facility has electronic medical records, the tracing is scanned into the patient's electronic chart or recorded directly into the patient's medical record.

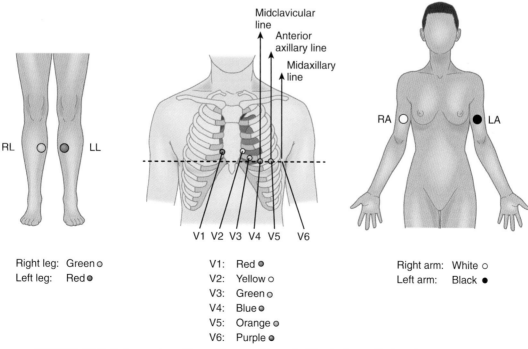

FIGURE 16.9 Color codes. (From Proctor D et al: *Kinn's the medical assistant: an applied learning approach*, ed 13, St. Louis, 2017, Saunders.)

1. Sanitize your hands.
2. Explain the procedure to the patient.
3. Ask the patient to disrobe to the waist (including the bra for women) and remove belts, jewelry, socks, stockings, or pantyhose as necessary. If the patient is already wearing a gown, ask the patient to position it so that it opens in the front.
4. Position the patient supine on the examination table and drape appropriately.
5. Turn on the machine to allow the stylus to warm up; this may not be necessary with newer machines.
6. Label the beginning of the tracing paper with the patient's name, the date, the time, and the patient's current cardiovascular medications, or input this information into the machine.
7. At each location where an electrode will be placed, clean the skin with an alcohol wipe.

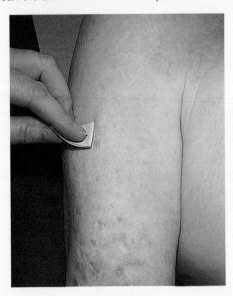

8. Apply the self-adhesive electrodes to clean, dry, fleshy areas of the extremities. Extremely hairy areas may need to be shaved to achieve adequate electrode attachment, or place a piece of tape over the electrode to ensure that it is secure.

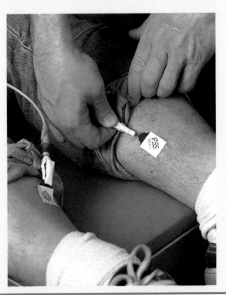

9. Apply the self-adhesive electrodes to the clean areas on the chest.

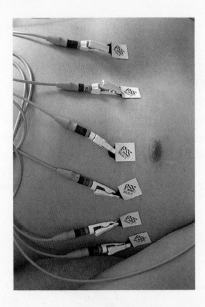

10. Carefully connect the lead wires to the correct electrode with the alligator clips on the end of each lead. Ensure that the lead wires are not crossed.
11. Press the AUTO button on the machine and run the ECG tracing. The machine automatically places the standardization at the beginning, and the 12 leads then follow in the three-channel matrix with a lead II rhythm strip across the bottom of the page.
12. Watch for artifacts during the recording. If artifacts are present, make appropriate corrections and repeat the recording to get a clean reading.
13. Remove the lead wires from the electrodes and then remove the electrodes from the patient.
14. Assist the patient with getting dressed as needed. Clean and return the ECG machine to its storage area.
15. Place the ECG recording in the patient's medical record for physician review.
16. Sanitize your hands.
17. Document the procedure in the patient's medical record.

Regardless of the particular method used, each ECG should be labeled with the following information:

- Patient's full name
- Gender
- Age
- Date and time of ECG
- List of all medications and/or supplements the patient takes
- Variations from normal sensitivity and normal speed

Additional notes should be recorded for any variation from the routine, such as the following:

- Very nervous or anxious patient
- Lack of rest before the test
- Smoking immediately before the test
- Failure to follow any pretest instructions

Telephone Transmission

An electrocardiograph with phone transmission capabilities can transmit a recording over a telephone to an ECG data interpretation center. The machine is equipped with a direct ECG fax transmitter. The recording is interpreted by a computer at the data center and verified by a cardiologist. Patient information that may be important to the interpretation, such as medications and vital signs, is sent with the ECG data. A printout with the computer-assisted interpretations is returned to the sender by fax or e-mail.

Interpretive Electrocardiographs

Interpretive electrocardiographs are equipped with a computer that analyzes the recording as it is being run. With this capability, immediate information on the heart's activity is available, which can be valuable for reaching an early diagnosis and initiating immediate treatment. Patient baseline data must be entered into the computer before the ECG is recorded. The computer analysis of the ECG and the reason for each interpretation are then printed on the top of the recording.

Artifacts

An artifact is an unwanted, erratic movement of the stylus on the paper caused by outside interference. The electrocardiograph is extremely sensitive to any kind of nearby electrical activity. Electrical artifacts on the tracing make accurate interpretation of the ECG difficult. The patient care technician should have a thorough understanding of the causes of and remedies for these artifacts. The main types of artifacts are wandering baseline, somatic tremor, alternating current (AC) interference, and interrupted baseline.

Wandering Baseline

With a wandering baseline, the stylus gradually shifts away from the center of the paper. This usually happens because of slight movement of the patient during the tracing or poor electrode attachment (Fig. 16.10). A wandering baseline is resolved by reminding the patient to remain as still as possible; this can be facilitated by keeping the patient comfortable. Ensure that electrodes are completely attached to each specific site to eliminate this artifact.

Somatic Tremor

The term *somatic tremor* means muscle movement. Any muscle movement, including movement of skeletal muscle, produces a measurable electrical impulse. This additional input causes unwanted stylus movement during the tracing; this shows up on the recording as jagged peaks of irregular height and spacing with a shifting baseline (Fig. 16.11). The most common causes include patient discomfort, apprehension, movement, or talking or a condition that causes uncontrollable body tremors. A patient with uncontrolled tremors must be as calm and comfortable as possible to minimize the somatic tremor artifact. The other causes all can be resolved after they have been identified correctly.

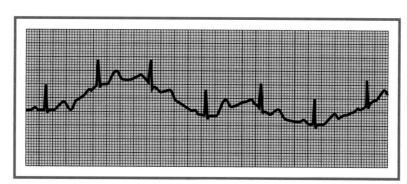

FIGURE 16.10 Wandering baseline. (From Proctor DB, Adams AP: *Kinn's The medical assistant: An applied learning approach,* ed 12, St. Louis, 2012, Saunders.)

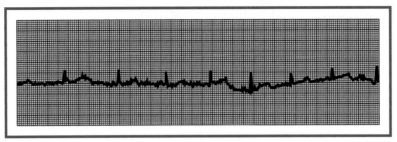

FIGURE 16.11 Somatic tremor. (From Proctor DB, Adams AP: *Kinn's The medical assistant: An applied learning approach*, ed 12, St. Louis, 2012, Saunders.)

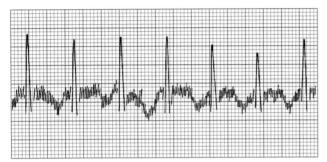

FIGURE 16.12 Sixty-cycle interference. (From Sanders M: *Mosby's paramedic textbook*, ed 4, Burlington, 2012, Jones & Bartlett Learning.)

Alternating Current Interference

AC interference appears as a series of uniform small spikes on the paper (Fig. 16.12). Electrical currents in nearby equipment or wiring can leak small amounts of electrical energy into the area where the ECG machine is located. The very sensitive electrocardiograph can easily pick up this additional electrical energy signal. This can be decreased by ensuring that the machine is plugged into a three-pronged, grounded outlet; keeping lead wires uncrossed; unplugging other electrical appliances in the room; moving the table away from the wall; and perhaps even turning off overhead fluorescent lights. If all these measures don't work, you may need to move to another examination room for the procedure, although this is not possible when the patient is admitted in the hospital. The last step is to call the manufacturer or your local service representative.

Interrupted Baseline

Baseline interruption occurs when the electrical connection has been interrupted. The stylus moves onto the margin of the paper erratically (Fig. 16.13). It moves violently up and down across the paper, or it may record a straight line across the top or bottom of the paper. Noticeable patient movement that dislodges the electrodes causes most baseline interruptions. This cause is virtually eliminated by using disposable, stick-on electrodes. Other causes include a broken cable wire and cable tips that are attached too loosely to the electrodes.

INTERPRETING AN ECG STRIP

Normal Appearance of ECG Complexes

When you examine the ECG recording, first look at the characteristics of each of the waves in the recording (Table 16.2). Are the P waves, QRS complexes, and T waves clearly present? Do they have a consistent appearance and do they occur at regular intervals? Are any odd beats present that do not fit in with the others? Is the rate normal, fast, or slow? Is the rhythm regular or irregular?

In NSR (see Fig. 16.1), each beat of the heart is initiated by an impulse from the SA node that travels without interruption along the normal conduction pathway of the heart. In NSR, each beat on the ECG shows a P wave followed by a QRS complex.

Rate

To calculate the heart rate from the ECG recording, count the number of P waves in a 6-second strip (30 large squares) and multiply by 10. In the same manner, you can count the number of P waves in a 3-second strip (15 large squares) and multiply by 20. To get the ventricular contraction rate, you can count the number of complete QRS complexes that occur within 6 seconds and multiply that number by 10 to get the number of ventricular contractions in 1 minute.

The heart rate also can be calculated by counting the number of small squares between two R waves and then dividing that number into 1500 (1 minute on an ECG strip passes 1500 small boxes). When the number of boxes from one cardiac event to the next same event is divided into 1500, the result is the patient's heart rate. You can use the ECG strips in Figs. 16.1 and 16.10 to practice these techniques.

Rhythm

The rhythm of a patient's heartbeat is either regular or irregular. You may pick up an irregular heartbeat when taking the patient's pulse. This same patient will show an

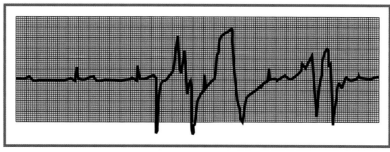

FIGURE 16.13 Interrupted baseline. (From Proctor DB, Adams AP: *Kinn's The medical assistant: An applied learning approach,* ed 12, St. Louis, 2012, Saunders.)

Table 16.2   Normal Appearance of ECG Waveforms and Complexes

Wave or Complex	Duration (Sec or Amplitude)	Characteristics to Examine
P wave	0.06-0.11	Are P waves present? Are they normal shape (not notched or peaked) and normal size (<3 mm)? Do all deflect upward (positive)? Is there one for each QRS? Are they evenly spaced from the QRS?
PR interval	0.12-0.20	Is it constant?
QRS complex	0.08-0.12	Are they evenly spaced from T waves? Do all point in the same direction? Do all QRS complexes appear the same? Is each preceded by a P wave? Does the Q wave have a pronounced negative deflection?
ST segment	On baseline (isoelectric line)	Is it on baseline? Is it constant? Is it elevated above the baseline?
T wave	≤5 mm in leads I, II, III ≤10 mm in V_1-V_6	Is T wave present? Are all the same? Do all show upward deflection (positive)?
QT interval	Should not be more than half the RR interval* if patient has a regular rhythm	Is it constant?
U wave	Rounded, upright deflection	Is it present?

*RR interval: from onset of one QRS complex to onset of next QRS complex.

irregularity (i.e., a difference in the length of time between cardiac cycles) when an ECG is recorded. If the patient's heart is beating in a regular rhythm, each cardiac cycle occurs within the same time frame, and individual cardiac cycles occur exactly the same length of time apart. To check for ventricular rhythm, you can measure the distance between two consecutive RR intervals. Atrial rhythm is determined by measuring the distance between two consecutive PP intervals. If the heart rhythm is regular, each of these interval measurements is the same.

Calculating a Patient's Heart Rate

To calculate the patient's heart rate from an ECG strip, remember the following:
- 5 large boxes on the graph paper = 1 second
- 15 large boxes = 3 seconds
- 30 large boxes = 6 seconds

Analyzing an ECG Strip

The ECG rhythm strip (lead II view) is evaluated from left to right. Each strip should be assessed for the following:
- Rate
- Rhythm
- P waves: There should be one P wave before each QRS complex; each is a positive deflection and similar in size and shape.
- Intervals: Assess for duration and distance.
- Appearance of the segments and waveforms: Are rhythmic PQRST cycles present? Are there any abnormalities, such as more than one P wave, QRS segments without a previous P wave, or an elevated ST segment? All of these abnormalities should be brought to the physician's attention immediately.

TYPICAL ECG RHYTHM ABNORMALITIES

Abnormalities in cardiac rhythm are called *arrhythmias.* These can result from disturbances anywhere along the electrical conduction pathway in the heart from the SA node through the right and left bundle branches. The best way to determine whether an arrhythmia is present is to know what the NSR looks like on an ECG. Study the NSR in the ECG in Fig. 16.1. NSR is a heart rate between 60 and 100 beats/min. Any deviations from this should be recognized during the ECG recording, and the patient care technician should notify the nurse immediately.

Cardiac arrhythmias commonly fall into one of four broad categories: sinus arrhythmias, atrial arrhythmias, ventricular arrhythmias, and biochemical arrhythmias. The characteristics of several arrhythmias in each of these categories are compared in Table 16.3.

Sinus Arrhythmias

Sinus rhythm is considered normal; the heart's electrical activity begins in the SA node and follows through the electrical system, ending in atrial and ventricular depolarization. In sinus arrhythmias, the pathway of the electrical charge is normal but the rate or rhythm of the heartbeat is altered. Sinus arrhythmias may be caused by the SA node firing too slowly or too quickly. In sinus bradycardia, the heart rate is below 60 beats/min. This can be a normal heart rate in well-conditioned athletes, but it is abnormal in other individuals. In sinus tachycardia, the heart rate is above 100 beats/min. This can be a normal heart rate in a person doing aerobic exercise, but it can be abnormal in a resting individual (Fig. 16.14).

Atrial Arrhythmias

Problems with electrical discharge of the atria are caused by faulty electrical impulse formation or conduction defects within the atria. Premature atrial contraction (PAC) occurs when the atria contract before they should for the next cardiac cycle. This can appear on the ECG as an abnormally shaped P wave or an extra P wave. PACs can be seen in smokers and people who consume large amounts of caffeine. Occasional PACs are not abnormal, but they become a medical concern if they

Table 16.3	Characteristics of Arrhythmias		
Type	**Signs and Symptoms**	**Cause**	**ECG Changes**
Sinus Arrhythmias			
Bradycardia	<60 beats/min	Vagal nerve stimulation; sleep; SA node ischemia; digitalis toxicity; drugs Can be normal in athletes	Essentially "normal" appearing, but slow
Tachycardia	Nonpathologic; heart rate >100 beats/min is pathologic	Increased demand for cardiac output; ectopic pacemaker	P wave can be obscured by ST segment (increasing the ECG speed can reduce this problem)
Atrial Arrhythmias			
PAC	Not pathologic if only several per minute	Increased SA node excitability, causing premature beats of atria Can be caused by nicotine or caffeine	"Extra" P waves
Flutter	200-350 beats/min	Many ectopic atrial pacemakers; normally unstable and progresses to atrial fibrillation if not corrected	Multiple, sawtoothed P waves before essentially normal-appearing QRS complexes
Ventricular Arrhythmias (See Fig. 16.15)			
PVC	Generally none	Ectopic pacemakers originating in ventricles from electrolyte imbalance, hypoxia, acute MI	Widened QRS complex
V-tach	Heart rate >100 beats/min, always pathologic	Damaged tissue around one of the "bundles," causing a difference in conduction speed between the two branches or ectopic pacemaker cells	Rapid rate, irregular pattern that includes "extra" or erratic, irregular, or wide QRS complexes
V-fib*	Shock, loss of consciousness, no pulse	Complete loss of synchronization of conduction system	Erratic deflections on the ECG (can be either coarse or fine) No identifiable ECG waves
Asystole	<5 beats/min	Death imminent	Flatline

IV, Intravenous; *MI,* myocardial infarction; *PAC,* premature atrial contraction; *PVC,* premature ventricular contraction; *SA,* sinoatrial.
*Most life-threatening arrhythmia; frequently precedes asystole if not reversed.

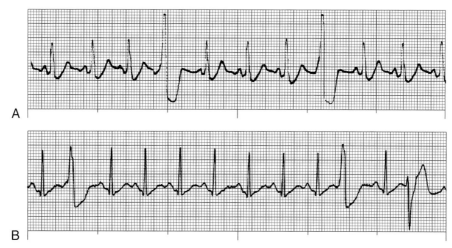

FIGURE 16.14 Sinus tachycardia with frequent, uniform PVCs (A) and with multiform PVCs (B). *PVCs,* premature ventricular contractions. (From Aehlert B: *ECGs made easy,* ed 5, St. Louis, 2013, Mosby.)

regularly occur more than six times a minute. In this situation, the PACs can indicate developing cardiac abnormalities.

Atrial flutter occurs when the atria beat at an extremely rapid rate, up to 300 beats/min. In atrial flutter the impulses come from many ectopic atrial locations but are blocked at the AV node, which prevents ventricular fibrillation. Atrial flutter is reversed with medication to slow the heart or with *cardioversion* (electrical shock).

Ventricular Arrhythmias

Premature ventricular contractions (PVCs Fig. 16.15A and B) occur when the ventricles contract before they should for the next cardiac cycle; that is, a QRS complex appears before a P wave. PVCs occur when an electrical charge originates in either ventricle. This can appear on the ECG as an absent P wave, an abnormally shaped T wave, and a widened QRS complex. This is followed by a pause before the initiation of the next cardiac cycle (see Fig. 16.14). PVCs can result from the use of tobacco, alcohol, medications containing epinephrine, and occasionally from anxiety. Infrequent PVCs are not abnormal, but they become a medical concern if they regularly occur more than six times a minute. Pathologic PVCs occur in patients with hypertension, coronary artery disease, and lung disease.

Ventricular tachycardia (commonly referred to as *V-tach;* Fig. 16.15C) is diagnosed when the ventricles beat at extremely rapid rates. It may be seen when multiple PVCs occur in a row or as a short run of fast beats, or it may persist longer than 30 seconds. The patient's heart rate may range from 101 to 250 beats/ min. V-tach can precede ventricular fibrillation if not reversed with drugs, cardioversion, or both. V-tach always reflects a pathologic state.

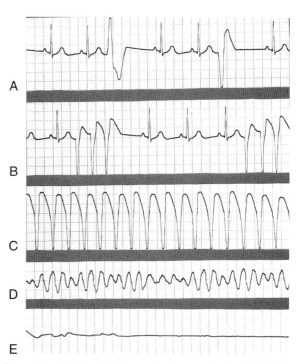

FIGURE 16.15 Ventricular arrhythmias. A, PVC. B, Three PVCs in a row. C, V-tach. D, V-fib. E, Asystole. *PVCs,* Premature ventricular contractions; *V-fib,* ventricular fibrillation; *V-tach,* ventricular tachycardia. (From Chester GA: *Modern medical assisting,* Philadelphia, 1999, WB Saunders.)

Ventricular fibrillation (commonly referred to as *V-fib;* Fig. 16.15D) is the most critical, life-threatening arrhythmia; it quickly results in death if not treated. V-fib is estimated to precede 85% of cases of *cardiac arrest* in adults. In V-fib, the electrical conduction system of the heart is in total dysfunction. The heart muscle quivers uncontrollably and is essentially ineffective at pumping any blood; therefore there is no pulse, and the patient is unresponsive and not breathing. Cardioversion with a *defibrillator* is necessary to restore normal function of the

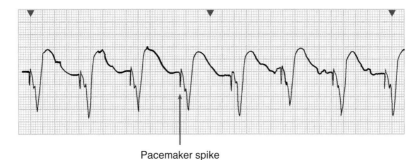

Pacemaker spike

FIGURE 16.16 Pacemaker rhythm strip. (From Lewis S et al: *Medical-surgical nursing,* ed 9, St. Louis, 2014, Mosby.)

electrical conduction system. Asystole is the result of absence of a heartbeat, or cardiac cessation, which shows as a flatline on the ECG (Fig. 16.15E).

Pacemaker Rhythms

A pacemaker is a device implanted under the skin that stimulates the electrical activity of the heart. It consists of a small metal pulse generator with a battery and electronic leads that extend from the generator to the myocardium. The entire pulse generator is replaced when the battery wears out, usually every 5 to 10 years. Current pacemakers are rate responsive, which means that they speed up or slow the heart rate based on such factors as the breathing rate and body temperature. Biventricular pacemakers, which stimulate both the right and left ventricles to enable more efficient cardiac contractions, may be implanted in patients with congestive heart failure.

Pacemakers are implanted in a hospital setting, and local anesthesia is used. Before the patient is discharged, the device is programmed to fire according to the needs of the individual patient. The patient is instructed to telephone the physician's office periodically to transmit pacemaker readings across the phone lines. The patient may use a transmission device attached to a wristband or a wand that is placed over the pacer. Pacemakers cause wide variations in the appearance of an ECG (Fig. 16.16).

Legal and Ethical Issues

An ECG is a valuable diagnostic tool, and it continues to be one of the most common procedures used in the diagnosis of cardiac diseases and conditions. The cardiologist measures the heart's activity and compares the results with known values by analyzing the ECG tracing. Comparing an ECG tracing with previous tracings can identify changes in the condition of the patient's heart.

The physician must be able to interpret the ECG tracing accurately and to establish its value in correctly diagnosing the patient's condition; the patient care technician, therefore, has the ethical obligation to complete the task as accurately and carefully as possible. Diagnostic procedures have a huge effect on a patient's next plan of action for treatment.

Delegation and Documentation Box 16.1

- When you are entrusted with performing testing procedures, you assume full responsibility for the accuracy and precision of each test you perform.
- This is a critical role in the patient care profession, so it is important to do it right.
- The results you submit make a difference in each patient's therapeutic treatment plan. No test is ever just routine.

CHAPTER SUMMARY

The heart beats in response to an electrical signal that originates in the SA node in the right atrium, spreads over the atria, and causes atrial contraction. This impulse continues to the AV node, through the bundle of His, through the right and left bundle branches, and into the Purkinje fibers, eventually causing ventricular contraction. *Polarization* is the resting state of the myocardial wall, when there is no electrical activity in the heart. When the electrical system of the heart stimulates a

myocardial cell, *depolarization* occurs, resulting in contraction of the stimulated heart muscle. The heart muscle cells must then return to a resting state; the process of reaching this resting state is *repolarization*.

The *P wave* shows atrial contraction, the beginning of cardiac depolarization; the *PR segment* is the return to baseline after atrial contraction; the *PR interval* is the time from the beginning of atrial contraction to the beginning of ventricular contraction; the *QRS complex* shows the contraction of both ventricles and the completion of cardiac depolarization; the *ST segment* is the time between the end of ventricular contraction and the beginning of ventricular recovery; the *T wave* is repolarization of the ventricles; the *QT interval* is the time between the beginning of the QRS complex through the T wave; a *U wave* occasionally can be seen as a small waveform just after the T wave in certain patients.

A six-channel ECG machine records all 12 leads simultaneously within seconds. Limb and chest electrodes with leads must be placed on the patient at specific anatomic locations before the recording starts. ECG paper is standardized to represent amplitude and time. The horizontal lines allow determination of the intensity of the electrical activity, and the vertical lines represent time; each of the large squares represents 0.2 second; five of them equals 1 second.

Recording an ECG requires a knowledge of where to place the electrodes and connect the leads to obtain the most accurate recording possible; the ability to recognize and correct the most common types of artifacts on the ECG recording; and proper use of the machine available.

An artifact is an unwanted, erratic movement of the stylus on the paper caused by outside interference. The main types include wandering baseline artifacts, in which the stylus gradually shifts away from the center of the paper because of slight movement or poor electrode attachment. Somatic tremor artifacts are a result of muscle movements in the patient that cause jagged peaks of irregular height and spacing and a shifting baseline. AC interference causes a series of uniform, small spikes on the paper because of electrical energy in the area. Interrupted baseline artifacts occur when the electric connection between the electrode and the lead is interrupted.

In sinus rhythm, the heart's electrical activity begins in the SA node and follows through the electrical system, ending in atrial and ventricular depolarization. In sinus bradycardia, the heart rate is less than 60 beats/min; in sinus tachycardia, the rate is more than 100 beats/min. A PAC occurs when the atria contract before they should for the next cardiac cycle. Atrial flutter occurs when the atria beat at an extremely rapid rate, up to 300 beats/min. PVCs occur when the ventricles contract before they should for the next cardiac cycle. V-tach causes the ventricles to beat at an extremely rapid rate, from 101 to 250 beats/min. V-fib is the most critical, life-threatening arrhythmia and results in death if not effectively treated. Asystole is the result of no heartbeat. Biochemical systemic problems also can cause arrhythmias.

Diagnostic procedures have a profound effect on a patient's subsequent treatment. When the medical assistant is entrusted with performing testing procedures, he or she assumes full responsibility for the accuracy and precision of tests performed. This is a critical role in the medical assisting profession. The results you submit strongly influence each patient's therapeutic treatment plan. No test is ever just routine.

Case Scenario

Martha Reyes has worked for almost 4 years at a local family practice office, but she has decided to take a new position in the cardiology practice next door, where she will be working for Dr. Julie Lee. Martha is very enthusiastic about the new position, but she realizes that she has a great deal to learn to provide the best patient service possible in Dr. Lee's practice. Although Martha is familiar with general cardiology practices from her previous employment, she must understand and be able to perform procedures performed for cardiac patients, especially electrocardiography.

- To fulfill her job description with Dr. Lee, what does Martha need to know about the electrical conduction system of the heart?
- How does an electrocardiography (ECG) machine work?
- How should a patient be prepared for an ECG?
- How will Martha perform an ECG diagnostic procedure?
- What is the normal appearance of ECG complexes?
- What are the characteristics of common ECG arrhythmias that Martha must be able to recognize?

REVIEW QUESTIONS

1. Which is the first wave seen on the ECG strip?
   a. P wave
   b. T wave
   c. QRS complex
   d. ST segment

2. If a person is extremely hairy, you may need to shave the area where the electrode will be placed.
   a. True
   b. False

3. How should the patient be positioned for the electrocardiography?
   a. Supine
   b. Prone
   c. Trendelenburg
   d. High-Fowler's

4. It is better for the patient to have a full bladder when conducting an ECG.
   a. True
   b. False

5. How many extremities are used for lead placement when obtaining a 12-lead ECG?
   a. 1
   b. 2
   c. 3
   d. 4

Patient Care and Comfort

Assisting With Admission and Discharge

1. Identify guidelines for admission, transfer, and discharge of a patient.
2. Discuss the concepts of the Health Insurance Portability and Accountability Act (HIPAA).
3. Describe common patient reactions to hospitalization.
4. Identify nursing interventions for common patient reactions to hospitalization and how they relate to tasks assigned to the patient care technician (PCT).
5. Discuss the PCT's responsibilities in performing an admission.
6. Describe how the PCT prepares a patient for transfer to another unit or facility.
7. Explain how the PCT prepares a patient for discharge.

admission Entry of a patient into the healthcare facility

continuity of care Continuing of established patient care from one setting to another

discharge The exiting of a patient from a healthcare facility; when a patient leaves the hospital to go home or to another facility

discharge planning The systematic process of planning for patient care after discharge from a hospital or healthcare facility

disorientation Mental confusion characterized by inadequate or incorrect perception of place, time, and identity

empathy Ability to recognize and to some extent share the emotions and state of mind of another and to understand the meaning and significance of that person's behavior

healthcare facility Any agency that provides healthcare

separation anxiety Fears and apprehension caused by separation from familiar surroundings and significant people

third-party payers Entities [people or elements] other than the giver or receiver of service responsible for payment; e.g., Medicare or insurance company

transfer Moving a patient from one unit to another [intraagency transfer] or moving a patient from one healthcare facility to another [interagency transfer]

COMMON PATIENT REACTIONS TO HOSPITALIZATION

Admission (entry of a patient into the healthcare facility) to a hospital or other healthcare facility (any agency that provides healthcare) is an anxious time for patients and their families. Patients are usually concerned about health problems or possible health problems and what could happen to them. Often the patient is having pain or other discomfort. The first contact with healthcare workers is important. It provides an opportunity to make them feel more comfortable and initiate a positive attitude regarding the care to be received.

A way to decrease the patient's anxiety and promote cooperation with treatment is to truly let them know that you are concerned for them while still going through the necessary admission routines. Admission routines the patient perceives as uncaring tend to make them more anxious and less willing to cooperate, and actually can prevent them from responding to treatment. It can also make their symptoms worse.

The patient care technician's (PCT's) responsibility is to assist the patient in maintaining dignity and a sense of control and in becoming comfortable in the new environment of the healthcare facility. This environment is different from a patient's home in that it has new sights, sounds, and smells that may interfere with the patient's comfort.

Each person's reaction to admission to a healthcare facility is unique. Some common reactions include fear of the unknown, loss of identity, disorientation (mental confusion characterized by inadequate or incorrect perception of place, time, and identity), separation anxiety (fears and apprehension caused by separation from familiar surroundings and significant people), and loneliness. These reactions are related to some of the needs described by Maslow (1970).

Fear of the unknown, which causes insecurity, is often the most common reaction. This is related to the need Maslow calls safety. Explanations about facility policies, information about medical orders and procedures, and simple direct answers to common questions from the patient or family help the person feel more comfortable and in control of the situation. Questions the patient may ask include the following: "How do I work the bed?"; "How do I call the nurse?"; "How or when do I get some food?"; "When can my family visit?"; and "What are they going to do to me next?" Orienting the patient to the new environment and answering these simple questions can take away much of the fear and anxiety felt by the patient on admission to the facility.

During the admission process to a healthcare facility, many patients feel a loss of identity that reflects a need for esteem, love, and belonging. Recognition, as described by Maslow, is part of this need. Sometimes putting the identification (ID) band on the patient's wrist reduces the patient to feeling like the number and name on the ID rather than a person. Explain that the ID is a necessary procedure to provide a positive means of identification and maintain the safety of the patient.

The PCT should learn new patient name quickly. Address patients with Mr., Mrs., Ms., or Miss with the last name, and only use a first name at the patient's request. Use of terms such as "honey," "dear," "sweetie," and "sugar" is never appropriate. These are known as terms of endearment, and should be avoided in the healthcare setting (Box 17.1).

Box 17.1   Life Span Considerations for Older Adults: Admission, Transfer, and Discharge

- The older adult admitted to the healthcare facility today is likely to be seriously ill.
- In a normally alert and oriented older adult, medical conditions that require admission to a healthcare facility often result in some level of disorientation or confusion.
- Older adults, who often have some limitation of vision or hearing, are more likely to become agitated or fearful on admission to a healthcare facility. Many experience relocation stress, from having to change locations from their home setting to the hospital setting.
- Transfers, even within the facility, tend to be confusing and upsetting to older adults.
- Hospitalized older adults frequently are concerned that they will be unable to return to their homes and will need institutional placement.
- Appropriate referrals for home nursing, therapy, homemaking, home nutrition programs, or other services are essential for older adults.
- Older adult patients need healthcare professionals to converse with them slowly and clearly because hearing may not be as sharp and information may take longer to process. Do not rush older patients; wait for patients to answer questions rather than letting family members answer.
- The change in environment and daily routine sometimes causes disorientation, loss of appetite, or reversal of sleeping-waking patterns.
- The stress of being in a healthcare facility sometimes is serious for the older patient because of a reduction in their ability to adapt. Helplessness, lack of control, and dependency often emerge, although a large degree of personal control possibly can be restored.
- When an older adult patient is transferred to a new facility, the relocation is also stressful. Ensure that significant support people are still accessible, the patient is thoroughly oriented to new surroundings, the patient is allowed to take along important memorabilia (items from home that have special meaning to them), and the patient has an opportunity to make decisions about care.

Separation anxiety and loneliness are reactions that reflect the needs Maslow identified as belongingness and love. Separation anxiety is very common in young children, but adults and older adults often have this reaction as well. In children, they usually react by crying; with adults, behaviors may include the patient being withdrawn or being very talkative; the older adult sometimes exhibits disorientation or depression.

The company of friends and loved ones is the best treatment for separation anxiety. Flexible visiting hours in healthcare facilities encourage family and friends to visit. Many facilities allow small children to visit relatives (facility policy and the patient's condition must be considered). Parents should be encouraged to stay with their hospitalized child to prevent the anxiety separation causes and to give the child a feeling of security. In some facilities, pets are allowed to visit. Many long-term facilities have pet-therapy visits from organizations or actually have pets that live in the facility.

The PCT has the ability to help reduce the severity of these common reactions to hospitalization with a warm, caring attitude and with courtesy and empathy (ability to recognize and to some extent share the emotions and state of mind of another and to understand the meaning and significance of that person's behavior). To help patients adjust, treat them with respect; maintain their dignity; involve them in the plan of care; and, whenever possible, adjust facility routines to meet their desires. Special considerations for the older adult are listed in Box 17.1.

CULTURAL CONSIDERATIONS FOR THE HOSPITALIZED PATIENT OR LONG-TERM CARE RESIDENT

If the patient does not speak English and is not accompanied by a bilingual family member on admission, contact the appropriate resource (usually the social services department) to secure an interpreter. Culture plays a vital role in the patient's ability to cope with stress and illness. The PCT should assist the patient with maintaining cultural practices as much as possible (Box 17.2).

ADMITTING A PATIENT

The admission procedure generally begins in the admitting department of the healthcare facility. The admission department representative is responsible for obtaining vital information from the patient, such as demographic information, insurance information, identifying information (social security number), and emergency contacts. Privacy and confidentiality must be maintained while this information is obtained. An interpreter should be used if the patient is non-English

Box 17.2   Cultural Considerations: Admission, Transfer, and Discharge

- Some Haitian-American patients are more likely to feel that they are receiving effective treatment when a nurse is physically involved in the care. In some Haitian cultures, a nurse is given more authority and status than a physician or assistive personnel. When interventions are implemented (e.g., taking the patient's blood pressure), tell the patient verbally what you are doing and that it is for the patient's benefit. If they request the nurse's presence, let your nurse know.
- Many Haitians believe that plant or tree leaves have a special significance in healing. The PCT may sometimes find leaves in the clothes and on various parts of the body. Leaves are thought to have mystical power related to regaining or keeping health.
- Some Haitian-Americans associate wheelchairs with sickness. Therefore the patient who is allowed to walk out of the hospital at discharge is more likely to feel that care has been effective.
- According to traditional Japanese belief, contact with blood, skin disease, and corpses causes illness. Some Japanese also believe that improper care of the body, including poor diet and lack of sleep, causes illness.
- Some Orthodox Jewish patients consider sundown Friday to sundown Saturday to be the Sabbath, which is a time of rest. These patients may avoid the use of any electronic equipment, so try to find alternatives to the use of this equipment if possible.
- Chinese-Americans often value personal relationships over rules and procedures. Be sure to consider the importance of loved ones when planning your care.
- Latino patients often use traditional healers within their cultural group who participate in alternative therapies such as aromatherapy and massage therapy. Latino women prefer to have a female care provider. These patients use time as a loose frame of reference and may not arrive right on time for an appointment. Instead, they use the appointment time as a guide.

speaking. Depending on the facility and the time of admission, the collection of this information may become the responsibility of the nurse.

Once the necessary identifying information has been collected, an ID band is placed on the patient's wrist. The ID band usually contains the patient's full name and date of birth. Some facilities may assign a facility number that is also included on the ID band. Patient allergies are typically identified on a separate red wristband. This information should be checked and verified by looking at the ID band and asking the patient to state this information (if capable) before procedures and medication administration. ID of the patient who is unconscious on admission to the facility is delayed until a family member or legal guardian is present.

On admission to a healthcare facility, the patient signs a consent form that gives permission for general treatment to be given. The Joint Commission and Medicare and Medicaid Services require that all hospitals and other healthcare facilities present a Patient's Bill of Rights to the patient or the patient's legal guardian at the time of admission. Facilities may also have other written forms that are presented, which contain policies and procedures that further inform patients of their rights and of the nurse's responsibilities in ensuring that these rights are honored.

The Patient Self-Determination Act of 1991 and the Health Insurance Portability and Accountability Act (HIPAA) are also presented on admission to a healthcare facility. Facilities that accept Medicare and Medicaid reimbursement are required to present information on The Patient Self-Determination Act. It addresses the patient's right to refuse or accept medical treatment and information regarding advance directives. The facility must refer the patient who requests information about advance directives to the appropriate resources. All patients, regardless of the type of healthcare facility, must be given and sign a document that verifies receipt of information regarding HIPAA (see Chapter 1 for an explanation of HIPAA).

People brought to the emergency department of a hospital are sometimes admitted directly to a patient care room or a special care unit (SCU), intensive care unit (ICU), coronary care unit (CCU), or burn unit. In these situations, a family member, usually the next of kin or the patient's healthcare representative, provides the admitting office with the necessary information.

When the unit staff is notified that a new patient is en route, they prepare the room for admission of the patient. A room that is neat and clean, with appropriate temperature and with lighting and personal care items in place, makes the patient feel expected and welcome. This makes a good first impression and facilitates the development of a therapeutic nurse–patient relationship.

If special equipment is needed by the new patient, such as oxygen, the PCT should have it in place and ready when the patient arrives. A patient who arrives on a stretcher needs the bed in the high position; the low bed position is best for a patient who arrives by wheelchair or walking.

Greeting the patient by name and making the patient feel welcome is one of the most important aspects of the admission procedure. Call patients by their last name unless otherwise directed by the patient. Your introduction consists of stating his or her first name and title. A person who is warmly welcomed is more comfortable in this new environment.

The patient's admission to the unit may occur at any time, which can include times when the unit is particularly busy. Regardless of the time or the activity occurring on the nursing unit, the staff needs to be courteous

---

Box 17.3	Patient Room Orientation

Orientation should include the following:
- The relationship of the room to the nurses' station
- The location of lounge areas
- The location of shower and bathroom facilities
- How to call the nurse from the bed and the bathroom
- How to use the intercom system if one is present
- How to adjust the bed and the lights
- How to operate the television
- How to operate the telephone and the radio
- Explanation of policies applicable to the patient (this is usually done by the nurse during the admission assessment)

---

to, interested in, and receiving of the new patient. The new patient needs to be given an orientation to the unit and the room (Box 17.3).

The routine of the facility must be explained to the patient and family. Knowing when meals are served (or in some facilities the time frame for the patient to call the dietary department to order food to be delivered), when family and friends are allowed to visit, when laboratory tests or diagnostic imaging evaluations are scheduled, when the healthcare provider usually makes rounds, and the policy on side rails gives the patient a sense of security and lessens anxiety. Many facilities have booklets for patients that explain these routine activities so that patients have a reference for this information. Some booklets include information about the availability of various social services, religious services, and facilities such as cafeteria, library, and gift shop. Some degree of patient teaching may also occur during the admission process.

The admitting procedure on the patient care unit is much more extensive than that in the admitting department (Procedure 17.1). Check the ID band and verify the information with the patient. If another patient is in the room, introduce the two patients.

Encourage the patient to give jewelry, money, and medications to the family to take home as long as the patient feels comfortable with doing so. If no family member is present, valuables are placed in the facility safe. Carefully follow the facility policy for patient valuables. Loss of a patient's valuables incurs serious legal implications for both the PCT and the facility. Documentation of disposition of valuables must be in the medical record.

In an Alzheimer's unit of a long-term care facility or in a mental health unit, the facility does assume some responsibility for patient belongings because the patient is not competent to do so. In this case, the careful listing and description of the patient's property become even more important. In some cases, hospitals are required to reimburse this patient for lost items. In these units, patients generally are not allowed to keep any jewelry

PROCEDURE 17.1

Admitting a Patient

1. Perform hand hygiene.
2. Prepare the room before the patient arrives: care items in place; bed at proper height and open (see Chapter 18 for an open bed); light on.
3. Courteously greet the patient and family. Introduce yourself. Project interest and concern. Introduce roommate.
4. Check the ID band and verify its accuracy.
5. Assess immediate needs for toileting.
6. Orient the patient to the unit, the lounge, and the nurses' station.
7. Orient the patient to the room. Explain the use of equipment, call system, bed, telephone, and television.
8. Explain facility routines, such as visiting hours and meal times.
9. Provide privacy if the patient desires or if abuse is suspected. Family members are sometimes asked to leave the room. Admission of an infant or small child requires emotional support for both child and parents. Parents are generally encouraged to stay with their child to prevent separation anxiety. The most reliable source of admission information is the parent.
10. Assist the patient to undress if necessary.
11. Follow facility policy for care of valuables, clothing, and medications.
12. Provide for safety: bed in low position; side rails up (unless admission is to a long-term care facility); call light within easy reach.
13. Begin care as directed by the nurse.
14. Invite family back into the room if they left earlier.
15. Perform hand hygiene.
16. Record the information on the patient's healthcare record according to agency policy.
17. Allow patient and family time alone together, if desired.

(other than a wedding ring) or any money at the bedside. Medications brought in by the patient should be sent home if possible. If this is not possible, these medications are typically locked in a designated area following the same process as valuables. Notify your nurse if the patient states that he or she brought medications with them.

Delegation and Documentation Box 17.1

The Joint Commission (TJC) requires each hospitalized patient to have an admission assessment prepared by a registered nurse (RN) within 24 hours of admission (TJC, 2008). The RN is then allowed to delegate aspects of the patient's care to the licensed practical nurse and the PCT. Admission requirements for long-term care facilities are directed by each state's governing agency.

The patient is usually asked to put on a hospital gown for the admission process so that a physical assessment can be completed. If the patient does not need help with dressing, the PCT provides privacy for the patient to change. An inventory is made of clothing along with other personal items the patient uses, such as glasses, contacts, dentures, prostheses, canes, or hearing aids. If the patient is keeping any jewelry or money in the room, these items must also be recorded. Fig. 17.1 shows sample clothing and valuables on an inventory checklist.

The healthcare provider is notified when the patient has been admitted. If no orders have been received to this point in the admissions process, the healthcare provider gives orders at this time. In some acute care

Box 17.4   Managing Emergency Admissions

- For the patient admitted through the emergency department (ED), immediate treatment takes priority over routine admission procedures. After ED treatment, the patient arrives on the nursing unit with a temporary ID bracelet, a physician's order sheet, and a record of treatment. Confer with the nurse to determine how you will be most helpful during this time to ensure continuity of care.
- Obtain and record the patient's vital signs. If family members accompany the patient, ask them to wait in the lounge while the nurse is assessing the patient and beginning treatment. Permit them to visit the patient after the patient is settled in the room.

settings, a hospitalist is assigned to the patient's care if the primary healthcare provider chooses not to follow patient care in the hospital setting.

Procedure 17.1 identifies the general steps to follow in admitting a patient. Specific facility policies and the patient's condition may necessitate some alterations to these steps. See Box 17.4 for managing emergency admissions.

TRANSFERRING A PATIENT

Changes in the physical or mental condition of a patient, whether they are improving or getting worse, may frequently require transfer (moving a patient from one unit to another [intraagency transfer] or moving a patient from one healthcare facility to another [interagency

Personal Belongings		
[ ] Clothing 　[ ] Belt 　[ ] Boots 　[ ] Bra 　[ ] Coat/jacket 　[ ] Dress/skirt 　[ ] Hat/gloves/scarf	[ ] Hose/Socks/Tights [ ] Jeans/Pants [ ] Luggage [ ] Pajamas [ ] Robe [ ] Shirt [ ] Shoes [ ] Shorts	[ ] Slippers [ ] Socks [ ] Sweat pants/sweat shirt [ ] Sweater [ ] Tie [ ] Undergarments [ ] Other **[ ] Clothing sent with Family** **[ ] No clothing items**
[ ] Personal Items 　[ ] Bible/Journal/Books 　[ ] Crutches 　[ ] Curling Iron/Straightener 　[ ] Hairdryer 　[ ] Upper dentures 　[ ] Lower dentures 　[ ] Partial dentures 　[ ] Retainer/Mouthguard 　[ ] Right hearing aid 　[ ] Left hearing aid	[ ] Laptop Computer [ ] Luggage [ ] MP3 Player/Headphones [ ] Phone/Charging cord [ ] Razor [ ] Toothbrush [ ] Walker [ ] Other personal items	**[ ] Personal items sent with family** **[ ] Personal items in storage on unit** **[ ] No personal items**
[ ] Valuables 　[ ] Bracelet 　[ ] Earrings 　[ ] Glasses/case 　[ ] Contacts 　[ ] Medals/Rosary/Cross 　[ ] Money {$_____}	[ ] Necklace/Earrings [ ] Purse [ ] Rings [#____} [ ] Wallet [ ] Watch [ ] Other Valuables	**[ ] Valuables sent with family** **[ ] Valuables sent to safe** **[ ] Valuables stored in locker number** _____
I assume full responsibility for retaining in my possession any items or clothing noted above and any others brought to me while I am a patient.		
Admission Signatures (signed at time of admission)		**Discharge Signatures (signed at time of discharge)**
Patient/Family: Date/Time:		Patient/Family: Date/Time:
Witness 1:	Date/Time:	Nurse: Date/Time:
Witness 2:	Date/Time:	

FIGURE 17.1 Example of a clothing and personal belongings list.

transfer]). Transfers are sometimes to another unit in the hospital and sometimes to another healthcare institution, such as a long-term care facility or rehabilitation hospital (Box 17.5).

Often a patient whose condition becomes critical while in the hospital is moved to special care areas, such as the ICU or the CCU. A patient whose condition improves is likely to be moved from a special care area to a general care area or a step-down unit. Other patients are transferred to a long-term care facility if they need continued care. Transfers may also be performed at the patient's request; for example, some patients wish to have a private room or a quieter room.

The patient transfer requires thorough preparation and careful documentation. Preparation includes an explanation of the transfer to the patient and family, discussion of the patient's condition and plan of care with the staff of the receiving unit or facility, and arrangements for transportation, if necessary. This is explained to the patient by the nurse assigned to the patient. Documentation of the patient's condition before and during transfer and adequate communication among nursing staff ensures continuity of care (continuing of established patient care from one setting to another) and provides legal protection for the transferring facility and its staff.

Transfer combines admission and discharge. The patient is discharged from one unit and received on the new unit, much like an admission. An order from the healthcare provider is necessary to begin the transfer process. An interagency transfer requires documentation from the accepting facility and healthcare provider and a signed consent from the patient indicating an understanding of the risks and benefits associated with the transfer. Failure to follow these procedures instituted may result in monetary fines to both facilities. Procedure 17.2 gives general steps to follow when transferring a patient. Box 17.6 lists special considerations for transferring patients.

DISCHARGING A PATIENT

Discharge Planning

Planning for a patient's discharge is just one aspect that aids in providing continuity of care for a patient in a healthcare facility. Discharge planning is defined as the systematic process of planning for patient care after discharge from a hospital or healthcare facility. The patient may be going home or to another facility, such as a long-term care facility.

Although discharge from a facility is usually considered routine, you still must plan carefully and ensure that the patient's needs are met during the discharge phase.

Delegation and Documentation Box 17.2

- It is important that a patient continues to receive care during the discharge phase.
- Continue to take vital signs according to the original order until the patient has exited the building.
- If discharge time is going to occur at or near a meal, ask patients if they would like you to order their tray early (if this is possible), or if they will have a meal ready for them when they reach their final destination.
- As you prepare them for discharge, be sure to attend to any hygiene needs. If they are incontinent, it is best practice to have them in a clean and dry undergarment at time of discharge.

Box 17.5 Long-Term Care Considerations

Admission to a long-term care facility sometimes occurs as a transfer from the hospital (see Procedure 17.2) and sometimes as a direct admission. Encourage the patient to bring clothing and other personal items, such as pictures; even personal furniture may be brought to place in the room to give a feeling of familiarity. Agency policies and requirements of third-party payers (entities [people or elements] other than the giver or receiver of service responsible for payment, e.g., Medicare or insurance company) must be followed so that benefits are not lost. Discharge from a nursing home is essentially the same as discharge from a hospital. There are more personal belongings to gather and pack.

Box 17.6 Special Considerations for Transferring Patients

- Arrange transportation via ambulance with social services department, if the patient requires it, for transfer to another facility. Ensure that the necessary equipment is assembled to provide care during transport.
- If the patient is being transferred to a different facility, be sure that all of the appropriate patient care measures have been performed (e.g., changing of soiled dressings, bathing of an incontinent patient, and emptying of collection devices).

PROCEDURE 17.2

Transferring a Patient

1. Perform hand hygiene.
2. Check healthcare provider's order for transfer and receive instruction from nurse.
3. Inform patient and family of the transfer.
4. Notify the receiving unit of the transfer and when to expect the patient.
5. Gather all the patient's belongings and necessary care items to accompany the patient.
6. Assist in transferring the patient, usually via stretcher or wheelchair. The nurse will tell you how to transfer the patient.
7. Introduce patient and family to nurses on new unit and to roommate.
8. Perform hand hygiene.
9. Record means of transfer. The nurse on the new unit also records an assessment of the patient's condition on arrival.
10. For an intraagency transfer, other departments, such as diagnostic imaging, laboratory, admission department, physical therapy, dietary, and business offices, must be notified of the transfer.
11. An interagency transfer is usually made via air or ground ambulance or via private car. Be sure that the patient is dressed or covered appropriately for environmental comfort. If oxygen is necessary, a small transport tank is usually used. A nurse generally accompanies a critically ill patient who is being transferred.
12. Infants are generally transported in an isolette that is later returned to the sending healthcare facility. Parents usually accompany their child during transfer unless the transfer is via air ambulance. In this case, the parents generally follow in family transportation.

Ideally, discharge planning begins shortly after admission. The healthcare team should always be working toward getting the patient ready for discharge. After all, hospitals are not designed for patients to remain there permanently. One should always begin with the end in mind. As the PCT, you may be asked to assist with the discharge planning. You may be asked to assist with arranging for transportation, scheduling follow-up appointments when necessary, and ensuring that there is someone available to pick up the patient's prescriptions.

The Joint Commission (TJC, 2008) requires the following instruction before patients leave healthcare facilities:

- Safe and effective use of medications and medical equipment
- Instruction on nutrition and modified diets
- Rehabilitation techniques to support adaptation to or functional independence in the environment
- Access to available community resources as needed
- When and how to obtain further treatment
- The patient's and family's responsibilities in the patient's ongoing healthcare needs and the knowledge and skills needed to carry out those responsibilities
- Maintenance of good standards for personal hygiene and grooming

The nurse is responsible for ensuring that the discharge teaching has been delivered in an effective way. It is not within the scope of practice for the PCT to provide patient discharge teaching. It is within the scope of the PCT to gather the necessary supplies and equipment the patient may need, but the nurse should provide the teaching on the supplies and equipment.

Discharge planning is a multidisciplinary process that involves participation by all members of the healthcare team, the patient, and the patient's family or significant others. Many larger hospitals have discharge planners or coordinators. The social worker is often in charge of discharge planning for the long-term care resident. Considered part of the healthcare team, these people orchestrate the discharge planning. This is especially important when the patient is considered at risk. Depending on the facility or acuity level of the patient, the staff or the charge nurse may be responsible for discharge planning. With the assistance of social workers or community-based nurses, the staff identifies and anticipates patient needs after discharge from the hospital and formulates a plan for meeting those needs.

Referrals for Healthcare Services

Often a patient who is discharged needs the further services of various disciplines (departments) within a facility, such as dietary, social work, or physical therapy. Referrals should be made as soon as possible after the patient's need is identified. This is usually done by the nurse, in communication with the physician or healthcare provider. In many facilities, a healthcare provider's order is needed for a referral, especially when specific therapies are planned (e.g., physical therapy) (see Injury & Illness Prevention Box 17.1).

The Discharge Process

Many facilities have a form with written instructions and teaching documentation for the patient to sign acknowledging understanding of the instructions. These instructions serve as a guide for the patient to use at home (see Fig. 17.2). Procedure 17.3 outlines the steps for discharging a patient.

Injury & Illness Prevention Box 17.1

Referrals and Discharge Planning

The following list summarizes the role that various health disciplines play in referrals during discharge planning.

Dietitian
- Provides proper nutrient and food source requirements in patients' diets
- Instructs patients on meal planning and diet restrictions

Social Worker
- Provides counseling for major life crises, such as terminal illness and family problems
- Assists in finding community resources, such as equipment for home healthcare or an agency that accepts patients after discharge from a facility
- Assists in finding financial resources to cover medical costs

Physical Therapist
- Assists in the examination and treatment of physically disabled people

- Assists in rehabilitating patients and restoring musculoskeletal function to a patient's greatest potential

Occupational Therapist
- Teaches patients to adapt to physical or cognitive challenges by learning new job skills or activities of daily living

Speech Therapist
- Assists patients with disorders that affect normal speech
- Assists patients with techniques that address swallowing disorders

Home Healthcare Nurse
- Provides follow-up discharge visits to a patient's home for the delivery of nursing services

Name: *Jane Doe*			Allergies: *Codeine*	
Diet:	Regular √	Soft	Liquid	Other:
Activity:	Walking √	Lifting (# of lbs)	Driving	Work
Bathing:	Shower	Tub	Sponge √	None until:
Wound Care:	Incision care:	Dressing Change:	Special Instructions: *Leave dressing intact until follow-up with physician*	
Tubes/Drains:	Special Instructions: *Physician will remove drain at follow-up appointment*			

Medications:	Drug	Dose	Route/Frequency	Special Instructions
	Ibuprofen	800 mg	Take 1 by mouth every 8 hours	Take with food or milk
	Amoxicillin	400 mg	Take 1 by mouth twice per day	Take until finished
	Colace	2 capsules	Take 1–2 by mouth at bedtime	Drink 6–8 glasses of water per day

Other Instructions: *Call physician if any redness, pain, or swelling around incision or drain occurs. Also call if temperature is greater than 100°F*

Follow-Up Appointment: *Call to schedule an appointment with the physician to be seen in two days.*

I have read these instructions and understand how I am to care for myself upon discharge. If I have further questions, I will ask the nurse.

Patient or Responsible Party Signature:	
Nurse's Signature:	
Date/Time:	Patient Label

WeCare Valley Hospital
Nowhere, USA
555-555-1234
Email: wecare@valleyhospital.org

FIGURE 17.2 Example of a discharge instruction sheet.

PROCEDURE 17.3

Discharging a Patient

1. Perform hand hygiene.
2. Be certain from the nurse that there is a discharge order.
3. Notify the family or the person who will be transporting the patient home.
4. Verify that the patient and the family or caregiver have their instructions for care from the nurse (e.g., medications, special diet, exercise, follow-up care).
5. Gather equipment, supplies, and prescriptions that the patient is to take home.
6. Assist the patient in dressing and packing items to go home.
7. Check clothing and valuables list made on admission according to policy.
8. Transfer the patient and belongings to the vehicle outside.
   a. Many facilities escort the patient via wheelchair.

b. Many patients are discharged via a stretcher.

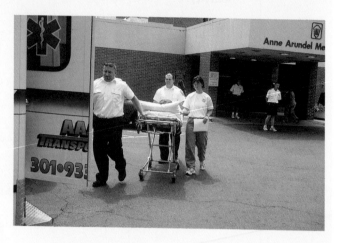

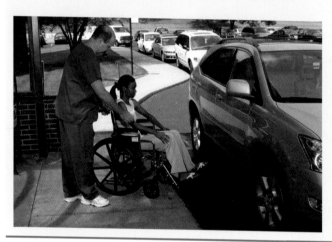

   c. Assist the patient into the vehicle. Help the family place personal belongings into car. As with all procedures, use good communication skills and wish patients well as they leave the facility.
9. Perform hand hygiene.
10. Report to the nurse the time the patient was taken out of the facility and using what method (wheelchair, etc.). Document the following:
   a. If the patient is an infant or child, he or she may be required to have a child restraint or car seat. This is determined by the state, and varies across states. If the family does not have an appropriate car seat, report this to the nurse before taking the patient off the unit.

CHAPTER SUMMARY

Admission into a healthcare facility begins with ensuring that patients are knowledgeable about routine procedures and activities that will occur during their stay. The Patient Self-Determination Act requires all Medicare-recipient and Medicaid-recipient hospitals to provide patients with information about their right to accept or reject medical treatment.

Common reactions to admission to a healthcare facility are fear of the unknown, loss of identity, disorientation, separation anxiety, and loneliness. An adult patient should always be addressed as Miss, Ms., Mrs., or Mr. (last name), unless the patient grants permission to do otherwise.

Discharge planning begins when a patient is admitted to a healthcare facility. Although discharge from a healthcare facility is usually considered routine, effective discharge requires careful planning and continuing assessment of patients' needs during their stay in the facility.

Every patient in a healthcare facility requires discharge planning.

Case Scenario

Molly is working as a PCT on a busy critical care floor. She has been asked by the charge nurse to assist with a transfer of a patient to the surgical floor. The nurse states that all paperwork for transfer has been completed, and the unit is awaiting the patient. The patient will be transferred by wheelchair to the surgical floor. Her belongings have been packed and are with her family members. Molly assists with taking the patient to the surgical floor by wheelchair. When she arrives to the unit, Molly stops at the nurse's station to let them know that the patient is here. The unit secretary looks at Molly with a somewhat puzzled look, and then asks the charge nurse whether she knows anything about this patient. The charge nurse responds to Molly, and says that she must have the wrong unit; they do not have any beds available on this unit and were unaware that this patient was being transferred. What should Molly do at this time? Should Molly leave the patient on the unit and go back to her unit to determine where she should take the patient? How should Molly handle this potential miscommunication? What step in the transfer process was probably omitted?

REVIEW QUESTIONS

1. A 90-year-old patient has been hospitalized with pneumonia and needs reorientation to his surroundings periodically. The nurse assisting him with his morning care hears the PCT refer to the patient as "Gramps." What action should the nurse take?
   a. Tell the PCT that it is okay to call him "Gramps" if he has grandchildren.
   b. Inform the PCT that it is acceptable if the Unlicensed Assistive Personnel (UAP) cannot remember his name.
   c. Explain that it is acceptable if the PCT feels comfortable calling him "Gramps."
   d. Educate the PCT that it is not acceptable to call the patient "Gramps" unless the patient has requested to be called so.

2. A patient has been transferred out of the ICU to a medical unit. A PCT has been asked to help the nurse complete the transfer. Which type of transfer is this?
   a. Patient-initiated transfer
   b. Interagency transfer
   c. Business office transfer
   d. Intraagency transfer

3. During the admission of a patient to a long-term care facility, what is the PCT most likely responsible for?
   a. Admission charting
   b. Admission interview
   c. Formulating nursing diagnoses
   d. Obtaining vital signs

4. Who is responsible for deciding whether the patient can be discharged from the hospital?
   a. Nurse
   b. PCT
   c. Physician
   d. Patient's family

5. What type of bed should be prepared for the patient who is being admitted from home?
   a. Open
   b. Closed
   c. Surgical
   d. Occupied

Bed Making and Hygiene

1. Discuss the therapeutic hospital room environment.
2. Describe personal hygienic practices.
3. Discuss variations of the bath procedure determined by a patient's condition and physician's orders.
4. Describe the procedure for a bed bath.
5. Identify nursing interventions for the prevention and treatment of pressure ulcers.
6. Describe the procedures for oral hygiene, and eye, ear, and nose care.
7. Outline the procedure for a back rub.
8. Summarize the procedure for perineal care for a male patient and a female patient.
9. Discuss the procedures for skin care.
10. Describe the procedure for making an unoccupied bed.
11. Describe the procedure for making an occupied bed.

KEY TERMS

axilla The underarm area or armpit
bedpan A shallow container used for urination or defection while in the bed
canthus Corner of the eye
cerumen Ear wax
circumorbital Circular area around the eye
dentures A set of artificial teeth not permanently implanted
febrile Condition characterized by an elevated body temperature
hygiene The principles of health
labia majora Larger fold or lip of tissue connecting to the vagina
labia minora Smaller fold or lip of tissue connecting to the vagina
medical asepsis The principles of using clean technique
oral hygiene Care of the oral cavity
pathogenic Disease-producing
perineal care Care of the genitalia
personal hygiene The self-care measures people use to maintain health and prevent disease
prone Lying face-down
supine Lying face-up
syncope Fainting
umbilicus The depressed point in the middle of the abdomen
urinal A container used by men to urinate in when in the bed
vertigo Dizziness

Hygiene (the principles of health) includes care of not only the skin but also the hair, the hands, the feet, the eyes, the ears, the nose, the mouth, the back, and the perineum. This chapter discusses the bath, components of the bath, and bed making. Many factors influence the practice of an individual's personal hygiene (Box 18.1 and Box 18.2).

When providing for the patient's hygiene needs, the patient care technician (PCT) has an opportunity to assist the patient with the performance of self-care. Assisting patients with hygiene care gives them the opportunity to maintain a degree of independence by allowing them to do what they can, and allows for some extra assistance if needed. Assisting a patient with bathing involves close contact with the patient and offers an opportunity to communicate with the patient to strengthen the relationship with the patient.

Patients often find themselves needing assistance from the PCT in performing their personal hygiene (the self-care measures people use to maintain health and prevent disease). The PCT's responsibility is to preserve the patient's well-being, encourage as much of the patient's independence as possible, and respect the patient's privacy when assisting with hygiene measures.

The different types of hygienic care are usually performed at certain times throughout the day. These times depend on various factors, including patient schedules and staff responsibilities (Box 18.3). Sometimes, scheduling of hygiene measures to be performed at the same

Box 18.1	Cultural Considerations and Personal Hygiene

- Touch or lack of touch has cultural significance and is a learned behavior. Cultural uses of touch vary. Sometimes touching a patient in a certain way is offensive to them. You may not always know how each culture feels about touch. It is always best to ask permission from the patient before touching him or her.
- Chinese Americans sometimes view tasks associated with closeness and touch as offensive. Vietnamese Americans are likely to feel very uneasy during a back rub. Ask patients what makes them most comfortable during a bath.
- Use good judgment when deciding how to use touch and avoid forcing touch on anyone. What may seem as a harmless, incidental touch may actually help to establish a positive, temporary bond between strangers, making them more compliant, helpful, positive, and giving.
- Consider the individual patient's beliefs, values, and habits.
- Usually you can incorporate a person's preferences into his or her plan of care without it causing much, if any, trouble.
- One culture that considers personal hygiene to be extremely important is that of the East Indian Hindus. A daily bath is part of their religious duty. Bathing after a meal is believed by some Hindus to cause injury. Likewise, a bath that is too hot has the potential to injure the eyes. Hot water may be added to cold water, but cold water is not to be added to hot water when one is preparing a bath. Once a bath is completed, the individual carefully dries the body thoroughly with a towel.

Box 18.2	Factors That Influence a Patient's Personal Hygiene

- *Social practices.* Social groups, family customs, age, friends, and work groups all influence practices of personal hygiene.
- *Body image.* Body image is a person's subjective concept of physical appearance. This body image affects the manner in which hygiene is maintained. The nurse will provide education to the unclean patient about the importance of hygiene. PCTs must be careful not to convey feelings of disapproval when caring for the patient whose hygiene practices differ from others.
- *Socioeconomic status.* The patient's economic resources often influence the type or extent of hygienic practices used.
- *Knowledge.* Knowledge alone is not enough. The patient also must be encouraged to maintain self-care. Often, learning about an illness or condition encourages patients to improve hygienic practices. For example, teaching the patient with diabetes the importance of foot care helps prevent infections. It is important to maintain a nonjudgmental attitude while providing hygiene for the patient.
- *Personal preference.* Individual patients have individual desires and choices as to when to bathe, shave, and shampoo. Patients choose different shampoos, deodorants, and toothpastes according to personal needs or selections. Do not try to change the patient's preferences unless the patient's health is affected.
- *Physical condition.* Patients in the late stages of terminal illness or those who have undergone surgery often lack the physical energy or dexterity to perform personal hygiene. Some disease conditions exhaust or incapacitate patients, thereby requiring you to perform all aspects of hygiene. Other disease conditions, such as serious cardiac or pulmonary problems, cause severe activity intolerance.
- *Cultural variables.* Patients from diverse cultural backgrounds follow different self-care practices. In North America, people typically take daily baths (tub or shower), but in many European countries, it is not unusual to bathe completely only once a week. Avoid being judgmental when caring for patients with different hygienic practices (see Cultural Considerations box).

Box 18.3	Hygiene Care Schedule

- *Early morning care.* The patient care technician provides basic hygiene to patients getting ready for breakfast, scheduled tests, or early morning surgery. "AM care" includes offering a bedpan or urinal if the patient is not ambulatory, washing the patient's hands and face, and assisting with oral care.
- *Morning care, or after-breakfast care.* This care is performed after breakfast. Offer a bedpan or urinal to patients confined to bed; provide a bath or shower; provide oral, foot, nail, and hair care; give a back rub; change the patient's gown or pajamas; change the bed linens; and straighten the patient's bedside unit and room. This is often referred to as complete AM care.
- *Afternoon care.* Because hospitalized patients often undergo many exhausting diagnostic tests or procedures in the morning, they tend to greatly appreciate afternoon care. This is also true for the long-term care resident. Many of these residents have participated in exercise, physical therapy, or activities throughout the day. Afternoon hygienic care includes washing the hands and face, assisting with oral care, offering a bedpan or urinal, and straightening bed linen.
- *Evening care, or hour-before-sleep (HS) care.* Before bedtime, offer personal hygienic care that helps a patient relax to promote sleep. "PM care," sometimes referred to as HS care, typically includes changing soiled bed linens, gowns, or pajamas; assisting the patient in washing the face, hands, and back; providing oral hygiene; giving a back massage; and offering the bedpan or urinal to nonambulatory patients.

Box 18.4	Personal Hygiene for Patient Care Technicians

- Take a daily bath or shower.
- Use a strong, odorless, and effective deodorant every day.
- Wear clean undergarments every day.
- Wear a clean uniform every day.
- Shampoo hair as often as necessary to maintain cleanliness.
- Keep hair off the collar or at least pulled back away from the face and in a contained hairstyle. Wear barrettes and bows that blend in with your hair.
- Wear clean, comfortable shoes that follow facility policy.
- Keep fingernails short, clean, and well-manicured. Nail polish and artificial nails are not allowed in many facilities. Pathogens get trapped underneath polish or artificial nails and have the potential to cause serious infections, especially in newborns.
- Wear makeup only in moderation.
- Wear only an engagement ring or wedding ring (or both) without stones (stones harbor microorganisms). In departments such as the operating and delivery rooms, rings are not worn at all.
- Wear only small unobtrusive earrings; wear only one pair. Large or dangling earrings are not recommended. These are considered hazardous because they can easily be pulled out and damage the ear.
- Avoid perfumes or colognes (many patients are allergic to these).
- Wear white-only T-shirts under uniform tops.
- Wear the standard departmental uniform.
- Keep beards and mustaches clean, short, and well-trimmed.
- Use breath mints; the smell of coffee, foods, or nicotine is often offensive to patients.

time as other care measures is most convenient. This is known as coordination of care.

The PCT's own practice of personal hygiene is essential (Box 18.4). The healthcare team should be a role model and teach by example. Hygienic practices promote medical asepsis, also known as clean technique. This technique inhibits the growth and spread of pathogenic (disease-producing) microorganisms.

PATIENT'S ROOM ENVIRONMENT

Many patients with limitations such as traction, casts, or monitoring equipment may not leave their rooms as often as other patients. Patients who are very sick may be confined to their rooms for an extended period. These rooms must be kept comfortable and safe (Fig. 18.1). By keeping the room comfortable and the noise down, the PCT can create a more therapeutic environment. Keeping the room clean, neat, and orderly contributes to a sense of well-being.

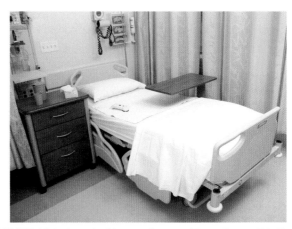

FIGURE 18.1 A typical hospital room. (From Potter PA, Perry AG: *Fundamentals of nursing: concepts, process, and practice,* ed 9, St. Louis, 2017, Mosby.)

Maintaining Comfort

Consider the age of patients, how bad their illness is, and whether they can tolerate activity in order to make them most comfortable. The recommended room temperature is 68° to 74°F (20° to 23°C). Infants, older adults, and the acutely ill are likely to need warmer temperatures. Physically active patients and patients with chronic respiratory problems tend to be more comfortable in a cooler environment.

Good ventilation is necessary to keep stale air and odors from lingering in the room. Take care to protect the patient from drafts. It is also important to ensure that odors are kept to a minimum. Promptly emptying and cleaning bedpans, urinals, and commodes helps in eliminating odors.

Noises are unpleasant intrusions. Ill patients are more sensitive to the noises commonly heard within the hospital environment. Work with other hospital personnel to monitor the noise level that results from the moving of metal equipment on and off the elevator and from televisions and radios, telephones ringing, loud talking, and laughter at the nurses' station. Manage equipment properly, answer phones immediately, and control voice volume. Ask patients to keep televisions and radios turned down.

Life Span Considerations for Older Adults

Hygiene Practices

- Older individuals are more likely to become chilled during bathing or when left uncovered. Maintain a warmer room temperature than for younger people, and keep drafts to a minimum.
- Drape older adults properly during care to prevent chilling and provide for modesty.
- Older adults with limited mobility need assistance in perineal care. Use of a side-lying position increases the patient's comfort and provides the PCT with opportunity to provide perineal care and inspect surrounding skin. Perineal care should be performed daily and after each episode of incontinence.
- Impaired circulation or neurologic changes sometimes decrease the older person's ability to sense temperature changes in water, so use caution to prevent burns during tub or shower bathing.
- Too-frequent bathing and use of detergent soaps have harmful effects on the skin of most older adults. Determine the kind of and frequency of baths and the choice of soap on individual needs.
- Rehydrate patient's skin with lotions and fluids; baths are drying to the skin.
- Immobility, incontinence, and poor nutrition increase the risk of skin impairment in older adults. Adequate diet, frequent change of position, use of pressure-reducing devices, regular toileting, and prompt cleansing of the skin after incontinence reduce the risks.
- Older adults with urinary incontinence need meticulous skin care to reduce skin irritation from urine and feces.
- The aging process contributes to changes in voiding (urinating) and defecating (stooling). Often, the aging patient needs immediate response to a request for the **bedpan** or **urinal** or assistance to the toilet. If they have to wait, they may have an accident.
- Incontinence of urine or stool is *not* an expected result of the aging process. This is a myth many do not understand.
- Decreased production of saliva in aging means that there is a need for more frequent oral hygiene. Good cleaning of the oral cavity and teeth or dentures helps reduce the alteration in taste common with aging.

- Good oral hygiene practices help older adults preserve their ability to eat. Patients with diabetes need to visit the dentist a minimum of every 6 months. Older adults, especially those at risk for oral problems, should avoid spicy, coarse, acidic, and sugary foods, which tend to cause dental caries.
- Treat older adults with respect. Keep grooming, including hair care and use of cosmetics, age appropriate.
- Because of normal changes in the nails and an increased incidence of circulatory problems or diabetes mellitus, older individuals are more likely to require special foot care.
- Changes in aging skin include thinning of epidermis and subcutaneous fat and dryness because of decreased activity of oil and sweat glands. These changes become visible in the feet. In addition, nails become opaque, tough, scaly, brittle, and hypertrophied.
- Individuals who have not participated in regular exercise often experience a relaxing of foot ligaments and musculature, which leads to instability and impaired mobility.
- Common foot problems of older adults include heel pain caused by tearing of plantar fascia and foot musculature, hammertoes and claw toes, corns and calluses, pathologic nail conditions (e.g., ingrown toenails, fungal infections), arthritis, and neuropathies that cause diminished sensation in the foot.
- Older persons are also more vulnerable to bunions because feet tend to spread with aging.
- Usually the facial hair of the older adult does not grow quickly; thus a shave is not necessarily a must every day.
- Older adults have fragile skin and require more protection. Be sure that bed linens are clean, dry, and free of wrinkles.
- Encourage older adults to spend as much time out of bed as possible.
- Use draw sheets and waterproof pads with caution. Accumulation of moisture creates a risk for skin breakdown, so these items must be changed as needed.

Proper lighting is necessary for the safety of both the PCT and the patient. Reduce lighting levels to encourage sleep, and brighten the room for stimulation. Adjust the lighting by closing or opening the drapes, adjusting over-bed and floor lights, and opening or closing room doors.

The PCT must help the patient conserve energy for the recovery process. Controlling stimuli within the patient's personal environment is one way to help conserve energy. This promotes a sense of security and enhances the patient's ability to gain needed rest and sleep.

Room Equipment

The usual hospital room contains certain basic furniture: bedside stand, bed, over-bed table, chairs, and lights (see Fig. 18.1). In addition, the standard hospital room has either a closet or drawer space. Room equipment and furniture for the long-term care facility differs somewhat, often incorporating more of the patient's own furniture and decorations.

The bedside stand serves to store the patient's personal articles and hygienic equipment, such as towels, the emesis and bath basins, toothpaste and toothbrush, and comb and brush. The telephone, the drinking glass, and the water pitcher are ordinarily kept on the patient's bedside stand.

The over-bed table is on wheels and is adjustable to various heights over the bed or a chair. Usually, a storage area is located under the tabletop. This tabletop is ideal to use as a working space when performing procedures. It also serves as a surface for meal trays, toileting items needed during hygienic care, and other objects frequently used by the patient. The tabletop should be cleaned before and after procedures, and before meals.

Chairs are a necessity in the hospital room. Both straight chairs and lounge chairs are typical. Both the patient and visitors make use of the lounge chair. Straight chairs are easier to move around than lounge chairs. They are also more convenient when temporarily transferring the patient from the bed, such as during bed making. Relatives who sit with the patient will typically want to use the recliner chairs.

Lights in each patient's room provide comfort, safety, and ease. A call light is available at each bedside. The call signal indicates that a patient needs assistance. Many facilities are designed so that the call light from a patient's bathroom flashes off and on quickly, denoting a call of a more serious nature. In contrast, the bedside call light typically does not flash. Respond as soon as possible when a patient indicates a need for assistance.

Critically ill patients often remain in bed for longer periods. Hospital beds are designed for comfort and safety, and their capacity to accommodate position changes (Table 18.1). The standard hospital bed has a firm water-repellent mattress on a metal frame that is raised and lowered horizontally as needed. An even surface provides for the greatest comfort. Bariatric beds are available in most facilities to accommodate the obese patient. Handles on the sides of the mattress serve to help with removing or turning the mattress.

Different bed positions are used to promote lung expansion, postural drainage, and other interventions. Most beds are powered by electricity, but some are operated manually. PCTs may find that these beds are convenient to raise while working at the bedside and then lower when the patient is being transferred or when leaving the patient's room. The bed is also constructed so that the PCT or patient is able to raise and lower the head and the foot independently. In most cases, the controls are conveniently situated on the side of the bed or in the side rail. Teach the patient the proper use of the controls, and caution the patient to leave the bed at its lowest level to prevent injuries from falls.

Hospital beds have a number of safety features. Locks on the wheels prevent unwanted movement. Side rails (adjustable metal frames that are raised and lowered by pushing or pulling a knob) are located on both sides of the bed. These side rails protect patients from falling, aid patients in positioning themselves, and provide upper extremity support as the patient gets out of bed. Never leave the bedside of a patient in bed if the side rail is lowered. Note that full side rails are considered a form of restraint in a long-term care setting. Another safety feature is the special removable headboard on some beds, which is important when the medical team needs easy access to the patient's head during cardiopulmonary resuscitation (CPR).

BATHING

How detailed the patient's bath is and how you bathe the patient depends on what the patient is capable of doing, the degree of hygiene required, and the physician's order, as in the case of therapeutic baths. The types of therapeutic baths are outlined in the following sections. Some hygiene skills are acceptable for PCTs and other unlicensed assistive personnel to perform (see Coordinated Care box on bathing and other hygienic care measures).

The PCT should maintain a bathing water temperature of 110° F (about 43° C) if the purpose is to apply heat to the affected area. If the purpose is to promote healing or to produce relaxation, use a water temperature of about 98° to 102° F (34° to 39° C). Remember to prevent chilling by covering the patient's legs with a bath blanket and the shoulders with a towel. Place a towel behind the patient's back for comfort.

Observe the patient for signs and symptoms of weakness, such as a rapid or weak pulse, tachypnea, or vertigo (dizziness) or syncope (fainting). If the patient

Table 18.1	Bed Positions	
Position	**Description**	**Uses**
Fowler's to high Fowler's	Head of bed raised to angle of 45 degrees or more (up to 90 degrees); semisitting to full upright sitting position	Appropriate position for eating or drinking to prevent aspiration; beneficial during breathing exercises to promote full lung expansion
Semi-Fowler's (also referred to as low Fowler's)	Head of bed raised approximately 30 degrees	Often used for patients who cannot tolerate Fowler's or high Fowler's; position sometimes ordered after lumbar puncture has been performed
Trendelenburg's	Entire bed tilted downward toward head of bed with no break in the middle of the bed	Facilitates removal of secretions with postural drainage; facilitates venous return in patients with poor peripheral circulation; sometimes used to aid in dilation of large vessels for central line placement
Reverse Trendelenburg's	Entire bed frame tilted downward toward foot of bed with no break in the middle of the bed	Not commonly used position; promotes gastric emptying and prevents esophageal reflux; facilitates arterial circulation to lower extremities
Flat	Entire bed frame parallel to floor	For patients with vertebral injuries, immediately after lumbar puncture, and in cervical traction; generally preferred by patients for sleeping

(Modified from Potter PA, Perry AG: *Basic nursing: a critical thinking approach*, ed 7, St. Louis, 2011, Mosby.)

Delegation and Documentation Box 18.1

Hygiene Care Measures

Bathing

Skills of bathing are often delegated to the PCT or Unlicensed Assistive Personnel (UAP). Keep these tips in mind when accepting the assignment of bathing the patient:

- Find out from the nurse what type of bath (e.g., complete, partial assist, tub, shower) is appropriate to the patient's diagnosis and needs.
- Notify the nurse of any skin integrity problems so that you will know of areas of impairment or potential impairment.
- Use an organized approach and reassuring tone of voice so that the patient feels safe and comfortable during bathing.
- Encourage the patient to report any concerns or discomfort during the bath.
- Encourage as much independence in the patient's self-care skills as appropriate and to provide positive feedback.

Oral Care

Skills of oral care, tooth brushing, and denture care are appropriate to delegate to the PCT, but the patient's gag reflex should be assessed by the nurse first.

- Position the patient if the patient is unconscious or debilitated.
- Report any changes in oral mucosa.
- Review the use of oral suction for cleansing oral secretions (if allowed by facility policy), if the patient is likely to need it.

Hair Care and Showering

The skills of shampooing and shaving are appropriate to be delegated to the PCT unless the patient has a trauma or injury of the cervical spine.

- Properly position individual patients and use any special products indicated.

Hygiene Care Measures

- Be sure that you know how to correctly use medicated shampoos for lice or other conditions and the appropriate steps to prevent transmission to other patients.
- Report how the patient tolerated the procedure and any changes that indicate possible inflammation or injury.

Hand, Foot, and Nail Care

The skill of care of the fingernails and foot care for patients without diabetes or any circulatory compromise or bleeding disorder is appropriate to delegate to the PCT.

- Use nail files and clippers correctly.
- Use warm water.
- Report any changes that indicate possible inflammation or injury.

Bed Making

Bed making is usually delegated to the PCT.

- Find out from the nurse whether an unoccupied or occupied bed is to be made.
- Review the safety precautions or activity restrictions for the patient; use the side rails in the acute care setting

and the call system in the event that staff assistance is needed.

- Notify the nurse immediately if wound drainage, dressing material, drainage tubes, or intravenous [IV] tubing is found in the linen or becomes dislodged.
- Allow the patient rest periods and notify the nurse if the patient becomes fatigued.

Care of the Patient With Incontinence

The skill of providing care for patients with incontinence is appropriate to delegate to the PCT. The following measures are all particularly important when assisting the patient with incontinence:

- Be aware of the patient's dignity and self-esteem needs and to take measures to prevent violating these needs.
- Know standard precautions guidelines related to handling of body fluids.
- Report information such as abdominal pain, increased episodes of incontinence, changes in appearance of urine or stool, and evidence of skin breakdown.

experiences any of these, notify the nurse at once. Never leave the patient alone unless you are sure that the patient is safe; a call signal should be placed within easy reach. Instruct the patient to stay out of drafts and to rest after a sitz bath.

Cool Water Tub Bath

The cool water tub bath is an option to relieve tension or lower body temperature. Measures should be instituted to prevent the patient from chilling. The water temperature is tepid, 98.6°F (37°C). Cold water should not be used because it promotes chilling and shivering.

Warm Water Tub Bath

A warm water tub bath is given primarily to reduce muscle tension. The recommended water temperature is 109.4°F (43°C).

Hot Water Tub Bath

The hot water tub bath helps relieve muscle soreness and muscle spasms. This procedure is not recommended for children. The proper water temperature for adults is 113° to 115°F (45° to 46°C). Keep in mind the danger of burns, and take precautions to prevent them. This bath is not used for patients with neurologic disorders or circulatory impairment because of the risk of causing burns.

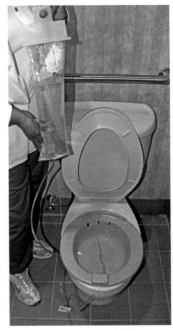

FIGURE 18.2 The portable sitz bath. (From Cooper K, Gosnell K: *Foundations of nursing*, ed 7, St. Louis, 2015, Mosby.)

Sitz Bath

A sitz bath cleanses and aids in reducing inflammation of the perineal and anal areas of the patient who has undergone rectal or vaginal surgery or childbirth. Discomfort from hemorrhoids or a fissure is also relieved with a sitz bath.

The appliance for the sitz bath is shown in Fig. 18.2. Depending on the patient's diagnosis and the healthcare provider's order, the desired results are possible to obtain from a tub bath. However, the tub is the least desirable method because heat is also applied to the legs and thereby reduces the effects on the pelvic region. Optimally, the sitz bath lasts from 20 to 30 minutes; it is usually ordered three times daily. The time seems to pass more quickly when the patient has reading material.

Other Baths

A complete bed bath is for patients who are totally dependent and require total assistance (Procedure 18.1). As the patient's condition improves, only partial assistance becomes necessary. Assist the patient to

Text continued on p. 342

PROCEDURE 18.1

Bathing the Patient and Administering a Back Rub

1. Refer to medical record, nurse, care plan, or Kardex for special interventions.
2. Assemble the necessary supplies.
3. Introduce self.
4. Identify patient.
5. Explain procedure to patient.
6. Perform hand hygiene and, as appropriate, don clean gloves. Know agency policy and guidelines from the Centers for Disease Control and Prevention (CDC) and Occupational Safety and Health Administration (OSHA).
7. Prepare patient for intervention.
   a. Close door or pull curtain.
   b. Drape for procedure as appropriate.
   c. Suggest use of bedpan, urinal, or bathroom.
   d. Arrange supplies.
   e. Adjust room temperature.
   f. Raise bed to comfortable working position.
8. Bed bath.
   a. Lower side rail; position patient on side of bed closest to you.

b. Loosen top linens from the foot of the bed; place bath blanket over the top linens. Ask patient to hold bath blanket while you remove top linens. If patient is unable, you need to hold bath blanket in place while removing linens.
c. Place soiled laundry in laundry bag; do not touch uniform with soiled laundry.
d. Assist patient with oral hygiene. If patient is unable, the PCT performs the procedure (see Procedure 18.3).
e. Remove patient's gown, all undergarments, and jewelry. If an extremity is injured or has reduced movement, begin removal of the gown from the unaffected side. If the patient has an IV tube, remove gown from the arm without IV first, then lower IV container or remove tubing from pump and slide gown covering down over the affected arm and over tubing and container. Rehang IV container and check flow rate or reset pump. Do not disconnect tubing.

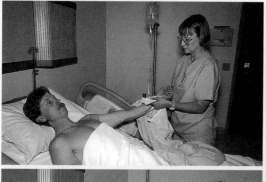
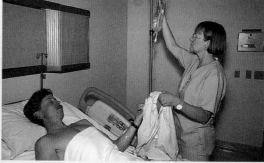
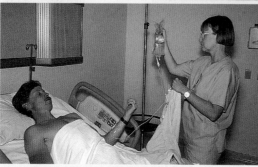
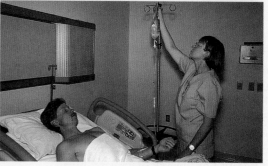

PROCEDURE 18.1
Bathing the Patient and Administering a Back Rub—cont'd

f. Raise side rail and fill washbasin two-thirds full with water at 110° to 115°F (43° to 46°C). To prevent spillage, do not overfill basin.

g. Remove pillow and raise head of bed to semi-Fowler position if patient is able to tolerate it.

h. Form mitt with bath cloth around your hand (see illustration); dip mitt and hand into bath water. Squeeze out excess water.

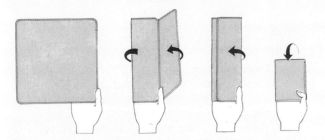

i. Wash around patient's eyes, using a different portion of washcloth for each eye. Cleanse from inner to outer **canthus** (corner of eye; see illustration). Dry gently.

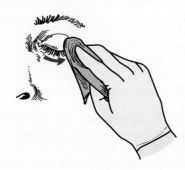

j. Rinse bath cloth (then continue to use as mitt) and finish washing face. (Ask patient about use of soap on face because some patients, especially female patients, do not use soap on face.) Wash ears and neck. Cleanse pinna (the projecting part of the external ear) with cotton-tipped applicators.

k. Expose arm farthest from you. Place towel lengthwise under patient's arm. To cleanse the hands, the PCT can place washbasin on towel and place patient's hand in basin of water, or the hands can be cleansed with the washcloth (be sure to clean between the fingers). Bathe arms with long, firm strokes; a firm stroke rather than a light stroke prevents tickling the patient. Supporting arm, raise it above patient's head to bathe the **axilla** (the underarm area or armpit). Rinse and dry well. Apply deodorant if desired.

l. Bathe arm closest to you. Follow step k.

m. Cover patient's chest with bath towel; fold bath blanket down to waist and wash chest with circular motion. Be certain to cleanse and dry well in skin folds and under breasts. Continue to observe the condition of the patient's skin, degree of mobility, and behavior and encourage the patient to verbalize concerns.

n. Fold bath blanket down to pubic area, keeping chest covered with dry towel. Wash abdomen, including **umbilicus** (the depressed point in the middle of the abdomen; wash umbilicus with cotton-tipped applicators), and skin folds. Dry thoroughly.

o. Raise side rail; empty basin into hopper or stool.

p. Rinse basin and washcloth. Refill basin two-thirds full with water at 110° to 115°F (43° to 46°C).

q. Expose leg farthest away from you, keeping *perineum* (the genital area) covered. Place bath towel lengthwise on bed under patient's leg. Place washbasin on towel and place patient's foot in basin. Patients with diabetes mellitus need special foot care. Be certain to support patient's leg properly; flex knee and grasp heel. If patient is unable to place foot in washbasin, wash leg and foot with mitted washcloth.

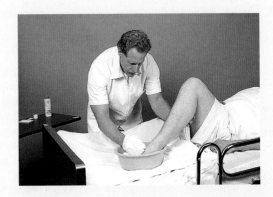

r. With long firm strokes, bathe the leg. However, note that bathing the lower extremities of patients with history of deep vein thrombosis (DVT) or hypercoagulation disorders with long firm strokes is contraindicated; use circular, gentle strokes for these patients so that the clot is not dislodged. After soaking, do nail care (may be done at a separate time; see Chapter 19). If skin is dry, apply lotion if desired. Do not massage legs. **Never massage lower extremities**.

s. Bathe leg and foot closest to you as in steps q and r. Raise side rail. Be sure that patient is covered with bath blanket. Be certain to expose only those body parts being bathed. Change water (see steps p and q). Lower side rail. If patient tolerates, position **prone** (lying face-down) or in **Sims's position** (side-lying position). Place towel

Continued

PROCEDURE 18.1

Bathing the Patient and Administering a Back Rub—cont'd

lengthwise on bed along back. Wash and dry back from neckline down to buttocks. If patient tolerates a massage action, do so while washing back.

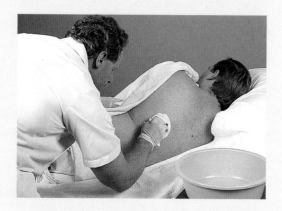

t. Reposition patient **supine** (lying face-up). Provide basin of water, soap, washcloth, and towel, and instruct patient to cleanse perineal area. (Give patient privacy to do this.) If patient is unable to finish bath, don new gloves and complete this step in patient care (see Procedure 18.2).

u. Be certain that patient is covered with blankets. Raise side rail. Empty, wash, and rinse basin. Replace basin in bedside stand. Place washcloth in laundry bag for soiled linen.

v. Position patient in Sims's or prone position close to you. Place towel lengthwise along patient's back. Give back rub. Never massage reddened areas.

w. Assist patient into clean gown. If ordered, assist patient to ambulate to chair; place towel over shoulders, and comb hair. Women sometimes wish to apply makeup at this time. While patient is in chair, make unoccupied bed (see Procedure 18.5). If patient is not ambulatory, you have to make the occupied bed (see Procedure 18.5).

x. Place all soiled linen into laundry bag. Be certain that all bath equipment is clean and put it away as necessary.

y. Place call light, overbed table, nightstand, and telephone within easy reach.

z. Position patient for comfort, and provide warmth.

aa. Remove gloves, if wearing any; discard them in proper receptacle, and perform hand hygiene. Maintain a neat, clean work area.

9. The partial bed bath differs from the bed bath only in that the patient does not need assistance bathing many anatomic regions. Help by bathing those areas that the patient cannot reach (e.g., feet, back, perineal area). All steps of the bath are followed, and the same considerations prevail. Place supplies within easy reach. Change water as noted in the bed bath procedure, and give back care, skin care, nail care, and hair care. A partial bath, in which face, neck, hands, axilla, and perineum are washed, is practiced in some agencies.

The feet might be included in a partial bed bath if necessary.

10. Towel bath.*

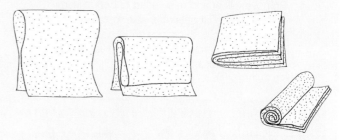

a. Prepare patient.

b. Remove patient's clothing and excess bedding (top linens, bedspread). Place patient on bath blanket, and cover patient with bath blanket.

c. Cover with plastic any surgical dressings, casts, or areas that are not to be gotten wet.

d. Fanfold a clean bath blanket at foot of the bed.

e. Position patient supine with legs partially separated and arms loosely at sides.

f. Prepare towel. Fold towel in half, top to bottom; fold in half again, top to bottom; fold in half again, side to side. Then roll towel–bath towel with bath towel and washcloths inside, beginning with folded edge.

g. Place rolled-up towel–bath towel (with bath towel and washcloths inside) in plastic bag with selvage edges toward open end of bag.

h. Draw 2000 mL of water at 115° to 120°F (46° to 49°C) into plastic pitcher. If the towel is not warm, the sauna-like effect is not produced and the patient is chilled. Measure 30 mL of concentrate with a pump (a single stroke measures 30 mL). Mix 2000 mL of water and no-rinse solution.

i. Pour mixture over towel in plastic bag.

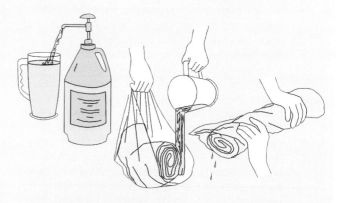

11. Knead the solution quickly into towel; position plastic bag with open end in sink and squeeze out excess water.

a. Bathe patient with the following procedure.

(1) Fold bath blanket down to waist. Remove warm moist towel from plastic bag and

place on patient's right or left chest with open edges up and outward. Unroll towel across chest.

(2) Open towel to cover entire body while removing top bath blanket. Tuck towel–bath towel in and around body (leave bath towel and washcloths in plastic bag to keep warm).

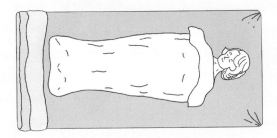

(3) Begin bathing at feet, with gentle massaging motion. Use clean section of towel for each part of body as you move toward patient's head.

(4) Fold lower part of towel upward away from feet as bathing continues. If you have an assistant, the bath is given more effectively.

(5) Continue to draw clean bath blanket upward and place over patient as you move upward. Leave 3 inches of exposed skin between towel and bath blanket. Skin dries in 2 or 3 seconds. If towel bath is given properly, the patient is refreshed and relaxed.

(6) Wash face, neck, and ears with one of the prepared washcloths.

(7) Turn patient onto side.

(8) Use prepared bath towel for back care.

(9) Use second washcloth for perineal care (don disposable gloves). Sometimes you need a basin of warm water, soap, washcloth, towel, and gloves to perform perineal care (see Procedure 18.2).

(10) When bath is completed, remove towel and place with soiled linens in plastic laundry bag.

(11) If top bath blanket is not soiled, fold for reuse later.

b. Make occupied bed (see Procedure 18.5).

12. Tub bath or shower.

a. Follow steps 1 and 3 to 7.

b. Determine whether activity is allowed by consulting patient's activity order.

c. Be certain that tub or shower appliance is clean. See agency policy. Place nonskid mat on tub or shower floor if necessary and disposable mat outside of tub or shower.

d. Assemble all items necessary for bathing.

e. Assist patient to tub or shower. Shower chairs are available in most facilities to transport patients from the bedside to the shower, bathe and dry patients, and return them to bed. Be certain that patient wears robe and slippers.

f. Instruct patient on how to use call signal. Place "in use" sign on tub or shower door if not using private bath.

g. If tub is used, fill with warm water, 109.4°F (43°C). Have patient test water, if able, then adjust temperature. Instruct patient on use of faucets—which is hot and which is cold. If shower is used, turn water on and adjust temperature.

h. Caution patient to use safety bars. Discourage use of bath oil in water. Safety must be maintained at all times. Check on patient every 5 minutes (q 5 min). Do not allow to remain in tub more than 20 minutes.

i. Return when patient signals with the call light. Make an unoccupied bed while the patient bathes unless patient condition is such that you are required to remain with the patient. Return to the tub or shower room and offer to wash the patient's back. Knock before entering.

j. Assist patient out of tub and with drying. Observe the patient for signs and symptoms of weakness, such as rapid pulse, paleness, diaphoresis, unsteady gait, tachypnea, vertigo, and syncope. If patient reports weakness, vertigo, or syncope, drain tub before patient gets out and place towel over patient's shoulders. Notify the nurse.

k. Assist patient into clean gown, robe, and slippers. Accompany to room, position for comfort, and give back rub (see step 14).

l. Make unoccupied bed if patient can tolerate sitting in chair. Perform back, hair, nail, and skin care.

m. Return to shower or tub. Clean according to agency policy. Place all soiled linens in laundry bag and return all articles to patient's bedside.

n. Perform hand hygiene.

13. Tepid sponge bath for temperature reduction.

a. Follow steps 1 and 3 to 7.

b. Assess patient for elevated temperature.

c. Explain to patient; outline steps of the procedure.

d. Assemble equipment.

e. Cover patient with bath blanket, remove gown, and close windows and doors.

f. Test water temperature. Place washcloths in water, and then apply wet cloths to each axilla and groin (the depressed area between the thigh and trunk). If patient is in tub, allow to stay in water for 20 to 30 minutes.

g. Gently sponge an extremity for about 5 minutes. If patient is in tub, gently sponge water over upper torso, chest, and back.

h. Continue sponge bath to other extremities and back, for 3 to 5 minutes each. Assess temperature and pulse q 15 min.

Continued

i. Change water and reapply freshly moistened washcloths to axilla and groin as necessary.

j. Continue with sponge bath until body temperature falls to slightly above normal. Keep body parts that are not being sponged covered. Discontinue procedure according to agency policy.

k. Dry patient thoroughly and cover with light blanket or sheet.

l. Avoid rubbing the skin too vigorously because that may cause an increase in heat production. Leave patient in comfortable position.

m. Clean and return equipment to storage, clean area, and change bed linens as necessary. Perform hand hygiene.

14. Back rub.

a. Prepare supplies.
   - Bath blanket (optional)
   - Bath towel
   - Skin lotion, powder. If powder is used, apply sparingly.

b. Follow steps 1 and 3 to 7 and provide quiet environment.

c. Lower side rail. Position patient with back toward you. Cover patient so that only parts to massage are exposed.

d. Warm hands if necessary. Warm lotion by holding some in hands. Explain that lotion often feels cool.

e. Begin massage by starting in sacral area using circular motions. Stroke upward to shoulders. Massaging over bony prominences is no longer recommended because this may cause skin breakdown.

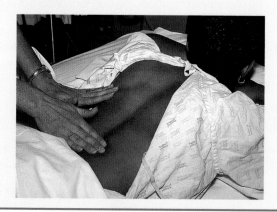

f. Use firm, smooth strokes to massage over scapulae. Continue to upper arms with one smooth stroke and down alongside of back to iliac crest. Do not break contact with patient's skin. Complete massage in 3 to 5 minutes.

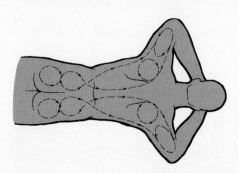

g. Gently but firmly knead skin by grasping area between thumb and fingers. Work across each shoulder and around nape of neck. Continue downward along each side to sacrum.

h. With long smooth strokes, end massage, remove excess lubricant from patient's back with towel, and re-tie gown. Position for comfort. Lower bed and raise side rail as needed and place call button within easy reach.

i. Place soiled laundry in proper receptacle, and perform hand hygiene.

15. Document.
   - Type of bath (e.g., sitz bath, medicated bath, or tepid sponge bath), water temperature, and solution used, when appropriate
   - Duration of treatment
   - Level of assistance required (how much the patient required assistance from you)
   - Vital signs if applicable (e.g., sponge bath for temperature reduction)
   - Patient's response

16. Report alterations in skin integrity to nurse in charge or physician.

---

*An alternative to towel bath is "bath-in-a-bag." This is similar to towel bath except that the washcloth is presoaked with no-rinse soap. The bag is placed in a warmer, and the patient is bathed. Some facilities use disposable cloths for bath-in-a-bag.

(Figures 8a, 8h, and 8i from Perry AG, Potter PA: Clinical nursing skills and techniques, ed 8, St. Louis, 2014, Mosby; Figures 8q and 8s from Potter PA, Perry AG: Fundamentals of nursing: concepts, process, and practice, ed 9, 2017; Figure 14e from Potter PA, Perry AG: Fundamentals of nursing: concepts, process, and practice, ed 9, 2017; Figure 14f from Perry AG, Potter PA, Ostendorf WR: Nursing intervention and clinical skills and techniques, ed 6, St. Louis, 2016, Mosby; Figures 10, 10i, 11a(2) from Cooper K, Gosnell K: Foundations of nursing, ed 7, St. Louis, 2015, Mosby.)

PROCEDURE 18.2

Perineal Care: Male and Female and the Catheterized Patient

1. Refer to medical record, care plan, or Kardex for special interventions.
2. Assemble supplies.
3. Introduce self.
4. Identify patient.
5. Explain procedure.
6. Examine patient for the following, wearing gloves when in contact with mucous membranes or secretions:
   - Accumulated secretions
   - Surgical incision
   - Lesions
   - Ability to perform self-care
   - Extent of care required by patient
7. Remove and dispose of soiled gloves and perform hand hygiene and don clean gloves according to agency policy and guidelines from the CDC and OSHA.
8. Prepare patient for interventions. Allow postpartum patients to perform this procedure by themselves while sitting on the stool, using a pericare squeeze bottle. Patients allowed tub or shower baths do this by themselves. Be certain supplies are close by.
   a. Close door or pull privacy curtain.
   b. Raise bed to comfortable working height and lower side rail.
   c. Arrange supplies at bedside.
   d. Assist patient to desired position in bed: dorsal recumbent for female or supine for male.
   e. Drape for procedure.
9. Female perineal care.
   a. Raise side rail and fill basin two-thirds full of water at 105° to 109°F (41° to 43°C).
   b. Position waterproof pad or towel under patient's buttocks with patient lying in the dorsal recumbent position in bed. Drape patient with bath blanket placed in the shape of a diamond. One corner is under the patient's chin; one corner is on each side of the patient, with the bath blanket wrapped around each foot and leg; and the last corner is between the patient's legs. This corner can be lifted to expose the patient's perineum.

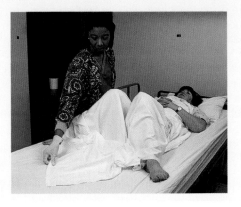

c. With a washcloth or disposable washcloth wrapped around one hand, wash and dry patient's upper thighs.
d. Wash both **labia majora** (larger fold or lip) and **labia minora** (smaller fold or lip). Wash carefully in skin folds. Cleanse in direction anterior to posterior. Use separate corner of washcloth for each skin fold.
e. Separate labia to expose the urinary meatus (opening) and the vaginal orifice. Wash downward toward rectum with smooth strokes. Use separate corner of washcloth for each smooth stroke.

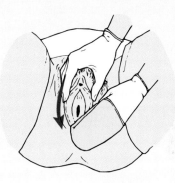

f. Cleanse, rinse, and dry thoroughly.
g. Assist patient to side-lying position and cleanse rectal area with toilet tissue, if necessary. Wash area by cleansing from perineal area toward anus. You may often need several washcloths. Many facilities have disposable wipes. If so, use them. Wash, rinse, and dry thoroughly.

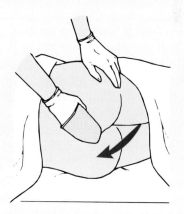

10. Male perineal care.
    a. Raise side rail and fill basin two-thirds full of water at about 105° to 109°F (41° to 43°C).
    b. Gently grasp shaft of penis. Retract foreskin of uncircumcised patient.
    c. Wash tip of penis with circular motion.

Continued

PROCEDURE 18.2

Perineal Care: Male and Female and the Catheterized Patient—cont'd

d. Cleanse from meatus outward. Two washcloths are often necessary. Wash, rinse, and dry gently.

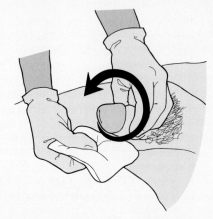

e. Replace foreskin, and wash shaft of penis with a firm but gentle downward stroke. Replace the

foreskin of the uncircumcised male patient after thorough cleansing.

f. Rinse and dry thoroughly.

g. Cleanse scrotum gently. Cleanse carefully in underlying skin folds. Rinse and dry gently.

h. Assist patient to a side-lying position. Cleanse anal area. Follow step 9f of female perineal care.

11. Remove gloves. Clean and store equipment. Dispose of contaminated supplies in proper receptacle. Perform hand hygiene.

12. Position patient for comfort.

13. Document:
   - Procedure
   - Pertinent observations such as the following:
     Character and amount of discharge and odor if present
     Patient's ability to perform own care

14. Report abnormal findings to nurse in charge or healthcare provider.

(Figures from Potter PA, Perry AG: Fundamentals of nursing: Concepts, process, and practice, *ed 9, St. Louis, 2017, Mosby.)*

---

bathe those body parts that are inaccessible to the patient.

If the patient's condition warrants it and ambulation has been ordered, the patient may be allowed to take a tub bath; however, in most facilities, a patient may take a shower. A tepid sponge bath is administered to reduce the elevated temperature of patients who are **febrile** (condition characterized by an elevated body temperature).

A medicated bath is sometimes ordered. This bath is likely to include agents such as oatmeal, cornstarch, Burow's solution (acid and aluminum solution), and soda bicarbonate (alkaline bath). The medicated bath helps reduce tension, relax the patient, and relieve the pruritus (itching) caused by certain skin disorders. When bathing patients who are confused or have dementia, the PCT may find it necessary to adjust the way they interact with those patients (Box 18.5).

Back Care and Back Rub

The PCT typically administers the back rub after the patient's bath. Offer this opportunity to the patient because it promotes relaxation, relieves muscular tension, and stimulates circulation. To give an effective back rub, massage for 3 to 5 minutes (see Procedure 18.1). During the back rub, observe the skin for abnormalities. Monitor pulse and blood pressure of those patients with a history of hypertension or dysrhythmias.

Box 18.5   Bathing Patients Who Have Dementia

- When caregivers maintain a more relaxed demeanor and smile frequently while bathing patients with dementia, the patients demonstrate greater degrees of calmness and cooperation. Use language appropriate to the patient's level of comprehension, and try to determine which words and phrases the patient uses in reference to bathing—some say "washing up" rather than "having a bath," for example. Explain what you intend to do. If the patient reports pain or discomfort, apologize and try to determine and address the cause: for example, "I'm sorry that I hurt you. I won't scrub as hard. Is that better?" Offer reassurance frequently, such as, "You are doing really well; we'll be finished soon," or "As soon as we're finished, I'm going to wrap you in a warm towel and put some of the lotion that you like on your skin."
- Use distraction and negotiation instead of demands.
- Minimize noise in the bathing area.
- Be sure that bathing environment is warm.
- Set priorities as to which body parts need bathing and which can be "skipped."
- Use as few staff as possible.

The back rub is contraindicated if the patient has conditions such as fractures of the ribs or vertebral column, burns, pulmonary embolism, or open wounds. Verify with the nurse that the patient can receive a back rub after the bath.

COMPONENTS OF THE PATIENT'S HYGIENE

Care of the Skin

When a person's physical condition changes, the skin often reflects this by alterations in color, thickness, texture, turgor, temperature, and hydration. As long as the skin remains intact and healthy, its function remains optimal. It is important to remember that intact skin is the first line of defense against infection by invasion of pathogenic organisms.

Data Collection

Determine the condition of the patient's skin by observing its color, texture, thickness, turgor, temperature, and hydration. Be certain to use ample lighting. Natural or halogen lighting is suggested. Normal skin has the following characteristics:

- Intact without abrasions
- Warm and moist
- Localized changes in texture across surface
- Good turgor (elastic and firm); generally smooth and soft
- Skin color variations from body part to body part

Pressure Ulcers

Preventing and treating skin breakdown is one of the highest priorities of care. Prevention is the ultimate goal, but when this is not possible, good interventions can result in (1) optimal healing of the impaired skin without complications; (2) a decrease in the patient's discomfort; (3) a decrease in length of stay in the facility if a discharge is planned; and (4) a decrease in the cost of ongoing care.

Approximately 2.5 million hospitalized patients have pressure ulcers develop each year despite national guidelines regarding their prevention and treatment. Of these 2.5 million patients, 60,000 die of complications, and the financial cost incurred from treating patients with pressure ulcers is estimated at $9 to $11 billion each year (AHRQ, 2016).

To encourage acute care facilities to become more aggressive in the prevention of pressure ulcer development, as of October 2008, the Centers for Medicare and Medicaid stopped covering the costs of treatment of pressure ulcers that develop during the patient's hospitalization. The goal is to prevent patients from experiencing the pain, loss of function, complications such as infection, prolonged hospital stays, and the increased costs associated with the development of pressure ulcers (www.cms.gov).

Pressure ulcers occur when pressure on the skin causes the blood vessels in an area to collapse. The flow of blood and fluid to the cells is impaired, resulting in ischemia, or lack of oxygen and nutrients, to the cells. When the external pressure against the skin is greater than the pressure in the capillary bed (network of capillaries), blood flow decreases to the adjacent tissue. If the pressure continues without relief for more than 2 hours, cells in the involved layers of skin tend to undergo necrosis (death of tissue). Pressure is usually most severe over bony prominences (e.g., sacrum, scapulae, ears, elbows, heels, inner and outer malleoli, inner and outer knees, back of head, trochanteric areas of the hips, and heels).

In addition to unrelieved pressure, two mechanical factors play a common role in the development of pressure ulcers. The first is *shearing force*. This occurs when the tissue layers of skin slide on each other, causing subcutaneous blood vessels to kink or stretch and resulting in an interruption of blood flow to the skin (Fig. 18.3).

The second mechanical factor is *friction*. The rubbing of skin against another surface produces friction, which may remove layers of tissue. This might occur when moving patients in bed by sliding them across the bed linen, when improperly lifting patients, and when improperly placing bedpans.

The appearance of pressure ulcers is a major cause of impaired skin integrity (Fig. 18.4). A patient who stays in one position without relief of pressure, especially over bony prominences, is at risk for development of a pressure ulcer. Patients especially at risk are chronically ill, debilitated, older, disabled, or incontinent and those with spinal cord injuries, limited mobility, circulatory impairment, or poor overall nutrition.

Individuals who are incontinent are at risk because constant contact of the skin with urine and feces often causes chemical irritation, which frequently leads to impaired skin integrity. Nutritional factors play a role for both those who are overweight and those who are underweight. Obesity increases the risk because the added bulk and weight increase the pressure on bony

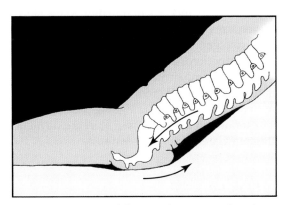

FIGURE 18.3 Diagram of shearing force exerted against sacral area. (From Potter PA, Perry AG: *Fundamentals of nursing: concepts, process, and practice*, ed 9, St. Louis, 2017, Mosby.)

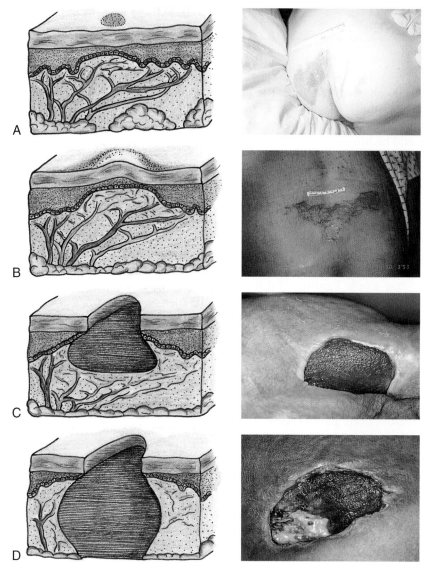

FIGURE 18.4 Stages of pressure ulcers. (From Elkin MK, Perry AG, Potter PA: *Nursing interventions and clinical skills,* ed 4, St. Louis, 2008, Mosby.)

prominences. Obesity also causes increased skin-on-skin contact, especially in skin folds. Underweight increases the risk because of a lack of cushion over the bones and muscles and lack of nutrition to the skin cells. In addition, any condition that results in a decreased supply of oxygen and nutrients to the cells, such as anemia, atherosclerosis, or edema (swelling), increases the risk of skin impairment because the cells are not adequately nourished. Patients who are at increased risk for any reason need careful ongoing assessment and a plan of care aimed at preventing skin impairment (see Coordinated Care box on skin care).

Oral Hygiene

Oral hygiene (care of the oral cavity) helps maintain a healthy state of the mouth, the teeth, the gums, and the lips. Brushing the teeth removes food particles, plaque, and bacteria; massages the gums; and relieves discomfort that results from unpleasant odors and tastes. Complete oral hygiene gives a sense of well-being and thus can stimulate appetite. Proper care prevents oral disease such as gingivitis or periodontitis and tooth destruction. Certain patients are at risk for oral disorders (Box 18.6).

Patients should brush their teeth on their own when possible. When the patient is unable to do so, the PCT needs to perform this procedure (Procedure 18.3).

Dentures (a set of artificial teeth not permanently fixed or implanted) are the patient's personal property. Dentures must be handled with care because they can be easily broken and they can be very expensive. Use an enclosed, labeled cup to soak dentures or to store them when they are not being worn (e.g., during surgery or a diagnostic procedure, or at night). Patients who return

Coordinated Care: Skin Care

Although assessment for the presence of skin impairment is a nursing responsibility and is not to be delegated, the PCT can provide hygienic care in many settings. The PCT should follow these guidelines when providing hygienic care.

- Report any changes in the patient's skin condition, such as redness, irritation, dryness, maceration, or discomfort.
- Provide care to prevent the patient from exposure to body fluids such as urine, feces, wound drainage, and gastric secretions.
- Observe bony prominences (e.g., sacrum, scapulae, ears, elbows, heels, inner and outer malleoli, inner and outer knees, back of head, ischial tuberosities, trochanteric areas of the hips, and heels) for any signs of redness, irritation, or skin breakdown.
- Observe and prevent any areas of pressure from external devices such as oxygen tubing, nasogastric tubing, casts, braces, urinary catheter tubing, or drainage tubing.
- Provide perineal care as needed and observe the area for any signs of skin breakdown. Apply protective barrier creams as allowed by facility policy.

Box 18.6 Conditions That Place Patients at Risk for Oral Disorders

- Not knowing about oral hygiene
- Not able to perform oral care
- Patients in hospitals or long-term care facilities often do not receive good oral care. Patients who are particularly at risk are those experiencing the following:
  - Paralysis
  - Serious illness
  - Upper-extremity activity limitations
  - State of unconsciousness
  - Disorientation
  - Diabetes
  - Nothing-by-mouth (NPO) status
  - Radiation therapy
  - Chemotherapy drugs
  - Oral surgery

from surgery or a diagnostic test and patients who have just woken up in the morning usually prefer to have their dentures reinserted as quickly as possible. Many people find the change in appearance that results when dentures are removed to be embarrassing.

Most patients prefer to clean their dentures themselves; encourage them to do so as often as for natural teeth to prevent infection and irritation. However, when the PCT must assist with denture care, always consider the patient's preference of cleanser and soaking (Procedure 18.4).

Provide oral care regularly; frequency of hygiene measures depends on the condition of the patient's mouth. The benefits of oral hygiene are probably not seen for several days. Repeated cleansing is often needed to remove thick, dried exudate of the tongue and to restore the mucosa's hydration to normal. For patients whose condition means that they need to be turned and repositioned by the staff on a scheduled basis (e.g., every 2 hours), it is helpful to go ahead and provide oral care at these times.

Perineal Care

Perineal care (pericare, or care of the genitalia) is part of the complete bed bath. Those patients most in need of meticulous pericare are those at risk for acquiring an infection: for example, patients with indwelling catheters, patients recovering from rectal or genital surgery, and postpartum patients (those just having a baby). If patients are able to do their own pericare, allow them to do so. A professional, dignified attitude helps diminish embarrassment when providing this care for patients who are unable to do so themselves. Be aware that often the genitalia may have an odor that is unpleasant before pericare being performed. Try to prevent facial expressions that may show that you are uncomfortable with the odor. Catheter care is performed at least two times daily on all patients with indwelling catheters, unless otherwise ordered by the healthcare provider.

Be alert for signs of vaginal or urethral exudate (discharge), skin impairment, unpleasant odors, reports of burning during urination, or localized tenderness or pain of the perineum. Also observe for skin impairment in the perineal area, especially in those patients with urinary or fecal incontinence, rectal and perineal surgical dressings, and indwelling urinary catheters (see Procedure 18.4).

Perineal Care for the Patient With an Indwelling Catheter

Catheter care is to be performed twice daily on all patients with indwelling catheters, unless otherwise ordered by the healthcare provider. Daily catheter care includes cleansing of the meatal–catheter junction with a mild soap and water and sometimes application of a water-soluble microbicidal ointment (only if ordered by the healthcare provider; this is not routinely performed).

Eye, Ear, and Nose Care

Special attention is given to cleansing the eyes, the ears, and the nose during the patient's bath. The PCT often has the responsibility of assisting patients in the care of

---

PROCEDURE 18.3
Administering Oral Hygiene

1. Refer to medical record, nurse, care plan, or Kardex for special interventions.
2. Assemble supplies.
3. Introduce self.
5. Identify patient. Explain procedure to patient.
6. Perform hand hygiene and don clean gloves according to agency policy and guidelines from the CDC and OSHA.
7. Prepare patient for intervention.
   a. Close door or pull privacy curtain.
   b. Raise bed to comfortable working position.
   c. Arrange supplies.
   d. If patient tolerates the activity, provide supplies in the bathroom and allow patient privacy.
   e. If patient is on bed rest but tolerates the activity while remaining in bed, arrange overbed table in front of patient; provide supplies, and allow patient privacy.
   f. If you are performing the procedure with an unconscious patient, position patient's head to the side toward you (dependent side if possible) and close to you.
8. Oral care
   a. Place towel under patient's face and emesis basin under patient's chin.

   b. Carefully separate patient's jaws.
   c. Cleanse mouth using brush, tongue blade, or toothette moistened with cleansing agent. Clean inner and outer tooth surfaces. Swab roof of mouth and inside cheeks. Use flashlight for better visualization of oral cavity. Gently swab tongue. Rinse and repeat. Rinse several times.

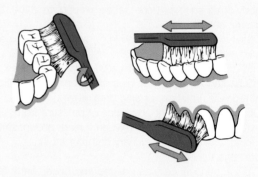

   d. Apply lubricant to lips.

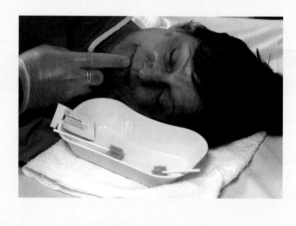

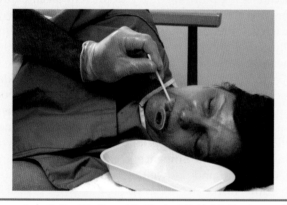

(Figures from Potter PA, Perry AG, Stockert P, Hall A: Fundamentals of nursing: concepts, process, and practice, ed 9, St. Louis, 2017, Elsevier.)

---

eyeglasses, contact lenses, or artificial eyes. For patients who wear eyeglasses, contact lenses, artificial eyes, or hearing aids, assess the patient's knowledge, preferences and methods used to care for the aids, and any problems caused by the aids. Patients who cannot pick up small objects, have limited mobility in the upper extremities, have reduced vision, or are seriously fatigued need the PCT's assistance. The eyes, ears, and nose are sensitive; therefore take extra care to prevent injury to these tissues.

Care of the Eyes

The **circumorbital** (circular area around the eye) area of the eyes is usually cleansed during the bath, typically by washing with a clean washcloth moistened with clear water. Do not use soap because it often causes burning and irritation. Cleanse the eye from the inner to the outer canthus. Use a separate section or corner of the washcloth each time to prevent spread of infection. If the patient has dried exudate that is not removed easily with gentle cleansing, try first placing a damp cotton ball or gauze on the lid margins to loosen secretions. Never apply direct pressure over the eyeball; doing so has potential to cause injury. Remove any exudate from the eyes carefully and as often as necessary to keep the eye clean.

The eyes are well protected with eyelashes, tearing, and a split-second blink reflex and usually do not need special care. However, the unconscious patient is likely to need frequent special eye care. Secretions often collect along the

PROCEDURE 18.4
Denture Care

1. Fill emesis basin half full of tepid water or place a washcloth in the bottom of the sink.
2. Ask patient to remove dentures and place in emesis basin. If patient is unable to remove own dentures, break suction that holds upper denture in place by using thumb and finger. With gauze, apply gentle downward tug and carefully remove from patient's mouth. Next, remove lower denture by carefully lifting up and turning sideways. Remove and place in emesis basin.
3. Cleanse biting surfaces. Cleanse outer and inner tooth surfaces. Be certain to cleanse lower surface of dentures.

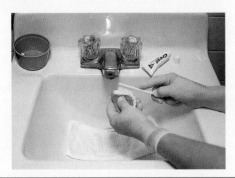

4. Rinse dentures thoroughly with tepid water.
5. Before replacing dentures in patient's mouth or after storing dentures properly, gently brush patient's gums, tongue, and inside of cheeks and rinse thoroughly.
6. Replace dentures either in patient's mouth or in container of solution placed in safe place.
7. When reinserting the dentures, replace the upper denture first if patient has both dentures. Apply gentle pressure to reestablish the suction. Moisten dentures for easier insertion. Be certain that dentures are comfortably situated in patient's mouth before leaving the bedside.
8. Dispose of gloves in proper receptacle. Clean and store supplies. Perform hand hygiene.
9. Position patient for comfort, raise side rail, and lower bed.
10. Assess for patient comfort.
11. Document:
    - Procedure.
    - Pertinent observations (bleeding gums, dry mucosa, ulcerations, or crust on tongue).
    - Most facilities have flow sheets for documenting activities of daily living (ADLs).
    - Report bleeding or presence of lesions to nurse in charge or to healthcare provider.

(Figure from Perry AG, Potter PA: Nursing interventions and clinical skills, ed 6, St. Louis, 2016, Mosby.)

margins of the lid and the inner canthus when the blink reflex is absent or when the eyes do not completely close.

Many patients wear eyeglasses. They cost the patient a lot of money; therefore use care when cleaning glasses and protect them from breakage or other damage when not worn.

Store eyeglasses in the case and place them in the drawer of the bedside stand when not in use to prevent accidentally breaking or damaging them. Eyeglasses may require special cleansing solutions and drying tissues. Washcloths, towels, tissue paper, and paper towels should not be used when cleaning eyeglasses. Cloth made of a soft microfiber material is generally preferred for cleaning eyeglass lenses.

Most patients prefer caring for their own contact lenses. A contact lens is a small, round, sometimes colored disk that fits on the cornea of the eye over the pupil. If the patient's condition does not permit self-removal of the lenses, seek assistance if necessary from someone who is familiar with the procedure (Box 18.7). The lenses need not be reinserted until the patient is more capable of caring for the lenses. The PCT must protect those patients who are unable to care for their lenses properly because wearing of contact lenses too long is likely to cause damage to the cornea. A large variety of products are available for lens care. Use only the products that are the preference of the patient.

Care of the Ears

The ears are cleansed during the bed bath. A clean corner of a moistened washcloth rotated gently into the ear canal works best for cleaning. Also, a cotton-tipped applicator is useful for cleansing the pinna or outside aspects of the external ear. Teach patients never to use bobby pins, toothpicks, cotton-tipped applicators, or any device to clean the internal auditory canal. These objects easily damage the tympanic membrane (eardrum) or cause cerumen (wax) to become affected in the canal.

Hearing Aids

Hearing loss is a common health problem. The ability to hear enables patients to communicate and react appropriately to things that arouse them in their environment. The care of the hearing aid involves routine cleanings, battery care, and proper insertion technique. Ask the patient how they normally clean their hearing aid. Determine whether the patient hears clearly with the use of the aid by talking slowly and clearly in a

Box 18.7   Contact Lens Removal and Care

Soft Lenses

- Wear gloves if drainage is suspected or present.
- If possible, have patient look straight ahead. Retract lower eyelid, and expose lower edge of lens.
- With pad of index finger, slide lens off cornea to white of eye.
- Pull upper eyelid down gently with thumb of other hand, and compress lens slightly between thumb and index finger.
- Gently pinch lens, and lift out without allowing edges to stick together.
- If lens edges stick together, place lens in palm and soak thoroughly with sterile saline or contact solution.
- Place lens in storage case with contact solution.
- Follow recommended procedure for cleansing and disinfecting.

Rigid Lenses

- Wear gloves if exudate is suspected or present.
- Be sure that lens is positioned directly over cornea. If it is not, have patient close eyelids. Place index and middle fingers of one hand beside the lens, and gently but firmly massage lens back over cornea.
- Place index finger on outer corner of patient's eye, and draw skin gently back toward ear.
- Ask patient to blink. Do not release pressure on lids until blink is completed.
- If lens fails to pop out, gently retract eyelid beyond edges of lens. Press lower eyelid gently against lower edge of lens.
- If patient is unable to assist, use a specially designed suction cup. Place cup on center of lens, and while applying suction, gently remove lens off patient's cornea.
- Place lens in storage case.
- Follow manufacturer's recommended procedure for cleansing and disinfecting.

Delegation and Documentation Box 18.2

Care of the Hearing Aid

The skill of caring for a hearing aid is appropriate to delegate to you as the PCT.

- Confirm that patient knows proper way to care for prosthetic device.
- Clarify communication tips to use for individual patient while aid is being cleaned.
- Report presence of any drainage to registered nurse (RN).
- The small size of hearing aids (see Fig. 18.4) frequently makes handling and manipulating the devices difficult for older adults. Have patients with this difficulty contact their hearing aid specialist for assistance. Family members are often able to assist with care of device.
- High-pitched signals associated with consonants f, p, t, k, ch, sh, and st are more difficult to hear clearly as people age.
- Avoid exposure of aid to extreme heat or cold. Do not leave in its case near stove, heater, or sunny window. Do not use it with hair dryer on hot settings or with sunlamp.
- Remove aid for bathing and when at hair stylist.
- Hair spray tends to clog hearing aid.
- Because of the typically high number of hearing aids in long-term care facilities, patients and their families need to clearly mark the hearing aid with identifying information.
- Always store the hearing aid according to facility policy.
- Instruct family to buy an extra battery to keep in patient's bedside table, whenever possible.
- Instruct patients not to remove their aids in common rooms of the facility (e.g., sunroom, recreation areas).

normal voice tone. Have the patient suggest any additional tips for care of the hearing aid. When not in use, see that the hearing aid is stored where it will not become damaged. Take care to turn off the hearing aid or remove the battery when not in use to prolong the life of the battery. Clean the outside of the hearing aid with a dry, soft cloth.

Care of the Nose

The patient is usually able to remove secretions from the nose by gently blowing into a soft tissue. This is often the only daily hygiene necessary. Teach the patient that harsh blowing causes pressure capable of injuring the tympanic membrane (eardrum), the nasal mucosa, and even sensitive eye structures. If the patient is not able to clean the nose, give assistance, using a saline solution–moistened washcloth or cotton-tipped applicator. Never insert the applicator beyond the cotton tip. If nasal

secretions are excessive, suctioning sometimes is necessary. When the patient receives oxygen per nasal cannula or has a nasogastric tube, cleanse the nares every 8 hours with a cotton-tipped applicator moistened with saline solution. Because secretions are more likely to collect and dry around the tube, the tube should be cleansed with water and a mild soap.

Bed Making

The patient's bed is usually made in the morning after the bath. When possible, make the bed while it is not occupied, when the patient is in the tub, showering, or out of the room for a diagnostic examination or procedure. When the patient is unable to be out of bed, you make an occupied bed (Procedure 18.5).

Patient safety is a top priority. Comfort and privacy are also important. Remember to use side rails, to keep the call light within easy reach, and to maintain the bed in the proper position: high position while working at the bedside, and low position when work is completed, to protect the patient from accidental falls.

PROCEDURE 18.5
Bed Making

1. Refer to medical record, nurse, care plan, or Kardex to determine potential for orders or specific precautions for mobility and positioning.
2. Gather supplies.
3. Introduce self.
4. Identify patient.
5. Explain procedure.
6. Perform hand hygiene and don gloves according to agency policy and guidelines from the CDC and OSHA.
7. Prepare patient.
   a. Close door or pull privacy curtain.
   b. Raise bed to appropriate height and lower side rail on the side closest to you.
   c. Lower head of bed (HOB) if patient tolerates it.
   d. Assess patient's tolerance of procedure. Be alert for signs of discomfort and fatigue.
8. Occupied bed.
   a. Remove spread and blanket separately and, if soiled, place in laundry bag. If linens will be reused, fold neatly and place over back of chair. (Keep linens away from uniform.) Do not fan or shake linens.
   b. Place bath blanket over patient on top of sheet.
   c. Request patient to hold onto bath blanket while you remove top sheet by drawing sheet out from under bath blanket at foot of bed. If patient is unable to assist, you need to hold bath blanket in place while removing sheet.
   d. Place soiled sheet in laundry bag.
   e. With assistance from coworker, slide mattress to top of bed.
   f. Position patient to far side of bed with the back toward you. Assure patient that he or she will not fall out of bed. Adjust pillow for comfort. Be sure that side rail is up.
   g. Beginning at head and moving toward foot, loosen bottom linens. Fanfold linen draw sheet, protective draw sheet, and bottom sheet, tucking edges of linens under patient.
   h. Apply clean linens to bed by first placing mattress pad (if used). Fold lengthwise, ensuring that crease is in center of bed. Likewise, unfold bottom sheet and place over mattress pad. Place hem of bottom sheet (if flat sheet is used) with rough edge down and just even with bottom edge of mattress (see illustration of step 9g).
   i. Miter corners (if flat sheet) at head of bed. Continue to tuck in sheet alongside toward front, keeping linens smooth.

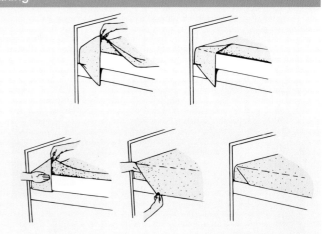

j. Reach under patient to pull out protective draw sheet (if used), and smooth out over clean bottom sheet. Tuck in. Unfold linen draw sheet and place center fold along middle of bed, smooth out over protective draw sheet, and tuck in. Tuck in folded linens in center of bed so that they are under patient's buttocks and torso.

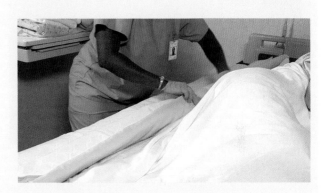

k. Keep palms down as linens are tucked under mattress.
l. Raise side rail and assist patient to roll slowly toward you over folds of linen. Go to opposite side of bed and lower side rail.

Continued

PROCEDURE 18.5

Bed Making—cont'd

m. Loosen edges of all soiled linens. Remove by folding into a bundle, and place in laundry bag. Perform hand hygiene and don a new pair of clean gloves.

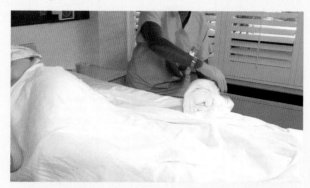

n. Spread clean linens, including protective draw sheet, out over mattress and smooth out wrinkles. Assist patient to supine position and position pillow for comfort.

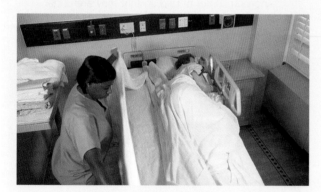

o. Miter top corner of bottom sheet, pulling sheet taut. Tuck bottom sheet under mattress all the way to foot of bed.

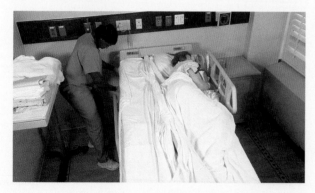

p. Smooth out draw sheets. Pulling sheet taut, tuck in protective draw sheet, and then tuck in linen draw sheet, first in center, then top, and bottom last.

q. Place top sheet over bath blanket that is over patient. Request patient to hold top sheet while you remove bath blanket. Place blanket in laundry bag. (Be sure that center fold of sheet is in center of bed.) If blanket is used, place over sheet and place spread over blanket. Form cuff with top linens under patient's chin.

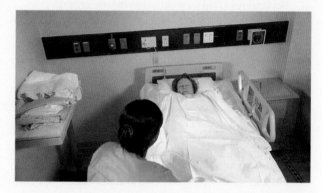

r. Tuck in all linens at foot of bed, making modified miter corner (see illustration). Raise side rail and make opposite side of bed. Remember to allow for toe pleat. Make toe pleat by placing fold either lengthwise down center of bed or across foot of bed.

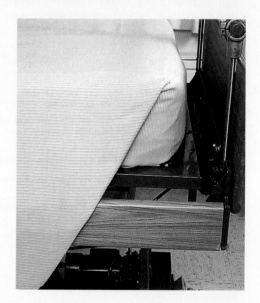

s. Change pillowcase. Grasp closed end of pillowcase, turning case inside out over hand. Now grasp one end of pillow with your hand in the case and smooth out wrinkles, ensuring pillow corners fit into pillowcase corners. *(Never place pillow on top of patient while changing its cover.)* As pillow is removed from under patient, support neck muscles. Never hold pillow under your chin.

PROCEDURE 18.5

Bed Making—cont'd

9. Unoccupied bed.
   a. Starting at head of bed, loosen linens all the way to foot. Go to opposite side of bed, loosen linens, roll all linens up in ball, and place in soiled laundry bag. Do not permit linens to come in contact with uniform. Do not shake or fan linens. Wash hands after handling soiled linens. Perform hand hygiene.
   b. If blanket and spread are to be reused, fold neatly and place over back of chair. Remove soiled pillowcase.
   c. Slide mattress to head of bed.
   d. If necessary, clean mattress with cloth moistened with antiseptic solution, and dry thoroughly.
   e. Begin to make bed standing on side where lines are placed. Unfold bottom sheet, placing fold lengthwise down center of bed. Be certain that rough edge of hem lies down away from patient's heels and even with edge of mattress. Smooth out sheet over top edge of mattress and miter corners (see step 8i). Tuck remaining sheet under mattress all the way to foot. Keep linens smooth.
   f. Place draw sheet on bed so that center fold lies down middle of bed. If protective draw sheet is to be used, place it on first. Smooth out over mattress and tuck in. Keep palms down.
   g. Place top sheet over bed and smooth out. Place blanket over top sheet. Smooth out. Place spread over blanket and smooth out. Make cuff with top linens.
   h. Allow for toe pleat. Make modified mitered corner by not tucking tip of sheet under mattress.
   i. Move to opposite side of bed and complete making bed as described in steps 9e to 9h. Pull linens tight and keep taut as linens are tucked in.
   j. Put on clean pillowcase (see step 8s). Place pillow at head of bed and position for comfort. Place call light within easy reach and lower bed level.
   k. If patient is to return to bed, fanfold top linens down to foot of bed. Be sure that cuff at top of linens is easily accessible to patient.
10. Arrange personal items on bed table or bedside stand and place within patient's easy reach.
11. Leave area neat and clean.
12. Place all soiled linens in proper receptacle. Remove gloves. Perform hand hygiene.
13. Assist patient to bed, and position for comfort.
14. Documentation:
    • Bed making does not have to be recorded in most facilities.
    • Record patient's vital signs only if changes occur.
15. Report any abnormal findings to nurse in charge.

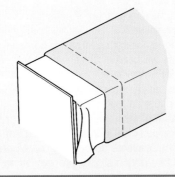

(Figure 8i from Elkin MK, Perry AG, Potter PA: Nursing interventions and clinical skills, ed 4, St. Louis, 2008; Figures 8j, m, n, o, q from Mosby's nursing assistant video skills, 4.O, St. Louis; Figures 8r, 9g from Elkin MK, Perry AG, Potter PA: Nursing interventions and clinical skills, ed 3, St. Louis, 2004.)

The PCT's responsibility is to keep the bed as clean and comfortable as possible. This means that you will need to check the bed frequently to ensure that bedding is clean, dry, and wrinkle-free. Look for food particles in the linens after meals and for urine incontinence or stooling. If linens are soiled with urine, feces, blood, or emesis, change them. Use waterproof pads with caution. Accumulation of moisture creates a risk for skin irritation and breakdown.

Follow basic principles of medical asepsis (Box 18.8).

Box 18.8 Principles of Medical Asepsis for Bed Making

• Keep soiled linens away from uniform.
• Wear gloves when handling soiled linen.
• Place soiled linens in hamper or plastic bag.
• Never fan linens in the air. *(This causes air currents, which spread microorganisms.)*
• Never place soiled linens on the floor. If clean linens touch the floor, place in laundry hamper immediately.
• Remove all unnecessary equipment and maintain a neat work area.

Use proper body mechanics while making the bed: for example, raise the bed to a working level to avoid bending down or stretching. Also, apply the principles of body mechanics while turning and repositioning the patient.

The two ways to make an unoccupied bed are open and closed. In the open bed, the top linens are fan-folded toward the foot of the bed to allow the patient to return to bed more easily. A closed bed is prepared after a patient's discharge or transfer, or when the patient dies, before another patient is admitted. Closed beds are frequently made in long-term care settings because many patients do not return to bed until night time. Housekeeping personnel clean the mattress and bed and apply fresh linens (see Procedure 18.5).

The postoperative bed is a form of the open bed. The top sheet and the spread are not mitered or tucked in at the corners. The top linens are usually fan-folded lengthwise or crosswise at the foot of the patient's bed. Arrange the top bed linens in such a way that they allow easy transfer of the surgical patient from the gurney to the bed. A complete linen change is done if the patient is returning from surgery (Fig. 18.5).

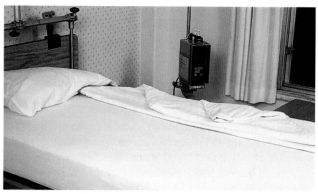

FIGURE 18.5 The postoperative bed. (From Potter PA, Perry AG: *Fundamentals of nursing: concepts, process, and practice,* ed 9, St. Louis, 2017, Mosby.)

Injury & Illness Prevention Box 18.1

In order to prevent injury to the patient, the PCT should follow these guidelines:

- Know how to assess temperature of the bath water, especially for elderly and other patients with reduced sensation (e.g., bath thermometer).
- Be sure to inspect surfaces between skin folds for signs of irritation or impairment (breakdown; e.g., erythema, scalding).
- Perform proper cleansing of the perineum (e.g., female patients: cleansing from front to back; uncircumcised males: retracting foreskin to adequately cleanse underneath, then replacing foreskin).
- Wash hands before and after performing catheter care or after urinating and defecating.
- Prevent or heal dry lips by applying lip ointment or lubricant and avoiding licking the lips.
- Practice proper storage methods for dentures, stressing techniques of cleaning that avoid damage to dentures (e.g., use brush with soft bristles; carry dentures in a container; hold dentures with cloth to avoid dropping).
- Remove patient's dentures at bedtime to give gums a rest and to store dentures in water or cleansing solution to prevent drying and warping.
- Encourage proper hair care: regular shampooing, avoidance of chemicals and hot combs for straightening hair (may result in scalp burns, hair loss, or allergic reaction).
- Perform proper foot care:
  - Wash and soak feet daily with lukewarm water; thoroughly pat feet dry and dry well between toes. Soaking the feet of a patient with diabetes or a patient with peripheral vascular disease is not recommended. This potentially leads to maceration (excessive softening of the skin), skin breakdown, and infection.
  - File nails; never clip them if patient is diabetic or has circulatory issues.
  - Be cautious against self-treating corns or calluses. The nurse will consult the physician to see if there is a need for a podiatrist.
  - If needed, apply a mild foot powder.
  - Inspect patient's feet daily.
  - Ensure that patients wear clean socks or stockings daily (change twice a day if feet perspire).
  - Ensure that patients do not walk barefoot.
  - Be sure that patients wear properly fitting shoes.
  - Wash and dry minor cuts immediately. Use only mild antiseptic (e.g., triple antibiotic ointment).
- Clean the eye by going from the inner corner or canthus to the outer corner or canthus.
- Never insert hairpins, toothpicks, cotton-tipped applicators, or any device into the ear canal. If necessary, consult a physician.
- Perform good skin care:
  - Process of wound healing and expected wound appearance.
  - Signs and symptoms of pressure ulcers to report to healthcare team.
  - Prevention guidelines to halt further breakdown.
  - Importance of good nutrition and adequate fluid intake.

CHAPTER SUMMARY

Hygiene is a personal matter; all factors that influence the personal hygiene routine must be considered. Be sure that the patient's room is comfortable, safe, and large enough to allow the patient and visitors to move around freely.

Assisting or providing the patient with daily hygienic needs allows you to use communication skills to develop a meaningful relationship with the patient. Consider the patient's personal preferences as you plan the daily hygienic care. Be sure to maintain the patient's privacy and comfort when providing daily care.

External pressure, shearing force, moisture, impaired peripheral circulation, edema, and obesity contribute to the development of pressure ulcers. When the external pressure against the skin is greater than the pressure in the capillary bed, blood flow decreases to the adjacent tissues. Pressure ulcers tend to occur initially in the superficial layers of the skin.

Preventive skin care is aimed at controlling external pressure on bony prominences and keeping the skin clean, well lubricated, hydrated, and free of excess moisture. Proper positioning reduces the effects of pressure and guards against shearing force.

Cleansing and topical agents used to treat pressure ulcers vary according to the stage of the ulcer. Wear gloves during hygienic care when there is risk of contracting body fluids.

Case Scenario

You are a female PCT and have been assigned to give a bed bath to a male patient who is of Asian descent. Knowing that this culture prefers caregivers who are of the same gender, how would you go about completing the task of the bed bath without offending the patient's cultural beliefs? Can you refuse the bed bath based on the patient's gender? What are the choices you have, considering the bed bath must get done, and the patient's rights must be protected?

REVIEW QUESTIONS

1. During the bed bath, the PCT covers the patient with a bath blanket. The patient asks what the bath blanket is for. What is the PCT's best response?
   a. "The bath blanket helps to prevent skin irritation."
   b. "The bath blanket is part of our bathing procedure."
   c. "The bath blanket is used to prevent the spread of microorganisms."
   d. "The bath blanket helps to prevent chilling."

2. A 64-year-old patient with terminal cancer is too weak to perform her own perineal care. The PCT includes bathing which areas as part of perineal care?
   a. Back and buttocks
   b. Eyes, ears, and nose
   c. Upper torso and thighs
   d. Upper thighs, genitalia, and anal area

3. A 52-year-old patient is in her second postoperative day after an abdominal hysterectomy. The PCT plans to give the patient a bed bath. Which action is most appropriate when caring for the patient's face?
   a. Use only water.
   b. Ask the patient her preference.
   c. Use soap in all areas except the eyes.
   d. Use a cleansing cream.

4. The PCT is providing oral care to an 82-year-old patient who is unconscious. The optimal position for providing oral hygiene to this patient is _____ to prevent choking.
   a. High Fowler position
   b. High Fowler position with head hyperextended
   c. Supine with the head lowered
   d. Side-lying with head facing to the side

5. A 72-year-old patient has pancreatitis. The PCT cleanses her ears while giving her a soothing bed bath. Which intervention for cleansing her ears is correct for this bath?
   a. Cleansing the outer ear with the washcloth during the bath
   b. Retracting the outer ear downward to loosen visible cerumen
   c. Irrigating to remove tenacious cerumen
   d. Using cotton-tipped applicators to remove cerumen

6. An 82-year-old patient is in his first postoperative day. As part of his morning care, the PCT removes and cleanses his dentures. Which of the following techniques is correct?
   a. Work over an open sink convenient to the water faucet.
   b. Rinse dentures thoroughly with hot water.
   c. Brush dentures with a soft toothbrush.
   d. Hold dentures securely in the palm of the hand.

Assisting With Grooming

LEARNING OBJECTIVES

1. Describe personal hygienic practices.
2. Describe the procedures for shaving, hair care, and nail care.
3. Discuss safety precautions to take when shaving the patient.
4. Discuss the procedures for dressing the patient.
5. Explain how to change the gown of a patient with an intravenous line.

KEY TERMS

alopecia An area of the scalp where there is hair loss or no hair; also known as baldness
anticoagulant therapy Medications that increase the tendency to bleed
dandruff An excessive amount of flaking skin that appears white in color
grooming Taking care of one's personal needs
hygiene The activities to maintain personal cleanliness
pediculosis capitis Head lice
podiatrist A doctor who specializes in the care of the feet
tinea capitis Also known as ringworm, a fungal infection of the skin

COMPONENTS OF THE PATIENT'S HYGIENE

Ensuring that the patient's hygiene needs are attended to is an important part of the care delivered by the patient care technician. A person's hair, skin, and nails, if left uncared for, can cause further illness or disease. Grooming, or the overall taking care of one's personal needs as they relate to hygiene, can affect how comfortable the person is.

Hair Care

Proper hair care is important to the patient's self-image. Combing, brushing, and shampooing are basic hygiene measures needed by all patients. Illness or disability often prevents patients from performing their own daily hair care, especially when their hands are affected. A patient who is confined to the bed will have hair that soon becomes tangled. Remember, most patients are aware of their appearance at all times. Good hair care should be performed routinely, at least daily, to meet the hygiene needs of the patient. If the patient is not able to carry out this part of self-care, the patient care technician needs to give assistance.

Brushing the Hair

When a patient stays in the bed throughout the day, his or her hair is easily tangled and becomes matted in the back. This can cause discomfort for the person, and may make them feel embarrassed to be seen. Personal hygiene is important to maintain in order to keep the person comfortable. Brushing their hair is one way to maintain that comfort.

If patients are able to brush their own hair, allow them to do so. This encourages independence and gives them some control. If they are unable to brush their own hair, then you as the patient care technician may need to assist them, or do it for them. Typically, brushing and combing the person's hair is done at the beginning of the day, although some prefer to do it just before bedtime. It may also be done during the day if the person is expecting family or friends to visit.

Brushing the hair is a healthy behavior because it promotes blood flow to the scalp and helps to move the oils located on the hair shaft throughout the head. It can be an uncomfortable procedure though when the person's hair is tangled or matted. To decrease their discomfort, start at the scalp of the head and work your way down to the ends. Brush or comb small sections of hair at a time. Some patients will prefer you to braid their hair once it is brushed, or to place it upon their head in the form of a bun or in an elastic band that will hold the hair together. This is completely up to the patient; it should not be forced upon them.

Some patients may have specific preferences when brushing their hair, such as use of special oils or conditioners. Be sure to ask patients of their preferences before beginning to comb or brush their hair.

There are a variety of combs and brushes that can be used on the hair. Take care when using a round brush to not cause further entanglement by rolling the hair onto the brush. It is easier to brush straight downward instead of using a rolling method. If a knot or entanglement does occur when brushing or combing, notify the nurse at once for assistance.

Some patients may experience dandruff, which is an excessive amount of flaking skin that appears white in color. You may notice this on the person's clothes, near the shoulder and neck area. It is not considered to be infectious or contagious. Often a specialized shampoo may help to provide extra moisture to the scalp.

Some patients may experience an area where there is hair loss, or they may be completely bald; this is known as alopecia. Patients who have recently undergone chemotherapy, a treatment for cancer, may experience areas of alopecia. If there is a small patch of hair loss noted by flaking of the skin, notify the nurse at once, as this may be a fungal infection known as tinea capitis, or ringworm. This is a contagious skin infection and one that needs to be treated with oral or topical medication.

If, while combing the patient's hair, you notice very small insects moving from one area to another, notify the nurse at once. Pediculosis capitis, or head lice, is the presence of very small parasites known as lice. They migrate to the scalp of the head for a blood supply in order to live, and they travel up and down the shaft of the hair throughout the day. Lice must return to the scalp every 24 hours to feed and grow. It is highly contagious, and easily spread from one patient to another if appropriate care measures are not taken.

Injury & Illness Prevention Box 19.1

- To prevent the spread of pediculosis capitis, or head lice, never share the brush or comb of one patient with another.
- All head coverings, such as hats, scarves, and hair pieces, should be labeled with the patient's name and used only with that patient.
- Sharing of any articles that touch the head can promote the spread of head lice.

Shampooing the Hair

If the patient is able to take a shower or tub bath, the hair can be easily shampooed at this time. One option is to use a portable chair in the shower, and another is to place a chair in front of a sink. For the bedfast patients who are unable to independently shampoo themselves, the shampoo must be performed with the patient in bed.

Sometimes there is a shampoo tray that can be used to shampoo the person in bed. The tray is directed to the side of the bed so that the water drains into a collecting basin and not on the patient's bed linens (Fig. 19.1).

Check whether a healthcare provider's order is necessary. Most facilities have portable blow dryers, curling irons, and shampoo boards available (Procedure 19.1). Shampoo caps are often available (cap with no-rinse shampoo inside). Dry shampoos are also available in most facilities.

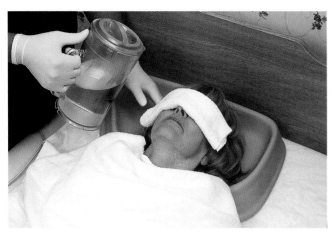

FIGURE 19.1 Shampoo tray. (From Sorrentino SA: *Mosby's assisting with patient care,* ed 2, St. Louis, 2004, Mosby.)

Injury & Illness Prevention Box 19.2

- Be careful when shampooing patients to keep the shampoo out of their eyes. It can cause burning and irritation.
- Be sure to rinse all of the shampoo out of the person's hair; if there is some left, it can cause irritation to the scalp.
- Always follow standard precautions when shampooing the person's hair, especially if any lesions or wounds are present.

Delegation and Documentation Box 19.1

- Verify with the nurse whether you are to shampoo the person's hair.
- Discuss with the nurse whether the person is able to assist with the shampooing or if he or she will need total assistance.
- Verify what type of shampoo the patient is to receive.
- Always follow safety precautions with maintaining the temperature of the water so that it will not burn the patient.
- Document any observations of lesions, scalp lice, bare spots, and whether or not the patient tolerated the procedure well.

PROCEDURE 19.1
Giving Hair Care

1. Verify with the nurse the need for a shampoo.
2. Introduce self.
3. Identify patient.
4. Explain procedure.
5. Perform hand hygiene and don clean gloves according to agency policy and guidelines from the Centers for Disease Control and Prevention (CDC) and the Occupational Safety and Health Administration (OSHA).
6. Prepare patient.
   a. Close door or pull privacy curtain.
   b. Raise bed to a comfortable working height.
   c. Arrange supplies at bedside or, if patient is able to perform procedure, have supplies available in the bathroom and offer assistance as needed.
7. Bed shampoo.
   a. Position patient close to one side of bed. Place shampoo board under patient's head and washbasin at end of spout. Ensure that spout extends over edge of mattress (see Fig. 19.1).
   b. Position rolled-up bath towel under patient's neck. Certain conditions such as cervical neck injuries, open incisions, and tracheostomy place the patient at risk for injury, in which case a modified position is used.

c. Brush and comb patient's hair. If hair is matted with blood, hydrogen peroxide is effective as a cleansing agent.
d. Obtain water in pitcher at about 110°F (43°C).
e. If patient is able, instruct patient to hold washcloth over eyes. Completely wet hair and apply small amount of shampoo.

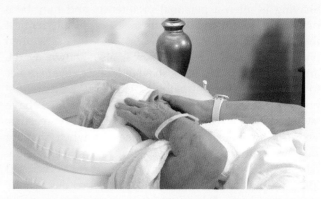

Continued

PROCEDURE 19.1

Giving Hair Care—cont'd

f. Massage scalp with pads of fingertips, not nails. Shampoo hairline, back of neck (lift head slightly), and sides of hair.

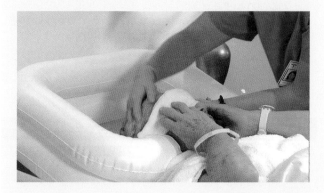

g. Rinse thoroughly and apply more shampoo, repeating steps e and f. Rinse, and repeat rinsing until hair is free of shampoo.
h. Wrap dry towel around patient's head. Dry patient's face, neck, and shoulders. Dry hair and scalp with second towel.

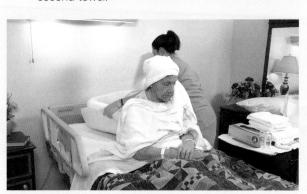

i. Comb hair and dry with hair dryer as quickly as possible.

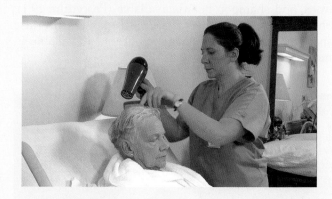

j. Complete styling hair and position patient for comfort.
k. Report abnormal findings (breaks in the skin or ulcerations) to nurse in charge.

(Figures from Mosby's nursing assistant video skills 4.0, St. Louis, 2015, Elsevier.)

Shaving the Patient

Shaving is often a personal preference, and may be a practice of both men and women. Men typically request their beard or upper lip to be shaved, whereas women typically request their axilla area, also known as the armpit, and their legs to be shaved. Many patients prefer to shave at the time of bathing. Although there are disposable razors that use a blade, most facilities have switched to electric razors because of safety reasons. There is an increased risk of bleeding when shaving someone with a razor blade. Electric razors decrease the risk significantly. An electric razor should always be used for those patients who have a bleeding disorder or who are undergoing anticoagulant therapy (medications that increase the tendency to bleed). Do not allow a disoriented or depressed patient to use a razor with a blade, to prevent accidental or self-inflicted injury. A male patient's beard, mustache, or sideburns are never removed without consent of the patient except for emergency purposes.

The patient needs to be shaved if unable to perform this himself or herself (e.g., the patient is too ill or has an arm immobilized in traction or a cast) (see Procedure 19.2).

HAND, FOOT, AND NAIL CARE

Hands and feet often need special attention to prevent infection, odors, and injury. Problems arise from abuse or poor care of the hands and feet (e.g., biting the nails or wearing ill-fitting shoes).

Administer care of the hands and feet during the morning bath, or at another time if desired (see

PROCEDURE 19.2

Shaving the Patient

Verify with the nurse the need for a shave.

1. Assemble supplies.
3. Introduce self.
4. Identify patient.
5. Explain procedure.
6. Assess patient for the following:
   - Contraindications to shaving (patients who are on blood thinners may be restricted from shaving)
   - Restrictions to positioning, conditions of the skin
   - Patient's ability to care for their own shaving needs.
7. Perform hand hygiene and don clean gloves according to agency policy and guidelines from the CDC and OSHA.
8. Prepare patient for intervention.
   a. Close door or pull privacy curtain.
   b. Raise bed to a comfortable working height.
   c. Arrange supplies at bedside or, if patient is able to perform procedure, have supplies available in the bathroom and offer assistance as needed.
9. Shaving the patient.
   a. Assist patient to sitting position if patient is able.
   b. Observe face and neck for lesions, moles, or birthmarks.
   c. Use shaving cream or soap if an electric razor is not available.

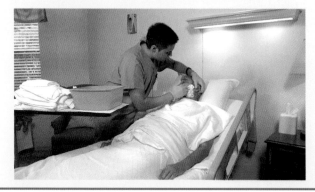

d. Shave in direction hair grows. Use short strokes. Start with upper face and lips, and then extend to neck. If patient is able, hyperextending (tilting backward) his head is helpful to shave curved areas.
e. Pull skin taut with nondominant hand above or below the area being shaved. *(Promotes uniform shaving.)*

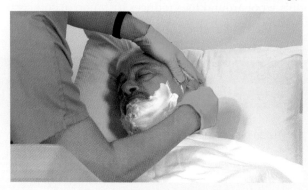

f. Rinse razor after each stroke if using a disposable razor.
g. Rinse and dry face.
h. If patient desires, apply lotion or cologne.
i. Dispose of blades in sharps container.

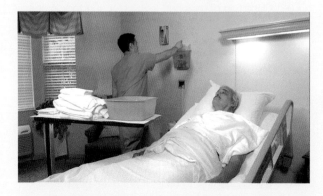

j. Report abnormal findings (breaks in the skin or ulcerations) to nurse in charge. *(Additional interventions are sometimes required.)*

(Figures from Mosby's nursing assistant video skills 4.0, *St. Louis, 2015, Elsevier.)*

Procedure 19.3). Many patients enjoy having their hands massaged with lotion. This increases blood flow to the fingers and provides comfort. Fingernails and toenails should be kept short to limit the number of bacteria that grow underneath the nail. Some patients prefer to have a nail polish painted on their nails. This is a personal preference. By taking the time to paint the patient's nails, you are showing them that you care for them. Remember that their physical presence is often very important to them. They are made to feel pretty or handsome by the way they look

to others. Your interest in ensuring that their nails are in good shape can make them feel cared for and loved.

Pay special attention to the toenails of both men and women. Some patients are prone, or more likely, to grow ingrown toenails; that is, the corner of the nail is growing down into the skin. This is often painful and can result in causing a skin infection. Be sure to notify the nurse if you notice any ingrown toenails.

Some patients who have diabetes, or a decreased circulation to their feet, are unable to have foot care given by the patient care technician. These patients are more likely to experience trauma or injury to their feet and therefore need the care of a nurse or podiatrist.

Some patients will choose alternative therapies to comfort their feet. Moleskin applied to areas on feet that rub together, or are under friction, is less likely to cause local pressure than corn pads; spot adhesive bandages guard corns against friction but do not have padding to protect against pressure; wrapping small pieces of lamb's wool around toes reduces irritation of soft corns between toes. These are all types of therapies that are typically patient preferred.

Financial constraints often make patients wear poorly fitted shoes, which can cause foot problems. If you notice that a patient does not have good-fitting shoes, notify the nurse so that appropriate referrals can be made. Many local churches and other organizations such as the Salvation Army may have resources available that can provide patients with a pair of good-fitting shoes once they are discharged. In the hospital, social

---

PROCEDURE 19.3
Giving Nail and Foot Care

Verify with the nurse the need for nail and foot care.
1. Assemble supplies.
2. Introduce self.
3. Identify patient.
4. Explain procedure.
5. Verify with nurse any of the following:
   - Contraindications to nail care. (In some facilities, only registered nurses are permitted to trim the toenails of a patient with diabetes. Follow agency policy.)
   - Restrictions to positioning.
   - Condition of nails and feet; color and temperature of toes, feet, and fingers.
6. Perform hand hygiene and don clean gloves according to agency policy and guidelines from the CDC and OSHA.
7. Prepare patient for intervention.
   a. Close door or pull privacy curtain.
   b. Raise bed to a comfortable working height.
   c. Arrange supplies at bedside or, if patient is able to perform procedure, have supplies available in the bathroom and offer assistance as needed.
8. Hand and foot care.
   a. Position patient in chair. If possible, place disposable mat under patient's feet.
   b. Fill basin with warm water and test temperature. Place basin on disposable mat and assist patient to place feet into basin. **Do not soak hands and feet of a patient with diabetes for extended periods; soaking increases risk of infection by skin breaking down from maceration.** Allow to soak 10 to 20 minutes. Rewarm water as necessary.
   c. Place overbed table in low position in front of patient. Fill emesis basin with warm water and test water temperature. Place basin on table, and place patient's fingers in basin. Allow fingernails to soak 10 to 20 minutes. Rewarm water as necessary.
   d. Using orangewood stick, gently clean under fingernails. (Orangewood stick removes debris that harbors microorganisms from under nails.) With clippers, trim nails straight across and even with tip of fingers.

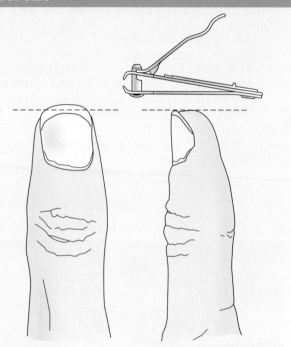

With emery board, shape fingernails. Push cuticles back gently with washcloth or orangewood stick.

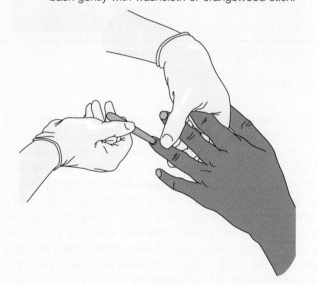

PROCEDURE 19.3

Giving Nail and Foot Care—cont'd

e. Don gloves, and with washcloth scrub areas of feet that are calloused.

f. Trim and clean toenails following step d instructions.

g. Apply lotion or cream to hands and feet. Return patient to bed and position for comfort. Dry fingers and toes thoroughly to impede fungal growth and prevent maceration (a softening and breaking down of tissue resulting from prolonged exposure to moisture). Do not apply lotion between toes of patients with diabetes.

h. On completion of procedure, observe the nails and the surrounding tissue for condition of skin and any remaining rough edges.

i. If the patient's nails are extremely hard or if the patient is unable to perform personal nail care, have a podiatrist (a person trained in the treatment of nail and foot problems) provide nail care.

j. Teach the patient with diabetes about appropriate foot care. The teaching plan includes inspecting the feet daily for breaks, wearing shoes at all times, wearing socks, drying feet completely, and noting any areas of numbness, tingling, or pain.

9. Dispose of gloves in proper receptacle. Clean and store supplies. Place soiled laundry in hamper. Perform hand hygiene.

10. Assess for patient's comfort, lower bed level, raise side rails, and place call button within easy reach.

11. Document:
   • Document the procedure.
   • Document pertinent observations (e.g., breaks in the skin, inflammation, or ulcerations).
   • Most facilities have flow sheets for Activities of Daily Living (ADLs); know agency policy.
   • Report abnormal findings (breaks in the skin or ulcerations) to nurse in charge. (Additional interventions are sometimes required.)

(Figures from Sorrentino SA: Mosby's assisting with patient care, *ed 2, St. Louis, 2004, Mosby.)*

services can often assist with locating a pair of fitting shoes for the patient.

DRESSING AND UNDRESSING THE PATIENT

Sometimes patients need assistance with dressing and undressing, as they may not be strong enough to remove their garments, or they may have disabilities that prevent them from having enough range of motion to dress themselves. As the patient care technician, it may be your role to assist patients with either removing their garments or dressing them. Typically this is done in the morning with AM care and in the evenings with PM care. In the hospital setting, many patients will wear only a hospital gown; however, they may need assistance with getting dressed in their street clothes when it comes time for discharge. In a long-term care facility, residents typically will dress in street clothes attire for the day and will change into pajamas at night. This is a personal preference and not typically something that is mandated, or required. In the long-term care facility, it is important to ensure that patients' clothes remain their own and are not given to another patient. Most facilities require that patients' clothing be labeled with their name and room number. When selecting clothes for the patient to wear, be sure to allow them to choose. This gives patients control when possible, and reminds them that they are in charge of their care somewhat. Encourage them to choose clothes that would be easier for them to manipulate for toileting, such as elastic waist. Use of belts is discouraged, as it often requires more fine motor skill and dexterity, which is sometimes challenging for the older adult. Regardless, support the patient in their choice of clothing for the day (see Procedure 19.4).

Changing the Gown of a Patient With an Intravenous Line

Changing the gown of a patient who has an intravenous (IV) line can be challenging if not performed correctly. It is important that the IV line not be disrupted while you are changing the gown. Some hospitals have gowns that have snaps at both shoulders of the gown, which make it much easier to change; however, this is not always the case. If the nurse is planning to change the IV solution container, the tubing, and the dressing, then that would be the ideal time to change the patient's gown. This reduces the risk of introducing bacteria into the system and cuts down on infections at the site. The patient care technician must never disconnect the tubing when assisting with a gown or clothing change. Instead, the IV solution container and tubing should be threaded through the sleeve of the patient's garment (see Procedure 19.5).

If the patient is allowed to shower, ensure that the IV insertion site and dressing is protected with a water-resistant covering. Verify with the nurse whether it is okay for the patient to shower with his or her IV line, and then be sure to cover it. After the patient showers, remove the covering and inspect the area around the IV insertion site to ensure that it remained dry. If the dressing appears to be wet, notify the nurse so that he or she may observe and change it if necessary.

PROCEDURE 19.4

Dressing and Undressing the Patient

1. Verify with the nurse the need for changing the patient's clothes.
2. Assemble supplies.
3. Introduce self.
4. Identify patient.
5. Explain procedure.
6. Verify with nurse any of the following: any existing drainage tubes, dressings.
7. Be sure to pull the curtain.
8. If the patient is able to assist you with dressing, ask the patient to stand at the bedside. If the patient is unable to provide any assistance, lower the bed rail and raise the bed to a height that is appropriate for good body mechanics.

Undressing the Patient

9. Untie the patient's gown from behind the neck and backside. If the patient is wearing street clothes, unfasten any snaps, buckles, or buttons. Take care to not drag the skin across the bed linens as you reach to the back to untie the gown. You may need to have the patient roll to one side of the bed while you untie the gown. Have the patient roll to the other side to remove the gown from the second side.

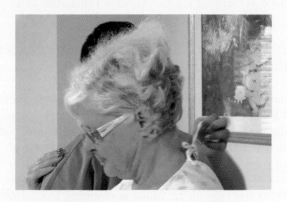

10. Raise the patient's top piece of clothing to the shoulders; ensure to support the patient's head if needed. Remove the strong arm from the sleeve of the garment first. Use the bath blanket to cover any areas that are revealed when removing the patient's top.
11. Remove the sleeve of the weak arm second.

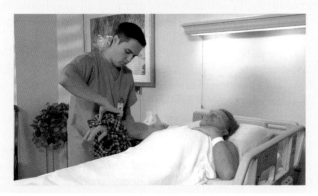

12. Place the new gown on and tie in the back and around the neck. If the top garment is a shirt or sweater, gently place over the patient's head and ensure to not twist their head and neck.
13. To remove the clothing from the lower part of the body, take any shoes off of the patient. Undo any buttons, unzip zippers, and unsnap any snaps.
14. If the person is lying in bed, ask to raise the hips slightly off of the bed.
15. If the person is unable to lift the hips off the bed, turn the patient toward you and gently slide the pants down the strong side until it is below the hip and buttocks. Roll the person to the other side and do the same. Once the patient is supine again, lower the pants to the patient's feet. Use the bath blanket to cover the person's lower extremities while removing the pants.
16. Gently slide the pants down over the buttocks and down to the feet.

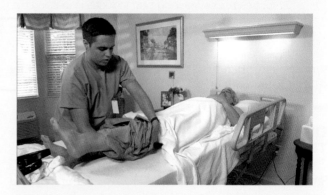

17. If the patient is able to stand, gently slide the pants down beneath the buttocks and hips to the ankles. Be careful to not allow the cuffs of the pants to get stuck around the foot as the person steps out of the pants.

Dressing the Patient

18. If the patient is lying supine in the bed, keep the bath blanket over top of the patient until he or she is completely dressed.
19. Be sure that buttons, zippers, and snaps are undone or opened before trying to dress the patient. For tops that open in the back, slide the arm of the weak side into the sleeve opening.

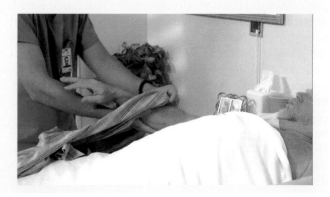

PROCEDURE 19.4

Dressing and Undressing the Patient—cont'd

20. Slide the arm of the strong side into the sleeve opening next.
21. If the patient is able to lift the head, pull the opening of the top over the patient's head and down over the chest.
22. Fasten the closure in the back.
23. For tops that open in the front, slide the sleeve of the top onto the arm that is on the weak side.
24. If the patient can raise the head and shoulders, bring the garment around the back to the other side. Then slide the sleeve on to the arm of the strong side.
25. If the patient cannot raise the head or shoulders, then have the patient turn toward you and lie on their side.
26. Take the top and tuck it underneath the patient.
27. Turn the patient to the other side, with the back toward you.
28. Pull the garment that was tucked underneath the patient out and then turn the person back onto the back, in a supine position.
29. Take the clothing top and place it on the arm of the strong side.
30. For pants or a skirt, slide the pants or skirt over the feet and onto the lower legs.
31. Once the person lowers the hips to the bed, fasten any closures, buttons, zippers, etc.
32. If the patient can lift the hips, have the patient raise them slightly off the bed. Lift the pants or skirt up the legs and to the waist.

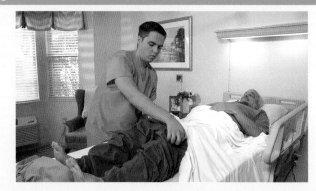

33. If the patient is standing, have the patient lift one foot at a time and place the opening of the pants onto the foot and pull the pant leg upward. Repeat for the second foot. Be sure to steady the patient by having him or her hold onto a bedrail or bathroom bar rail.
34. Assist the patient with fastening any closures, buttons, zippers, etc.
35. Put socks and shoes on the patient if he or she will be walking; if the patient will remain in bed, place socks only on the feet.
36. Always lower the bed back to the original position.
37. Place the patient's call light within reach.
38. Remove the privacy curtain.

(Figures from Mosby's nursing assistant video skills 4.0, *St. Louis, 2015, Elsevier.)*

PROCEDURE 19.5

Changing the Gown of a Patient With an IV Line

1. Verify with the nurse the need to change the gown.
2. Assemble supplies.
3. Introduce self.
4. Identify patient.
5. Explain procedure.
6. Examine the location of the venipuncture site to ensure changing the gown will not disturb it.
7. Raise the patient's bed to a level that is appropriate for you.
8. Maintain the patient's privacy by covering the patient with a sheet or bath blanket.
9. Untie the patient's gown from behind the neck or unsnap any snaps across the top sleeve seam.
10. Slide the gown down the arm that does not have the IV line.
11. Take the sleeve of the arm with the IV line and pull it gently over the IV site and tubing, taking care to not catch or pull on the IV site.

12. Holding the material of the gown with one hand, remove the patient's hand from the sleeve of the gown with the other hand.
13. Take the IV bag, keeping it at as close to the same height as it was on the pole as possible, and pull it through the sleeve of the gown. If the IV bag is on a pump or electronic infusion device, ensure the roller clamp is slowed or clamped before removing to prevent an infusion of a large volume of solution or medication.
14. The clean gown is passed through the opening of the arm sleeve in the gown from the opening up toward the shoulder of the gown and then replaced on the pole. See image below. Next, place the arm without the IV line through the gown sleeve.

Continued

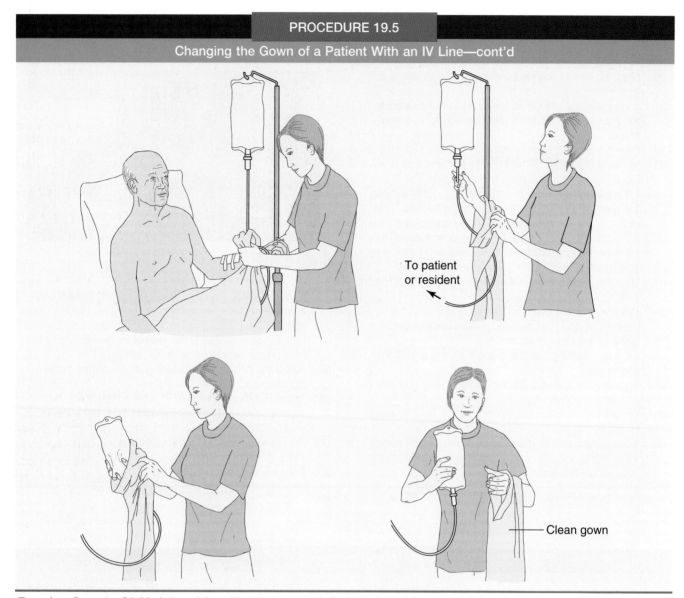

To patient
or resident

Clean gown

(Figure from Sorrentino SA: Mosby's assisting with patient care, *ed 2, St. Louis, 2004, Mosby.)*

CHAPTER SUMMARY

Providing for the grooming needs of a patient can be comforting for them and can reduce their pain. It also increases their feeling of self-esteem if they are comfortable with the way they look. Being sick often makes one feel bad and guilty for not being able to take care of him- or herself; therefore, by providing for basic grooming needs, the patient care technician can make the patient feel better.

Special attention should be given to the care of the patient's hair. Prevention of tangling and matting is the best treatment; once the hair is tangled, it is difficult to clear and often uncomfortable for the patient. Shaving can provide a sense of cleanliness for the patient; however, it can be harmful for the patient if a razor blade is used. Electric razors are safer for the patient and work just as well.

Caring for the patient's nails actually decreases the risk of infection, as bacteria often like to reside under the nailbeds. Take great care to keep nails long enough that the skin is not cut when trimming. Cut toe nails straight across to prevent growth of ingrown toenails.

Case Scenario

Jill is working on the long-term care unit today as a patient care technician. She is going to provide foot care to all of the patients on her wing. Before she begins, what items does she need to gather from the supply closet? What information does she need to obtain from the nurse before providing foot care? Are there any exclusions, or reasons she should not provide foot care to anyone? One of the patients has requested red nail polish on her toes. Is this allowed? Why or why not?

REVIEW QUESTIONS

1. To brush the patient's hair, you should start at which location?
   a. The ends of the hair strands
   b. In the middle of the hair strands
   c. At the scalp
   d. The front of the forehead

2. How often should the hair of the patient be brushed?
   a. Daily
   b. Twice a day
   c. As often as the hair needs it to keep from tangling
   d. Once per week

3. When brushing the patient's hair, you notice something very small moving from one hair strand to another. What should you do?
   a. Notify the nurse
   b. Ask the patient if he or she has been itching more lately
   c. Wash the patient's hair again
   d. Attempt to remove the moving object with your fingers

4. A patient has diabetes and complains of decreased feeling in the feet. What should you do?
   a. Use cold water when washing the feet so as to not burn them
   b. Verify with the nurse whether you should wash the feet
   c. Avoid the feet when bathing the patient
   d. Ask the patient to adjust the temperature of the water to his or her preference before washing the feet

5. The patient requests to take a shower with the IV line still in the arm. What should you do?
   a. Notify the nurse to see whether the IV line could be covered before allowing the patient to take a shower
   b. Cover the IV line with a Band-Aid before allowing the patient to take a shower
   c. Tell the patient that he or she is not allowed to take a shower with the IV line still in the arm
   d. Remove the IV line and place a dressing on the site so that the patient can shower

Assisting With Nutrition and Fluids

LEARNING OBJECTIVES

1. Explain the purpose of water and its importance in maintaining hydration.
2. Outline the variations in nutrition according to developmental stage.
3. Discuss cultural factors that may affect a person's nutrition status.
4. Discuss the proper procedure for calculating a patient's intake and output.
5. Discuss the elements to consider when feeding the patient.
6. Outline the procedure for discontinuing an intravenous line.
7. Discuss the patient care technician's role in assistance with nutrition and fluid balance.

KEY TERMS

anorexia Lack of appetite.
basal metabolic rate (BMR) The body's use of energy to maintain bodily functions.
dehydration When the body loses more water than it takes in.
dysphagia Difficulty swallowing.
glomerular filtration rate (GFR) A test used to check how well the kidneys are working; specifically, it estimates how much blood passes through the glomeruli in each minute.
homeostasis The process of keeping body fluids in balance.
infiltration Leaking of intravenous fluid into the tissue surrounding the vein.
intravenous (IV) Taking place in, or being administered into, a vein.
peripheral Veins that are not in the chest or abdomen; this includes the arms, legs, hands, and feet.
phlebitis Inflammation, or swelling, of the walls of a vein.
skin turgor The degree of elasticity of skin.
therapeutic diet A diet used as a medical treatment.

Nutrition is the sum of all body processes involved in taking in nutrients and using them to maintain body tissue and provide energy. It is one of the foundations for life. In the past century, much progress has been made to improve the general level of health in all people, and healthcare providers have come to realize that good nutrition is essential for optimal health throughout all stages of life. Eating the right kinds and amounts of food and following good dietary habits throughout the entire life yields a healthier body and mind, greater energy, and greater protection against disease. For patient care technicians (PCTs), it is important to always consider the patient's nutritional state when providing care to them.

ROLE OF THE PCT IN PROMOTING NUTRITION

Because the PCT spends a considerable amount of time caring for patients, there are many opportunities for the PCT to help the patients meet their nutrition requirements. The PCT may be responsible for assisting a patient to eat, for recording a patient's intake, and for communicating any dietary concerns to the nurse.

Infancy

The time from birth to 1 year of age is of rapid growth and development. The infant's birth weight doubles by 6 months and triples by 1 year of age. Nutrition plays an important part in this rapid growth.

Breast milk or iron-fortified infant formula is recommended for the entire first year of life. Breast milk contains antibodies and easily digested fats. This composition tends to lead to a lower incidence of infections in breastfed infants and fewer episodes of gastrointestinal (GI) upset. Regular cow's milk (whole, low-fat, or skim) should be avoided during the first year of life. Introduction of regular cow's milk before 1 year of age could lead to iron-deficiency anemia and increase the risk for developing milk allergies later in life. Also, the fat in cow's milk is more difficult for the infant to digest and could create GI disturbances. The large amounts of protein, sodium, and potassium found in cow's milk could also overwhelm the infant's system and cause damage to the kidneys. Acceptable alternatives to cow's milk during the first year of life are breast milk and iron-fortified infant formula. Whole milk is acceptable after the first year, but skim and low-fat milk are inappropriate until the child is 2 years of age because the fat content is insufficient. In the first 6 months, water, juice, and other solid foods are generally unnecessary for infants. In most cases, breast milk or formula provides adequate nutrition for about the first 4 to 6 months. At approximately 4 to 6 months of age, depending on the

infant's development, it is possible to introduce solid foods into the diet. Solid feedings are usually started with iron-fortified rice cereal because rice cereal is less allergenic than most other foods. Infants should start with 1 to 2 teaspoons, and the amount is gradually increased. Fruits are added next, then vegetables, and then meats. Single-ingredient foods should be introduced one at a time at weekly intervals. This allows sufficient time to detect any food-related allergies. If the family has a history of food allergies, it is generally best to withhold wheat cereal, wheat products, and egg whites until the child is 1 year of age. Infants younger than 12 months of age should also never be given honey, especially wild honey, because of the potential for botulism. Wild honey is a potential source of *Clostridium botulinum* spores and can easily cause botulism in the infant.

Most commercially prepared baby foods in the United States are nutritious, safe, and of high quality. However, it is important to read labels and use foods without added salt, sugar, or honey. If baby foods are prepared at home, it is important to take care to reduce the risk of foodborne illness by having a sanitary preparation area and proper storage conditions.

There is no nutritional benefit to feeding juice to infants younger than 6 months. Offering juice before solid foods are introduced into the diet may cause the infant to prefer juice over breast milk or infant formula and tends to reduce the intake of important nutrients such as protein, fat, vitamins, and minerals.

Childhood

At approximately 1 year of age, appetite generally reduces, and the growth rate slows. Children still need adequate nutrition, although nutrient needs relative to weight are generally less than that in infancy. The website www.ChooseMyPlate.gov offers an appropriate guide for children's diets. Younger children typically need smaller serving sizes than adults, and as a child grows, serving sizes should increase. By the toddler years, the child's digestive system should be able to handle all the nutrients found in the normal family diet, and by school age, the child's taste preferences should be emerging. Most children prefer simple, plain foods and will eat what they need if they are not coaxed, nagged, bribed, rewarded, or influenced by television commercials. Childhood is a critical time for encouraging good dietary habits. It is also a time for children to test their independence. Food is often a source of frustration at mealtime, with the parents resorting to bribing the child to eat or arguing with the child to gain compliance. Often the more pressure that is placed on the child at mealtime, the more negative the experience (see Injury & Illness Prevention Box 20.1). It is important to carefully supervise children's eating habits and offer

Injury & Illness Prevention Box 20.1

Ways to Encourage Good Dietary Habits in Children

- Encourage children to eat meals and snacks at regular times and at the table. By having set eating times, children will learn that they cannot eat continually all day.
- Try to make meals relaxed and enjoyable. Children need time to eat, and mealtimes should be a positive experience. Do not act rushed when you are feeding a child.
- Offer a variety of foods from all food groups, and allow children a choice of food, with reason.
- Do not force children to eat more than they want to eat.
- Give small servings, or teach children how to serve themselves small servings. Then let them have seconds if they are still hungry.
- Offer new foods, but do not force children to eat foods they dislike. If the child will not eat a new food, quietly remove the food and offer it again at another time.
- Encourage children to help with food selection and preparation.
- Keep nutritious snacks available, such as fruits, cheese, crackers, raw vegetables, and bread. Most children need to snack.
- Limit sweets, and do not use sweets and foods as rewards or bribes.
- Encourage children to be physically active.
- As adults, set a good example by practicing sound dietary and exercise habits.

nutritious meals and snacks, but they must also allow the child the freedom to decide what and how much to eat.

Adolescence

Puberty is another time in the child's life when growth is very rapid and nutrition becomes more important for proper development. Even though adolescents may understand good nutrition concepts, they may not relate this understanding to their own dietary habits. They usually are more willing to follow the nutritional teaching if it applies to them directly. Adolescents may be more likely to practice good nutrition if they consider factors such as how nutrition helps skin (facial appearance), strength (for any athlete), and the ability to concentrate in school. Because of the fast growth rate and participation in sports, adolescents may need more food to supply their energy requirements. Because adolescents are seeking to establish their independence, their food choices are sometimes not wise and tend to be influenced by peer preference rather than by parental advice. Their diets are often filled with calorie-rich and nutrient-poor snack foods. The era of fast food has given the adolescent access to high-calorie, nutritionally unbalanced meals. Too many fast food meals and too much snacking on empty calorie foods can lead to nutritional deficiencies. When good nutritional habits have been established earlier in life, adolescent nutrition is likely to be better balanced. Being part of a family that practices good nutrition ensures that occasional lapses into sweets, fast foods, and other peer group food preferences will not create serious deficiencies. Another nutritional factor to consider is that during adolescence, many teenagers experiment with alcohol and drugs, and these substances may have dangerous effects on their nutritional status as well.

Obesity in young people is a common problem in the United States today. The years associated with adolescence are a time of growth, and although obesity is not ideal, restrictive diets sometimes cause harm by suppressing development and can even leading to eating disorders. Encourage adolescents to develop healthy eating habits and to use moderation when they consume soft drinks and sugar- and fat-laden snack foods. Emphasize adequate physical activity, and suggest limiting television viewing and computer usage.

Adulthood

During adulthood, nutrient needs change little in comparison with those of the adolescent. However, metabolism gradually slows, and the caloric needs decrease. At the same time, the activity level of many adults tends to decrease. The combined effects of decreased energy (caloric) needs and reduced physical activity often result in weight gain. As adults advance in years, it is important to remind them to eat nutrient-dense foods, so that they can maintain adequate nutrition with fewer kilocalories, and to maintain an active lifestyle.

Aging is associated with increased health concerns. Older adults suffer from conditions such as heart disease, arthritis, osteoporosis, diabetes, kidney disease, and other disorders with increased frequency. Special conditions may mean differing nutrient needs that may vary greatly from person to person (Box 20.1). It is important to educate each patient about his or her particular dietary needs and explain the importance of any restrictions.

Nutritional Concerns of Adults in Long-Term Care Facilities

Malnutrition is a common problem among residents in long-term care facilities and greatly influences physical health and quality of life. Poor nutritional status in these residents is related to a number of factors:

- Residents of long-term care facilities may experience cognitive or physical impairment, disease processes,

| Box 20.1 | Life Span Considerations for Aging and Nutrition in Older Adults |

Aging and Nutrition

- Aging often affects the eating process. Changes in dentition, decreased saliva production, and alterations in swallowing all have the potential to affect nutrient intake. It is sometimes necessary to adjust food consistency to facilitate food intake. Chopped, ground, pureed, and liquid diets tend to be less appealing to older people; serve them in as palatable a manner as possible.
- The smell and taste of foods are sometimes affected by normal changes of aging. In addition, many older adults are on special diets that restrict the use of salt, sugars, and fats. This could lead to inadequate nutrient intake. The use of flavorings, seasonings, and spices to enhance flavor and aroma is often helpful.
- Older adults experience changes in digestive secretions, gastrointestinal mucosa, and enzyme production. This affects how food is digested, absorbed, and excreted. Water, dietary fiber, and adequate physical activity play an important role in preventing constipation in older adults.
- Aging often leads to loss of muscle mass, thereby reducing BMR.

- Because of illness, limited mobility, or financial limitations, or a combination of these, some older adults have difficulty obtaining and preparing nutritious food.
- Age-related social and mental changes such as forgetfulness, loneliness, and apathy are likely to affect the eating habits of older adults.
- Chronic medical conditions often mean that they have to use therapeutic diets. The most common of such conditions in older adults include diabetes mellitus, cardiovascular disease, renal insufficiency, osteoporosis, diverticulosis, anemia, and lactose intolerance. Older adults who have long-standing dietary preferences and eating habits often find diet modification difficult.
- Some older adults have difficulty in feeding themselves because of inflammation of the joints, or chronic pain. They may need assistance with opening their cartons or condiments on their dietary trays. They may use assistive devices, such as utensils with longer handles or a larger grip so that they do not have to squeeze as hard to hold on to their utensils. Assist the patient when needed, but allow for independence when possible.

| Box 20.2 | Life Span Considerations: Dehydration in Older Adults |

Older adults are at increased risk of dehydration because of several factors. The following factors should be kept in mind when dehydration in an older adult is considered:

- Fat replaces lean muscle as aging progresses, leading to a decrease in total body fluid.
- The aging kidney is less able to concentrate urine, so more fluid is lost.
- Decreases in mobility and a diminished sense of thirst often result in decreased fluid intake.
- Incontinent older individuals sometimes restrict fluid intake to reduce the frequency of urination and incontinence.
- To compensate for changes in taste, older adults often oversalt their food, which results in electrolyte and fluid imbalances.

- Physiologic changes in the skin and mucous membranes decrease their reliability as indicators of dehydration.
- Mild disorientation may be the first indication of dehydration.
- Signs and symptoms of dehydration include thirst, dry mucous membranes, increased heart rate, decreased blood pressure, poor **skin turgor,** and flat neck veins.
- Dehydration increases the risk of orthostatic hypotension.
- Decreased fluid intake increases the likelihood of constipation.
- Because the aging kidney is less efficient at excretion, giving intravenous infusions or supplements containing sodium or potassium increases the risk of electrolyte imbalance.

and emotional disturbances, all of which have an effect on nutritional intake and status.

- Many residents in the long-term care environment need some assistance or encouragement with eating and drinking. PCTs working within a long-term care facility must be educated and trained on how to feed the patients to ensure that they get adequate nutrition.
- Restricted diets may be prescribed for residents of long-term care facilities. Common modifications include sodium and fat restrictions. Diabetic features

may be instituted for groups of residents. Dietary restrictions can affect the palatability of the food and thereby hinder nutritional intake.

- Inadequate fluid intake and dehydration are sometimes secondary to decreased thirst sensation, decreased independence, dysphagia (difficulty swallowing), and incontinence (Box 20.2).

All members of the healthcare team must work together to coordinate care to ensure that the nutritional needs of the facility residents are met. Concerns need to be identified quickly and treatment planned to ensure that nutritional compromise does not occur.

Offering familiar foods and incorporating cultural preferences within the prescribed diet is important. Long-term care facilities have begun to embrace these principles in their dietary offerings. The diet that tries to control intake of potentially unhealthy substances has mild salt, fat, and concentrated sweet restrictions but avoids severe restrictions when possible. These dietary policies promote a sense of control and independence. Liquid nutritional supplements may help increase kilocalorie, protein, and nutrient intake if the resident's intake is less than optimal; however, these supplements should not be used as a substitute for regular food.

Fluids should be offered to residents at all meals and between meals to ensure adequate intake. It is important for healthcare providers to watch for signs of dehydration in long-term care residents and to correct any deficits quickly. Family involvement and socialization at mealtime may help increase residents' dietary intake; encourage it whenever possible.

MEDICAL NUTRITION THERAPY AND THERAPEUTIC DIETS

Medical nutrition therapy is the use of specific nutritional variations to build good health. It may simply involve modifying a nutritionally inadequate diet so that it becomes nutritionally adequate, or it may involve changing the texture or calorie content of the diet. A diet used as a medical treatment is called a therapeutic diet (Box 20.3). Modifying a diet usually means adding or taking away specific nutrients or calories in a diet or a change in the consistency of a diet, such as a pureed or soft diet. If a patient needs a special diet, the healthcare provider prescribes the diet, and it is up to the nurse to ensure that the patient understands and follows the diet, as well as to record how the patient reacts to it. When therapeutic diets are considered, it is important to account for the patient's cultural and religious preferences in order to increase compliance with the diet (Box 20.4). The PCT is responsible for making sure that the patient receives the type of diet that has been ordered by the physician. If the tray contains the incorrect type of diet, report it at once to the nurse.

Box 20.3 Consistency, Texture, and Frequency Modifications

The term *therapeutic diet* often brings to mind nutrient-modified diets such as low-fat or low-sodium diets. Modifications in textures, consistencies, and meal frequency, however, are also therapeutic in some cases. Most hospitals have standard diets based on consistency; these may include liquid, soft, and regular diets.

Liquid Diets

There are two types of liquid diets: clear liquid and full liquid. The clear liquid diet is nonirritating and consists of liquids that are easily digested and absorbed and leave little residue, or waste, in the GI tract. Because of that, very little stool is formed on a liquid diet. The clear liquid diet is typically used before diagnostic tests, particularly tests on the GI tract, and before surgery. It is frequently used postoperatively until peristalsis returns and is sometimes used during episodes of vomiting or diarrhea. The clear liquid diet is low in kilocalories, protein, and most nutrients. It is to be used temporarily, preferably for 2 to 3 days or less. Foods on a clear liquid diet include any type of liquid that you can see through, such as apple juice or white grape juice, fat-free broth or bouillon, plain gelatin, tea, or black coffee. When patients are on a clear liquid diet, they are usually given small meals more frequently, usually every 2 to 3 hours (Box 20.5).

The full-liquid diet is used as a transition diet after a clear liquid diet. It is more nutritionally complete than a clear liquid diet but is still lacking in some nutrients, such as iron, zinc, and fiber. A liquid dietary

---

Box 20.4 Cultural Considerations Culture and Nutrition

There is much to consider in dealing with patients of varied cultural, social, or religious backgrounds:

- Food habits are among the oldest and most deeply rooted aspects of many cultures.
- Food plays an important role in quality of life. The loss of culturally related foods during hospitalization or long-term care has great potential to affect the patient both emotionally and physically.
- Never make assumptions. Be specific when asking questions regarding the patient's dietary preferences. Ask patients to provide a list of foods they like and dislike.
- The patient is likely to need help in marking the menu if he or she speaks another language or is unfamiliar with foods on the menu. Pictures of food are often helpful when there is a language barrier.
- Communication between the staff and nutrition services is key to maintaining an adequate diet for the patient.
- Patients often have strong beliefs regarding certain foods or food combinations. Unless these beliefs are harmful to the patient, attempt to respect the patient's beliefs.
- In long-term care facilities, it is important to make every effort to work with the patient or family to provide special foods for observance of holidays, festivals, and other occasions.
- Occasionally, the family of a patient is permitted (with the healthcare provider's approval) to bring in food for the patient if the facility is unable to provide that food. Take special care to ensure food safety.

| Box 20.5 | Foods Included in Liquid Diets |

Clear Liquids
- Bouillon
- Fat-free broth
- White grape, apple, cranberry juice
- Popsicles
- Gelatin
- Tea, coffee
- Ginger ale, lemon-lime soda
- Supplemental formulas

Full Liquids
- All clear liquids
- Strained cereals
- Strained soups
- Fruit and vegetable juices
- Milk, milk shakes
- Ice cream, sherbet
- Custard
- Puddings
- Supplemental formulas

supplement, or vitamins, may be added to increase the nutritive value of the diet. This diet too is best used only temporarily. Examples of foods on a full-liquid diet are ice cream, creamy soups, gelatin, pudding, milk, and juices.

Soft and Low-Residue Diets

Soft diets often serve as an intermediate step when a patient is progressing from a liquid to a regular diet. Soft diets and low-residue diets are also used for many people with conditions affecting the GI tract, such as acute diverticulitis, inflammatory bowel disease, gastritis, and during periods of indigestion or diarrhea.

A soft diet is generally low in fiber and is similar to a regular diet. It includes foods from all food groups, including meat, fish, poultry, eggs, milk, grains, fruits, and vegetables, but foods with strong spices are avoided. Mechanical soft diets are often ordered for patients who have difficulty chewing or swallowing. All meats are ground, and fruits and vegetables are cooked and pureed. This diet is nutritionally adequate, but supplements may be added.

The low-residue diet is similar to the soft diet but also includes restrictions on milk and milk products because they leave more residues in the colon. If milk is omitted, the patient needs to get adequate calcium from other sources.

High-Fiber Diets

The high-fiber diet is a variation of the regular diet and is sometimes used therapeutically. High-fiber diets are often used in the treatment of constipation. With adequate fluids, fiber has the capacity to reduce constipation

in young and older patients alike, which helps reduce or eliminate the need for laxatives. A high-fiber diet is also recommended for patients with diverticulosis and often helps lessen the severity of symptoms and inflammation (diverticulitis).

Patient instructions concerning high-fiber diets should include recommendations promoting higher fiber options such as whole grains. Fiber intake should be increased gradually to prevent excess gas formation. Fresh cooked or raw fruits and vegetables are preferred over processed foods, which have lesser nutritional values and contain high levels of sodium and other preservatives.

Kilocalorie Modifications

The body requires a specific amount of energy each day to carry out its tasks. This energy comes from the intake of food and fluids. The body uses this energy to maintain necessary, involuntary body functions, also called basal metabolic rate (BMR), to digest nutrients, or diet-induced thermogenesis, and for physical activity. When energy intake equals energy output, the body is in zero energy balance, or equilibrium. During zero energy balance, weight remains constant. If energy intake exceeds energy output, the energy balance becomes positive. Positive energy balance results in weight gain. On the other hand, if energy intake is less than energy output, the energy balance becomes negative, leading to weight loss.

High-Kilocalorie and High-Protein Diets

During times of physiologic stress—such as after surgery, during sepsis, or in the presence of bone fractures, burns, or pressure ulcers—the body's energy and protein needs are increased. Medical trauma has the potential to greatly increase the BMR, so if energy needs are not met by diet, the patient will lose protein stores and weight, and both energy balance and nitrogen balance will become negative.

In addition to the increased energy and protein needs, many patients with trauma and cancer suffer from anorexia, or lack of appetite. This adds to the already difficult task of maintaining adequate nutrition. High-kilocalorie and high-protein diets provide increased amounts of kilocalories and protein in a small volume and are used to help the compromised patient maintain adequate nutritional intake. Suggestions to help increase intake of kilocalories and protein are listed in Box 20.6. Always ask the nurse before adding anything to the patient's diet, even if the patient requests something be added.

Some patients suffer from certain eating disorders. When a patient is suffering from anorexia, the appearance of the food and how it is served may be the factors

Box 20.6	Suggestions for Increasing Kilocalories and Protein

- Add powdered milk or protein powder to milkshakes, beverages, soups, puddings, and cooked cereals.
- Spread peanut butter on crackers, fruit, or celery.
- Add cheese to casseroles, soups, and sauces.
- Use extra meat, chicken, or fish in casseroles and soups.
- Add sugar to foods when reasonable (this adds only kilocalories).
- Use generous amounts of calorie-dense foods such as butter, vegetable oils, mayonnaise, cream cheese, sour cream, and cream in recipes, as spreads, or as dips.
- Add nuts and dried fruits to cereals, breads, or desserts.
- Have snacks available at all times.
- Encourage the patient to eat high-calorie foods first and eat the low-calorie foods if still hungry.

that decide whether the patient eats it. Therefore it is important to maintain a positive attitude and provide encouragement when serving meals. Make meals as attractive as possible, and serve beverages, especially liquid nutritional supplements, in glasses, not cans. Make sure to serve meals promptly and at the correct temperature. Refrigerate snacks and supplements if necessary.

Fat-Modified Diets

Research has shown that modifying the amount of fat in the diet may reduce risk of heart and vascular disease by about 14% and that the risk for some cancers can be reduced as well. There are many foods available that are low in fat and are reasonably priced.

Low-Fat Diets

A low-fat diet has limited amounts of total fat, saturated fat, and *trans* fatty acids. This type of diet is often used for the prevention and treatment of *atherosclerosis* (a disorder characterized by buildup of cholesterol and lipids on the artery walls), heart disease, and *hyperlipidemia* (elevated levels of blood lipids).

To help Americans reduce the risk of cardiovascular disease, the American Heart Association has recommended dietary guidelines for the general population to decrease the amount of fat in the diet. The National Cholesterol Education Program has also developed the Therapeutic Lifestyle Changes (TLC) diet to help decrease the amount of fat and cholesterol ingested (Table 20.1).

Many patients have a difficult time complying with a low-fat diet because they think the required foods lack flavor and are not as satisfying. Even though they need

to reduce saturated and *trans* fatty acids in the diet, patients are still able to choose low-fat foods from all the food groups. Encourage them to choose low-fat dairy products, lean meats, skinless poultry, and fish. Advise limiting eggs to four or fewer per week and limiting organ meats, such as liver, to one serving or less per week. Limits are also necessary on added fats, such as butter, stick margarine, mayonnaise, cream, and sour cream.

Keep in mind that fat possesses many good qualities and offers much pleasure when eaten. Many Americans tend to rebel against a low-fat diet because they believe that it is necessary to completely eliminate all fatty foods. Choosing a low-fat and low-cholesterol diet does not mean "never eat cheese because it contains fat" or "never eat egg yolks because they contain cholesterol." It is the *total* amount of fat, saturated fat, and cholesterol that matters. Besides, foods such as cheese and egg yolks contribute nutrients necessary to the diet, and sometimes eliminating all high-fat foods compromises the diet's overall nutritional value. Rather than totally eliminating high-fat foods, patients should be encouraged to use moderation. Patients should balance high-fat foods with other foods that contain less fat and cholesterol. By adhering to balance, variety, and moderation, patients are still able to enjoy some of their favorite foods while following a healthy, fat-controlled diet.

Fluid-Modified Diets

Fluid is a big part of the diet and can be found in many foods. Of course, all beverages add fluid to the diet, as do gelatins, ice cream, sherbet, puddings, popsicles, fruit ices, and soups. While in good health, most adults need between 2 and 3 liters of water a day to keep themselves hydrated; in the presence of certain illnesses, however, the amount of water the patient is allowed to intake may be restricted.

During end-stage renal disease and other kidney diseases with low urine output, fluid is restricted to 500 to 750 mL/day (approximately 2 to 3 cups) plus an amount equal to any daily urine output. Fluid restrictions are also common with patients diagnosed with congestive heart failure, directly after a myocardial infarction, in hepatic coma, or in the presence of ascites.

In the hospital, fluid restrictions are often divided between the nursing and the dietary departments. For example, if a patient has a 1000-mL fluid restriction, the dietary department is sometimes allowed to provide the patient with 600 mL/day, and the nursing department gives 400 mL/day. The amount of fluid allowed for nursing depends on the patient's intravenous (IV) and medication needs.

While patients have fluid restrictions, they often experience excessive thirst. Some suggestions to help

Table 20.1	Guidelines for Following the Therapeutic Lifestyle Changes (TLC) Diet	
Food Groups	**Choose …**	**Go Easy on …**
Meat, poultry, and fish (<5 oz/day; 2 servings of fish/week) Eggs (<2 egg yolks/week) Dry beans and nuts	• Lean fresh meats, extra-lean ground beef, and lean deli meats* • Poultry without the skin, ground turkey made from white meat • Fish and shellfish • Eggs (limit yolks to 2/wk; substitute 2 egg whites for 1 egg in recipes) • Dry beans and peas, fat-free refried beans, tofu • Nuts* (in moderation)	• Meats with visible fat and marbling • Regular ground beef • Processed meats: sausage, bacon, frankfurters, cold cuts • Organ meats • Duck and goose • Deep-fried meats, poultry, or fish • Shellfish (some are high in cholesterol; use moderate portions)
Milk, yogurt, and cheese (2 to 3 servings/day)	• Fat-free (skim) or 1% milk, buttermilk, soy milk • Fat-free or reduced-fat cheeses* (3 g of fat or less per oz) • Low-fat or nonfat cottage cheese* • Low-fat or fat-free yogurt	• Whole or 2% milk, half-and-half • Whole-milk yogurt • Full-fat cheese with more than 3 g fat per oz
Fruits and vegetables (5 or more servings/day)	• Fresh, frozen, canned, or dried fruits and vegetables • Add more vegetables to meat dishes, casseroles, or soups • Keep fresh fruits and vegetables readily available for snacks • Use fruit as dessert	• Vegetables with high-calorie sauces • Fruits with added sugar • Deep-fried vegetables (including French fries) • Limit juices, instead choosing whole fruits and vegetables for more fiber
Breads, cereals, rice, pasta, and other grains (6 or more servings/day depending on energy needs)	• Breads, bread products, and cereals made from whole grains such as whole wheat, buckwheat, bulgur (cracked wheat), oats, rye, millet, quinoa, bran • Brown rice, wild rice • Whole-grain pastas • Popcorn	• White breads and products made with refined grains that are lower in fiber (check label) • Baked goods made with added fat and eggs, such as muffins, biscuits, croissants, and butter rolls
Fats and oils (limited total amount; replace saturated fats with unsaturated fats; read labels to identify saturated and *trans*-fat content)	• Liquid vegetable oils (canola, corn, olive, peanut, safflower, sesame, soybean, and sunflower) • Margarines with liquid vegetable oils as first ingredient (soft tub, liquid, or vegetable oil spreads) • Light or nonfat mayonnaise and salad dressing • Reduced-fat sour cream, cream cheese, and whipped toppings	• Butter, lard, fatback, bacon drippings • Margarines with hydrogenated or partially hydrogenated oil as the first ingredient (read label for *trans*-fat) • Solid shortening • Coconut milk; coconut, palm and palm-kernel oils • Full-fat sour cream, cream cheese, whipped cream
Sweets, snacks, condiments (to be used occasionally on basis of caloric needs)	• Low-fat ice cream, frozen yogurt, sorbet, sherbet, or low-fat puddings • Angel food cake; low-fat brownies • Fat-free or low-fat cookies such as animal crackers, vanilla wafers, gingersnaps, graham crackers • Whole-grain snack crackers*	• Regular ice cream; pudding made with whole or 2% milk • Doughnuts and pastries • Pie, regular cakes, and cookies • Snack crackers with high fat content

*Sometimes contain high levels of sodium.
(Adapted from U.S. Department of Health and Human Services: Lowering your cholesterol with TLC. Retrieved from www.nhlbi.nih.gov/health/public/heart/chol/chol_tlc.pdf.)

alleviate thirst include rinsing the mouth with cold mouthwash, putting lemon into cold water to make it more refreshing, freezing fluid so that it takes longer to consume, eating cold fruits and raw vegetables, chewing gum, sucking on breath mints or hard candies (in moderation), brushing teeth often, and limiting sodium intake.

Feeding the Patient

Patients who are weak, are paralyzed, have a cast, or have some other form of physical or neurological limitation may not be able to feed themselves or may need assistance with feeding. It may be the responsibility of the PCT to assist these patients with meals.

When assisting patients to eat, it is necessary to create a relaxed mood so that patients do not feel rushed. It is also important to allow them time for their usual before-meal rituals. Many people pray before eating; others need to wash their hands and face. Provide the time and privacy for whatever routine a patient is used to during the preparation to take a meal. This demonstrates caring and respect for the patient. Before feeding, ask the patient about the order he or she wants food and fluids offered. Also ensure that the temperature of the food is not hot enough to burn the patient. When feeding a patient, it is best to use a spoon because spoons are less likely than forks to cause injury. Give the patient small bites, and allow for chewing and swallowing the food without being rushed.

Patients who are not able to feed themselves sometimes believe that they are losing control over their lives and feel angry, humiliated, and embarrassed. Some of them do not like depending on others. Some may be depressed and resentful, and others may refuse to eat. Allow these patients to try to feed themselves as much as possible, and offer assistance as needed. Ensure that they do not exceed activity limits ordered by the healthcare provider, but provide them positive reinforcement and support.

Many visually impaired patients are keenly aware of food aromas. Often they can identify foods being served. Always tell a visually impaired patient what foods and fluids are on the tray and indicate their location on the tray by referring to the numbers on a clock (Fig. 20.1). When feeding a visually impaired patient, identify what food or fluid is being offered before placing the food or drink in the patient's mouth.

Meals are often considered by many people to be a social activity, and many patients may not have family or friends visiting at mealtime. Engage the patient in pleasant conversation while giving the patient enough time to chew and swallow food. Also, sit facing the patient. Sitting with the patient is more relaxing and shows the patient that the staff cares and is not too busy to help him or her. Standing communicates nonverbally that the staff does not have time and that they really are not interested in the patient. By facing the patient, the PCT is also able to see how well the patient is eating and whether the patient has problems swallowing. Procedure 20.1 describes techniques to use in assisting patients with eating.

Keep in mind that odors, unpleasant equipment, an uncomfortable position, the need for oral hygiene, the need to void, and the presence of pain may affect appetite. To improve a patient's appetite, remove any offensive odors or equipment and offer to help the patient void or wash up before meals. It is also important to serve the meal as quickly as possible so that the food is at the correct temperature and more appetizing to the patient.

PCTs play an important role in promoting good nutrition. Nutrients are necessary for the proper functioning of all life processes in the body. For healthy Americans, a well-planned diet is able to provide adequate nutrition without supplementation.

Nutrient needs change throughout the life cycle, and people need to adjust their diet to meet those needs. Diets are often altered in consistency or frequency when GI function precludes the use of a regular diet.

Fat-controlled and low-fat diets emphasize reduction of total fat, saturated fat, and *trans*-fatty acids. They are used in the treatment of a variety of diseases, including heart disease, atherosclerosis, obesity, diabetes, metabolic syndrome, malabsorption syndromes, and gallbladder disease.

Fluid restrictions are necessary when urine output is decreased, when edema is present, or during heart failure. Adequate fluid is necessary to prevent dehydration, particularly in older adults. In feeding a patient or resident, ask about the preferred order in which to offer foods and fluids, and allow sufficient time for the patient to chew and swallow the food. Remove any offensive odors or equipment and then serve meals promptly to maintain appropriate temperature and increase nutritional intake.

WATER

Water is the nutrient that is most vital to life; humans can survive longer without food than they can without water. Lack of this nutrient brings about detrimental changes in the body quicker than being without any other nutrient. Water makes up approximately 60% of adult body weight and 80% of infant weight and is responsible for performing many functions in the body. It provides form and structure to body tissues, acts as a solvent, and is necessary for most of the body's chemical processes. Water transports nutrients from foods and other substances throughout the body by way of the blood, body secretions, and tissue fluids; it lubricates and protects moving parts of the body, such as joints; it aids in digestion; and it is necessary for regulating body temperature. If fluid needs are not met, in relation to inadequate intake or through abnormal losses such as vomiting, hemorrhage, burns, or an increase in perspiration (sweat) or urination, dehydration results. Severe dehydration (more than 10% of body weight lost) could become a life-threatening situation. Signs of dehydration include poor skin turgor; flushed, dry skin; dry

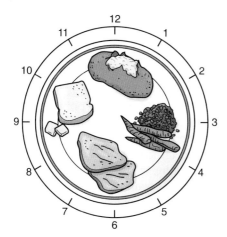

FIGURE 20.1 For the visually impaired patient: "The potato is at the 12 o'clock position." (From Sorrentino SA, Remmert LN: *Mosby's essentials for nursing assistants,* ed 5, St. Louis, 2014, Mosby.)

PROCEDURE 20.1

Assisting Patients With Eating

1. Complete or delay care that will interfere with eating.
2. Provide a period of rest or quiet before meals.
3. Offer the patient a bedpan or urinal before mealtime.
4. Provide the patient with an opportunity for hand washing, and offer mouth care before the meal.
5. Remove soiled articles or clutter from room.
6. Make the patient comfortable for eating; give pain medication at least 30 minutes before a meal.
7. Raise the head of the bed to a sitting position.
8. Cover the patient's upper chest with a napkin or some form of clothing protector.
9. Sit beside the patient to assist with feeding.
10. Encourage patients to feed themselves as much as possible.
11. Provide a flexible straw for patients who are unable to use a cup or glass.
12. Serve manageable amounts of food in each bite.
13. For a patient who has had a stroke, direct the food toward the side of the mouth not affected by the stroke.
14. Serve food in the order of the patient's preference.
15. Give the patient time to chew and swallow food.
16. Provide drinking water between bites of food and when the patient requests it.
17. Modify utensils and texture of food if the patient has to remain flat while eating. Use a training cup or a large syringe with flexible rubber tube. Puree or grind foods.
18. During the feeding, do not leave the patient until he or she has finished eating. Do not interrupt the meal.
19. Carry on pleasant conversation with patient during the meal.
20. Remove the tray from the patient's room as soon as the meal is completed.

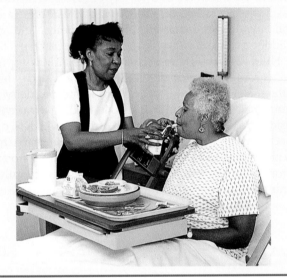

mouth; cracked, dry lips; decreased urine output; irritability; and disorientation. Dehydration in infants is evidenced by sunken fontanels, a decrease in the number of wet diapers, and no tears when the child cries.

About 80% of total water intake comes from drinking water and other beverages, and 20% comes from the water contained in foods. The need for water varies, depending on factors such as body size, age, activity level, metabolic needs, and temperature, and so it is not possible to give a specific recommendation for the drinking of fluids; however, a suggested daily intake of 9 cups (women) to 13 cups (men) of fluids from drinking water and other beverages is adequate for most adults. Pregnant and breastfeeding women have increased water needs (up to 3 L/day). Infants tend to be at greater risk for dehydration because they have a higher percentage of body water and are more susceptible to greater

skin losses of water. In young infants, breast milk and formula normally provide adequate fluid, but extra fluids may be needed in warmer weather. Older adults have decreased sensitivity to thirst and are also at greater risk for dehydration. It is necessary to pay special attention to these two population groups to make certain that fluid needs are met and that dehydration does not become a problem. The PCT is an active member of the healthcare team in ensuring that patients have adequate water to drink.

Unless the patient is on fluid restrictions, each patient should have a pitcher of water available in their room at all times. The water should be kept fresh; usually it is the responsibility of the PCT to provide fresh water at least twice per shift. Some patients prefer water at room temperature and some prefer it on ice. Ask patients of their preference rather than just assuming they want ice water.

If you are trying to encourage children to drink water, you may have to be creative. Fun, colorful drinking straws may make the water seem more appealing to the child. Playing a game such as tea party or Simon Says may also make the child more willing to drink water. Pouring smaller amounts more often may encourage the child to drink more often instead of pouring a tall glass of water.

Intake and Output

As water moves through all parts of the body, it is constantly being lost and must be replaced. Fluid leaves the body through the kidneys, the lungs, the skin, and the GI tract. Homeostasis is the process of keeping body fluids in balance. The body is equipped with several mechanisms to keep the composition and volume of body fluid within narrow limits of normal. The average adult fluid intake is approximately 2200 to 2700 mL/day. Oral intake of fluids should be approximately 1100 to 1400 mL/day; solid foods contribute approximately 800 to 1000 mL/day; and fluid produced from cellular metabolism provides approximately 300 mL/day (Table 20.2).

Fluid intake is regulated mainly through the thirst mechanism. Receptors in the hypothalamus called *osmoreceptors* measure the concentration of the blood. When the amount of particles (solutes) in the blood is higher than normal, the sensation of thirst is present, and the person drinks to satisfy that sensation. Anyone who is unable to respond to or perceive the thirst mechanism is at increased risk for dehydration and may require fluids administered by way of tube feedings, IV infusion, or total parenteral nutrition (TPN).

Fluid loss from the body is considered either sensible (measurable) or insensible (not measurable). Sensible losses are seen in urine, feces, vomiting, and wound drainage. Insensible fluid losses include those from perspiration and expiration. Because it is difficult to accurately measure insensible fluid losses, approximations are acceptable. However, because measurement of sensible losses is possible, it is very important to keep accurate records of fluid intake, what the patient is taking in, and output, what the patient is putting out, in order to help determine a patient's fluid needs.

The kidneys play an extremely important role in fluid balance. If the kidneys are not functioning properly, the body has great difficulty regulating fluid balance. The nephrons are the functioning units of the kidneys, and they filter blood at a rate of 125 mL/minute, or about 180 L/day. This is called the glomerular filtration rate (GFR) and leads to an output of 1 to 2 L (1000 to 2000 mL) of urine per day. The nephrons reabsorb the remaining fluid on the basis of bodily needs. If the body loses even 1% to 2% of its fluid, the kidneys conserve fluid by reabsorbing more water from the renal filtrate, which results in less water excreted and more concentrated urine. In order to effectively eliminate waste products from the body, it is necessary for the kidneys to excrete a minimum of 30 mL/hour of urine. In the presence of fluid excesses, the kidneys react by excreting more dilute urine, thus ridding the body of excess fluid and conserving electrolytes.

One simple and accurate way to determine water balance is by weighing the patient under controlled conditions: for example, at the same time of day, with the same amount of clothing, and when attached to the same equipment, such as electrodes, IV tubing, braces, or splints. It is important to empty all drainage bags before the patient is weighed, in order to get an accurate measurement. One liter of fluid equals 2.2 pounds (1 kg); therefore a weight change of 2.2 pounds reflects a loss or gain of 1 L of body fluid (Procedure 20.2).

Delegation and Documentation Box 20.1

- Be as accurate as possible when documenting intake and output.
- Use measuring devices that have markers on the container to indicate how much the patient has taken in.
- If the patient is drinking from a can in which you are unable to see inside to determine how much the patient has drunk, pour what is remaining into a measured cup. Subtract what is left from how much was there in the beginning.
- Do not estimate in obtaining urine output. Obtain a specimen hat that has measurements marked on the inside of the urine container (Fig. 20.2)

Table 20.2	Normal Fluid Intake and Output in an Adult Eating 2500 Calories/Day (Approximate Statistics)		
Type of Content	**Gain (mL)**	**Route**	**Amount of Loss (mL)**
Water in food	1000	Skin	500
Water from oxidation	300	Lungs	350
Water as liquid	1200	Feces	150
		Kidney	1500
Total	2500	Total	2500

Urine specific gravity is a measurement of urine concentration. It is also a good indicator of fluid balance. A urine specific gravity value of more than 1.030 indicates that the urine is concentrated, as in conditions of dehydration, whereas a measurement of less than 1.003 to 1.000 indicates that the urine is dilute, as in conditions of overhydration.

PROCEDURE 20.2
Measuring Intake and Output

1. Identify patient.
2. Explain procedure.
3. Instruct patient to inform staff of all oral intake. Provide a marked intake and output (I&O) container.
4. Instruct patient not to empty any output collection receptacles and to notify the nurse after elimination.
5. Alert all staff and remind patient of need to measure I&O.
6. Measure and record all fluids taken orally, gastric tube feedings, and all fluids administered parenterally.

7. Wash hands and don gloves.
8. Measure and record output in Foley drainage system, diarrhea stools, nasogastric suction, emesis, ileostomy, and surgical wound receptacles such as Davol, Jackson-Pratt, and Hemovac drains. Measure and record output from chest tube drainage in water-sealed container by marking with felt-tip pen.
9. Remove gloves and wash hands.
10. Compute I&O, and document it on patient's record.

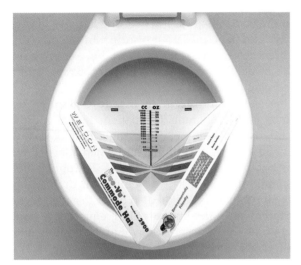

FIGURE 20.2 Specimen hat for urine measurement. (Courtesy Welcon, Inc., Fort Worth, Texas. IN Sorrentino SA: *Mosby's assisting with patient care,* ed 2, St. Louis, 2004, Mosby.)

Delegation and Documentation Box 20.2

- The skills of basic IV needle insertion, adjusting IV flow rate, administering IV medications, and maintaining an IV site require the knowledge of a nurse. Many states include this skill in the scope of practice for licensed practical (vocational) nurses. Delegation of these tasks to unlicensed assistive personnel (UAP), such as the PCT, is inappropriate.
- It is acceptable for PCT to inform the nurse when a fluid container is almost empty, when the patient complains of any discomfort at the IV site, and when an electronic controlling device sounds an alarm.
- In the clinical setting, the registered nurse (RN) is responsible for supervising infusion therapy and may delegate the task of IV insertion, adjusting IV flow rate, administering IV medications, and maintaining an IV site to the Licensed Practical Nurse (LPN)/Licensed Vocational Nurse (LVN) if those tasks are within the LPN/LVN's scope of practice for that state.

INTRAVENOUS THERAPY

The body's fluid and electrolyte balance must be maintained to keep all body systems healthy and functioning properly. When there is an imbalance either in fluid intake and output or in electrolyte concentration, complications can arise. To help prevent these complications, the healthcare provider may order IV therapy (infusion of medication or other liquid therapeutic agents).

There are many reasons why IV therapy may be ordered. It may be needed to maintain fluid volume if a patient is not taking in fluid or nutrients by mouth, or it can be used as replacement for fluid lost through prolonged nausea or vomiting. It can also be used to give medications, blood, or blood products and to provide the patient with nutritional support. The IV route provides faster absorption and more rapid distribution of medications, solutions, or nutrients and can be used for either long-term or short-term applications.

Each state's nurse practice act determines the legal guidelines for IV administration, and facility policy further defines the nurse's role in the administration of IV medications, fluids, blood, or blood products. Only specially trained nurses who meet the legal qualifications and facility guidelines should be involved in IV administration (see Delegation and Documentation Box 20.2).

Maintaining and Discontinuing an Intravenous Site

Complications sometimes occur with peripheral IV infusions. Infiltration of the site, phlebitis of the vessel, and local or systemic infections are possible. Appropriate management of IV sites helps prevent or minimize these complications (Procedure 20.3).

Keeping the IV insertion site covered and dry helps prevent the introduction of microorganisms and reduces

PROCEDURE 20.3
Discontinuing a Peripheral IV Site

Discontinuing a Peripheral Intravenous Dressing

1. Assemble equipment
2. Perform hand hygiene.
3. Explain to the patient what you are going to do.
4. Remove any overlying tape. Then remove transparent membrane dressing by picking up one corner and pulling the side laterally while holding catheter hub. Repeat for other side.

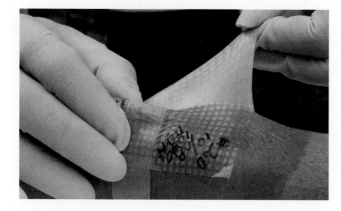

   a. Alternative is to remove gauze dressing and tape from site one layer at a time by pulling toward the insertion site. Tape securing catheter to skin should be left intact.
5. Site evaluation:
   a. Review healthcare provider's orders or verify with the nurse for discontinuation of IV therapy.
   b. Determine patient's understanding of the need for removal of peripheral IV catheter.
6. Explain procedure to patient.
7. Turn IV tubing roller clamp to "off" position. Remove tape securing tubing.
8. Remove IV site dressing and tape while stabilizing catheter.

9. With dry gauze held over site, apply light pressure and withdraw the catheter, using a slow steady movement, keeping the hub parallel to the skin.

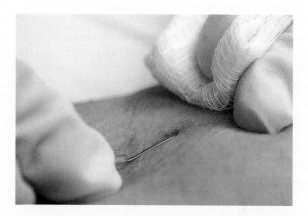

10. Apply pressure to the site for 2 to 3 minutes, using a dry, sterile gauze pad. Secure the tape over the gauze snugly.
11. Inspect the catheter for intactness, noting tip integrity and length.
12. Discard used supplies.
13. Remove and discard gloves, and perform hand hygiene.
14. Instruct patient to report any erythema, pain, drainage, or edema that occurs after catheter removal.
15. Document and record the following:
   • Time peripheral IV infusion was discontinued
   • Condition of site
   • Gauge and length of catheter
   • Whether catheter is intact

(Figure 4 from Elkin MK, Perry AG, Potter PA: Nursing interventions and clinical skills, ed 3, St. Louis, 2004, Mosby. Figure 9 from Perry AG, Potter PA: Nursing Interventions and clinical skills, ed 6, St. Louis, 2016, Mosby.)

the possibility of infection. Most often, a gauze dressing or a transparent dressing is used to cover the insertion site. Transparent dressings make seeing the site easier and keep the site dry. Gauze dressings do not allow visualization of the site and can become soiled or damp; therefore their use is limited.

It is important that the IV solution not run out or become completely empty. This could make the IV site clot, which would prevent any further fluids from being able to enter the bloodstream and would often require the patient to have an additional needle stick. If you

note during your hourly rounds that the IV solution bag is nearing empty, notify the nurse at once.

The nurse may delegate to the PCT discontinuation of an IV site. It is within the scope of practice for the PCT to discontinue a peripheral IV site. A peripheral IV needle is inserted into the peripheral veins, that is, the ones closer to the skin surface. Other lines, such as central lines, or peripherally inserted central catheters (PICC), must be initiated, monitored, and discontinued by a licensed nurse. See Procedure 20.3 for detailed instructions on discontinuing an IV site.

CHAPTER SUMMARY

Water is the primary fluid in the body and is necessary for life. One can live longer without adequate food than they can without water. As a PCT, it is important to ensure that each patient has an adequate supply of fresh water.

Sometimes patients do not eat well; this can be when they are ill, in a strange environment, or just do not have an appetite. Encourage patients to eat what is on their plate, but do not become frustrated or pushy with them. Oftentimes, patients are lonely and just want someone to sit with them while they eat. If time allows, provide an opportunity to sit with patients while they eat. Patients who have limited vision may need additional assistance with eating. Those with chronic pain or inflammation in their hands may have difficulty in opening their cartons and condiments on their tray. Assist them as needed. Some patients may use assistive devices to allow them to feed themselves easier. Promote independence as much as possible.

Some patients require IV therapy. As the PCT, you may be asked to discontinue the IV line, either when the patient no longer requires IV fluids or when they are being discharged. Be sure to verify the order for discontinuation of an IV site before performing the procedure.

Accurate record keeping is vital when managing fluid balance in a patient. It is important to be as specific as possible when determining how much a patient drank or ate at each meal, as well as during other times when it is requested by the nurse or ordered by the physician. Keep good notes, and document as soon as possible.

Case Scenario

You have been asked by the nurse to discontinue the IV sites of four patients who will be discharged that day. The nurse has given you the patients' names and room numbers. You gather your supplies and proceed to the first patient's room. When you explain the procedure to the patient, the patient replies, "But the doctor just left my room, and he said he's decided to keep me another day. You go ahead though; I've been wanting to get that thing out of my arm for days." What should you do at this point? Should you proceed with discontinuing the IV site because the nurse told you to do so? Should you move on to the next three patients and then come back to this patient when you are done? Explain your answer and give the reason for your decision.

REVIEW QUESTIONS

1. Normal daily water intake and output (I&O) is approximately how many milliliters?
   a. 1500
   b. 2500
   c. 3500
   d. 6500

2. How many milliliters of urine per hour must the kidneys secrete in order to eliminate waste products from the body?
   a. 30
   b. 60
   c. 20
   d. 100

3. Which of the following statements best describes the risk of fluid and electrolyte imbalances in the older adult?
   a. Most older adults can maintain fluid and electrolyte balance just as well as younger adults.
   b. Older adults have unlimited reserves to maintain fluid balance when abnormal losses occur.
   c. Body water increases with age, which puts the older adult at risk for fluid volume excess.
   d. Physiologic changes in the skin and mucous membranes decrease their reliability as indicators of dehydration.

4. Which of the following is the most important in preventing the introduction of microorganisms to the patient when an IV infusion is discontinued?
   a. Hand hygiene
   b. Checking the identification of the patient
   c. Ensuring the six rights of medication administration
   d. Carefully checking the order for discontinuation

5. When collecting information on a patient's intake, IV fluids should not be included.
   a. True
   b. False

Assisting With Urinary Elimination

1. Discuss assisting a patient in the use of the bedpan, the urinal, and the bedside commode.
2. Discuss the different types of urinary catheters.
3. Explain the purpose in using a urinary catheter.
4. Outline the steps for catheterization of a male and female patient.
5. Discuss management of the patient who has an indwelling Foley catheter.

bedpan A device for receiving feces or urine from either male or female patients confined to bed
bladder training The achievement of voluntary control over voiding
catheterization A procedure used to drain the bladder and collect urine
defecation The act of eliminating feces
incontinence The inability to control urine or bowel elimination
residual urine Amount of urine left in the bladder after a patient void
urinal A device for collecting urine from male patients; urinals for female patients are also available
urinary catheter A flexible tube that is passed through the urethra and into the bladder to drain urine
urination The act of emptying the bladder

URINARY ELIMINATION

Urinary elimination is a natural process that clears the body of waste material and aids in maintaining electrolyte balance. Therefore conditions that interfere with urinary function have the potential to create a health crisis. The urinary tract can be affected by a problem with the kidneys, the ureters, the bladder, the urethra, or surrounding organs. It is also very susceptible to infection.

Patients at risk for problems with urine elimination include those who have undergone surgical procedures of the bladder, the prostate, or the vagina; those patients who have recently experienced childbirth; patients with primary urologic problems; and those who are critically ill with multisystem problems. When there is a problem with the urinary system, the healthcare provider often orders a urinary catheter to be inserted to monitor urinary output and the urinary system. Most often the nurse caring for the patient is responsible for inserting and monitoring the catheter and output; however, this can be delegated to the patient care technician (PCT) who has received training on the skill (see Delegation and Documentation Box 21.1).

Assisting the Patient With Elimination

A patient who is unable to get up to the bathroom or bedside commode for the purpose of urination (the act of emptying the urinary bladder) or of defecation (the act of eliminating feces) uses a bedpan (a device for receiving feces or urine from either male or female patients confined to bed) or urinal (a device for collecting urine from male patients; urinals for female patients are also available). Use of a bedpan or urinal is a private and personal procedure. Be sure to give patients as much privacy as possible. Of course, this is depending on their safety; if they are unable to be left alone, give them privacy as you are able.

Offer the bedpan or urinal often throughout the day because patients may have an accident if their elimination needs are not met. Patients often procrastinate using a bedpan because it is uncomfortable and embarrassing. Some have difficulty using a bedpan because it seems so unusual to use the bathroom while in bed. Patients sometimes try to get to the bathroom without help even if they are not supposed to be walking on their own. Remind patients of the possibility of accidents or falls (Box 21.1).

Report to the nurse and record in the flow sheet any abnormalities in urine or stool (Box 21.2). Flow sheets are usually provided for documentation of normal voiding and stools.

Bedpans used to be made of stainless steel or porcelain so that they could be sanitized for repeated use. This is no longer considered to be best practice; now

---

| Box 21.1 | **Assisting the Patient With Elimination** |

- Allow the patient enough time for elimination. Ignoring the urge to defecate or urinate or not taking time to eliminate completely is a common cause of constipation or urine retention.
- Be prompt when called to assist the patient to the bathroom or onto the bedpan or bedside commode.
- When the patient shares a room with another patient, be certain to curtain off the patient's area. This enables the patient to relax, knowing that interruptions will not occur.
- Close the bathroom door. If it is necessary to remain nearby, stand outside door or curtain.
- For those patients unable to assume the normal squatting position, stool risers can be used, which call for less effort to sit or stand.

| Box 21.2 | **Characteristics of Normal Urine and Normal Stool** |

Normal Urine
- Ranges from a pale to straw color
- Is transparent at the time of voiding
- Has a characteristic odor: faintly aromatic
- Yields negative results when tested for protein, glucose, ketone bodies, red blood cells, white blood cells, and bacteria

Normal Stool
- Brown
- Odor affected by food types
- Has soft, formed consistency
- Frequency ranging from once a day to two or three times a week
- Resembles the shape of the rectum
- Contains undigested food, dead bacteria, fat, bile pigment, living cells, intestinal mucosa, and water

---

they are made of plastic and are disposable upon the patient's discharge from the facility. There are two types of bedpans: one type has a high back, and the second type is flat and smaller and is called a fracture pan (Fig. 21.1A).

A urinal is made of plastic; there are two types of urinals. One type serves the male patient for urinating, or voiding (see Fig. 21.1B). The other type is called a *female urinal,* which has an adapter that accommodates the female anatomy.

Empty the bedpan and the urinal immediately after use, and cleanse and store it properly. If the patient's intake and output are being monitored, measure the urine and record the result. Remember to use a calibrated specimen container so that your amount is accurate. Estimate liquid stool on the appropriate form

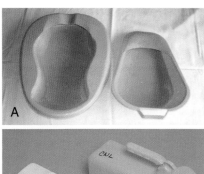
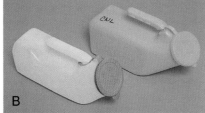

FIGURE 21.1 Selected equipment and supplies for elimination. A, Regular bedpan *(left)* and fracture pan *(right)*. B, Male urinals. (From Perry AG, Potter PA: *Clinical nursing skills & techniques,* ed 8, St. Louis, 2014, Mosby.)

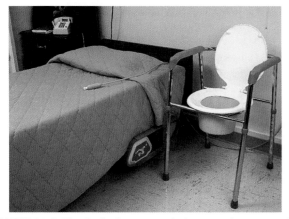

FIGURE 21.2 The bedside commode has a toilet seat with a container underneath. The container slides out from under the toilet seat for emptying and cleaning.

according to the agency's policy. See Procedure 21.1 for positioning the bedpan.

Another option for elimination, in lieu of the bedpan or the urinal, is the bedside commode (Fig. 21.2). It is useful at night and for the patient who is not able to easily walk far to the bathroom easily.

Care of the Incontinent Patient

Incontinence is a very common problem, especially among older adults and adults who are debilitated. Regardless of the cause, incontinence is psychologically distressing and socially disruptive.

Urinary incontinence occurs because pressure in the bladder is too great, because the muscle sphincters are weak, or because neurologic function has been compromised as a result of illness or injury. Collaborate with other members of the healthcare team to determine the cause and the extent of incontinence and to assist in managing the problem. The physical therapist, for example, is prepared to assess the extent of musculoskeletal involvement and determine methods of treatment. The nurse will be able to direct you in how you can assist patients in meeting their incontinence needs.

Patients who are aware and alert may need an incontinence product that is discreet and promotes self-care. Some incontinence products are designed for small amounts of leakage. Persistent urge, stress, or overflow incontinence most likely necessitates referral for urologic evaluation. Incontinence products often resemble sanitary napkins women use for their monthly menstrual cycle; the difference is the absorbent material is located near the front so as to collect the urine and prevent leaking through to their clothes. Always respect a patient's privacy by keeping these products out of sight of visitors. This is a very personal situation and one that deserves privacy.

When patients are incontinent of either urine or stool, and they are unable to determine when this will occur, it often means that they will need to use disposable adult undergarments or underpads as the primary means of managing their incontinence. Urine and feces are very irritating to the skin because of the acidic substances that are produced as a part of food digestion. Skin that is continually exposed quickly becomes inflamed and irritated. Cleanse the skin thoroughly after each episode of incontinence with warm soapy water and dry it thoroughly to help prevent skin impairment. Many facilities use a protective barrier cream for patients with incontinence to prevent skin breakdown. The nurse will direct you on a particular barrier cream to use after changing the patient's undergarments.

When urinary incontinence results from the patient's decreased perception of bladder fullness or impaired voluntary motor control, bladder training may be helpful. Bladder training consists of assisting the patient to the bathroom or commode at certain time intervals in an attempt to strengthen the urinary sphincter muscles, typically every 2 hours initially for the first several times, and then at increased time intervals as the patient tolerates until the point of bladder control is reached.

Urinary Catheters

Most urinary catheters are made of soft plastic or rubber, are disposable, and can be used for both treatment and diagnosis. Urinary catheters are used to maintain urine flow, to divert urine flow to help with healing postoperatively, to give medications by irrigation, and to dilate or prevent narrowing of some portions of the urinary tract. Catheters are used for both intermittent and continuous urinary drainage. Urinary catheters can be placed in the bladder, the ureter, or the kidney. Catheterization of the bladder, which can be delegated to the

PROCEDURE 21.1

Positioning the Bedpan

1. Refer to medical record, care plan, or Kardex.
2. Assess patient's needs.
3. Assemble supplies according to patient's needs.
4. Introduce self.
5. Identify patient.
6. Explain procedure.
7. Prepare patient.
   a. Close door or pull privacy curtain.
   b. Arrange supplies close to the bedside.
   c. Place protective pad under patient's buttocks, if necessary.
8. Perform hand hygiene and don clean gloves according to agency policy and guidelines from the Centers for Disease Control and Prevention (CDC) and the Occupational Safety and Health Administration (OSHA).
9. When patient is able to assist self onto bedpan, the PCT positions patient in supine position with knees flexed and bottom of feet flat on bed surface. As patient raises hips, the PCT supports patient's lower back with arm and positions bedpan under patient. When patient has finished with elimination, the PCT removes bedpan in same manner.
10. For patient unable to assist self on bedpan:
    a. Turn patient away from the PCT toward opposite side rail, moving linens out of way.
    b. Fit bedpan to patient's buttocks.

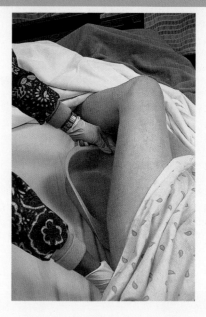

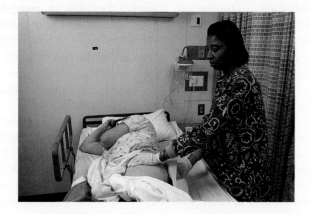

   c. Assist patient to turn over onto bedpan while the PCT secures bedpan.
   d. Raise head of bed 30 degrees.
   e. Place toilet tissue and call light within easy reach.
11. If the male patient is unable to place a urinal for himself, you need to assist him.
    a. Request that the patient abduct his legs a slight distance.
    b. Holding the urinal by the handle and directing the urinal at an angle, place the urinal between the patient's legs, making certain that the long flat side, which is opposite the handle of the urinal, is resting on the bed.
    c. Gently raising the penis; placing it fully within the urinal.
    d. Provide for privacy while the man urinates.
    e. Once he signals he is finished, provide toilet paper to dry the tip of the penis.
    f. Rinse the urinal with water before returning to its storage area (usually in the bottom cabinet of the bedside cabinet).
12. For those patients who can be out of bed but are unable to ambulate far, the bedside commode can be used (see Fig. 21.2). Some are equipped with wheels, which allow the patient to be moved to the bathroom.
13. When transferring a patient to the commode, assist the patient in the same manner as if assisting to a chair.
14. Provide a means for the patient to wash hands; either assisting to the sink or providing hand washing while patient is in the bed.
15. Remove your gloves and practice hand hygiene.
16. Provide for the patient's comfort by returning the bed to its original position.
17. Place the call light within reach.
18. Lower the bed to its original position.
19. Document the procedure, noting any abnormal observations.
20. Document according to agency policy:
    - Amount
    - Color
    - Consistency
    - Abnormal findings such as blood, unusual odor, or color
21. Report unusual findings.

(Figures from Perry AG, Potter PA: Clinical nursing skills & techniques, ed 8, St. Louis, 2014, Mosby.)

Delegation and Documentation Box 21.1

- Urinary catheterization is a task that can be delegated to unlicensed assistive personnel (UAP), such as the PCT (check facility policy). In some facilities, first-time catheterization, catheterization of patients in an acute care setting, or catheterization of patients with urethral trauma requires the critical thinking and knowledge of a nurse, and delegation of this task to UAP is inappropriate.
- The task of removing a urinary catheter can also be delegated to the PCT in some facilities; however, patient evaluation and teaching must be performed by the nurse. After removal of the catheter, the PCT should measure the amount of urine in patient's first voiding and to report time and amount to the nurse.
- It is acceptable for the nurse to delegate the task of obtaining urine specimens from a catheter to the PCT in some settings (check facility policy). Initial patient evaluation and coordination of repeated specimens require the knowledge of a nurse, and delegation of this task to PCT is inappropriate.
- The skill of catheter irrigation requires knowledge of a nurse. Delegation of this task to the PCT is inappropriate.
- The skill of caring for a newly established suprapubic catheter requires the knowledge of a nurse. Delegation of this task to the PCT is inappropriate.

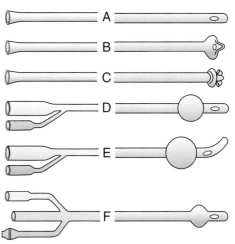

FIGURE 21.3 Different types of commonly used urinary catheters. A, Simple urethral catheter. B, Mushroom, or de Pezzer, catheter (can be used for suprapubic catheterization). C, Winged-tip, or Malecot, catheter. D, Indwelling catheter with inflated balloon. E, Indwelling catheter with Coudé tip, or Tiemann catheter. F, Three-way indwelling catheter (the third lumen is used for irrigation of the bladder).

PCT by the nurse, involves introducing a rubber or plastic tube (a urinary catheter) through the urinary meatus and the urethra into the urinary bladder. Catheterizing the ureters or kidneys is the responsibility of properly trained healthcare providers and not the PCT. Catheters are measured using the French sizing system and range in size from 14 to 24 Fr for adult patients.

Types of Catheters

Several types of catheters are used for different purposes (Fig. 21.3). The type and size of urinary catheter used are determined by the location being catheterized and the cause of the urinary tract problem. The Coudé type of catheter has a tapered tip and is used when enlargement of the prostate gland is suspected. The curved stylet of the Coudé catheter is used to assist the healthcare provider with the insertion of a urethral catheter in a male patient with prostate enlargement. The Foley catheter has a balloon near its tip that is inflated after insertion to hold the catheter in the urinary bladder for continuous drainage. This is the type of catheter most often inserted by the PCT. Malecot and de Pezzer (mushroom) catheters are used to drain urine from the renal pelvis of the kidney, and the Robinson catheter has multiple openings in its tip to facilitate intermittent drainage. Catheters designed to be inserted into the

ureters are long and slender to pass into the ureters more easily. In patients with blood in their urine, a whistle-tip catheter may be used because it has a slanted, larger orifice, or opening, at its tip. The cystostomy, the vesicostomy, or the suprapubic catheter is inserted through the abdominal wall above the symphysis pubis to create a urinary diversion in cases of obstruction, strictures, or injury to the bony pelvis, the urinary tract, or surrounding organs. The catheter is inserted surgically, is connected to a sterile closed drainage system, and is secured to avoid accidental removal; the wound is covered with a sterile dressing. When the lower urinary tract has healed, the patient's ability to urinate, or void, is tested, and when the patient's residual urine (amount of urine left in the bladder after the patient void) is low enough, according to the healthcare provider, the catheter can be removed. Sometimes, the problem causing the need for a suprapubic catheter is permanent, and the catheter is left in place.

Another form of urinary drainage system that many refer to as a catheter is the condom, or Texas, catheter. This device is not a catheter but rather a drainage system connected to the external male genitalia (Fig. 21.4). This noninvasive appliance is used for incontinent men to minimize skin irritation from urine. One drawback to using this device is that it can become too constrictive, or tight around the skin. It is therefore important to remove the appliance daily for cleansing and inspection of the skin. Use of the external condom catheter allows for a more normal lifestyle for the patient and limits the risk for infection that an indwelling catheter may cause.

Text continued on p. 394

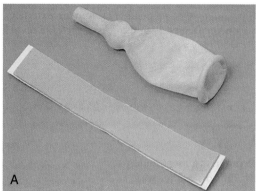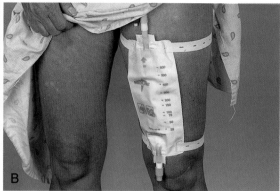

FIGURE 21.4 A, Condom catheter. B, Condom catheter attached to leg bag. (A, From Elkin MK, Perry AG, Potter PA: *Nursing interventions and clinical skills,* ed 4, St. Louis, 2008, Mosby; B, From Elkin MK, Perry AG, Potter PA: *Nursing interventions and clinical skills,* ed 3, St. Louis, 2004, Mosby.)

Injury & Illness Prevention Box 21.1

Interventions for the patient with a urinary drainage system are aimed at early detection and prevention of infection and trauma (Procedures 21.2, 21.3, and 21.4 and Fig. 21.5). When caring for urinary drainage systems, the nurse should take the following actions:

1. Follow sterile technique when inserting the catheter, and keep the collecting bag off the floor. This prevents the introduction of microorganisms into the body from the environment (Fig. 21.6).
2. Record fluid intake and urinary output (I&O), and check the drainage system for proper placement and function regularly (Fig. 21.7).
3. Encourage the patient to drink plenty of fluids to flush the urinary tract.
4. Do not open the drainage system after it is in place except with a specific order from the healthcare provider. It is important to maintain a closed system to prevent urinary tract infections (Fig. 21.8).
5. Perform catheter care twice daily and as needed, according to standard precautions (see Procedure 21.3). Inspect insertion site for blood or exudate that could indicate infection or trauma.
6. Check the drainage system daily for leaks. Know facility policy on replacing the system. Observe characteristics of the urine noting blood or sediment. Note odor when draining collection bag.

7. Avoid placing the urinary drainage bag above the level of the catheter insertion. This will cause urine to reenter the drainage system and contaminate the urinary tract (see Fig. 21.6).
8. Secure the catheter to the patient to prevent tension on the system or backflow of urine.
9. Have the patient ambulate, if possible, to facilitate urine flow. If it is necessary to restrict the patient's activity, turn and reposition patient every 2 hours.
10. Avoid kinks or compression of the drainage tube to prevent pooling of urine within the system. Gently coil excess tubing and secure to the bottom bed linens with a clamp or pin to avoid dislodging the catheter. Remember to release the tubing before transferring or repositioning the patient.
11. When urine specimens are ordered, collect specimens from the catheter by cleansing the drainage port with alcohol and then withdrawing the urine by using a sterile needle and 10-mL syringe according to standard precautions.
12. Be sensitive to the patient's feelings regarding the catheter and the constant drainage from the system, and answer patient's questions and concerns when presented (see Box 21.3)

PROCEDURE 21.2

Catheterization: Male and Female Patients

1. Refer to medical record, care plan, or Kardex.
2. Assess patient's needs.
3. Assemble supplies according to patient's needs.
4. Introduce self.
5. Identify patient.
6. Explain procedure.
7. Prepare patient.
8. Close door or pull privacy curtain.
9. Arrange supplies close to the bedside.

10. Place protective pad under patient's buttocks, if necessary.
11. Perform hand hygiene and don clean gloves according to agency policy and guidelines from the CDC and OSHA.
12. Determine the following:
    a. When patient last voided
    b. Patient's level of awareness
    c. Mobility and physical limitation of patient

PROCEDURE 21.2

Catheterization: Male and Female Patients—cont'd

d. Patient's sex and age

e. Whether patient's bladder is distended

f. Presence of any pathologic conditions that are likely to impair passage of catheter (especially enlarged prostate gland in men)

g. Allergies (to antiseptic [iodine], tape, rubber, and lubricant)

h. Patient's knowledge of the purpose of catheterization

13. Arrange for extra assistive personnel to assist if needed.

14. Position patient.

a. Male patient: supine position with thighs slightly abducted

b. Female patient: supine position with knees flexed and knees about 2 feet apart (see illustration)

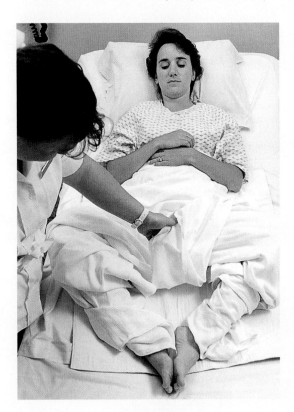

15. Drape patient with bath blanket, covering upper body and shaping over both knees and legs but leaving genital area exposed.

16. Place waterproof absorbent pad under patient's buttocks.

17. Arrange supplies and equipment on bedside table. Provide a good light.

18. Don clean gloves, and wash perineal area with mild soap and warm water.

19. Remove disposable gloves, and place them in proper receptacle.

20. Facing patient, stand on left side of bed if right-handed (on right side if left-handed).

21. Open packaging with the use of sterile technique. Don sterile gloves.

22. If indwelling catheter is used, test balloon by injecting normal saline or sterile water into balloon lumen until balloon is inflated; then aspirate saline or sterile water out of balloon. *(This determines integrity of balloon. If balloon fails to inflate, obtain another sterile catheter. This step is omitted if the manufacturer indicates that balloon testing has already occurred before shipment of the equipment.)*

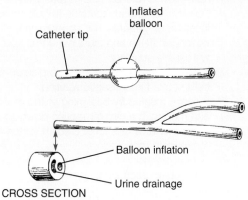

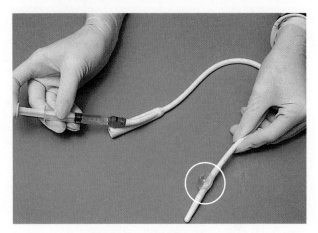

CROSS SECTION

23. Add antiseptic to cotton balls; open lubricant container. Lubricate catheter approximately 1.5 to 2 inches (3.5 to 5 cm) for female patient and approximately 6 to 7 inches (15 to 18 cm) for male patient.

Continued

PROCEDURE 21.2

Catheterization: Male and Female Patients—cont'd

24. Wrap edges of sterile drape around gloved hands, and request patient to raise hips; then slide drape under patient's buttocks.
25. Cleanse perineal area with forceps to hold cotton balls soaked in antiseptic solution.
    a. Male: If male patient is not circumcised, retract foreskin with nondominant hand. Be certain to replace foreskin when procedure has been completed. If erection occurs, discontinue procedure momentarily. This is normal but often embarrassing to patient. React in a professional manner.

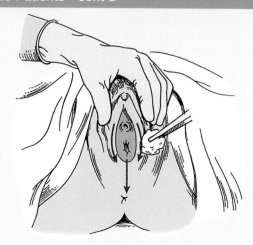

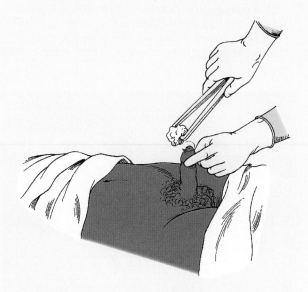

26. Pick up catheter with dominant sterile-gloved hand near the tip; hold remaining part of catheter coiled in hands; place distal end in basin.
27. Insert catheter gently, about 6 to 7 inches (15 to 18 cm) for male patient or 2 to 4 inches (5 to 10 cm) for female patient. Once urine flow is established, insert catheter 1.5 inches (3.5 cm) farther. *(Advancement of catheter ensures correct bladder placement.)* Inflate balloon with 10 mL of sterile water. Gently pull back on catheter until resistance is felt as balloon rests at orifice of urethra (see illustration and Fig. 21.6A). In a female patient, if no urine returns in a few minutes, observe whether catheter has been inserted by mistake into vagina. If so, leave catheter in place as landmark indicating where not to insert, and insert another sterile catheter.

    (1) Grasp penis at shaft below glans with nondominant hand; continue to hold throughout insertion of catheter. The nondominant hand is no longer sterile and must not come in contact with sterile supplies.
    (2) With other hand, use forceps to pick up cotton balls soaked in antiseptic solution.
    (3) Cleanse meatus by beginning at top of penis and moving in a circular motion down and around meatus one time. Discard cotton ball in appropriate receptacle.
    (4) Repeat cleansing two more times with sterile cotton balls each time.
    b. Female:
    (1) Spread labia minora with thumb and index finger of nondominant hand to expose meatus; continue to hold throughout insertion of catheter. The nondominant hand is no longer sterile and must not come in contact with sterile supplies.
    (2) With other hand, use forceps to pick up cotton balls soaked in antiseptic solution.
    (3) Cleanse area from clitoris toward anus. Use a different sterile cotton ball each time: first to the right of the meatus, then to the left of the meatus, then down the center over meatus.

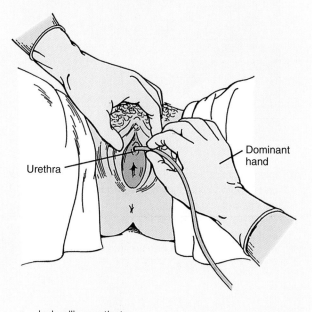

Urethra

Dominant hand

a. Indwelling catheter:
    (1) Inflate balloon with required amount of normal saline or sterile water (see Fig. 21.6A).

PROCEDURE 21.2

Catheterization: Male and Female Patients—cont'd

(2) Pull gently to feel resistance.

(3) Collect urine specimen, if needed, by placing open lumen end of catheter into specimen container.

(4) Attach open lumen of catheter to collecting tube of drainage system, holding drainage bag below bladder level. *(Some catheters are presealed to the collecting tube of the drainage system. If catheter is not presealed, clean both the catheter and tubing end with antiseptic before reconnecting them, to maintain sterility of catheter and tube.)*

(5) Attach collection bag to a stationary part on the side of bed (see Fig. 21.6B).

(6) Secure catheter to patient.

  (a) Male patient: Tape catheter to inner aspect of thigh or up over pubis, or apply leg strap (depends on healthcare provider's order); allow slack for body movement.

  (b) Female patient: Tape catheter to inner thigh or apply leg strap; allow slack for body movement.

(7) Clip drainage tubing to bed linen; allow slack for body movement.

b. Straight catheter:

(1) Once urine flow is established, hold open lumen of catheter over basin.

(2) Empty bladder (approximately 700 to 1000 mL). Refer to facility policy to determine whether urine should be allowed to continue draining.

(3) Collect urine specimen, if needed, by placing open lumen end of catheter into specimen container.

(4) Withdraw catheter slowly.

28. Wash and dry perineal area.

29. Label urine specimen with patient's name, date, healthcare provider's name, and other information as required by facility. Ensure that urine is transported to laboratory.

30. Check flow of urine and drainage tubing.

31. Remove your gloves and practice hand hygiene.

32. Provide for the patient's comfort by returning the bed to its original position.

33. Place the call light within reach.

34. Lower the bed to its original position.

35. Document the procedure, noting any abnormal observations.

- Date and time of procedure
- Type and size of catheter
- Amount of solution used to inflate balloon
- Characteristics of urine
- Amount of urine
- Color of urine and consistency of urine (note particles in urine)
- Specimen collected
- Patient's response to procedure (any resistance met)

36. Report any unusual findings immediately:

- No urine output
- Bladder discomfort despite catheter patency
- Leakage of urine from catheter
- Inability to insert catheter *(If it is not possible to advance catheter, report immediately. Discomfort indicates possible infection or trauma. Leakage around catheter indicates possibility of improper catheter placement or inflation of balloon.)*

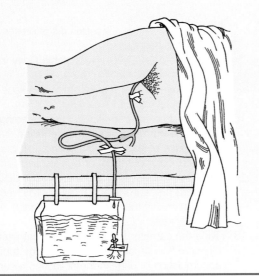 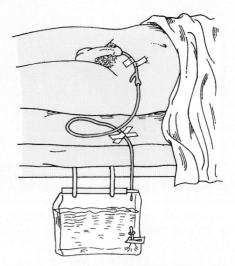

(Figures from Potter PA, Perry AG, Stocket PA, et al.: Fundamentals of nursing: concepts, process, and practice, ed 8, St. Louis, 2013, Mosby.)

PROCEDURE 21.3

Performing Routine Catheter Care

1. Refer to medical record, care plan, or Kardex.
2. Assess patient's needs. *(Allows nurse to note any potential problems with patient's environment.)*
3. Assemble supplies according to patient's needs (see Fig. 21.1).
4. Introduce self.
5. Identify patient.
6. Explain procedure.
7. Prepare patient.
   a. Close door or pull privacy curtain.
   b. Arrange supplies close to the bedside.
   c. Place protective pad under patient's buttocks, if necessary.
8. Perform hand hygiene and don clean gloves according to agency policy and guidelines from the CDC and OSHA.
9. Assemble equipment.
10. Evaluate patient for the following:
    a. Length of time catheter has been in place
    b. Encrustations or discharge around urethral meatus
    c. Complaints of pain and for allergies to antiseptic ointment
    d. Patient's temperature (check temperature every 4 hours for 24 hours if odor or exudate is present)
    e. Patient's intake (maintain adequate fluid intake to ensure free-flowing urine)
11. Position patient.
    a. Male: supine position in bed with thighs slightly abducted
    b. Female: supine position in bed with knees flexed and knees about 2 feet apart
12. Place waterproof disposable pad under patient's buttocks.
13. Drape patient with bath blanket, exposing only perineal area.

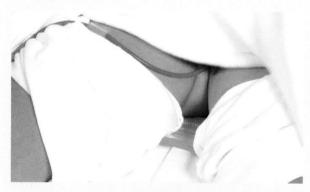

14. If sterile catheter care kit is to be used, perform the following:
    a. Open supplies with sterile technique, and arrange them on bedside table.
    b. Don sterile gloves.
    c. Place cotton balls in sterile basin near the nurse, and saturate with antiseptic solution.

d. With one hand, expose urethral meatus:
   (1) Male: Retract foreskin if it is present, then hold penis erect; hold position.
   (2) Female: Gently retract labia minora away from urinary meatus and hold in position.
e. Wash the area at the meatus and around catheter with cotton balls soaked in antiseptic solution.
   (1) Male:
       (a) With one cotton ball, cleanse around meatus and catheter in a circular motion, starting at top of penis.
       (b) Repeat twice more, using different cotton balls each time.
   (2) Female:
       (a) With one cotton ball, swab to one side of labia minora from anterior to posterior.
       (b) Repeat with second cotton ball on opposite side.
       (c) Repeat with third cotton ball down middle over meatus and around catheter; do not bring cotton ball back up once descent has begun.
f. Discard soiled cotton balls in other basin in kit.
g. With forceps, pick up cotton ball soaked in antiseptic solution, or use mild soap and water, and cleanse around catheter from urethral opening to approximately 4 inches (10 cm) of the catheter from the urethral opening.
15. If a collection of sterile supplies is to be used, perform the following:
    a. Open separate sterile packages, observing sterile technique.
    b. Don clean gloves.
    c. Arrange small plastic bag for used, contaminated supplies.
    d. Cleanse the perineal area with mild soap and warm water. Pat dry.
       (1) Male: Retract foreskin if it is present; then hold the penis erect.
       (2) Female: Gently retract labia away from urinary meatus.
    e. Release labia of female patient; replace foreskin of male patient after cleaning.
16. Observe meatus, catheter, and surrounding tissue to determine normal or abnormal condition. Note presence or absence of inflammation, edema, malodorous exudate, color of tissue, or burning sensation.
17. Dispose of equipment and linens, according to standard precautions and facility policy; remove gloves and dispose of them in proper receptacle. Perform hand hygiene.
18. Tape the catheter to thigh or use a catheter strap.
19. Observe flow of urine through drainage tubing; note the accumulation of urine in the collecting receptacle. If the drainage tubing becomes cloudy or stained, change

PROCEDURE 21.3

Performing Routine Catheter Care—cont'd

the tubing to aid accurate observations of urine. Empty drainage receptacle at least every 8 hours or as necessary to prevent backup of urine into the tubing or bladder.

20. Remove your gloves and practice hand hygiene.
21. Provide for the patient's comfort by returning the bed to its original position.
22. Place the call light within reach.
23. Lower the bed to its original position.
24. Document the procedure, noting any abnormal observations.

25. Document the following:
    - Date and time
    - Procedure
    - Assessment of urinary meatus
    - Character of urine
    - Patient's response
    - Patient teaching
26. Report any unusual findings immediately.

(Figure from Mosby's nursing assistant video skills 4.0, *St. Louis, 2015, Elsevier.)*

PROCEDURE 21.4

Changing a Leg Bag to a Drainage Bag and Emptying a Drainage Bag

1. Refer to medical record, care plan, or Kardex.
2. Assess patient's needs.
3. Assemble supplies according to patient's needs.
4. Introduce self.
5. Identify patient.
6. Explain procedure.
7. Prepare patient.
8. Close door or pull privacy curtain.
9. Arrange supplies close to the bedside.
10. Place protective on bed under patient's buttocks, if necessary.
11. Perform hand hygiene and don clean gloves according to agency policy and guidelines from the CDC and OSHA.
12. Assemble equipment.
13. If able, have the person to sit on the edge of the bed.
14. Don clean gloves, and gain access to the catheter and leg bag.
15. Clamp the catheter using the clamp on the leg bag; urine below the clamp will continue to drain into the leg bag.

17. Raise the bed to a height that promotes good body mechanics.
18. Using the bedside table to organize your supplies, place a towel across the surface.
19. Open the antiseptic wipes, sterile cap and plug, as well as the package with the drainage bag and tubing; do not touch the sterile cap or plug. These should be on the bedside table.
20. Attach the drainage bag to the bed frame.

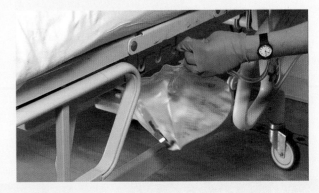

21. Disconnect the catheter from the drainage tubing, taking great care to not touch the tip or opening of either.

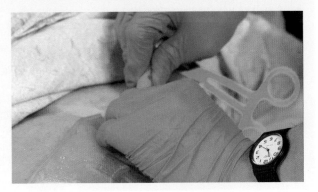

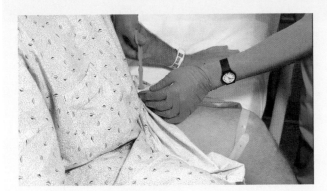

16. Have the person to lie down on the bed in a supine position; cover the patient with the bath blanket.

Continued

PROCEDURE 21.4

Changing a Leg Bag to a Drainage Bag and Emptying a Drainage Bag—cont'd

22. Pick up the sterile plug by the package and not the exposed tip, and insert it into the catheter end.
23. Attach the sterile cap onto the end of the leg bag drainage tube.

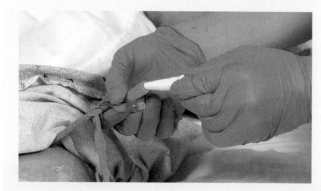

24. Remove caps from the tubing of the new drainage bag, and the sterile plug, and connect the two by inserting one into the other.

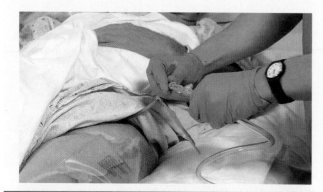

25. Release the clamp on the catheter that is currently clamped; urine should begin to flow through the tubing.
26. Discard of the leg bag once you have drained and measured the urine.
    a. To empty the urinary drainage bag, open the clamp on the drain.
    b. Let all urine drain from the bag into a graduated cylinder.
    c. Reclamp the drain so that no remaining urine leaks onto the floor.
    d. Measure the amount of urine obtained in the graduated cylinder.
    e. Take the graduated cylinder to the bathroom to dispose of the urine in the toilet.
    f. Rinse the graduated cylinder with clean water.
    g. Return it to its storage location (usually located in the bathroom)
27. Remove the bath blanket and return the patient's covers or gown.
28. Take the bedpan and other disposable supplies to the bathroom.
29. Dispose of any urine in the toilet once it has been accounted for.
30. Dispose of any disposable supplied in the trashcan.
31. Rinse the bedpan and return to its location in the lower portion of the bedside cabinet.
32. Remove your gloves and practice hand hygiene.
33. Provide for the patient's comfort by returning the bed to its original position.
34. Place the call light within reach.
35. Lower the bed to its original position.
36. Document the procedure, noting any abnormal observations.

(Figures from Mosby's nursing assistant video skills 4.0, *St. Louis, 2015, Elsevier.)*

Box 21.3   Life Span Considerations

Postpartum Women/Need for Catheterization

- A patient who has just delivered a baby vaginally may experience significant swelling in the perineal area. This may make voiding extremely difficult.
- The area of the perineum may have experienced significant trauma, resulting in the need for sutures. This makes the area extremely sensitive to the touch and sore.
- If a patient has had epidural anesthesia during childbirth, where the patient has experienced decreased sensation to the lower extremities, this can make voiding after childbirth difficult.

- At times, the patient needs to be catheterized to receive relief of bladder fullness.
- Take extreme care to be gentle when catheterizing the postpartum women who has given birth vaginally.
- Sometimes the landmarks are distorted because of the swelling; if you have difficulty visualizing the urethra, notify the nurse for assistance.
- Sometimes the patient complains of intense vaginal pain after childbirth. This can be a complication from childbirth; if the patient is complaining of intense pain, notify the nurse before attempting to perform a catheterization.

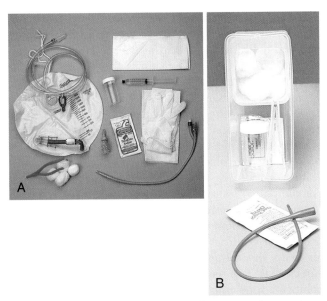

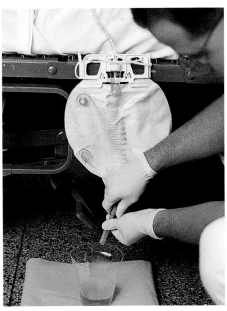

FIGURE 21.5 A, Urinary drainage device, sterile specimen cup, sterile drape, sterile gloves, indwelling catheter, sterile cleanser, sterile saline, and sterile cotton balls with forceps. B, Catheter kit with straight catheter and iodine cleanser used for an indwelling catheter placement. (From Elkin MK, Perry AG, Potter PA: *Nursing interventions and clinical skills*, ed 2, St. Louis, 2000, Mosby.)

FIGURE 21.7 Empty and record urine output from Foley catheter into clean graduated container. Clean the drainage port before draining and before recapping. (From Potter PA, Perry AG, Stocket PA, et al.: *Fundamentals of nursing: concepts, process, and practice*, ed 9, St. Louis, 2017, Mosby.)

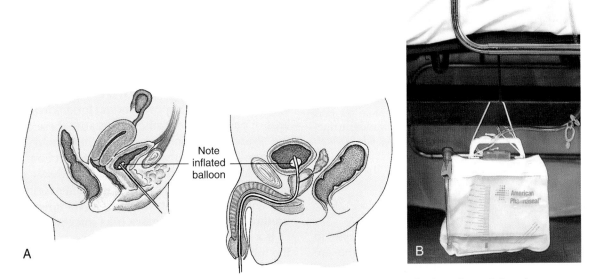

FIGURE 21.6 Urinary drainage system. A, Balloon inflation in both male and female patients. B, It is essential to keep drainage system below the level of the bladder. Do not place bag on side rails or allow it to rest on the floor. Attach drainage bag to bed or, while patient is ambulating, to intravenous pole. (From Potter PA, Perry AG: *Basic nursing: essentials for practice*, ed 7, St. Louis, 2011, Mosby.)

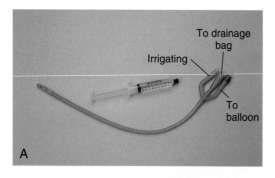

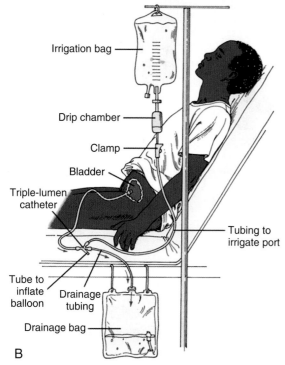

FIGURE 21.8 Bladder irrigation. A, Triple-lumen catheter with sterile syringe to inflate catheter balloon. Note the port for inflating the balloon. B, Continuous sterile bladder irrigation setup. (From Perry AG, Potter PA: *Nursing interventions and clinical skills*, ed 6, St. Louis, 2016, Mosby.)

Older Adults/Catheterization

A patient with a catheter is especially vulnerable to urinary tract infections. Older adult patients who are physically compromised run the additional risk of developing septicemia, a potentially life-threatening infection that has spread to the blood. Therefore do not routinely catheterize an older patient who is incontinent.

Encourage adequate oral fluid intake of at least 2000 mL/day, and assist the older adult to the bathroom on a regular, timed basis. This will help with bladder retraining and may prevent the need for excessive catheterization.

When catheters are required, an older adult may be more cautious when ambulating. Encourage as much ambulation as tolerated, and remove the urinary drainage device as soon as the nurse tells you to.

If a condom catheter is used on an older person, close monitoring is necessary. The skin of an older patient is frail and delicate, and the adhesive used on the condom catheter could damage the skin.

After the urinary catheter is removed, some patients may have difficulty voiding as a result of poor bladder tone and decreased sensation. If the patient complains of urinary retention or a full bladder, the PCT should try stimulating urination by running water, placing the patient's hands in warm water, or pouring warm water over the perineum. Female patients should be encouraged to sit on a bathroom stool or commode and male patients to stand to void. Some patients may experience some dribbling of urine after voiding as a result of dilation of the sphincter from the catheter. Such patients should be reassured that this is normal and should improve as sphincter tone improves. The PCT should record the time of urination, the amount of urine output, and the color of the urine.

Routine Catheter Care

Routine catheter care is an important aspect of an indwelling urinary drainage system. Patients should receive routine catheter care and perineal hygiene at least every 8 hours to prevent urinary tract infections (see Procedure 21.3). During catheter care, it is necessary to cleanse the first 2 inches of the catheter to remove any secretions or encrustations from the catheter. It is also important to look for inflammation or swelling at and around the urethral meatus, in addition to checking for swelling or discharge from the urethra. Some facilities discourage the use of powders and lotions in the perineal area of patients with catheters because these can lead to the growth of microorganisms that could enter the urinary tract and cause urinary tract infections. It is also important to perform perineal and catheter care after bowel movements, especially if the patient is incontinent of stool. The bacteria in stool can travel upward into the urethra and cause a urinary tract infection.

If a catheter strap or adhesive tape is used to secure the tubing to the abdomen or leg, it should be replaced after catheter care is given. If the tubing and collection device must be changed because of leakage, odor, or collection of sediment in the tubing or collection device, the PCT must be sure to follow sterile technique (see Box 21.4).

Incontinence and Its Management

Incontinence—the inability to control urine or bowel elimination—can be a psychologically distressing and socially disruptive problem, especially among older adults.

Box 21.4	Teaching Indwelling Urinary Drainage System Care to Patients

- Explain the procedure and expected sensations associated with the procedure to the patient before you insert the catheter.
- Answer patient's questions about the procedures.
- Explain the need for the patient to drink fluids to flush the urinary system.
- Instruct the patient about proper transfer from a bed, chair, or stretcher with the catheter bag.
- Caution the patient not to lie on tubing and to keep the drainage bag below the level of the bladder.
- Discourage the use of lotions or powder during perineal care.
- Encourage using a leg bag during the day and a bedside drainage bag at night.
- Instruct patient to wear loose-fitting clothing to promote adequate drainage.

Urinary incontinence can occur because pressure in the bladder is too great or because the sphincters are too weak. It can involve a small leakage of urine when the person laughs, coughs, or lifts something heavy (stress incontinence), or it can be a constant leakage whenever the bladder contains urine (urge incontinence). Collaborating with other members of the healthcare team is important to identify the cause and the extent of incontinence and to assist in managing the problem. The PCT can play an important role in managing the patient's incontinence.

Patients with urinary incontinence may be referred to a urologist for evaluation, and treatment may involve teaching the patient exercises to strengthen muscles around the external sphincters or employing bladder training. The nurse would be responsible for teaching the patient these exercises. If a paralyzed patient has overflow incontinence or incontinence related to an overfull bladder, the Credé maneuver is helpful. This involves applying manual pressure over the lower abdomen to express urine from the bladder at regular intervals. When this technique is used, care must be taken to prevent injury to the bladder from excess pressure. The nurse would be responsible for teaching the patient this method of urine expression.

Fecal incontinence may result from diarrhea or constipation, muscle damage or weakness, nerve damage, or even inactivity. Patients with urinary or fecal incontinence may require disposable adult undergarments or underpads to help prevent soiling of clothing and embarrassment. Use of discreet incontinence products helps promote self-care, as well as self-esteem.

Urine and feces are also highly irritating to the skin. Skin that is continuously exposed becomes inflamed and irritated quickly. To help prevent skin impairment, the nurse should make sure to change the undergarments or underpads frequently; cleanse the skin thoroughly after each episode of incontinence with warm, soapy water, and dry it completely. The PCT should cleanse the perineum in a professional, caring, and matter-of-fact manner. The patient must not be reprimanded, scolded, or humiliated for having an "accident."

Bladder Training

Bladder training is the achievement of voluntary control over voiding; it often involves developing the use of muscles in the perineum. When urinary incontinence results from decreased perception of bladder fullness or impaired voluntary motor control, bladder training is often helpful.

Before the removal of a urethral catheter, bladder training may be ordered by the healthcare provider and involves a clamp-unclamp routine to improve bladder tone. Kegel exercises may also be used to improve perineal muscle tone and sphincter control as part of a bladder training regimen. The patient is instructed by the nurse to perform Kegel exercises by trying to stop the flow of urine during voiding. Once the patient has identified the correct muscles and the feeling of their contraction, the patient can perform these exercises when not voiding by tightening the muscles of the perineum, holding the tension for 10 seconds, and then relaxing for 10 seconds. This should be done multiple times, several times a day. Because muscle control develops gradually, it sometimes takes 4 to 6 weeks to slow or stop urinary leakage.

Habit training is also a part of bladder training and involves establishing a voiding schedule. This provides cooperative patients with the opportunity to achieve continence by voiding at regular intervals (every 1.5 to 2 hours). The nurse may ask you to monitor the patient's voiding for a few days to identify patterns, or schedule voiding times to correlate with the patient's activities. Typical voiding times are upon rising, before each meal, and at bedtime. The PCT should assist the patient to void as scheduled, check the patient for wetness periodically, and remind or assist the patient to the toilet as scheduled. After a few days, the nurse evaluates the scheduled voiding pattern by identifying its effectiveness in keeping the patient continent. Then the schedule is modified until continence is established. Fluid intake and medications typically influence voiding patterns. Limiting fluids after the evening meal reduces the need for nighttime voiding and helps keep the patient dry.

Removal of an Indwelling Catheter

It is always best to remove an indwelling catheter as soon as possible because its presence increases the risk for urinary tract infection (Procedure 21.5). After surgery, the healthcare provider usually orders the catheter removed after 8 to 24 hours, depending on the type of surgery. In some situations, the catheter remains in place for days or even weeks. The longer a catheter has been in place, the greater is the risk that an infection will develop. Urinary tract infections are one of the most common types of *iatrogenic* (caused by treatments or diagnostic procedures) infections in healthcare. Symptoms of a urinary tract infection may not appear for 2 or more days after the catheter is removed. This means that the patient may already be home before he or she begins displaying symptoms. For that reason, it is

necessary to inform the patient of the risk for infection, how to prevent it, signs and symptoms to watch for, and when to call the healthcare provider.

Sometimes patients have difficulty voiding after the removal of a urinary catheter because the sphincter muscles are weakened. Patients with a distended, or very full bladder, or who have altered feeling because of regional anesthesia, such as a spinal or epidural block, are likely to have difficulty voiding after catheter removal. Most patients should void adequately within 8 hours after catheter removal. If they do not, the nurse needs to notify the healthcare provider and receive further orders.

PROCEDURE 21.5
Removing an Indwelling Catheter

1. Refer to medical record, care plan, or Kardex.
2. Assemble supplies according to patient's needs.
3. Introduce self.
4. Identify patient.
5. Explain procedure.
6. Prepare patient.
7. Close door or pull privacy curtain.
8. Arrange supplies close to the bedside.
9. Place protective pad under patient's buttocks, if necessary.
10. Perform hand hygiene and don clean gloves according to agency policy and guidelines from the CDC and OSHA.
11. Assemble equipment: 10-mL syringe or larger (depending on volume of fluid used to inflate balloon) without a needle.

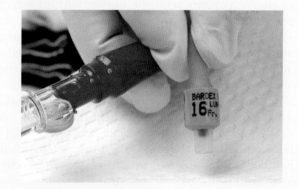

12. Determine the following:
    a. Length of time catheter has been in place.
    b. Patient's knowledge of procedure and what to expect.
13. Provide privacy. Position the patient supine, and place a waterproof pad under the patient's buttocks. Female patients need to abduct their legs with the drape between their thighs. For male patients, it is acceptable for drape to lie on the thighs.

14. Insert hub of syringe into inflation valve (balloon port), and aspirate until tubing collapses or resistance is felt.
15. Remove catheter steadily and smoothly (in female patients, the catheter is in about 2 to 3 inches [5 to 7.5 cm] and in male patients, about 6 to 7 inches [15 to 18 cm]). Catheter usually slides out very easily. Do not use force. If any resistance is noted, repeat step 5 to remove remaining water.
16. Wrap catheter in waterproof pad. Unhook collection bag and drainage tubing from the bed.
17. Measure urine, and empty drainage bag.
18. Record output.
19. Cleanse the perineum with soap and warm water, and dry area thoroughly.
20. Explain the following to patient, as directed by the nurse:
    a. It is important to have a fluid intake of 1.5 to 2 L/day unless contraindicated.
    b. The patient must void within 8 hours, and each voiding should be measured. Some facilities and healthcare providers determine how much the patient should void to verify adequate emptying of the urinary bladder.
    c. Mild burning sensation or discomfort with first voiding is anticipated. Instruct patient to notify the nurse if it does not subside with subsequent voidings.
    d. Signs of urinary tract infection are urinary urgency, burning sensation, urinary frequency, excretion of only small amount, and continued pain or discomfort. These symptoms may develop 2 to 3 days after removal of catheter.
21. Place the urine measuring device on the toilet seat.
22. Document and report the following:
    • Date and time of catheter removal
    • Time, amount, and characteristics of first voiding after catheter removal
    • Complete input and output record

CHAPTER SUMMARY

There are times when patients need your assistance in meeting their elimination needs. This is a very personal and private experience for the patient and often has feelings of embarrassment attached to it. No one wants to ask for help with going to the bathroom. Always respect the right to privacy for the patient who needs assistance with elimination.

Sometimes the patient is unable to urinate independently and may need further assistance. This may mean the use of intermittent catheterization to drain the bladder periodically, or it may mean that insertion of a urinary catheter is necessary. If a urinary catheter is necessary, you may be asked to insert it. Because of the risk of infection, it is important that only sterile technique is used when catheterizing someone in the hospital setting. There are many types of bacteria and viruses that are present in the hospital setting even though it is thoroughly cleaned daily. Use of sterile technique will help to decrease the risk of a urinary tract infection from an indwelling urinary catheter. Patients, especially the fragile older adult, can die from a urinary tract infection. Whether or not bacteria enter the urinary tract can be related to how well you perform strict sterile technique when you are inserting a urinary catheter. Third-party payers have stopped paying for urinary tract infections that are caused by extended use of a urinary catheter. To assist with keeping costs down at the medical facility where you are employed, as well as to decrease the rate of infection specifically related to the use of urinary catheters, always follow the nurse's delegation of discontinuing a urinary catheter as soon as possible. This is not something you want to put off to the end of your shift. The sooner the urinary catheter is discontinued, the less the risk of the patient developing a urinary tract infection. You can make a difference!

Case Scenario

You are working as a PCT on the postpartum unit. You are caring for a mother who has given birth 8 hours ago, and has been unable to urinate on her own. The nurse has asked you to perform intermittent, straight catheterization at this time. When you go into the room and prepare the area for the catheterization, you note that the patient is crying out in discomfort, complaining "her bottom hurts so bad." As you inspect her perineum to determine your landmarks for inserting the catheter, you note the area to be swollen, a bluish color, and difficult to visualize. What should you do? Should you proceed with attempting the straight catheterization? Why or why not? Should you ask for additional assistance in locating the urethra, or should you notify the nurse? Explain the reasoning for your next step.

REVIEW QUESTIONS

1. The bedpan is given to the patient for defecation only.
   a. True
   b. False

2. A man's urinal should be stored
   a. in the bed.
   b. on top of the bedside table.
   c. at the nurse's station.
   d. in the lower section of the bedside cabinet.

3. A urinary catheter should be removed as soon as the nurse gives the direction to for which of the following reasons?
   a. The longer the catheter stays in, the more bleeding it will cause.
   b. Patients who have a urinary catheter are unable to defecate because of the pressure.
   c. The longer the catheter stays in, the more chance there is for an infection.
   d. Urinary catheters are put in place only during a surgical procedure; once the person is awake, they should be removed.

4. A 50-year-old patient was discharged home with a Foley catheter. The PCT demonstrates the proper procedure on how to cleanse the female perineal area with which of the following directions?
   a. Cleanse the area in circular motions around the rectum.
   b. Cleanse from the rectum toward the pubis.
   c. Cleanse from the pubis toward the rectum.
   d. Cleanse in circular motions around the vaginal area.

5. To insert a Foley catheter, the PCT should use which kind of technique?
   a. Clean technique
   b. Sterile technique
   c. Aseptic technique
   d. Surgical technique

Assisting With Bowel Elimination

LEARNING OBJECTIVES

1. Identify the procedures for promoting bowel elimination.
2. Administer an enema.
3. Discuss factors that can interfere with bowel elimination.
4. Describe the various types of enemas used to promote bowel elimination.
5. Discuss the care necessary to maintain an ostomy.
6. Identify the potential complications of an ostomy.

KEY TERMS

cathartics Drugs that stimulate bowel evacuation (see laxatives)

colostomy Surgical creation of a stoma on the abdominal wall to where the colon is surgically attached

defecation Elimination of bowel wastes

enema Instillation of a solution into the colon via the anus

fecal impaction A collection of feces in the rectum in the form of a mass that becomes so large or hard that the patient is unable to pass it voluntarily

flatulence The presence of air or gas (flatus) in the intestinal tract

ileostomy Opening in the ileum; the distal part of the small intestine

laxatives A drug that stimulates the evacuation of the bowels (see cathartics)

ostomy An artificial opening

BOWEL ELIMINATION

Elimination of bowel wastes (defecation) is a basic human need and is essential for normal body function. Patients may refer to this as defecating, having a bowel movement, or stooling. Normal bowel elimination depends on several factors: a balanced diet, including high-fiber foods; a daily fluid intake of 2000 to 3000 mL; and activity to promote muscle tone and peristalsis (movement of digested food through the intestine). Each patient has an individual pattern of defecation, but every patient should have a bowel movement at least every 1 to 3 days. This pattern should be determined on hospital admission, and an abdominal evaluation should be completed by the nurse. The nurse will usually ask about any alterations in bowel elimination to determine nursing diagnoses related to elimination.

To promote a normal pattern of elimination, establish a routine time for defecation, encourage the patient to heed the urge to defecate, and allow the patient to sit on a commode or, if he or she is in bed, in a Fowler's position because this is the customary position for defecation. Bowel elimination is a private activity. Give the patient as much privacy as possible, and avoid continually "checking on" the patient because this may make the patient uncomfortable and will not provide an environment that makes defecation easier to accomplish. Some patients may not want to use a bedpan because of discomfort and lack of privacy. Reassure the patient as much as possible and ensure that the bed is in Fowler's position. Sometimes playing soft music will help the patient relax enough to have a bowel movement. There is research to show that those who are stressed or tense may have difficulty with defecation.

Many people have their own established ritual to promote elimination, such as drinking warm water with lemon juice or drinking black coffee with breakfast. Some habits are dangerous and actually prevent normal bowel function, such as long-term, routine use of laxatives and cathartics. Eventually these habits may cause the intestines to lose the ability to respond to the presence of stool in the rectum, which often results in chronic constipation. Overcoming dependency on laxatives and cathartics is often difficult to accomplish and requires cooperation and compliance from the patient (Box 22.1).

Delegation in Bowel Elimination

Delegation is an important skill that can assist nurses in performing efficient patient care. It involves assigning patient care tasks to unlicensed assistive personnel (UAP), such as the patient care technician (PCT), providing safe, timely, quality care. Delegation requires knowledge of the patient's needs and the ability to use nursing judgment. If used properly, delegation can improve nursing efficiency and helps coordinate patient care. Delegation

Box 22.1	Life Span Considerations for Altered Bowel Elimination in Older Adults

- In many older adults, constipation results from insufficient dietary bulk, inadequate fluid intake, laxative abuse, diminished muscle tone and motor function, decreased defecation reflex, mental or physical illness, and the presence of tumors or strictures.
- For an older adult, a diet including at least 6 to 10 g of dietary fiber per day adds bulk, weight, and form to stool and improves defecation.
- Older adults should develop a regular toileting routine in response to the urge to defecate.
- The older adult patient or a family member should keep a week's diary of meals and fluid intake. The nurse should determine whether dietary pattern contributes to constipation. The nurse should recommend an increase in fiber if it is needed.
- Encourage as much activity as tolerated to maintain peristalsis and decrease the risk for constipation.

is based on each state's nurse practice act. The PCT should have a complete knowledge of which tasks can be delegated even though the nurse delegating the task is ultimately responsible for the outcome.

Activities that are generally delegated are those that occur frequently during the daily care of a patient. These activities are predictable, and the procedures are standard and unchanging in terms of the facility's policies. PCTs are not qualified to exercise nursing judgment; therefore a task that requires this type of clinical judgment should not be delegated to PCTs. Bowel elimination is an area that is often delegated to the PCT and is an appropriate skillset for the PCT to perform.

Care of the Patient With Hemorrhoids

Hemorrhoids are swollen and inflamed veins in the anus and lower rectum. They may result from straining during bowel movements or from increased pressure during pregnancy or with heavy lifting. Hemorrhoids can be internal (inside the rectum) or external (around the anus). They are frequently a source of discomfort and have the capacity to cause an alteration in elimination. The goal for patients with hemorrhoids is to decrease pain, prevent elimination problems, and prevent damage to the already swollen tissue. To achieve this, it is necessary for the patient to maintain a proper diet high in fiber, ensure adequate fluid intake, and participate in regular exercise. If the hemorrhoids are particularly troublesome, localized heat in the form of a sitz bath or witch hazel pads often provides some relief. In these patients, rectal thermometers and rectal tubes should not be used.

Flatulence

Flatulence, or the presence of air or gas (flatus) in the intestinal tract, typically occurs when a person consumes gas-producing liquids and foods such as carbonated beverages, cabbage, or beans; swallows excessive amounts of air; or is constipated. It can also be caused by decreased peristalsis, abdominal surgery, some narcotic medications, and decreased physical activity. Flatulence may cause distention of the stomach and abdomen and, in some cases, mild to moderate abdominal cramping, which can be painful. To promote peristalsis and passage of flatus, encourage the patient to ambulate.

Administering an Enema

An enema is the instillation of a solution into the colon via the anus. The primary reason for an enema is promotion of defecation in a patient with constipation. Enemas can be given for a number of reasons, such as cleansing the colon before a diagnostic procedure or abdominal surgery, management of constipation or fecal impaction, and administration of medication. The volume and type of enema administered depends on the reason for it and the healthcare provider's order.

A cleansing enema stimulates peristalsis (intestinal movement) by introducing large volumes of fluid to distend the bowel. This type of enema helps empty the colon completely and is used frequently before surgery or a gastrointestinal diagnostic procedure.

An oil retention enema is used to soften the stool and lubricate the bowel to make defecation easier. It is used when a fecal impaction is suspected. A fecal impaction is a collection of feces in the rectum in the form of a mass that becomes so large or hard that the patient is unable to pass it voluntarily. Medicated enemas can be used for a variety of reasons but are used most frequently to bring down an extremely high potassium level.

No matter what type of enema is used, caution patients to limit the number of enemas they use. The defecation reflex may become dependent on enemas with repeated use, which can cause constipation. It is better to determine the cause of bowel irregularity or constipation and treat the cause rather than relying on enemas (Procedure 22.1).

PROCEDURE 22.1
Administering an Enema

1. Check the healthcare provider's order.
2. Introduce yourself to the patient; include your name and title or role.
3. Identify the patient by checking his or her identification bracelet and requesting that the patient state his or her name or birth date, or both.
4. Explain the procedure and the reason it is to be done in terms that the patient is able to understand. Advise the patient of any unpleasantness that may be involved with the procedure. Give the patient time to ask questions.
5. Determine need for and provide patient education before and during procedure.
6. Evaluate the patient. Each skill box contains an assessment section that includes specific data to evaluate.
7. Perform hand hygiene and don clean gloves according to agency policy and guidelines from the Centers for Disease Control and Prevention (CDC) and the Occupational Safety and Health Administration (OSHA).
8. Assemble equipment, and complete necessary charges.
9. Prepare the patient for the procedure:
   a. Close the door or pull the privacy curtain around the patient's bed.
   b. Raise the bed to a comfortable working height, and lower the side rail on the side nearest the PCT.
   c. Position and drape the patient as necessary. Descriptions of specific positions are included in each skill.

10. Assemble equipment.

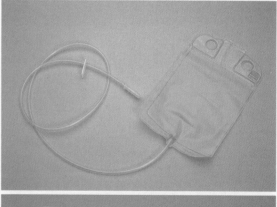

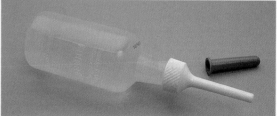

11. Determine the following:
   a. Most recent bowel movement
   b. Presence or absence of bowel sounds

Continued

PROCEDURE 22.1

Administering an Enema—cont'd

c. Ability to control rectal sphincter
d. Presence or absence of hemorrhoids
e. Presence of abdominal pain
f. Patient's level of understanding and previous experience with enemas

12. Prepare solution. There are several types of enema solutions. Cleansing enemas include tap water, normal saline, low-volume hypertonic solutions, and soapsuds solution.
13. Arrange equipment at patient's bedside.
14. Assist patient to the Sims's position. When an enema is given to a patient who is unable to contract the external sphincter, position the patient on the bedpan. Avoid giving the enema with the patient sitting on the toilet; it is possible for the inserted rectal tubing to abrade the rectal wall, and the enema solution is forced uphill, which makes the enema less effective.
15. Place waterproof pad under patient.
16. Place bath blanket over patient and fanfold linen to foot of bed; adjust patient's gown to keep it from being soiled while it still provides privacy.
17. Clamp tubing; fill container with correctly warmed solution (usually 750 to 1000 mL at 105°F [41°C]) and any additives ordered. Administer a child's enema using appropriate equipment at 100°F to avoid burning rectal tissue; read disposable package for instructions. *(Hot water has capacity to burn intestinal mucosa. Cold water has capacity to cause abdominal cramping and is difficult to retain.)* Release clamp, allowing solution to flow through tubing to remove any air from the tubing; reclamp. Suggested maximal volumes are as follows:
    * Infant: 150 to 250 mL
    * Toddler: 250 to 500 mL
    * School-aged child: 500 mL
    * Adolescent: 500 to 700 mL
    * Adult: 750 to 1000 mL
    a. For commercially prepared enema, perform the following:
       (1) Remove cover from tip of enema (tip is prelubricated, but add additional lubricant if needed); insert entire tip into anus.
       (2) Squeeze container until it is empty. Usually a small amount of solution will remain in container. Most containers hold about 250 mL. Continue to squeeze the container to prevent siphoning solution back into the container.
       (3) Encourage patient to retain solution at least 5 minutes.
    b. For standard enema, implement the following:
       (1) Lubricate 4 inches (10 cm) at end of tubing; spread patient's buttocks to expose anus; while rotating tube, gently insert it 3 to 4 inches (7 to 10 cm). Instruct patient to breathe out slowly through mouth.
       (2) Elevate container 12 to 18 inches (30 to 45 cm) above level of anus (see illustration).

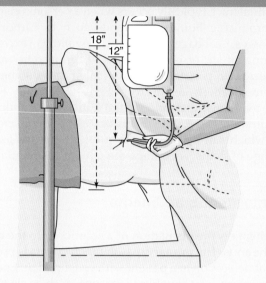

       (3) Release clamp, and allow solution to flow slowly. Usually solution will flow for 5 to 10 minutes.
       (4) Lower container or clamp tubing if patient complains of cramping; encourage slow, deep breathing. Do not remove tubing tip. If severe cramping, bleeding, or sudden severe abdominal pain occurs and is unrelieved by temporarily stopping or slowing flow of solution, stop enema and notify healthcare provider.
       (5) Clamp and remove tube when all of the solution has been administered. Encourage patient to retain solution at least 5 minutes.
18. When patient is no longer able to retain solution, assist patient to bedpan, bedside commode, or bathroom.
19. Instruct patient to call to inspect results before stool is flushed. Observe characteristics of feces or solution. When enemas are ordered "until clear" in preparation for surgery, enemas are repeated until patient passes fluid that is clear and contains no fecal matter. Usually three consecutive enemas are adequate. If after three enemas the water is highly colored or contains solid fecal material, notify the nurse before continuing.
20. Promote patient involvement as much as possible.
21. Determine the patient's tolerance of the procedure, and be alert for signs and symptoms of discomfort and fatigue. If the patient cannot tolerate a procedure, describe this inability in the nursing notes.
22. Provide for patient hygiene; assist patient to bed or chair.
23. Document the following:
    * Date and time
    * Type and volume of enema
    * Temperature of solution
    * Characteristics of results
    * How patient tolerates procedure

PROCEDURE 22.1

Administering an Enema—cont'd

24. Assist the patient to a position of comfort, and place needed items within easy reach. Ensure that the patient has a means to call for help and knows how to use it.
25. Raise the side rails, and lower the bed to the lowest position.
26. Remove gloves and all protective barriers such as gown, goggles, and masks. Store appropriately or discard. Remove and dispose of soiled supplies and equipment according to agency policy and guidelines from the CDC and OSHA.
27. Perform hand hygiene after removing gloves.
28. Document the patient's response to the procedure, expected or unexpected outcomes, and all patient teaching.
29. Report any unexpected outcomes. Specific notes for reporting unexpected outcomes are included in each skill.

(Figure 10 from Perry AG, Potter PA: Nursing interventions and clinical skills, ed 6, St. Louis, 2016, Mosby; Figure 17a(2) adapted from Sorrentino SA: Mosby's textbook for nursing assistants, ed 9, St. Louis, 2017, Mosby.)

Ostomies

An ostomy, by definition, is an artificial opening. The site of the opening is called a *stoma*. Ostomies can be created because of trauma to the intestine, severe inflammation, or diseases such as cancer that involve part of the intestine. They can be temporary or permanent, depending on the reason they are present, and the characteristics of the fecal material vary according to where the ostomy is located along the intestine. Fecal material in the ileum is liquid, and fecal matter in the rectum is solid. Therefore the closer the ostomy is to either end determines what type of stool will be in the ostomy. Material coming out of the stomach contains many enzymes that increase the acidity of the material. Therefore stool in the ileum, cecum, and ascending colon tends to be more acidic and irritating to the skin surrounding the ostomy. As the material moves through the large intestine, water is removed, and the material becomes more solid and less acidic, causing less irritation to the skin surrounding the stoma. The lower the ostomy is on the intestinal tract, the less acidic and irritating it is to the skin surrounding the ostomy.

An ileostomy is an opening in the ileum (the distal part of the small intestine). An ileostomy is needed when the entire colon needs to be removed or bypassed, as in cases of congenital defects, cancer, inflammatory bowel disease, or bowel trauma.

A colostomy is the surgical creation of a stoma on the abdominal wall to where the colon is normally attached. The colostomy then diverts stool through the stoma. Again, the stool may be liquid, semiformed, or formed, depending on the area of the colon incised. The procedure is performed for patients with cancer of the colon, intestinal obstructions, intestinal trauma, or inflammatory diseases of the colon. Some colostomies are permanent, and some are temporary measures used until intestinal healing occurs.

Colostomy Care

To provide the patient with optimal colostomy care, it is important for the PCT to know the correct use of various products used for colostomy care and to educate the patient about appropriate care. There are various types of pouching systems and skin barriers available to patients. One-pouch systems have a skin barrier (wafer) that is preattached to the pouch; two-piece systems have a pouch that is separate from the wafer. Some skin barriers are precut, whereas others must be cut to fit the stoma. When skin barriers are cut to fit the stoma, ensure that the ostomy appliance opening is small enough to form a proper seal, 1/16 inch larger than the stoma, and does not cause pressure on the stoma because there is a blood and nerve supply in the stoma but no sensation. An ill-fitting appliance can cause a pressure sore and lead to gangrene (Fig. 22.1 and Procedure 22.2; see Illness & Injury Prevention Box 22.1 and Delegation and Documentation Box 22.1).

Illness & Injury Prevention Box 22.1

- Avoid hot water and harsh soaps when washing the skin around the ostomy.
- Perform ostomy care any time the bag is leaking to prevent skin breakdown surrounding the ostomy site.
- The cost of ostomy supplies and reimbursement are often an important concern for older patients with limited incomes; referral to community resources by the nurse may be necessary.
- Some patients acknowledge a stoma with minimal emotional difficulty; some never completely adjust to it. Individualize care according to the patient's situation and circumstances.
- In most cases, patients are able to wear their normal clothes; snug clothing does not interfere with ostomy function.

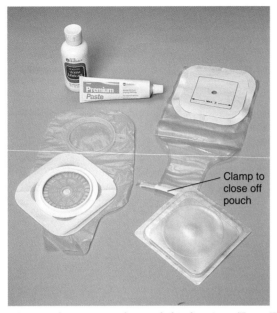

FIGURE 22.1 Ostomy pouches and skin barriers. (From Elkin MK, Perry AG, Potter PA: *Nursing interventions and clinical skills,* ed 4, St. Louis, 2008, Mosby.)

- The skill of applying a pouch to a fresh stoma requires the critical thinking and knowledge of a nurse. Some facilities permit delegation of the task of pouching of an established ostomy to the PCT. Gather the following information from the nurse before performing ostomy care: the expected amount, color, and consistency of drainage from the ostomy. Report changes in the stoma and surrounding skin integrity. Review facility policy.

PROCEDURE 22.2

Performing Colostomy, and Ileostomy Care

Ostomy Care

1. Check the healthcare provider's order.
2. Introduce yourself to the patient; include your name and title or role.
3. Identify the patient by checking his or her identification bracelet and requesting that the patient state his or her name or birth date, or both.
4. Explain the procedure and the reason it is to be done in terms that the patient is able to understand. Advise the patient of any unpleasantness that may be involved with the procedure. Give the patient time to ask questions.
5. Determine need for and provide patient education before and during procedure.
6. Evaluate the patient. Each skill box contains an assessment section that includes specific data to evaluate.
7. Perform hand hygiene and don clean gloves according to agency policy and guidelines from the CDC and OSHA.
8. Assemble equipment, and complete necessary charges.
9. Prepare the patient for the procedure:
   a. Close the door or pull the privacy curtain around the patient's bed.
   b. Raise the bed to a comfortable working height, and lower the side rail on the side nearest the PCT.
   c. Position and drape the patient as necessary. Descriptions of specific positions are included in each skill.

10. Observe for the following:
    a. Pouch leakage and length of time in place. *(Pouches must be changed every 3 to 7 days to prevent skin impairment.)*
    b. Stoma for healing and color. *(Proper stoma appearance is moist and reddish pink.)*
    c. Abdominal incision
11. Arrange supplies and equipment at patient's bedside or in bathroom (see Fig. 22.1).
12. Position patient supine and comfortable.
13. Carefully remove wafer seal from skin (adhesive solvent is sometimes needed).

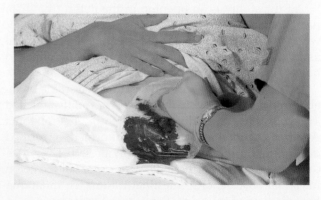

14. Place reusable pouch in bedpan or disposable pouch in plastic bag.

PROCEDURE 22.2

Performing Colostomy, and Ileostomy Care—cont'd

15. Cleanse skin around stoma with warm water; pat dry.

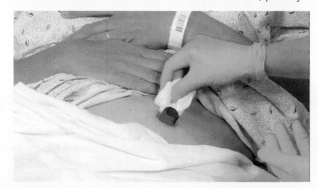

16. Measure stoma opening.
17. Place toilet tissue over stoma; use gauze for ileostomy. Note color and viability of stoma. If skin sealant is to be used, apply to skin and allow to dry.
18. Apply protective skin barrier about 1/16 inch from stoma.
19. Cut an opening in the center of wafer to 1/16 inch larger than stoma, and apply protective wafer with flange.
20. Gently attach pouch to flange by compressing the two together.
21. Remove tissue or gauze from stoma and backing from protectant wafer; center opening over stoma, and press against skin for 1 to 2 minutes.
22. Fold over bottom edges of pouch once to fit clamp. Secure clamp. If bottom edge of pouch is folded over more than once, the plastic will be too thick for the clamp, thus springing the clamp and causing spillage of fecal matter.
23. If patient uses belt, attach at this time.

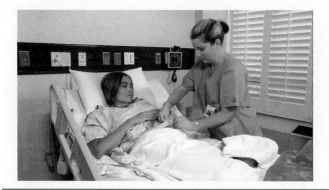

24. Assist patient to comfortable position in bed or chair; remove equipment from bedside.
25. Empty, wash, and dry reusable pouch.
26. Promote patient involvement as much as possible.
27. Determine the patient's tolerance of the procedure, and be alert for signs and symptoms of discomfort and fatigue. If the patient cannot tolerate a procedure, describe this inability in the nursing notes.
28. Document the following:
    - Date and time
    - Procedure
    - Type of pouch
    - Type of skin barrier
    - Amount and appearance of feces
    - Condition of stoma and peristomal skin
    - Patient's level of participation
29. Assist the patient to a position of comfort, and place needed items within easy reach. Ensure that the patient has a means to call for help and knows how to use it.
30. Raise the side rails, and lower the bed to the lowest position.
31. Remove gloves and all protective barriers such as gown, goggles, and masks. Store appropriately or discard. Remove and dispose of soiled supplies and equipment according to agency policy and guidelines from the CDC and OSHA.
32. Perform hand hygiene after removing gloves.
33. Document the patient's response to the procedure, expected or unexpected outcomes, and all patient teaching. Specific areas of documentation are indicated in each skill box.
34. Report any unexpected outcomes.

(Figures from Mosby's nursinng assistant video skills, 4.0, *St. Louis, 2015, Elsevier.)*

CHAPTER SUMMARY

The PCT uses many skills to assist the nurse in the care of the patient. Bowel elimination is one area where the PCT's knowledge and expertise can be used. By being aware of each patient's individualized needs and adapting care to meet those needs, the nurse can provide safe, effective nursing care so that the patient can reach his or her highest level of functioning.

Proper administration of an enema consists of the slow instillation of the correct volume of a warm solution. Emotional support of the patient with an ostomy is important to foster eventual acceptance of the change in body image. Consistency of the feces is directly affected by which portion of the colon is brought out to the stoma. Check with the nurse to determine the consistency of feces to expect.

Even when an ostomy pouch is adhering well, it is best to change it at least every 3 to 5 days or according to pouch recommendations to allow for observation of the stoma and the skin around the stoma. The nurse may delegate to you the skill of changing an ostomy pouch.

Skin impairment is possible after repeated exposure to liquid stool. This is especially true in patients who have a stoma. Be especially careful to protect the skin surrounding the stoma from acid, such as from liquid stool.

Case Scenario

Pat is working on a busy postoperative surgical unit. Her nurse has delegated to her the skill of changing a colostomy bag for a patient. The patient has had this colostomy for several years. When Pat enters the patient's room with the necessary supplies, the patient's family requests that Pat leave the supplies on the counter, stating that they will perform the colostomy bag change themselves. How should Pat respond to the family? If the skill has been delegated to Pat to perform, does Pat have a responsibility to perform the skill herself, or can Pat pass it along to the patient's family members? What is one way Pat can involve the family in the changing of the colostomy bag, yet still meet her obligation of performing this delegated task?

REVIEW QUESTIONS

1. If the patient is suspected of having a fecal impaction, which type of enema would the PCT anticipate the healthcare provider to order?
   a. Soapsuds enema
   b. Medicated enema
   c. Oil retention enema
   d. Tap water enema

2. A patient with a colostomy continues to worry about odor. Which statement would be appropriate for the PCT to tell the patient about colostomy odor?
   a. "It occurs only when the colostomy appliance is changed."
   b. "It is caused by certain foods that can be omitted from the diet."
   c. "It is mainly caused by poor hygiene and can be remedied."
   d. "It is far more noticeable to the patient than to others."

3. The PCT is administering a cleansing enema. Before administering the enema, the PCT assists the patient into which position?
   a. Supine
   b. On right side
   c. Left Sims's position
   d. Left side with head of bed elevated 45 degrees

4. The PCT is administering a routine enema to an adult patient. The patient complains of cramping and the urge to defecate. Which is best to do in this situation?
   a. Quickly finish instilling the rest of the solution
   b. Briefly stop the instillation
   c. Instruct the patient to hold his or her breath and bear down
   d. Immediately discontinue the instillation and withdraw the enema tubing from the rectum

5. When the PCT is changing the ostomy bag, an odor is noted of fecal material. What should the PCT do?
   a. Notify the nurse
   b. Continue with emptying the ostomy bag
   c. Ask the patient what he or she ate for lunch
   d. Ask the patient whether he or she has any room deodorizer

Assisting With Oxygen Needs

LEARNING OBJECTIVES

1. Identify the need for deep-breathing and coughing exercises for the postoperative patient.
2. Discuss interventions and related procedures for the patient receiving oxygen therapy.
3. Discuss care necessary for the patient receiving oxygen therapy.
4. Discuss care of (procedures for) a patient with a tracheostomy.
5. Describe the procedure for oropharyngeal suctioning.
6. Describe the procedure for coughing and deep breathing.

KEY TERMS

hypoxia Reduced oxygen content in tissue and cells.
nasal cannula A simple, two-pronged plastic device that is used to deliver low concentrations of oxygen.
tracheostomy Creation of an opening where the skin is cut to insert the breathing tube.

Promoting an open airway is one of the most important skills a patient care technician (PCT) will perform. There are many factors that may interfere with an airway being open or patent, such as choking on food, having a relaxed airway because of medications, or having an obstruction of tissue, such as obstructive sleep apnea. When the patient does not breathe slow and deep, oxygen-rich blood is not delivered to the brain. In a short duration, a few minutes to be more exact, brain damage can occur. It is important that you as the PCT promote an open airway at all times. One way to encourage an open airway in a patient is with coughing and deep-breathing procedures. When patients are coughing, they are fully expanding their lungs and are moving air, oxygenating the blood flow. When patients are breathing deeply, their lungs are expanding to include the entire area of the lung. Short and shallow breaths mean that the patient is not fully expanding the lungs. This can lead to complications in the lower bases of the lungs. Surgery or injury can cause someone to not want to breathe deeply or cough because of the medications—used to place the patient in a state of sleep—or because of the pain the patient may be experiencing before or after a procedure. Placing the patient in the side-lying position is the best position to keep the patient in if you are concerned about an obstructed or blocked airway. Older patients, those who smoke, and those who have a history of respiratory disease such as asthma or chronic obstructive pulmonary disease (COPD) are more likely to develop complications such as pneumonia.

To prevent respiratory complications, begin encouraging coughing and deep breathing early on in the recovery phase of a patient who has had surgery. Encourage coughing every 1 to 2 hours while patients are awake (Procedure 23.1). The nurse will manage the patient's pain control so that they are able to cough and deep breathe. You will want to provide good oral hygiene to help the patient expectorate, or cough up, excess mucus. This also helps to maintain a clear airway. The mucus is often what blocks, or plugs, the airway.

PROCEDURE 23.1

Assisting With Deep-Breathing and Coughing Exercises

1. Verify with the nurse the procedure to be performed.
2. Introduce yourself to the patient; include your name and title or role.
3. Identify the patient by checking his or her identification bracelet and requesting that the patient state his or her name or birth date, or both.
4. Explain the procedure and the reason it is to be done in terms that the patient is able to understand. Advise the patient of anything uncomfortable that may be involved with the procedure. Give the patient time to ask questions.
5. Determine need for and provide patient education before and during procedure. Notify the nurse of any additional educational needs.
6. Perform hand hygiene and don clean gloves according to agency policy and guidelines from the Centers for Disease Control and Prevention (CDC) and the Occupational Safety and Health Administration (OSHA).
7. Assemble equipment, and complete necessary charges.
8. Prepare the patient for the procedure:
   a. Close the door or pull the privacy curtain around the patient's bed.
   b. Raise the bed to a comfortable working height, and lower the side rail on the side nearest to the PCT.
   c. Position and drape the patient as necessary. Descriptions of specific positions are included in each procedure.
9. Assist patient in a semi-Fowler's position or sitting on the side of the bed or standing position. *(Upright positions facilitate diaphragmatic movement.)*
10. Stand or sit facing the patient. *(This allows patient to observe the breathing exercise.)*

11. Instruct the patient to place palms of hands across from each other, down and along lower borders of their anterior rib cage. Place tips of fingers lightly together.

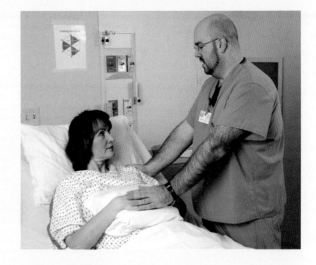

12. Show patient how to take slow, deep breaths, inhaling through nose and pushing abdomen against hands. Have him or her feel middle fingers separate during inhalation. Explain that the patient will feel normal downward movement of the diaphragm while inhaling and that abdominal organs move down and chest wall expands.
13. Instruct patient to avoid using chest and shoulders while inhaling.
14. Repeat complete breathing exercise 3 to 5 times.

Assisting With Deep-Breathing and Coughing Exercises—cont'd

15. Have patient practice exercise. Instruct him or her to take 10 slow, deep breaths every hour while awake.
16. Next, explain the importance of maintaining an upright or sitting position for the patient to be able to produce an effective cough.
17. If the patient has a surgical incision on either the throat or the abdomen, teach the patient to place a pillow or bath blanket over the incisional area and place hands over pillow to splint the incision. During breathing and coughing exercises, have the patient press gently against the incisional area for splinting and support.
18. Demonstrate coughing. Instruct patient to take two slow, deep breaths, inhaling through nose and exhaling through mouth.

19. Show the patient how to inhale deeply a third time and hold breath to a count of three. Cough fully for two or three coughs without inhaling between coughs. Tell the patient to push all air out of the lungs.
20. Caution patient against just clearing the throat instead of coughing.
21. Have patient practice coughing exercises 2 to 3 times every 2 hours while awake.
22. Instruct patient to look at sputum, or mucus, each time for consistency, odor, amount, and color changes. Have the patient report any noted changes to either you or the nurse.

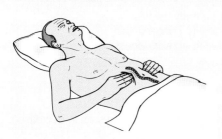
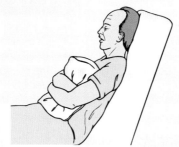
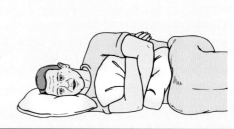

(Figures from Potter PA, Perry AG, Stocket PA, et al.: Fundamentals of nursing: concepts, process, and practice, *ed. 8, St. Louis, 2013, Elsevier.)*

OXYGEN THERAPY

The patient who has had surgery or an injury may need to have oxygen therapy in order to assist with oxygen-rich blood delivery to the brain. Oxygen is needed by all cells of the body to metabolize nutrients and produce energy needed to function. When hypoxia (reduced oxygen content in tissue and cells) occurs, cell metabolism slows down, and cells begin to die. Oxygen therapy is one method used for preventing or relieving tissue hypoxia. Oxygen therapy must be ordered by a healthcare provider and closely monitored by the nurse to ensure proper administration. As a PCT, it may be within your role to monitor a patient on oxygen. Oxygen is treated as a drug; therefore it is important to follow the nurse's direction and not alter the rate.

There are many safety issues involved in the administration of oxygen. It is a colorless, odorless, and tasteless gas that does not burn or explode, but it does support combustion; that is, if it is combined with other factors, such as an electrical spark or fire, oxygen enables combustion, and nearby objects ignite. Smoking, wool blankets, and friction toys should be avoided when oxygen is administered. The PCT must observe all safety precautions (Box 23.1). Oxygen therapy can also be very drying to mucous membranes of the mouth and oropharynx, which increases the risk of tissue cracking and

Delegation and Documentation Box 23.1

Oxygen Administration

- Oxygen administration requires the critical thinking skills of a nurse. The nurse is responsible for ensuring that the oxygen is administered in the correct manner, adjusting oxygen flow rate, and evaluating the patient's response to oxygen therapy. The PCT may assist with oxygen administration under the direction of the nurse.
- Correct placement and adjustment of oxygen devices may be delegated to unlicensed assistive personnel such as the PCT after the care provider is instructed about the possible complications and outcomes associated with oxygen delivery and the need to report these to the nurse immediately if they occur.

opening and of infection. Dry mucous membranes can cause an increase in the number of nosebleeds for the patient. In addition, oxygen toxicity, or an overdose of oxygen, can cause scarring of the respiratory tract tissue and blindness.

Oxygen therapy may be started by a respiratory therapist (CRT/RRT), a nurse, an emergency medical technician (EMT), or any other licensed healthcare provider with an appropriate order for the oxygen. In some facilities, there is a respiratory care department staffed by respiratory therapists who assume the responsibility of administering oxygen and delivering treatments that will improve a patient's ventilation and oxygenation.

Patients in need of oxygen may show various symptoms depending on how deprived of oxygen they are (Box 23.2). When caring for a patient having difficulty breathing or showing any symptoms of hypoxia, the PCT should notify the nurse immediately and ask whether he or she needs to assist with oxygen administration as soon as possible. Failure to act quickly can result in brain damage occurring from the loss of oxygen-rich blood delivery to the brain. There are several ways to deliver oxygen. Delivering through a nasal cannula (device consisting of small tubes inserted into the nares) is the most common way to administer oxygen; however, oxygen can also be delivered by a mask, by an oxygen hood or halo, and by way of an oxygen tent (Procedure 23.2 and Fig. 23.1). Many elderly patients and patients with chronic lung disease require oxygen in the home setting.

Box 23.1   Safety Precautions During Oxygen Use

- Place "No Smoking" or "Oxygen in Use" signs, or both, in the patient's room and where easily seen.
- Instruct the patient, the family, and visitors that smoking is not permitted because oxygen supports combustion (burning).
- Avoid the use of electrical appliances, such as razors, blankets, and heating pads while oxygen is administered.
- Secure portable oxygen delivery systems, such as cylinders, to prevent falling or tipping.
- Avoid placing oxygen cylinders near sources of heat, such as lamps or radiators.
- Avoid clothing that is not fire resistant.
- Ensure that all electrical equipment is functioning appropriately and is well grounded (three-prong plug). Avoid frayed, tangled, or cluttered cords, and do not overload circuits.
- Know the facility's fire procedure and the locations of fire extinguishers.
- Administer oxygen by the method and rate ordered by the healthcare provider.
- Avoid use of petrolatum products such as petroleum jelly when oxygen is administered.

Box 23.2   Signs and Symptoms of Hypoxia

- Apprehension, anxiety, restlessness
- Decreased ability to concentrate
- Decreased level of consciousness
- Increased fatigue
- Vertigo
- Behavioral changes
- Increased pulse rate: as hypoxia advances, bradycardia results, which in turn results in decreased oxygen saturation
- Increased rate and depth of respiration: as hypoxia progresses, respirations become shallow and slower, and apnea develops
- Elevated blood pressure
- Cardiac dysrhythmias
- Pallor
- Cyanosis
- Digital clubbing (with chronic hypoxia)
- Dyspnea

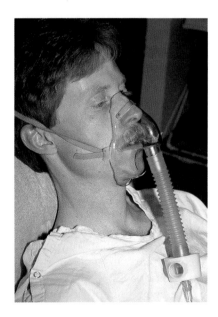
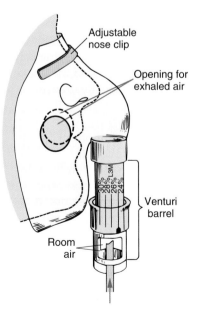

FIGURE 23.1 Venturi mask. (From Potter PA, Perry AG, Stocket PA, et al: *Fundamentals of nursing: concepts, process, and practice*, ed 8, St. Louis, 2013, Mosby.)

Transtracheal Oxygen Delivery

A newer method of oxygen delivery is the transtracheal catheter, which is inserted directly into the trachea between the second and third tracheal cartilages.

Unlike a tracheostomy tube, a transtracheal catheter (Fig. 23.2) does not interfere with drinking, eating, or talking. With a nasal cannula, oxygen is delivered only during the inhalation phase of breathing. With the transtracheal oxygen delivery system, oxygen is delivered throughout the entire respiratory cycle to include both inhalation and exhalation. No oxygen is lost to the atmosphere; therefore oxygen delivery is less expensive. Additional humidification is unnecessary

---

PROCEDURE 23.2
Oxygen Administration

1. Verify with the nurse the procedure to be done.
2. Introduce yourself to the patient; include your name and title or role.
3. Identify the patient by checking his or her identification bracelet and requesting that the patient state his or her name or birth date, or both.
4. Explain the procedure and the reason it is to be done in terms that the patient is able to understand. Advise the patient of anything uncomfortable that may be involved with the procedure. Give the patient time to ask questions.
5. Determine need for and provide patient education before and during procedure. Notify the nurse of any additional educational needs.
6. Perform hand hygiene and don clean gloves according to agency policy and guidelines from the CDC and OSHA.
7. Assemble equipment, and complete necessary charges.
8. Prepare the patient for the procedure:
   a. Close the door or pull the privacy curtain around the patient's bed.
   b. Raise the bed to a comfortable working height, and lower the side rail on the side nearest to the PCT.
   c. Position and drape the patient as necessary. Descriptions of specific positions are included in each procedure.
9. Assemble equipment.
10. Explain necessary precautions during oxygen therapy.
11. Position patient in Fowler's or semi-Fowler's position.
12. Auscultate lung sounds, and observe for signs and symptoms of hypoxia or respiratory distress (see Box 23.2). Review laboratory reports of arterial blood gas levels. Suction any secretions obstructing the airway, and listen to lung sounds after suctioning (see Procedure 23.4).
13. Fill humidifier container to designated level. Humidify oxygen if flow rate is greater than 4 L/min. Use only sterile water in humidifier.
14. Attach flowmeter to humidifier, and insert in proper oxygen source: central oxygen outlet, portable oxygen cylinder, or oxygen concentrator. Verify that water is bubbling.
15. Administer oxygen therapy:
   a. Nasal cannula: A simple, two-pronged plastic device that is used to deliver low concentrations of oxygen. A nasal cannula allows patient to eat and talk normally, and its use is appropriate for all age groups.

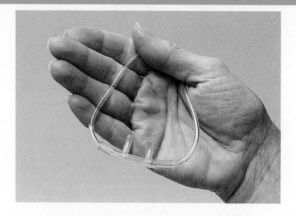

(1) Attach nasal cannula tubing to flowmeter.
(2) Adjust flowmeter to 6 to 10 L/min to flush tubing and prongs with oxygen.
(3) Adjust flow rate to prescribed amount; 1 to 6 L/min may be ordered.
(4) Place a nasal prong into each nostril of the patient.

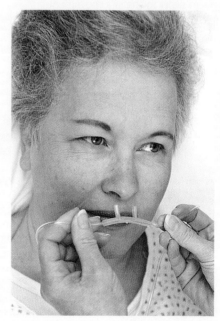

Continued

PROCEDURE 23.2

Oxygen Administration—cont'd

(5) Place cannula tubing over the patient's ears, and tighten under the chin.

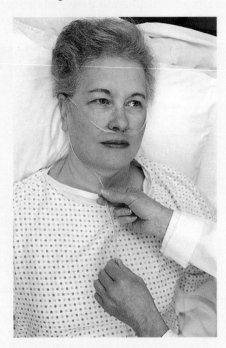

(6) Place padding between strap and ears if needed. Use lamb's wool, gauze, or cotton balls.
(7) Ensure that the cannula tubing is long enough to allow for patient movement.
(8) Regularly evaluate equipment and patient's respiratory status.
  (a) Evaluate cannula frequently for possible obstruction.
  (b) Observe external nasal area, nares, and superior surface of both ears for skin impairment every 6 to 8 hours.
  (c) Observe nares and cannula prongs at least once a shift for irritation or breakage. Cleanse skin with cotton-tipped applicator as needed.
  (d) Apply water-soluble lubricant to nares if needed.
  (e) Refer to the nurse for any prescribed changes in flow rate.
  (f) Maintain solution in humidifier container, if used, at appropriate level at all times.
b. Face mask: Depending on patient's respiratory condition, the healthcare provider may prescribe delivery of oxygen mask. The mask is designed to fit snugly over the patient's nose and mouth. Different types of masks are used according to patient's needs, such as the Venturi mask

(see Fig. 23.1), the partial-rebreathing mask, the nonrebreathing mask, and the simple face mask.

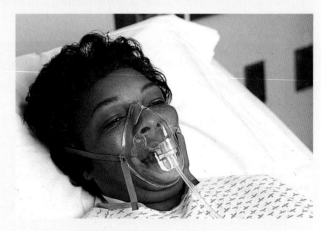

(1) Adjust flow rate of oxygen according to what the nurse told you. Usually 6 to 10 L/min, which is measured in percentages (35% to 95%), is prescribed. In some facilities, the respiratory therapist assumes responsibility for maintaining proper flow. Observe for fine mist or bubbling in humidifier.
(2) Explain to the patient the need for oxygen mask.
(3) Allow patient to hold the oxygen mask over the bridge of the nose and mouth, if he or she is able. Assist as necessary.
(4) Adjust straps around patient's head and over ears. Place cotton ball or gauze over ears under elastic straps.
(5) Observe reservoir bag for appropriate movement if one is attached to mask.
  (a) Partial-rebreathing mask: When functioning properly, the reservoir fills on exhalation and almost collapses on inhalation.

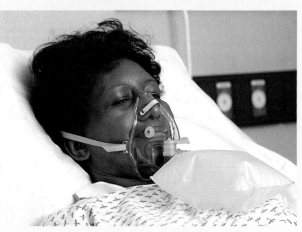

PROCEDURE 23.2

Oxygen Administration—cont'd

(b) Nonrebreathing mask: When functioning properly, the reservoir, or bag, fills on exhalation but never totally collapses on inhalation.

(6) Evaluate equipment function regularly.

(a) Remove mask and evaluate skin every 2 to 4 hours. Clean and dry skin as needed.

(b) Refer to the nurse for prescribed flow rate and any changes.

(c) Maintain solution in humidifier container, if used, at appropriate level at all times. Always use sterile water; never use tap water.

After the Procedure

16. Assist the patient to a position of comfort, and place needed items within easy reach. Ensure that the patient has a means to call for help and knows how to use it.

17. Raise the side rails, and lower the bed to the lowest position.

18. Remove gloves and all protective barriers such as gown, goggles, and masks. Store appropriately or discard. Remove and dispose of soiled supplies and equipment according to agency policy and guidelines from the CDC and OSHA.

19. Perform hand hygiene after removing gloves.

20. Report any unexpected outcomes to the nurse. Specific notes for reporting unexpected outcomes are included in each procedure.

21. Document the following:
- Date
- Time
- Flow rate
- Method of oxygen delivery
- Evaluation of respiratory status
- Patient's response to oxygen therapy
- Changes in healthcare provider's orders
- Adverse reactions or side effects of oxygen therapy

(Figures from Potter PA, Perry AG: Fundamentals of nursing: concepts, process, and practice, *ed 7, St. Louis, 2009, Mosby.)*

Illness & Injury Prevention Box 23.1

Oxygen Therapy

- If oxygen is used at home, the patient's family should have posted a "No Smoking" sign on all entry doors of the house.
- When oxygen cylinders are used, the family should secure them so that they will not fall over. Oxygen cylinders are stored upright, chained on appropriate holders.
- In home settings, oxygen tubing is sometimes as long as 50 feet (15.2 m). The patient is at a greater risk of falling because the tubing is long.
- Patients should have two complete sets of tubing so that one set of equipment is available for use while the other is being cleaned or repaired.
- There should be a three-pronged outlet to use for the compressor to prevent electric shock.
- The nurse may instruct the patient and family on deep-breathing and coughing exercises; as the PCT you can encourage the patient to perform those exercises.
- Because oxygen can be drying, it is important that the patient stays hydrated with fluids.

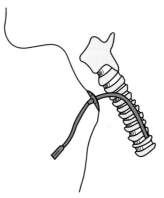

FIGURE 23.2 A transtracheal catheter is inserted into the trachea between the second and third tracheal cartilages. (From Cooper K, Gosnell K: *Foundations of nursing,* ed 7, St. Louis, 2015, Mosby.)

For transtracheal oxygen delivery, a small oxygen tube is inserted through the transtracheal tract opening through which oxygen is administered. This creation of an opening is a surgical procedure in which the skin is cut to insert the tube, known as a tracheostomy. After the insertion tract has matured (healed), it is possible for the patient or a family member to remove the tube for cleaning. A single transtracheal catheter may last up to 3 months. After that period, the catheter is likely to become brittle and must be replaced. This method of oxygen delivery is especially suited for home use. It allows the individual to be more active and can be concealed under a shirt. Some transtracheal oxygen delivery systems even have a beaded chain necklace attached to help disguise the catheter. The patient should be instructed to inspect the transtracheal tract opening

because the nasopharynx, or the nose area, is the area most in need of supplemental humidity, and this area is bypassed. This delivery system also allows the flow rate to be decreased for some patients. Patients who require 2 L/min with a cannula may need only 1 L/min with a transtracheal catheter because they are getting pure oxygen that is not lost to the air. The low flow rates also enable patients to use portable oxygen delivery systems longer between refills.

regularly for redness, edema, or excessive drainage, or exudate. Small amounts of clear exudate are expected. The area is cleaned twice daily with a cotton-tipped applicator. Hydrogen peroxide may be used to wash the neck and remove dried exudate. The transtracheal tract (like a tracheostomy) never truly heals as long as it is kept open with an oxygen delivery catheter. If the catheter is removed and not replaced within a timely manner, the opening may close over. This is the body's natural response of healing. If this occurs, the surgical procedure must be repeated.

Care of the Tracheostomy

A tracheostomy is an artificial opening made by a surgical incision into the trachea. A tracheostomy may be created for patients who are experiencing apnea (episodes in which they stop breathing) or some form of respiratory obstruction. It may also be used to prevent aspiration of secretions and blood or to provide easier access to the lower airways. Many types of tracheostomy tubes are available; the one chosen depends on why it is being used and the condition of the patient. A tracheostomy is a sterile surgical procedure in which the healthcare provider makes an incision into the patient's trachea and inserts a tracheostomy tube into the opening. The tube is then secured in place by cotton tape wrapped around the patient's neck. This provides the patient with a patent, or open, airway. Sterile gauze is placed around the opening in the neck, under the flange, or plastic rims of the outer tube. This protects the skin during the healing process and decreases the risk for infection. A tracheostomy tube provides a direct route for introduction of pathogens into the lower airway, which increases the risk of infection.

The primary responsibilities of the PCT for maintaining a tracheostomy tube are to keep the airway clear, keep the inner cannula (inner tube) clean, prevent breakdown of surrounding skin and tissue, and provide the patient with a means of communicating with you and others (Procedure 23.3, and Figs. 23.3 and 23.4). The care that follows enables the PCT to meet those respon-

---

PROCEDURE 23.3

Tracheostomy Suctioning and Care

1. Verify with the nurse the procedure to be done.
2. Introduce yourself to the patient; include your name and title or role.
3. Identify the patient by checking his or her identification bracelet and requesting that the patient state his or her name or birth date, or both.
4. Explain the procedure and the reason it is to be done in terms that the patient is able to understand. Advise the patient of anything uncomfortable that may be involved with the procedure. Give the patient time to ask questions.
5. Determine need for and provide patient education before and during procedure. Notify the nurse of any additional educational needs.
6. Perform hand hygiene and don clean gloves according to agency policy and guidelines from the CDC and OSHA.
7. Assemble equipment, and complete necessary charges.
8. Prepare the patient for the procedure:
   a. Close the door or pull the privacy curtain around the patient's bed.
   b. Raise the bed to a comfortable working height, and lower the side rail on the side nearest to the PCT.
   c. Position and drape the patient as necessary. Descriptions of specific positions are included in each procedure.
9. Assemble equipment.
10. Check patient's tracheostomy for exudate, edema, and respiratory obstruction.
11. Position patient in semi-Fowler's position.
12. Provide paper and pencil or a communication board for patient.

13. Position self at head of bed facing patient. Always face patient while cleaning or suctioning a tracheostomy.
14. Auscultate lung sounds.
15. Place towel or prepackaged drape under tracheostomy and across chest.
16. Perform hand hygiene. Prepare equipment and supplies on over the bed table. Check suction equipment and machine.

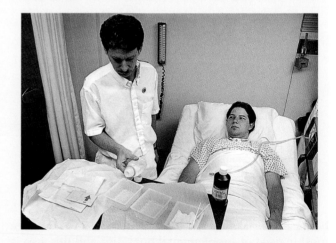

a. Open suction catheter kit but maintain sterility of contents, leaving the tip in its wrapper. Don sterile gloves. Open basin for sterile saline. Attach end of suction catheter to suction machine tubing, and pick up tubing from the machine with the nondominant hand. Fanfold or wrap suction catheter around dominant hand.

   b. Use nondominant hand to pour rinsing solution (sterile normal saline) into basin.

   c. Turn on suction machine with nondominant hand.

17. Preoxygenate patient by having patient take several deep breaths. If patient is receiving oxygen, wait to remove oxygen delivery system until just before suctioning.

18. Suction tracheal cannula.

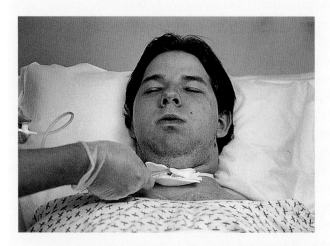

   a. Place thumb over suction control vent; place tip of suction catheter in container of sterile rinse solution. Withdraw sterile rinsing solution through catheter by placing thumb over suction control.

   b. Remove thumb from suction control; advance catheter until resistance is met, and then withdraw catheter approximately 1 cm. *(Depth of catheter approximately equals the length of outer cannula, the distal end of which protrudes from the opening approximately 1 to 2 inches.)*

   c. Apply intermittent suction by placing thumb on and off suction control, and gently rotate catheter as it is withdrawn.

   d. Suction for a maximum of 10 seconds at a time, never longer.

   e. Rinse catheter with sterile solution by suctioning sterile solution through it. Repeat steps 18b through 18d if needed.

   f. Allow patient to rest between each suctioning effort. If patient was previously receiving oxygen, reapply it at the prescribed rate between each suctioning episode.

   g. Turn off suction, and dispose of catheter appropriately. Perform hand hygiene.

   h. Auscultate lung sounds.

After the Procedure

19. Assist the patient to a position of comfort, and place needed items within easy reach. Ensure that the patient has a means to call for help and knows how to use it.

20. Raise the side rails, and lower the bed to the lowest position.

21. Remove gloves and all protective barriers such as gown, goggles, and masks. Store appropriately or discard. Remove and dispose of soiled supplies and equipment according to agency policy and guidelines from the CDC and OSHA.

22. Perform hand hygiene after removing gloves.

23. Report any unexpected outcomes to the nurse. Specific notes for reporting unexpected outcomes are included in each procedure.

24. Document the following:
- Date
- Time
- Tracheostomy suctioned
- Characteristics of material that was suctioned
- Amount
- Color
- Consistency
- Adverse reactions
- Patient's response
- Flow rate and method used if oxygen is administered

Tracheostomy Care

1. Refer to standard steps 1 to 9.

2. Check patient's tracheostomy for sanguineous exudate, edema, and respiratory obstruction.

3. Perform suctioning if it is needed before performing tracheostomy care.

4. Position patient in semi-Fowler's position.

5. Perform hand hygiene; then position self at head of bed, facing patient. Always face patient while cleaning or suctioning a tracheostomy.

6. Don, or put on, clean glove on nondominant hand. Remove old dressing from around tracheostomy stoma, and discard it in appropriate receptacle.

7. Prepare equipment and supplies on over the bed.

   a. Open tracheostomy cleaning kit with aseptic technique.

   b. If basins are packed with sterile gloves, apply one sterile glove to dominant hand. Separate basins with dominant hand. Use nondominant hand to pour cleansing solution (hydrogen peroxide) in one basin and rinsing solution (sterile saline) in another basin. In some facilities, a third solution of half hydrogen peroxide and half normal saline is used to clean around the tracheostomy stoma. Check facility policy.

8. With nondominant hand, unlock and remove inner cannula; place in hydrogen peroxide cleansing solution. Never remove outer cannula. If it is expelled by patient, use hemostat to hold tracheostomy open, and call for assistance. Always have a sterile packaged hemostat,

Continued

PROCEDURE 23.3

Tracheostomy Suctioning and Care—cont'd

as well as an extra sterile tracheostomy set, available at bedside.

9. Apply second sterile glove, or apply new pair of sterile gloves if contamination has occurred.
10. Clean inner cannula.
    a. Use brush to clean inside and outside of inner cannula.
    b. Place inner cannula in sterile normal saline solution.
    c. At some facilities, pipe cleaners are used to dry inside of inner cannula. Check facility policy.
    d. Inspect inner and outer areas of inner cannula. Remove excess liquid.
    e. Insert inner cannula and lock in place.

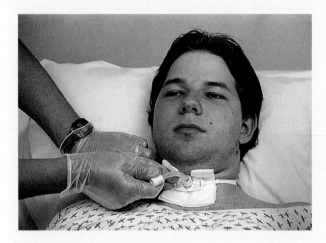

11. Clean skin around tracheostomy and tabs of outer cannula with hydrogen peroxide (or half-and-half mixture) and cotton-tipped swabs; clean away from the opening. Use wipes that are free of lint around the tracheostomy opening.
12. It may be necessary to rinse cleansing solution from skin. If so, use sterile 4 × 4 gauze. Place dry, sterile dressing around tracheostomy faceplate.

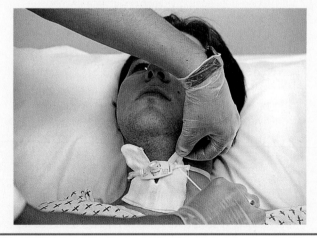

13. Change cotton tapes holding tracheostomy in place if necessary.
    a. If assistance is not available, thread clean tie through opening in flange of outer cannula alongside old tie. If assistance is available, untie one side of cotton tape from outer cannula and replace with clean one while the assistant stabilizes the tracheostomy tube.
    b. Bring clean tape under back of neck.
    c. If assistance is not available, thread tie through opening in opposite flange of outer cannula alongside old tie. If assistance is available, remove other side from outer cannula and replace with clean tape.
    d. Tie ends of clean cotton tapes together in a knot at side of neck.
14. Auscultate lung sounds.
15. Provide mouth care.

After the Procedure

16. Assist the patient to a position of comfort, and place needed items within easy reach. Ensure that the patient has a means to call for help and knows how to use it.
17. Raise the side rails, and lower the bed to the lowest position.
18. Remove gloves and all protective barriers such as gown, goggles, and masks. Store appropriately or discard. Remove and dispose of soiled supplies and equipment according to agency policy and guidelines from the CDC and OSHA.
19. Perform hand hygiene after removing gloves.
20. Report any unexpected outcomes to the nurse. Specific notes for reporting unexpected outcomes are included in each procedure.
21. Place call light, paper, and pencil within easy reach of the patient.
22. Reassess patient's tracheostomy for signs of bleeding, edema, and respiratory obstruction.
23. Document the following:
    - Date/time of tracheostomy care
    - Type of tracheostomy care performed
    - Patient's response
    - Evaluation of respiratory status
    - Adverse reactions
    - Condition of tracheal stoma and peristomal skin
    - Flow rate and method used if oxygen is administered

(Figures from Elkin MK, Perry AG, Potter PA: Nursing interventions and clinical procedures, ed 4, St. Louis, 2008, Mosby. Step 18–20 figures from Perry A, Potter P, Ostendorf W: Nursing interventions and clinical skills, ed 6, St. Louis, 2016, Mosby.)

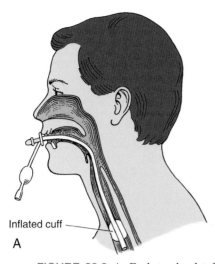

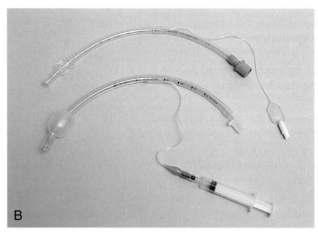

Inflated cuff

A   B

FIGURE 23.3 A, Endotracheal tube with inflated cuff. B, Endotracheal tubes with unin-flated cuffs and syringe for inflation. Patient is unable to speak while tube is in place because air cannot flow through the vocal cords. (From Cooper K, Gosnell K: *Foundations of nursing*, ed 7, St. Louis, 2015, Mosby.)

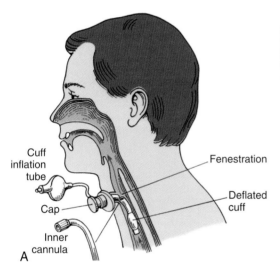

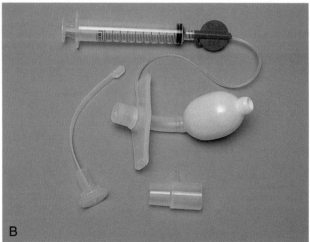

Cuff inflation tube

Cap

Inner cannula

A

Fenestration

Deflated cuff

B

FIGURE 23.4 A, Tracheostomy tube (fenestrated) with inner cannula removed and cap in place to allow speech. B, Tracheostomy tube with obturator for insertion and syringe for inflation of cuff. (From Elkin MK, Perry AG, Potter PA: *Nursing interventions and clinical skills,* ed 4, St. Louis, 2008, Mosby.)

sibilities and adequately care for a patient with a tracheostomy tube.

- Minimize infection risk.
- Evaluate the patient for excess secretions and suction as often as necessary.
- Provide constant airway humidification.
- Change all respiratory therapy equipment every 8 hours.
- Remove water that condenses in equipment tubing.
- Provide frequent mouth care (apply moisturizing agents to dry, cracked lips).
- Maintain nutritional levels.

- Patients with endotracheal tubes are allowed nothing by mouth (NPO). It is necessary to provide parenteral or enteral nourishment.
- Patients with a tracheostomy are not limited in regard to drinking fluids and eating. If a patient is able to eat, a cuffless tracheostomy tube is best. Not all patients have cuffless tracheostomy tubes. If the tracheostomy tube has a cuff, there is controversy about whether or not the cuff should be inflated or deflated during eating. Cuffs that are inflated when a patient is eating food create a problem with swallowing. Food must pass by an inflated cuff in the trachea, which is directly in front of the esophagus.

This may create a blockage and cause the potential for regurgitation and aspiration. Therefore some healthcare providers recommend that the cuff be deflated during meals.

- Turn and reposition the patient every 2 hours for maximal ventilation and lung expansion.
- The room should be set up with a spare tracheostomy tube at the bedside.
- Organize questions so that the patient is able to give simple "yes" or "no" responses by nodding the head or using hand signals.
- Talk to the patient and explain all procedures.
- Reorient the patient frequently if necessary.
- Encourage family and friends to talk to the patient.
- Keep a call light (or tap bell) within patient's reach.

There are many types of tracheostomy tubes available. With modern knowledge and technology, these tubes can be as specific as the patient who needs them. Tubes are available in cuffed and cuffless styles; some have only a single cannula, and others have an outer cannula and an inner cannula that can be easily removed

for cleaning. Being able to remove and clean the inner cannula reduces the risk of occlusion from a buildup of secretions (see Fig. 23.4).

Cuffed tracheostomy tubes are routinely used in patients who require mechanical ventilation. A cuffless tube may be used for patients who require a long-term tracheostomy and for those in the process of discontinuing use of a tracheostomy tube. A single-cannula tracheostomy tube has one tube or cannula for both airflow and suctioning of secretions. Uncuffed, single-cannula tubes are usually for neonates, infants, and young children. A double-cannula tube has both a hollow outer cannula and a removable inner cannula. A fenestrated tube has holes (fenestrations) for air to flow upward through the vocal cords and mouth. This type of tracheostomy tube lets the patient talk and breathe naturally.

Although interventions for patients with endotracheal and tracheostomy tubes are similar, patients with tracheostomies have additional care needs and considerations related to respiratory status and suctioning (Procedure 23.4).

PROCEDURE 23.4
Oropharyngeal Suctioning

1. Verify with the nurse the procedure to be done.
2. Introduce yourself to the patient; include your name and title or role.
3. Identify the patient by checking his or her identification bracelet and requesting that the patient state his or her name or birth date, or both.
4. Explain the procedure and the reason it is to be done in terms that the patient is able to understand. Advise the patient of anything uncomfortable that may be involved with the procedure. Give the patient time to ask questions.
5. Determine need for and provide patient education before and during procedure. Notify the nurse of any additional educational needs.
6. Perform hand hygiene and don clean gloves according to agency policy and guidelines from the CDC and OSHA.
7. Assemble equipment, and complete necessary charges.
8. Prepare the patient for the procedure:
   a. Close the door or pull the privacy curtain around the patient's bed.
   b. Raise the bed to a comfortable working height, and lower the side rail on the side nearest to the PCT.
   c. Position and drape the patient as necessary. Descriptions of specific positions are included in each procedure.
9. Assemble equipment.
10. Evaluate need for suctioning.
    - Gurgling respirations
    - Restlessness

- Vomitus in mouth
- Drooling

11. Explain procedure to the patient and that coughing, sneezing, or gagging is expected.
12. Position patient.
    a. If patient is alert and conscious, place in semi-Fowler's position with head to one side.
    b. If patient is unconscious, place in side-lying position facing nurse.
       (1) Place towel lengthwise under patient's chin and over pillow.
13. Pour sterile normal saline solution into sterile container.
14. Perform hand hygiene and don clean gloves. Turn on suction machine, and select appropriate suction pressure. (Check facility policy.) Never suction with any more vacuum pressure than needed to remove the secretions, and use the smallest catheter that will remove the secretions well. Connect suction catheter to tubing.
    a. Common vacuum settings for wall suction units:
       (1) Infants: 60 to 80 mm Hg
       (2) Children: 100 to 120 mm Hg
       (3) Adults: 120 to 150 mm Hg
    b. Common catheter sizes:
       (1) Infant: 6 to 8 Fr
       (2) Children: 10 to 12 Fr
       (3) Adults: 12 to 14 Fr
15. Suction solution through catheter by placing thumb over open end of connector or over vent.

PROCEDURE 23.4

Oropharyngeal Suctioning—cont'd

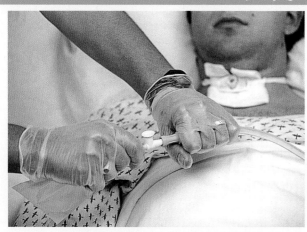

16. Remove thumb from open end of connector or vent, or pinch catheter with thumb and index finger.
17. Proceed with suctioning.
    a. Oropharyngeal suctioning:
       (1) Don clean gloves if those are not already on.
       (2) Gently insert Yankauer or tonsillar tip suction catheter into one side of mouth and glide it toward oropharynx without suction.

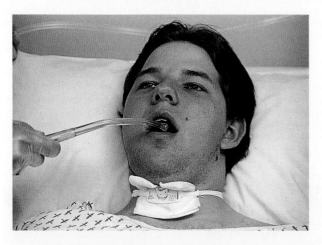

       (3) Place thumb over open end of connector or vet to apply suction. Move Yankauer or tonsillar tip catheter around mouth until secretions are cleared.
       (4) Encourage patient to cough.
       (5) Rinse Yankauer or tonsillar tip catheter with water in cup or basin until connecting tubing is cleared of secretions. Turn off suction.
       (6) Repeat procedure as necessary.

18. Observe patient closely, and limit suction to 10 to 15 seconds.
19. Repeat suctioning if it is needed.
20. Allow 1 to 2 minutes of rest between suctioning if it is necessary to repeat procedure. If oxygen is administered by nasal cannula, mask, or other means, reapply oxygen during rest period.
21. If patient is alert and is able to cooperate, instruct patient to breathe deeply and cough between suctioning attempts.
22. When suctioning of catheter is complete, suction between cheeks and gum line and under tongue; suction mouth last to prevent contaminating catheter.
23. Place catheter in solution and apply suction.
24. Discard catheter and used suction catheters: wrap catheter around gloved hand; pull glove off hand and over catheter. Remove face shield, if worn. Perform hand hygiene.
25. Place sterile, unopened catheter at patient's bedside.
26. Provide mouth care.
27. Evaluate patient's breathing patterns, fatigue, vital signs, level of consciousness, and color. Determine whether patient has a decrease in anxiety.

After the Procedure
28. Assist the patient to a position of comfort, and place needed items within easy reach. Ensure that the patient has a means to call for help and knows how to use it.
29. Raise the side rails, and lower the bed to the lowest position.
30. Remove gloves and all protective barriers such as gown, goggles, and masks. Store appropriately or discard. Remove and dispose of soiled supplies and equipment according to agency policy and guidelines from the CDC and OSHA.
31. Perform hand hygiene after removing gloves.
32. Report any unexpected outcomes to the nurse. Specific notes for reporting unexpected outcomes are included in each procedure.
33. Place call light, paper, and pencil within easy reach of the patient.
34. Document the following:
    • Date
    • Time
    • Method of suctioning
    • Amount, consistency, color, and odor of secretions
    • Respiratory assessment before and after procedure
    • Patient's response

(Figures from Perry A, Potter P, Ostendorf W: Nursing interventions and clinical skills, ed 6, St. Louis, 2016, Mosby.)

Illness & Injury Prevention Box 23.2

- Suctioning a patient may be performed by the PCT if delegated by the nurse and allowed by your facility's policy.
- Suction is performed as often as necessary, possibly every 5 minutes during the first few postoperative hours. (Whenever respirations are noisy and the pulse and respiratory rates are increased, the patient needs suctioning.)
- Patients who are conscious are usually able to let you know when they need suctioning.
- A patient who is able to cough up secretions requires less suctioning.
- The amount of mucus decreases gradually, and the PCT performs suctioning less frequently. A patient who remains anxious may require constant attendance and reassurance (Box 23.3).

Delegation and Documentation Box 23.2
Suctioning a Tracheostomy

- The task of oropharyngeal suctioning can be delegated to unlicensed assistive personnel (UAP), such as the PCT, including the patient and family when appropriate. Check facility policy.
- In special situations, the task of performing a permanent tracheostomy tube suctioning can be delegated to the PCT. These situations include those in which stable patients have permanent tracheostomy tubes and patients are receiving mechanical ventilation at home.
- The nurse is responsible for evaluating the patient's airway *patency* (openness) and response to airway suctioning.

Box 23.3   Life Span Considerations for Oxygen Therapy in Older Adults

- For patients with a chronic lung disorder, such as COPD, flow rates higher than 2 L/min could eliminate the respiratory drive to breath, and breathing may stop altogether. Pay close attention to the flow rate of patients with COPD.
- The older adult is often at increased risk for skin impairment. Therefore frequent monitoring for redness

and skin breakdown over the ears is necessary when a nasal cannula is being used for oxygen delivery. Early interventions such as loosening the straps, repositioning the tubing, or adding padding over the ears often prevent impairment.

CHAPTER SUMMARY

Maintaining a patient's oxygen level is as important as life itself. As the PCT, you can assist with maintaining oxygenation through applying oxygen, suctioning their airway, and encouraging coughing and deep breathing. Breathing should not be taken for granted. Many patients struggle with breathing after having surgery or experiencing an injury to the chest wall. When someone is in pain, he or she naturally wants to take short and shallow breaths to avoid the discomfort.

Oxygen therapy improves tissue oxygenation. Delivery devices for oxygen may include nasal cannula, or various types of oxygen masks. By teaching the patient effective coughing techniques and with the use of suctioning, a patient's airway will be kept open, or patent.

Case Scenario

Mrs. Campana has just returned to the floor from the operating room after having a right colectomy, which is a large bowel resection. Her vital signs are stable; however, she is taking short and shallow breaths. She is complaining of discomfort in the incisional area and is crying. She complains that she cannot take a deep breath because it hurts too much. She says that it is just easier to breathe shorter breaths. What can you, as the PCT, do to encourage deep breathing? Why is deep breathing better for her than breathing short and shallow breaths? Is there any danger in not deep breathing? How can the nurse assist in getting the patient comfortable so that she will be more likely to cough and deep breathe?

REVIEW QUESTIONS

1. The PCT is suctioning a patient through an endotracheal tube. What indicates proper technique? *(Select all that apply.)*
   a. Hyperventilating the patient before suctioning
   b. Dipping the suction catheter into sterile saline before suctioning
   c. Using a clean catheter with each suctioning attempt
   d. Withdrawing the catheter with the thumb covering the suction control vent
   e. Suctioning the tube for at least 30 seconds with each suctioning attempt

2. What is the maximum time suction should be applied during tracheal suctioning?
   a. 10 seconds
   b. 20 seconds
   c. 30 seconds
   d. 45 seconds

3. Which position should the postoperative patient assume before coughing and deep breathing?
   a. Prone
   b. Flat
   c. Semi-Fowler's
   d. Side-lying

4. Who is responsible for ordering the rate of oxygen for the patient?
   a. Nurse
   b. Patient care technician
   c. Pharmacist
   d. Physician

5. What are the dangers of having someone who is on oxygen around cigarette smoke?
   a. Combustion
   b. Toxicity
   c. Fire
   d. Sickness

Blood and Specimen Collecting and Testing

Blood Collecting and Processing

1. List the equipment needed for venipuncture.
2. Explain the purpose of a tourniquet.
3. Explain how to apply a tourniquet and the consequences of improper application.
4. Explain why the stopper colors on evacuated blood collection tubes differ.
5. State the correct order in which samples for various types of tubes should be collected.
6. Describe the types of sharps used in phlebotomy.
7. Explain why a syringe rather than an evacuated blood collection tube would be chosen for blood collection.
8. Discuss the use of sharps with engineered sharps protection.
9. Summarize postexposure management of needle sticks.
10. Describe and name the veins that may be used for blood collection.
11. List in order the steps of a routine venipuncture.
12. Collect a venous blood sample using the syringe method.
13. Collect a venous blood sample using the evacuated blood collection tube method.
14. Summarize typical problems that may be associated with venipuncture.
15. Identify the major causes of hemolysis during venous blood collection.
16. List situations in which capillary puncture would be preferred over venipuncture.
17. Discuss proper dermal puncture sites.
18. Describe containers that may be used to collect capillary blood.
19. Describe handling and transport methods for blood after collection.
20. Explain chain of custody procedures when drawing blood samples.

KEY TERMS

hemoconcentration A condition in which the concentration of blood cells is increased in proportion to the plasma.

hemolysis The destruction or dissolution of red blood cells, with subsequent release of hemoglobin.

phlebotomy The practice of drawing blood.

plasma The liquid portion of whole blood that contains active clotting agents.

serum The liquid portion of whole blood that remains after the blood has clotted.

stat The medical abbreviation for "immediately"; "at this moment".

thixotropic gel A material that appears to be a solid until subjected to a disturbance, such as centrifugation, whereupon it becomes a liquid.

Phlebotomy, the practice of drawing blood, began in the ancient practice of restoring the four body humors: blood, phlegm (mucus), yellow bile, and black bile. The foundation of all medical treatment was to keep these humors in balance by purging, starving, vomiting, or bloodletting.

The art of bloodletting was flourishing by the Middle Ages, and both barbers and surgeons performed it. Barbers advertised with a red-and-white striped pole; red represented blood, and white represented the tourniquet. The pole itself represented the stick the patient squeezed during the procedure. Typically, 16 to 30 ounces (1 to 4 pints) of blood was drained to treat an illness. When the patient became faint, the "treatment" was stopped. Often, bleeding over large areas of the body was accomplished by multiple incisions. George Washington is reported to have died in 1799 after being drained of 9 pints of blood within 24 hours to cure a throat infection. In Washington's day, it was believed that the blood was a carrier of the impurities of disease, and with bleeding, new and healthy blood would replace what was lost. By the end of the nineteenth century, bloodletting was declared quackery.

Today phlebotomy is performed primarily to diagnose and to monitor a patient's condition. According to the American Society of Clinical Pathologists (ASCP), nearly 80% of physicians' decisions are based on laboratory tests, most of which are blood tests. As a patient care technician, you may be responsible for phlebotomy procedures. Phlebotomy is an important role for the patient care technician, and must be completed correctly.

There is a certification available for those who would like to become certified in phlebotomy. The facility you work for may be able to help you become certified by providing payment for your certification examination. Certifying agencies include the National Health Careers Association (NHA), International Academy of Phlebotomy Sciences, the National Certification Agency (NCA), and the National Phlebotomy Association (NPA). Continuing education often is required to maintain certification. California and Louisiana were the first states to create state certification requirements. It is important that patient care technicians become familiar with the guidelines of their home states because not all states require a certificate to perform phlebotomy.

The most common method of obtaining blood is venipuncture, in which the blood is taken directly from a vein that is close to the surface of the skin. The vein is punctured with a needle, and the blood is collected either in a syringe or in a stoppered tube. The procedure is safe when performed by a trained professional, such as a patient care technician, but it must be performed with care. Much practice is required to become skilled and confident in the technique of venipuncture.

VENIPUNCTURE EQUIPMENT

Proper collection of blood requires specialized equipment. A complete list of materials used in routine venipuncture is shown in Box 24.1. Phlebotomists generally carry the equipment in a portable tray (Fig. 24.1). A physician's office laboratory often has a permanent location where venipuncture is performed. In such cases, you likely will seat the patient in a venipuncture chair, which has an adjustable locking armrest to protect the patient if he or she should faint (Fig. 24.2). However, if the patient has a history of syncope (fainting), it is best to perform phlebotomy while the patient is lying on an examination table.

Gloves

Employers must provide employees with gloves, including the hypoallergenic, powderless, and vinyl types, as needed. Remember, even though an employee may not have a latex allergy, the patient may be

Box 24.1	Equipment Used in Routine Venipuncture

- Double-pointed safety needles
- Evacuated, stoppered blood collection tubes
- Needle holder
- Sharps container
- Syringes
- Tourniquet
- Marking pen
- Alcohol swabs
- Gauze pads
- Bandages
- Gloves

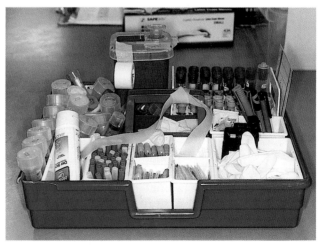

FIGURE 24.1 A fully stocked venipuncture tray. (From Stepp CA, Woods MA: *Laboratory procedures for medical office personnel*, Philadelphia, 1998, Saunders.)

allergic. Therefore it is important to ask patients about allergies each time they have blood drawn. Allergies can develop in between visits or hospitalizations. If the patient is allergic to latex, alternative gloves (e.g., vinyl) must be worn; in addition, the patient care technician must consider other necessary supplies, such as tourniquets and adhesive bandages, which may have to be exchanged for versions that do not contain latex. Many facilities stock only latex-free supplies because of the potential for allergic responses in workers and patients.

The Occupational Safety and Health Administration (OSHA) requires healthcare workers to wear gloves during venipuncture; however, the agency does not specify when during the course of the procedure the gloves must be put on. Because veins can be difficult to locate with gloved fingertips, the site may be palpated (fingertip pressure to locate a vein) before gloves are put on. The standard procedure for venipuncture

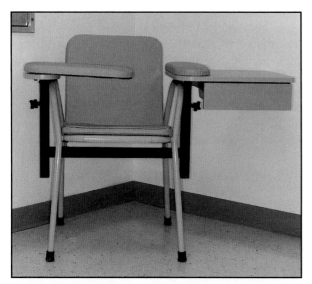

FIGURE 24.2 A phlebotomy chair. (From Stepp CA, Woods MA: *Laboratory procedures for medical office personnel*, Philadelphia, 1998, Saunders.)

established by the Clinical and Laboratory Standards Institute (CLSI, 2007) states that gloves should be put on after vein palpation but before preparation of the site. Those who need the final assurance of one last palpation before the needle is inserted must remember that touching the prepared site, even with gloves, contaminates the area. To help find the vein after cleansing the area, look for certain skin markers, such as creases, freckles, or scars. If the area is touched, it must be cleansed again. Keep in mind that the tourniquet should be tied for no longer than 1 minute at a time.

Tourniquets

Before blood can be drawn, a vein must be located. Application of a tourniquet (Fig. 24.3) is the most common way to do this; it prevents venous flow out of the site, causing the veins to bulge. The tourniquet is tied around the upper arm so that it is tight but not uncomfortable and can be released easily with one hand. Latex tourniquets are inexpensive, but they may become contaminated, and some patients are allergic to latex. Other tourniquets with Velcro closures are available and may be more comfortable for the patient, but they are difficult to release. Single-use, nonlatex tourniquets are available and currently are recommended for reducing cross-contamination between patients and healthcare workers, preventing nosocomial infection, and preventing latex exposure.

Tourniquets are tied 3 to 4 inches above the elbow immediately before the venipuncture procedure begins. Because a tourniquet delays blood flow, leaving it on for longer than 1 minute greatly increases the possibility of hemoconcentration and altered test results. The tourniquet should not be tied so tightly as to impede arterial blood flow; this restricts venous blood return, resulting in poor venous distention. Checking the pulse at the wrist ensures that arterial flow is not restricted. Tourniquets also are used when blood is drawn from hand and foot veins and are tied on the wrist or ankle, respectively.

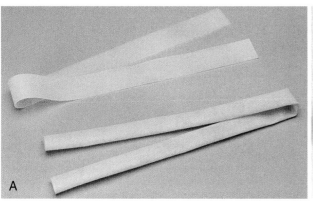
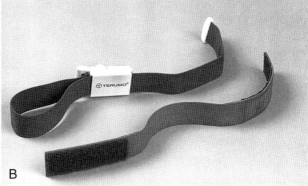

FIGURE 24.3 Examples of tourniquets. (B, From Flynn JC Jr: *Procedures in phlebotomy,* ed 3, Philadelphia, 2005, Saunders.)

Tourniquets can be uncomfortable for patients, especially those with heavy-set or hairy upper arms, if they are not applied correctly. Ensure that the tourniquet is flat against the skin, and if necessary, tie it over the clothing if it is causing the patient discomfort. This may be especially important when blood is drawn in an aging individual because of the fragility of the skin.

Antiseptics

To prevent infection, a venipuncture site must be cleansed with an antiseptic. The most commonly used is 70% isopropyl alcohol, also known as *rubbing alcohol.* Prepackaged alcohol "prep pads" are the most commonly used product. The square prep pad is rubbed on the skin in a circular motion, and the alcohol is allowed to dry. Alcohol does not sterilize the skin; it inhibits the reproduction of bacteria that might contaminate the sample. To be most effective, the alcohol should remain on the skin 30 to 60 seconds. However, isopropyl alcohol should not be used when a sample for a blood alcohol test is drawn. Sterile soap pads, benzalkonium chloride, or povidone-iodine (Betadine) can be used instead. Betadine swabs may be used if a sample for a blood alcohol test needs to be drawn (Fig. 24.4).

If a blood culture is ordered, additional preparation is needed at the venipuncture site to eliminate contaminating bacteria. Povidone-iodine solution is commonly used, and chlorhexidine gluconate or benzalkonium chloride can be used for patients allergic to iodine. More vigorous cleansing is required for a blood culture sample than for a routine venipuncture. Blood cultures must be drawn into a sterile tube or a bottle specifically designed for the test (Fig. 24.5). These bottles are typically made of glass; take care to not drop them when transporting them.

Evacuated Blood Collection Tubes

The evacuated tube (Vacutainer) system is the most common collection system in use. It consists of evacuated tubes of various sizes that have color-coded tops, which indicate the tube's contents (Table 24.1). Tubes are available in both glass and shatter-resistant glass. The tube contents include anticoagulants, clot activators, and/or thixotropic gel. The vacuum in each tube draws a measured amount of blood into the tube. Tube volumes range from 2 to 15 mL, which is up to one tablespoon of blood. Be sure to match the needle gauge to the size of the tube; the larger the tube, the greater the vacuum and the more likely it is that the blood will hemolyze if a high-gauge needle with a small lumen is used.

The size of the tube to be used depends on several factors. Each test performed in the laboratory requires a specific amount of blood. Consult the manual provided by the laboratory to ensure that you are drawing the right amount of blood for the test. Tests can often be combined, which reduces the number of tubes that must be drawn. For example, both a complete blood count and an erythrocyte sedimentation rate test are performed on a sample from a lavender-topped tube; you do not need to draw two tubes, because the 7-mL volume is sufficient for both tests. When in doubt, call the laboratory. Keep in mind that blood is approximately half cells and half liquid. If a test requires 3 mL of serum, 6 mL

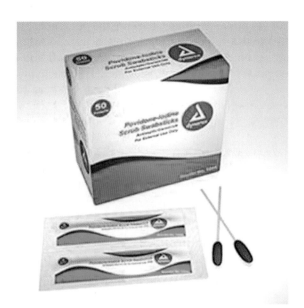

FIGURE 24.4 Betadine swabs. (Courtesy of Dynarex Corporation, Orangeburg, NY.)

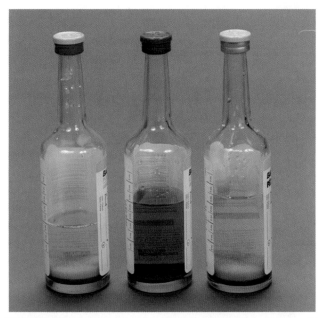

FIGURE 24.5 Bactec blood culture bottles. (From Proctor D, Adams A: *Kinn's the medical assistant: an applied learning approach*, ed 12, St. Louis, 2014, Saunders.)

| Table 24.1 | Common Stoppers and Additives and Their Laboratory Uses | | | |

Vacutainer Color*	Color	Hemogard Color†	Additive and Its Function	Laboratory Use	Optimum Volume/ Minimum Volume
Adult Tubes					
Yellow		Yellow	SPS; prevents blood from clotting and stabilizes bacterial growth	Blood or body fluid cultures	5 mL/NA
Red		Red	None	Serum tests; chemistry studies, blood bank, serology	10 mL/NA
Red-gray (marbled)		Gold	None, but contains silica particles to enhance clot formation	Serum tests	10 mL/NA
Light blue		Light blue	Sodium citrate; removes calcium to prevent blood from clotting	Coagulation testing	4.5 mL/4.5 mL
Green		Green	Heparin (sodium/lithium/ ammonium); inhibits thrombin formation to prevent clotting	Chemistry tests	10 mL/3.5 mL
Green-gray (marbled)		Light green	Lithium heparin and gel for plasma separation	Plasma determinations in chemistry studies	2 mL/2 mL
Yellow-gray (marbled)		Orange	Thrombin	Stat serum demonstrations in chemistry studies	2 mL/2 mL
Lavender		Lavender	EDTA; removes calcium to prevent blood from clotting	Hematology tests	7 mL/2 mL
Gray		Gray	Potassium oxalate and sodium fluoride; removes calcium to prevent blood from clotting; fluoride inhibits glycolysis	Chemistry testing, especially glucose and alcohol levels	10 mL/10 mL
Royal blue		Royal blue	Sodium heparin (also sodium EDTA); inhibits thrombin formation to prevent clotting	Chemistry trace elements	7 mL
Pediatric Tubes					
Red		Red	Gel plus clot activator	Serum tests	2 mL/NA 3 mL/NA 4 mL/NA
Lavender		Lavender	EDTA	Hematology tests	2 mL/0.6 mL 3 mL/0.9 mL 4 mL/1 mL
Green		Green	Lithium heparin	Chemistry tests	2 mL/2 mL
Light blue		Light blue	Sodium citrate	Chemistry tests	2.7 mL/2.7 mL

EDTA, Ethylenediamine tetraacetic acid; *SPS*, sodium polyanethol sulfonate.
*Stopper colors are based on BD Vacutainer tubes.
†Hemogard closures provide a protective plastic cover over the rubber stopper as an additional safety feature.
Additives, additive functions, and laboratory uses for pediatric tubes obtained from www.avena-medica.com/en/Catalogue/1-8-pediatric-blood-collection-tubes.html.
(Modified from Rodak BF: Diagnostic hematology, Philadelphia, 1995, Saunders.)

of blood must be collected. So, you will double the amount of blood you draw to obtain the amount of serum you need.

Patients are often concerned when several tubes of blood must be drawn. You can help reduce their fears by explaining that the average adult has a little less than 10 pints of blood (5 L). Most adults can relate to donating a unit of blood, which is around a pint (400 to 500 mL). Because the red-topped tube contains 10 mL, you would have to draw 40 to 50 tubes before you have removed a pint. Even though it looks like a lot when you are drawing multiple tubes of blood, it is not really that much blood; it is less than a tablespoon in each tube.

Tube Additives

All tubes except the red-topped one contain an additive. Anticoagulants are added to prevent blood from clotting. Tubes may be glass or plastic, and the additive may be a powder, a liquid visible in the tube, or a liquid sprayed inside the tube by the manufacturer and allowed to dry. The choice of anticoagulant depends on the test to be done.

Ethylenediaminetetraacetic acid (EDTA), found in the lavender-topped tube, prevents platelet clumping and preserves the appearance of blood cells for microscopic examination; however, it is incompatible with the testing reagents used in coagulation (clotting) studies. Consult the manual provided by the laboratory before obtaining a specimen from the patient.

Clot activators promote blood clotting. Silica particles enhance clotting, for example, by providing a surface for platelet activation. Thrombin quickly promotes clotting and is used in tubes drawn for stat (emergency; drawn immediately) chemistry testing or in the event a sample is needed from a patient taking a prescribed anticoagulant, such as heparin.

Anticoagulants prevent blood from clotting, which allows the contents of the tube to be used in two ways. First, the sample can be used as whole blood; second, the sample can be centrifuged, and the liquid portion, called plasma, can be retrieved. Whole blood is used for tests such as complete blood counts and blood typing, whereas plasma is used for stat chemistry testing and coagulation studies.

Once the blood is taken to the laboratory, it is centrifuged, or spun down, to separate the contents of it (Fig. 24.6). This is usually performed by laboratory personnel. If blood is allowed to clot and then is centrifuged, the liquid portion is referred to as *serum*. Without a clot activator, blood clots in 30 to 60 minutes, after which it must be centrifuged. The serum must be separated from the cells quickly, because cells may continue to metabolize substances such as glucose or may release metabolites that interfere with testing. Thixotropic gel can be found in some tubes, including the serum separation tube (SST; red-gray–topped tube) and the plasma separation tube (PST; green-gray marbled-topped tube) by Becton, Dickinson and Company (Franklin Lakes, New Jersey). This synthetic gel has a density between that of red cells and plasma or serum, and it settles between the two during centrifugation, forming a barrier that facilitates retrieval of the liquid portion without cellular contamination (see Fig. 24.7 for the different types of tubes).

It is important to mix the contents of the tube well after collection by inverting it several times (do not shake the tube) and also to avoid a short draw (i.e., a tube that is not completely filled) (Table 24.2 & Table 24.3). Having the proper ratio of blood to additive is crucial. Always be sure to check the tube for an expiration date. Outdated tubes may have diminished vacuum, or the additive may have degraded.

Table 24.2	Effects of Underfilling Collection Tubes
Stopper Color	**Effect**
Yellow	Reduces possibility of bacterial recovery
Red	Insufficient sample
Red-gray	Poor barrier formation; insufficient sample
Light blue	Coagulation test results falsely prolonged
Green	False results because of excess heparin
Green-gray	False results because of excess heparin
Lavender	Falsely low blood cell counts and hematocrits; morphologic changes to red blood cells; staining alteration
Yellow-gray	False results
Gray	False results
Royal blue	False results

Table 24.3	Stopper Color and Inversion Mixing
Stopper Color	**Mix by Inversion**
Yellow	8–10 times
Light blue	3–4 times
Red or red speckled	5 times
Green	8–10 times
Lavender	8–10 times
Gray	8–10 times

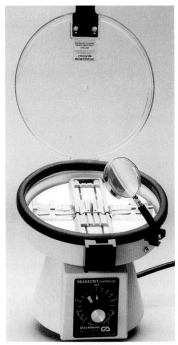

FIGURE 24.6 Centrifuge with capillary tube placement indications. (From Proctor D, Adams A: *Kinn's the medical assistant: an applied learning approach*, ed 12, St. Louis, 2014, Saunders.)

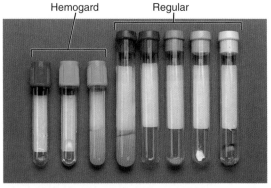

FIGURE 24.7 Types of tubes. (From Warekois RS, Robinson R: *Phlebotomy: worktext and procedures manual*, ed 4, St. Louis, 2016, Saunders.)

Order of Collection

If samples for more than one tube must be drawn during a venipuncture, a specified order must be followed so that material from a previous tube is not transferred to the next tube. Carryover of additives from one tube to the next could cause sample alteration and erroneous results. Because you are using the same needle, it matters the order that you collect the blood samples. CLSI (formerly the National Committee for Clinical Laboratory Standards [NCCLS]) developed a set of standards outlining the order of blood drawn for a multitube collection. The same order applies to the filling of tubes when blood is collected in a syringe and takes into account the use of newer plastic tubes:

1. *Yellow* blood culture tubes are filled first because they are sterile.
2. *Light blue*–topped tubes with sodium citrate are next because other anticoagulants might contaminate the sample collected for coagulation studies. If no blood culture has been ordered, CLSI (2010) recommends that blood for the light blue–topped tube should be drawn first if routine coagulation testing has been ordered (i.e., prothrombin time [PT] and activated partial thromboplastin time [APTT]). For testing other than routine PT and APTT, a red-topped "waste" tube may be filled. When a winged infusion set is used, CLSI currently recommends that blood be drawn into a red-topped tube even if the order does not call for it. This is done to fill the tubing's dead space with blood and to prevent any thromboplastin released during venipuncture from contaminating the light blue–topped tube and interfering with coagulation testing. It is not necessary to fill the tube to be discarded.
3. *Red* serum tubes without clot activator (red stopper) or with clot activator (*red-gold* or *speckled stopper*) are filled next. Although CLSI notes that glass, nonadditive serum tubes can be drawn before the light blue–topped tubes, the draw order has been simplified to function for all serum tubes, regardless of their composition.
4. *Green*-topped tubes are next, because heparin is less likely to interfere with EDTA than vice versa.
5. *Lavender*-topped tubes follow. Because EDTA binds with calcium, blood for this tube is drawn near the end.
6. The *gray*-topped tube is last, because the contents can elevate electrolyte levels or damage cells if passed into another tube.

Types of Sharps and Supplies Used in Phlebotomy

A critical part of phlebotomy is the knowledge of which needle and which tube or syringe should be used in each situation. All needles used in phlebotomy are sterile, disposable, and used only once. Each is kept in a cover, which should be inspected before use to ensure that sterility has not been compromised (i.e., the seal should be intact), and that the needle has no manufacturing defects, such as burrs or nicks. Needles have two parts: the hub and the shaft. Shafts differ in length, ranging from ¾ to 1½ inches. The length of the shaft has no bearing on the venipuncture procedure, but some prefer a longer needle because it is less likely to slip out of the vein, whereas others prefer a shorter needle because it makes patients less uneasy. One end of the shaft is cut at an angle and forms the bevel, which creates a very sharp point. The hole in the bevel is called the *lumen* (Fig. 24.8).

Lumen size is important in venipuncture and is referred to as the *gauge*. The gauge is designated by a numeric value; the higher the number, the smaller the lumen. A blood bank uses a 16-gauge needle to collect pints of blood for transfusions, because the lumen is wide, which reduces the chance of hemolysis. The smallest-gauge needles (23 gauge) are used to collect blood from small or fragile veins, such as those found in elderly and very young patients. Routine adult venipuncture requires a 20- to 21-gauge needle. The hub is the point where the needle attaches to the syringe or the needle holder.

Multisample Needles

Multisample needles are commonly used in routine adult venipuncture. They are used when several tubes are to be drawn during a single venipuncture. These needles are double-pointed (Fig. 24.9). One point enters the patient's vein, and the other punctures the rubber stopper of the collection tube. The point that enters the tube is sheathed with a retractable rubber sleeve that allows tubes to be changed without blood leaking into the needle holder or tube holder.

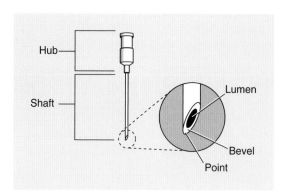

FIGURE 24.8 Parts of a needle. (From Warekois RS, Robinson R: *Phlebotomy: worktext and procedures manual*, ed 4, St. Louis, 2016, Saunders.)

Syringes

Syringes are used when there is concern that the strong vacuum in a stoppered tube might collapse the vein. The syringe needle fits on the end of the barrel and comes in different sizes. The amount of blood drawn into the barrel depends on how much is to be transferred to stoppered tubes. When blood is drawn into a syringe, it must be transferred immediately to another tube, because the blood will clot in the syringe barrel. In these situations, a syringe with a sharps injury prevention feature and safe work practices should be used to prevent a needle stick. The blood must be transferred from the syringe to the test tube with a needleless blood transfer device, as required by OSHA. A special transfer tube adapter is used to transfer the blood to the Vacutainer tube. The adapter connects to the top of the syringe once the needle cover is in place and the needle is removed. The adapter contains an enclosed needle that punctures and delivers the blood into the Vacutainer tube (Fig. 24.10).

Needle Holders

Double-pointed needles must be firmly placed into a needle adapter or tube holder (Fig. 24.11). Usually they are clear plastic cylinders, and they come in different sizes to accommodate the tube used. The cylinders often have a ring that indicates how far the tube can be pushed onto the needle without losing the vacuum. OSHA requires that, to prevent accidental needle sticks, needle holders must be discarded after a single use. In most cases the entire needle and holder are disposed of at the same time; needles are not removed from the needle holder, and the safety feature on the needle must be activated before disposal.

Needle Safety

Healthcare workers who use or may be exposed to needles are at increased risk of needlestick injury. Such injuries can lead to serious or fatal infections with blood-borne pathogens such as hepatitis B virus (HBV), hepatitis C virus (HCV), or human immunodeficiency virus (HIV). An estimated 600,000 needlestick injuries occur each year, and nursing staff members are most frequently injured. Needlestick injuries account for up to 80% of accidental exposures to blood. Used needles should never be recapped.

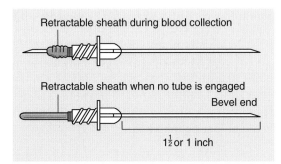

FIGURE 24.9 Multisample needles. (From Proctor D, Adams A: *Kinn's the medical assistant: an applied learning approach,* ed 12, St. Louis, 2014, Saunders.)

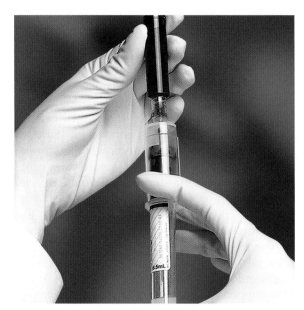

FIGURE 24.10 BD Vacutainer blood transfer device. (Courtesy Becton, Dickinson and Company, Franklin Lakes, New Jersey.)

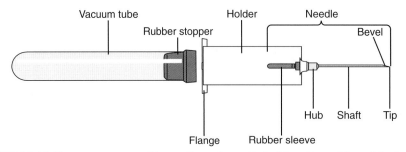

FIGURE 24.11 Vacuum system with needle and needle holder. (From Hunt SA: *Saunders fundamentals of medical assisting—revised reprint,* St Louis, 2007, Saunders.)

According to OSHA, the best practice for preventing needlestick injuries after phlebotomy is to use a sharp (needle) with engineered sharps injury protection (SESIP) attached to a needle holder. SESIPs, or safety needles, eliminate the need to remove the needle from the needle holder and in some way shield the needle immediately after use. The U.S. Food and Drug Administration (FDA), which is responsible for approving medical devices marketed and sold in the United States, recommends devices that provide a barrier between the hands and the needle after use in which the patient care technician's hands remain behind the needle at all times. Safety shields that can be activated before or immediately after removal of the needle from the vein and that keep the needle covered after disposal also should be an important part of the device. Finally, these devices should be as simple as possible, requiring little or no training to use. Some examples of SESIPs include the following:

- *Self-sheathing safety devices* (Fig. 24.12): These devices have sliding needle shields attached to disposable syringes and vacuum tube holders. Before activation, the sleeve is positioned over the barrel of the syringe. After the procedure, the phlebotomist slides the sleeve forward over the needle, where it locks into place, protecting the needle.
- *Retractable safety devices* (Fig. 24.13): After the needle has been used and removed from the vein, a plunger is pushed to retract the needle into the syringe or needle holder. The entire unit is disposed of in the sharps container.
- *Needle-blunting safety mechanisms* (Figs. 24.14 and 24.15): After the venipuncture, a blunt tube is moved through the needle, covering the sharp point. With the needle in the needle holder, the vacuum tube is removed and then is pushed forward again while the needle is still in the vein. This moves the blunt-tipped needle forward through the needle, past the sharp needle point. The blunt point tip of the needle can be activated before it is removed from the patient.
- *Hinged or sliding safety mechanisms* (Fig. 24.16): These devices, which are attached to the phlebotomy needle or to a winged infusion needle, are manually engaged after the needle has been removed from the vein. The plastic sheath covers the needle, and the entire unit is disposed of in the sharps container.

Injury & Illness Prevention Box 24.1

The following steps should be taken to protect against needlestick injuries:

- Do not use needles when safe, effective alternatives are available.
- Help your employer select and evaluate devices with safety features.
- Use devices with safety features provided by your employer.
- Never recap a contaminated needle.
- Plan for safe handling and disposal before beginning any procedure using needles.
- Dispose of used needles and needle holders promptly in appropriate sharps disposal containers.
- Report all needlestick and other sharps-related injuries promptly to ensure that you receive appropriate follow-up care.
- Tell your employer about hazards from needles that you observe in your work environment.
- Participate in blood-borne pathogen training and follow recommended infection prevention practices, including obtaining hepatitis B vaccination.

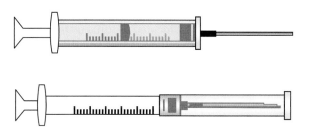

FIGURE 24.12 Self-sheathing device. (From Proctor D, Adams A: *Kinn's the medical assistant: an applied learning approach,* ed 12, St. Louis, 2014, Saunders.)

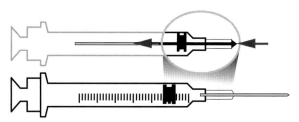

FIGURE 24.13 Retractable safety device. (From Proctor D, Adams A: *Kinn's the medical assistant: an applied learning approach,* ed 12, St. Louis, 2014, Saunders.)

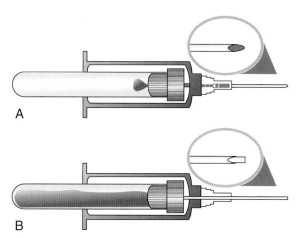

FIGURE 24.14 Needle-blunting sharp with engineered sharps injury protection (SESIP) for the needle holder. A, Needle while collecting specimen before activation. B, Needle with blunting device activated. (From Proctor D, Adams A: *Kinn's the medical assistant: an applied learning approach,* ed 12, St. Louis, 2014, Saunders.)

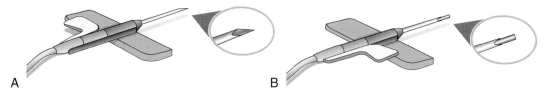

FIGURE 24.15 Needle-blunting sharp with engineered sharps injury protection (SESIP) for winged infusion sets. A, Before activation, with needle in vein. B, After activation. (From Proctor D, Adams A: *Kinn's The Medical Assistant: an applied learning approach,* ed 12, St. Louis, 2014, Saunders.)

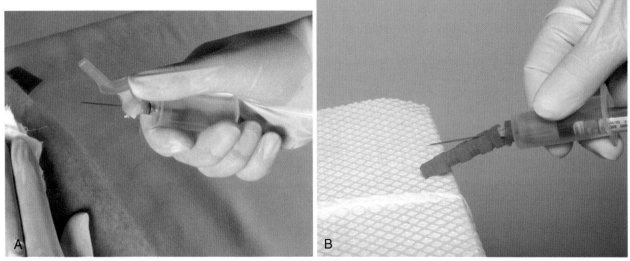

FIGURE 24.16 Hinged or sliding sharp with engineered sharps injury protection (SESIP). A, Before venipuncture. B, After activation. (Modified from Garrels M, Oatis C: *Laboratory testing for ambulatory settings,* ed 2, St. Louis, 2011, Saunders.)

OSHA requires employers to establish and maintain a sharps injury log for recording injuries from contaminated sharps. This log should contain information about the device involved in the incident and the department or work area where the incident occurred, as well as an explanation of the incident. Employee confidentiality must be maintained.

Postexposure Management of Needlesticks

An accidental needlestick is a medical emergency. Effective management of an accidental sharps exposure includes the following:

- Immediately after injury, the wound is inspected for foreign material, which is removed. The site is washed for 10 minutes with an antimicrobial soap, 10% iodine solution, or chlorine-based antiseptic.
- The injury is reported to the supervisor and an incident report is completed.
- The employee is referred to a physician for confidential assessment and follow-up. Baseline testing for HBV, HCV, and HIV is recommended for both the employee and the source individual. If the employee has been immunized for HBV and has a

positive postimmunization titer, there is no risk of acquiring HBV and no source testing is needed. If the worker has not been immunized, source testing for infection with HBV is recommended if the source is known and can be located. Source testing involves having the patient you were drawing the blood from tested to determine whether he or she has any infection or contagious illness in the bloodstream. If the source patient tests positive for HBV, the employee should receive HBV immune globulin (HBIG), and the series of HBV immunizations should be initiated. If the source tests negative, no treatment is indicated. If the source patient cannot be tested, the employee should be treated as if the source patient were positive for HBV. The source should also be tested for HCV. If positive, the employee should be monitored for signs and symptoms of hepatitis for 6 months. No postexposure prophylaxis is recommended for HCV infection. For HIV exposure, most employers recommend a 4-week regimen of antiretroviral drugs. To best protect the victim, antiretroviral therapy should be administered within hours of exposure. HIV treatment involves potentially serious side effects; therefore the employee decides whether medications are started. If the source is found to be negative, antiretroviral therapy can be discontinued.

- Interim testing may be performed if the healthcare worker experiences symptoms of acute HIV exposure or hepatitis. For HIV, antibody testing should be repeated at 6 weeks, 12 weeks, and 6 months if either the source was HIV positive or the source's status remains unknown. Confidential follow-up care must include provisions for emotional support and counseling for the healthcare worker.

ROUTINE VENIPUNCTURE

Your appearance and actions reflect your laboratory or facility. A patient's first impression of the facility often comes from you. Clean laboratory coats or scrubs tell the patient that the facility is clean; wearing gloves tells the patient that you will treat him or her with care; and speaking knowledgeably provides the impression that the facility is staffed with professionals.

Venipuncture involves several important steps with which the patient care technician must be thoroughly familiar before attempting the procedure. The first step is to select the proper method for venipuncture (syringe or evacuated tube). Next, the patient must be prepared for the procedure. Patient preparation is followed by the actual venipuncture and specimen collection. The final step is care of the puncture site before the patient is discharged.

Patient Preparation

All blood collections begin with a requisition, a form from the patient's physician requesting a test (Fig. 24.17). Requisitions may be computer generated or handwritten and at minimum must include the following information:

- Patient's name
- Date of birth
- Identification number
- Name of the physician making the request
- Type of test requested
- Test status (timed, fasting, stat, and so forth)

Currently, many facilities use computer-generated stickers to label the patient's blood samples (Fig. 24.18). It is important to take these stickers in the room with you before you draw the blood sample so that the tubes can be labeled in front of the patient and before you leave the room.

Venipuncture begins with greeting and identifying the patient. According to CLSI, proper identification includes asking outpatients to provide their full name and address, and an identification number or birth date. This information must be compared with the written information on the requisition. With inpatients, CLSI

Delegation and Documentation Box 24.1

- When you receive a requisition to perform a laboratory draw, examine it to ensure that it has all the necessary information, such as patient's full name, date of birth, ordering physician, and patient location.
- Check for duplicates; if there are several requisitions for one patient, group them together so that all collections can be made with a single puncture, or needlestick.
- Prioritize the requisitions; perform STAT immediately timed collections at that particular time ordered, and routine collections as soon as you can. Discuss with your nurse if there are any questions regarding which order patient laboratory draws should be done.
- Collect all the equipment you need for the collections you will be performing.

---

recommends asking for the same information and comparing it with the information on the requisition and on the identification bracelet. If the patient speaks a different language, has limited language skills (such as a child), or is otherwise unable to communicate, a family member, caregiver, or translator must provide the information. The name of this person should be documented.

Introduce yourself and briefly explain the purpose and procedure of the venipuncture. If the patient has questions about the ordered tests, politely request that the patient speak to the physician, and ask whether the individual would like to do so before you collect the sample. Obtain verbal consent to perform the procedure simply by asking whether you have permission to take some blood from the patient's arm. Always ask the patient whether he or she has experienced problems during routine venipuncture in the past, and take steps to prevent such problems. Your self-confidence in the procedure will be evident to the patient and will help allay any fears. Instilling confidence in your patients means acting and speaking professionally. Refer to the patient as "sir" or "ma'am" or "Mr. Jones" or "Ms. Smith," not "honey," "sweetie," "Bill," or "Margaret." Terms of endearment, such as "honey" or "sweetie," can be offensive to some. Being friendly is important, but ensure that your patients feel respected and understand that you take your role in their care seriously.

Preparing for the Venipuncture

Seat the patient in a chair or have the person lie down on an examination table, if the patient has a history of syncope, and ask the patient to extend the arm. Inspect both arms and ask whether the patient has a preference. In general, veins in the forearm or the elbow (antecubital

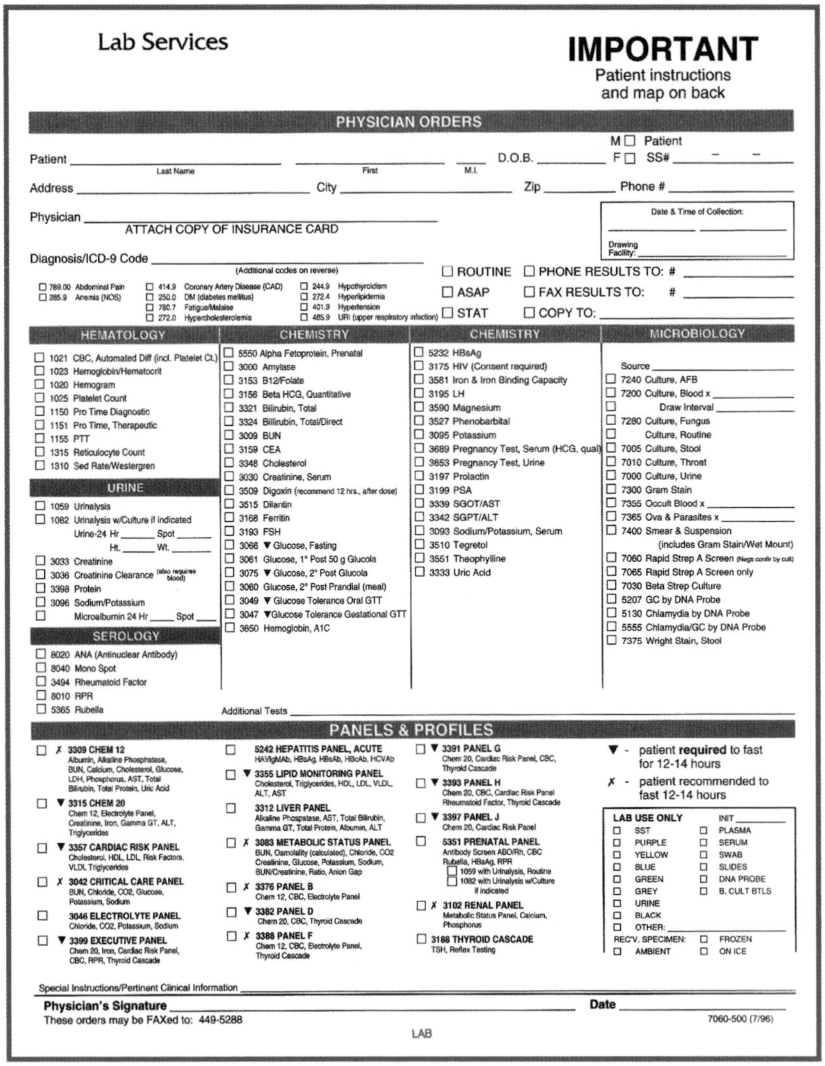

Lab Services

IMPORTANT
Patient instructions and map on back

PHYSICIAN ORDERS

Patient ______ (Last Name) ______ (First) ___ (M.I.) D.O.B. ______ M ☐ F ☐ Patient SS# ___ – ___ – ___

Address ______ City ______ Zip ______ Phone # ______

Physician ______
ATTACH COPY OF INSURANCE CARD

Date & Time of Collection: ______ ______
Drawing Facility: ______

Diagnosis/ICD-9 Code ______
(Additional codes on reverse)

☐ 789.00 Abdominal Pain
☐ 285.9 Anemia (NOS)
☐ 414.9 Coronary Artery Disease (CAD)
☐ 250.0 DM (diabetes mellitus)
☐ 780.7 Fatigue/Malaise
☐ 272.0 Hypercholesterolemia
☐ 244.9 Hypothyroidism
☐ 272.4 Hyperlipidemia
☐ 401.9 Hypertension
☐ 485.9 URI (upper respiratory infection)

☐ ROUTINE ☐ PHONE RESULTS TO: # ______
☐ ASAP ☐ FAX RESULTS TO: # ______
☐ STAT ☐ COPY TO: ______

HEMATOLOGY
☐ 1021 CBC, Automated Diff (incl. Platelet Ct.)
☐ 1023 Hemoglobin/Hematocrit
☐ 1020 Hemogram
☐ 1025 Platelet Count
☐ 1150 Pro Time Diagnostic
☐ 1151 Pro Time, Therapeutic
☐ 1155 PTT
☐ 1315 Reticulocyte Count
☐ 1310 Sed Rate/Westergren

URINE
☐ 1059 Urinalysis
☐ 1082 Urinalysis w/Culture if indicated
Urine-24 Hr ______ Spot ______
Ht. ______ Wt. ______
☐ 3033 Creatinine
☐ 3036 Creatinine Clearance (also requires blood)
☐ 3398 Protein
☐ 3096 Sodium/Potassium
☐ Microalbumin 24 Hr ____ Spot ____

SEROLOGY
☐ 8020 ANA (Antinuclear Antibody)
☐ 8040 Mono Spot
☐ 3494 Rheumatoid Factor
☐ 8010 RPR
☐ 5365 Rubella

CHEMISTRY
☐ 5550 Alpha Fetoprotein, Prenatal
☐ 3000 Amylase
☐ 3153 B12/Folate
☐ 3156 Beta HCG, Quantitative
☐ 3321 Bilirubin, Total
☐ 3324 Billirubin, Total/Direct
☐ 3009 BUN
☐ 3159 CEA
☐ 3348 Cholesterol
☐ 3030 Creatinine, Serum
☐ 3509 Digoxin (recommend 12 hrs., after dose)
☐ 3515 Dilantin
☐ 3168 Ferritin
☐ 3193 FSH
☐ 3066 ▼ Glucose, Fasting
☐ 3061 Glucose, 1° Post 50 g Glucola
☐ 3075 ▼ Glucose, 2° Post Glucola
☐ 3060 Glucose, 2° Post Prandial (meal)
☐ 3049 ▼ Glucose Tolerance Oral GTT
☐ 3047 ▼Glucose Tolerance Gestational GTT
☐ 3650 Hemoglobin, A1C

CHEMISTRY
☐ 5232 HBsAg
☐ 3175 HIV (Consent required)
☐ 3581 Iron & Iron Binding Capacity
☐ 3195 LH
☐ 3590 Magnesium
☐ 3527 Phenobarbital
☐ 3095 Potassium
☐ 3689 Pregnancy Test, Serum (HCG, qual)
☐ 3653 Pregnancy Test, Urine
☐ 3197 Prolactin
☐ 3199 PSA
☐ 3339 SGOT/AST
☐ 3342 SGPT/ALT
☐ 3093 Sodium/Potassium, Serum
☐ 3510 Tegretol
☐ 3551 Theophylline
☐ 3333 Uric Acid

MICROBIOLOGY
Source ______
☐ 7240 Culture, AFB
☐ 7200 Culture, Blood x ______
☐ Draw Interval ______
☐ 7280 Culture, Fungus
☐ Culture, Routine
☐ 7005 Culture, Stool
☐ 7010 Culture, Throat
☐ 7000 Culture, Urine
☐ 7300 Gram Stain
☐ 7355 Occult Blood x ______
☐ 7365 Ova & Parasites x ______
☐ 7400 Smear & Suspension (includes Gram Stain/Wet Mount)
☐ 7060 Rapid Strep A Screen (Negs confir by cult)
☐ 7065 Rapid Strep A Screen only
☐ 7030 Beta Strep Culture
☐ 5207 GC by DNA Probe
☐ 5130 Chlamydia by DNA Probe
☐ 5555 Chlamydia/GC by DNA Probe
☐ 7375 Wright Stain, Stool

Additional Tests ______

PANELS & PROFILES
☐ ✗ 3309 CHEM 12 — Albumin, Alkaline Phosphatase, BUN, Calcium, Cholesterol, Glucose, LDH, Phosphorus, AST, Total Bilirubin, Total Protein, Uric Acid
☐ ▼ 3315 CHEM 20 — Chem 12, Electrolyte Panel, Creatinine, Iron, Gamma GT, ALT, Triglycerides
☐ ▼ 3357 CARDIAC RISK PANEL — Cholesterol, HDL, LDL, Risk Factors, VLDL Triglycerides
☐ ✗ 3042 CRITICAL CARE PANEL — BUN, Chloride, CO2, Glucose, Potassium, Sodium
☐ 3046 ELECTROLYTE PANEL — Chloride, CO2, Potassium, Sodium
☐ ▼ 3399 EXECUTIVE PANEL — Chem 20, Iron, Cardiac Risk Panel, CBC, RPR, Thyroid Cascade
☐ 5242 HEPATITIS PANEL, ACUTE — HAVIgMAb, HBsAg, HBsAb, HBcAb, HCVAb
☐ ▼ 3355 LIPID MONITORING PANEL — Cholesterol, Triglycerides, HDL, LDL, VLDL, ALT, AST
☐ 3312 LIVER PANEL — Alkaline Phospatase, AST, Total Bilirubin, Gamma GT, Total Protein, Albumin, ALT
☐ ✗ 3083 METABOLIC STATUS PANEL — BUN, Osmolality (calculated), Chloride, CO2 Creatinine, Glucose, Potassium, Sodium, BUN/Creatinine, Ratio, Anion Gap
☐ ✗ 3376 PANEL B — Chem 12, CBC, Electrolyte Panel
☐ ▼ 3382 PANEL D — Chem 20, CBC, Thyroid Cascade
☐ ✗ 3388 PANEL F — Chem 12, CBC, Electrolyte Panel, Thyroid Cascade
☐ ▼ 3391 PANEL G — Chem 20, Cardiac Risk Panel, CBC, Thyroid Cascade
☐ ▼ 3393 PANEL H — Chem 20, CBC, Cardiac Risk Panel Rheumatoid Factor, Thyroid Cascade
☐ ▼ 3397 PANEL J — Chem 20, Cardiac Risk Panel
☐ 5351 PRENATAL PANEL — Antibody Screen ABO/Rh, CBC Rubella, HBsAg, RPR
☐ 1059 with Urinalysis, Routine
☐ 1082 with Urinalysis w/Culture if indicated
☐ ✗ 3102 RENAL PANEL — Metabolic Status Panel, Calcium, Phosphorus
☐ 3188 THYROID CASCADE — TSH, Reflex Testing

▼ - patient **required** to fast for 12-14 hours
✗ - patient recommended to fast 12-14 hours

LAB USE ONLY INIT ______
☐ SST ☐ PLASMA
☐ PURPLE ☐ SERUM
☐ YELLOW ☐ SWAB
☐ BLUE ☐ SLIDES
☐ GREEN ☐ DNA PROBE
☐ GREY ☐ B. CULT BTLS
☐ URINE
☐ BLACK
☐ OTHER: ______
REC'V. SPECIMEN: ☐ FROZEN
☐ AMBIENT ☐ ON ICE

Special Instructions/Pertinent Clinical Information ______
Physician's Signature ______ **Date** ______
These orders may be FAXed to: 449-5288
7060-500 (7/96)
LAB

FIGURE 24.17 Requisitions may be used for outpatients. (From Warekois RS, Robinson R: *Phlebotomy: worktext and procedures manual*, ed 4, St. Louis, 2016, Saunders.)

area) are used for venipuncture (Fig. 24.19). The puncture site should be carefully selected after both arms have been inspected. Alternative sites may be indicated if the area is cyanotic, scarred, bruised, edematous, or burned. You may use veins on the lower forearm, the back of the hand, or the wrist. Use of foot or ankle veins is not typically within the scope of the patient care technician without further training. Never draw blood from this area if the patient is diabetic.

To apply a tourniquet, place the tourniquet 3 to 4 inches above the patient's elbow, ensuring that it is not twisted (Fig. 24.20). Grasp the tourniquet ends, one in each hand, at the part of the tourniquet that is closest to the patient's skin. Pull the ends apart to stretch the rubber material, and then cross one end over the other while maintaining the tension. Tuck the top end of the tourniquet underneath the bottom piece, creating a loop with the upper flap free so that it can be released with one hand. The tourniquet should be tight without being twisted or pinching the patient's skin. Both ends of the tourniquet should be pointing upward so that they do not contaminate the blood draw site.

When the tourniquet is in place, ask the patient to make a fist, and palpate for an acceptable vein using your ungloved index finger. If you are able to palpate the vein through gloved fingers, you can continue with the phlebotomy process. A thorough inspection of both arms should be done before the venipuncture site is chosen. Veins bounce lightly when palpated. The medial veins generally run parallel or at a slight angle to the fold in the antecubital area, whereas the cephalic veins run lateral or to the outside of the antecubital area. These veins are the veins of choice. The basilic vein, which lies on the inside part of the antecubital area, is very close to the brachial artery and median nerves and should be used only if the medial or cephalic veins are inaccessible. The most common injury patients suffer from phlebotomy is nerve injury. If the patient complains

FIGURE 24.18 Computer-printed label for specimen tube. (From Warekois RS, Robinson R: *Phlebotomy: worktext and procedures manual*, ed 4, St. Louis, 2016, Saunders.)

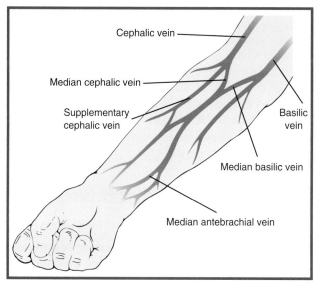

FIGURE 24.19 The veins of the forearm. (From Stepp CA, Woods MA: *Laboratory procedures for medical office personnel*, Philadelphia, 1998, Saunders.)

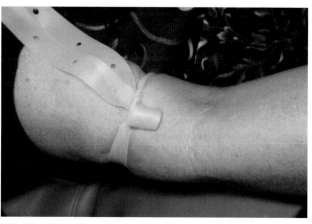

FIGURE 24.20 Placement of a tourniquet. (From Rose L, et al: *Periodontics*, St. Louis, 2004, Mosby.)

of tingling, numbness, or a shooting pain, discontinue the procedure and choose another site before continuing. Do not probe with the needle under this condition; any attempt at relocating the needle puts the patient at great risk of nerve injury.

Performing the Venipuncture

When you have located a vein, remove the tourniquet. A tourniquet can remain in place for 1 minute. After its removal, you must wait 2 minutes before reapplying it. Assemble the appropriate equipment, ensuring that everything is within easy reach, that the sterile packets are torn open, and that the contents are easily accessible. Sanitize your hands.

Reapply the tourniquet and quickly relocate the vein. Put on your gloves and cleanse the antecubital area with the alcohol, working outward in a circular motion. Do not touch this area after cleansing. Ask the patient to clench the hand into a fist. Do not have the patient pump the fist, because this may temporarily increase the level of potassium and ionized calcium in the blood. Anchor the vein by stretching the skin downward below the collection site with the thumb of the nondominant hand, and swiftly insert the needle into the vein at a 15-degree angle. The bevel should be facing up. If the needle is inserted at an angle greater than 15 degrees, it quickly penetrates the other side of the vein and enters other structures, such as nerves or the brachial artery, and very likely will cause a hematoma or an injury. Pull back on the syringe plunger or push the evacuated tube into the double-pointed needle. When blood enters the tube or barrel, ask the patient to unclench the fist.

Completing the Venipuncture

Continue to draw the specimen, checking periodically on the patient's condition. As you remove each tube from the needle holder, gently invert (not shake) it several times before you place it in the rack. Tubes with clot activator should be inverted 5 times, light-blue–topped tubes for coagulation studies should be inverted 3 or 4 times, and all other anticoagulant tubes should be inverted 8 to 10 times. If the tubes are not inverted immediately after collection, small clots can form in the specimen. When you are nearing the end of the draw and the last tube to be collected has been filled, carefully release the tourniquet without jarring the needle, and remove the final vacuum tube. Remove the needle quickly and apply gauze with pressure to the puncture site. Ask the patient to apply direct pressure to the gauze but not to bend the arm. Immediately activate the safety device to cover the needle, and dispose of the entire needle/needle holder unit into a sharps container. Before putting on the bandage, ensure that the vein is

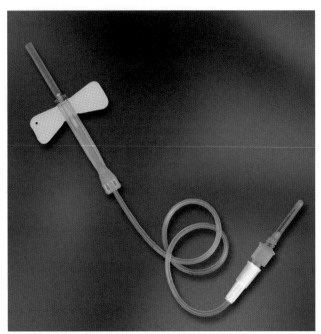

FIGURE 24.21 Winged infusion set attached to an evacuated tube holder with a Luer needle holder. (Courtesy and © Becton, Dickinson and Company, Franklin Lakes, New Jersey.)

not leaking. Observe the site for 5 to 10 seconds after releasing pressure and removing the gauze. If visible bleeding occurs, or if the tissue around the puncture site rises, continue applying pressure until the bleeding has stopped. Special precautions must be taken for patients receiving anticoagulants because the phlebotomy site will bleed longer than is the norm. Put on a bandage and dispose of the gauze in a biohazard waste container. Clean gauze, not a cotton ball, can be taped over the site in lieu of a bandage. Label all tubes by the patient's side. Never leave the room or release an outpatient until the tubes have been labeled. Assess the patient's status one last time, and then dismiss the patient or leave the room.

Procedures 24.1 and 24.2 outline the proper procedures for collecting a venous blood sample using a syringe and the evacuated tube method. Certain patients, such as those with narrow veins, young children, and aging adults, may require a winged infusion set (butterfly needle) rather than the previously mentioned methods. Butterfly units also can be used to draw blood from the hands of adults. Nurses or phlebotomists from the laboratory typically use the butterfly units (Fig. 24.21).

PROBLEMS ASSOCIATED WITH VENIPUNCTURE

Failure to obtain blood can occur because of a number of factors. Determining the cause of the problem may help you decide whether a second attempt would be

Text continued on p. 443

PROCEDURE 24.1

Collecting a Venous Blood Sample With a Syringe

1. Check the requisition form to determine the tests ordered. Gather the appropriate tubes and supplies.
2. Sanitize your hands and put on nonsterile gloves.
3. Identify the patient, explain the procedure, and obtain permission to perform the venipuncture.
4. Assist the patient to sit with the arm well supported in a slightly downward position.
5. Assemble the equipment. The choice of syringe barrel size and needle size depends on your inspection of the patient's veins and the amount of blood required for the ordered tests. Attach the needle to the syringe. Pull and depress the plunger several times to loosen it in the barrel. Keep the cover on the needle.
6. Apply the tourniquet around the patient's arm 3 to 4 inches above the elbow. The tourniquet should never be tied so tightly that it restricts blood flow in the artery. The tourniquet should remain in place no longer than 1 minute.

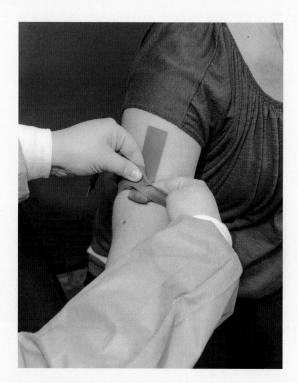

7. Ask the patient to make a fist.
8. Select the venipuncture site by palpating the antecubital space (if you have difficulty palpating the vein with gloves, you can remove the gloves, palpate the vein and visibly mark its location, and then put on new gloves before continuing); use your index finger to trace the path of the vein and to judge its depth. The vein

most often used is the median cephalic vein, which lies in the middle of the elbow.

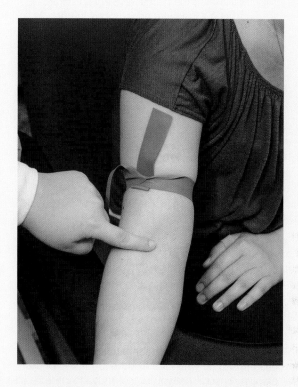

9. Cleanse the site, starting in the center of the area and working outward in a circular pattern with the alcohol pad. Allow the area to dry before proceeding.

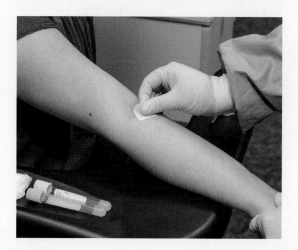

10. Hold the syringe in your dominant hand. Your thumb should be on top and your fingers underneath. Remove the needle sheath.
11. Grasp the patient's arm with the nondominant hand and anchor the vein by stretching the skin downward

Continued

below the collection site with the thumb of the nondominant hand.

12. With the bevel of the needle up, aligned parallel to the vein, and at a 15-degree angle, insert the needle through the skin and into the vein rapidly and smoothly. Observe for a "flash" of blood in the hub of the syringe. Ask the patient to release the fist.

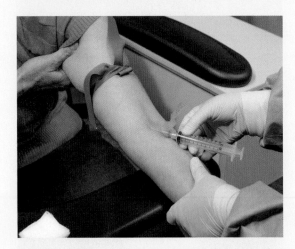

13. Slowly pull back the plunger of the syringe with the nondominant hand. Do not allow more than 1 mL of head space between the blood and the top of the plunger. Ensure that you do not move the needle after entering the vein. Fill the barrel to the needed volume.

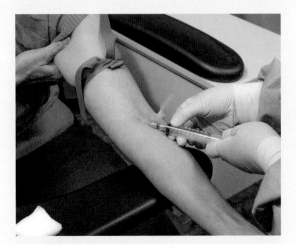

14. Release the tourniquet when venipuncture is complete. It must be released before the needle is removed from the arm.

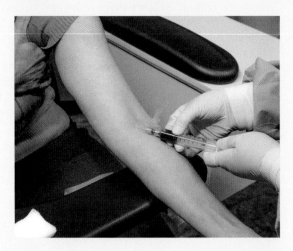

15. Place sterile gauze over the puncture site at the time of needle withdrawal. Immediately activate the needle safety device.

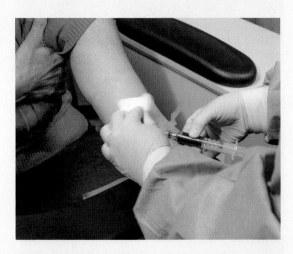

16. Instruct the patient to apply direct pressure on the puncture site with sterile gauze. The patient may elevate the arm but should not bend it.

17. Transfer the blood immediately to the required tube or tubes using a syringe adapter. Do not push on the

PROCEDURE 24.1

Collecting a Venous Blood Sample With a Syringe—cont'd

plunger during transfer. Discard the entire unit in the sharps container when transfer is complete. Invert the tubes after the addition of blood and label them with the necessary patient information.

18. Inspect the puncture site for bleeding or hematoma.
19. Apply a hypoallergenic bandage.

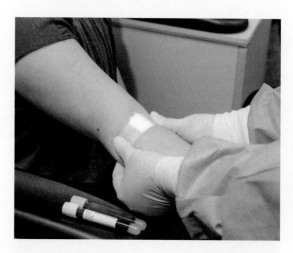

20. Disinfect the work area, dispose of any blood-contaminated materials (e.g., gauze) in the biohazard container, remove your gloves, and sanitize your hands.
21. Complete the laboratory requisition form and route the specimen to the proper place. Record the procedure in the patient's record.

(Figures from Warekois RS, Robinson R: Phlebotomy: worktext and procedures manual, ed 4, St. Louis, 2016, Saunders.)

PROCEDURE 24.2

Collecting a Venous Blood Sample Using an Evacuated Tube

1. Check the requisition form to determine the tests ordered. Gather the appropriate tubes and supplies.
2. Sanitize your hands and put on nonsterile gloves.
3. Identify the patient, explain the procedure, and obtain permission for the venipuncture.
4. Assist the patient to sit with the arm well supported in a slightly downward position.
5. Assemble the equipment. The choice of needle size depends on your inspection of the patient's veins.

Attach the needle firmly to the Vacutainer holder. Keep the cover on the needle.

6. Apply the tourniquet around the patient's arm 3 to 4 inches above the elbow. The tourniquet should never be tied so tightly that it restricts blood flow in the artery. Tourniquets should remain in place no longer than 60 seconds.

Continued

PROCEDURE 24.2

Collecting a Venous Blood Sample Using an Evacuated Tube—cont'd

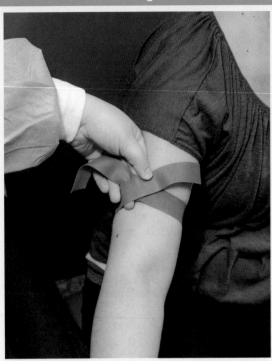

9. Cleanse the site, starting in the center of the area and working outward in a circular pattern with the alcohol pad.

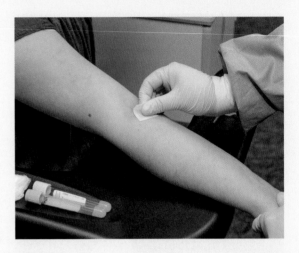

7. Ask the patient to make a fist.
8. Select the venipuncture site by palpating the antecubital space and use your index finger to trace the path of the vein and to judge its depth. The vein most often used is the median cephalic vein, which lies in the middle of the elbow.

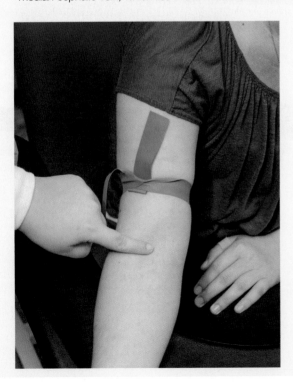

10. Dry the site with a sterile gauze pad or allow the area to dry before proceeding.
11. Hold the Vacutainer assembly in your dominant hand. Your thumb should be on top and your fingers underneath. You may want to position the first tube to be drawn into the needle holder, but do not push it onto the double-pointed needle past the marking on the holder. Remove the needle sheath.
12. Grasp the patient's arm with the nondominant hand and anchor the vein by stretching the skin downward below the collection site with the thumb of the nondominant hand.
13. With the bevel of the needle up, aligned parallel to the vein, and at a 15-degree angle, insert the needle through the skin and into the vein rapidly and smoothly.

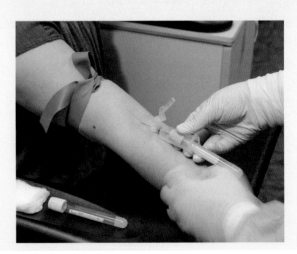

PROCEDURE 24.2

Collecting a Venous Blood Sample Using an Evacuated Tube—cont'd

14. Place two fingers on the flanges of the needle holder and use the thumb to push the tube onto the double-pointed needle. Ensure that you do not change the needle's position in the vein. When blood begins to flow into the tube, ask the patient to release the fist.

15. Allow the tube to fill to maximum capacity. Remove the tube by curling the fingers underneath and pushing on the needle holder with the thumb. Take care not to move the needle when removing the tube.

16. Insert the second tube into the needle holder, following the instructions in the previous steps. Continue filling tubes until the order on the requisition has been filled. Gently invert each tube immediately after removing it from the needle holder to mix anticoagulants and blood. As the last tube is filling, release the tourniquet.

17. Remove the last tube from the holder. Place gauze over the puncture site and quickly remove the needle, engaging the safety device. Dispose of the entire unit in the sharps container.

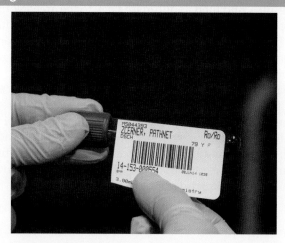

20. Check the puncture site for bleeding and hematoma formation.
21. Apply a hypoallergenic bandage.

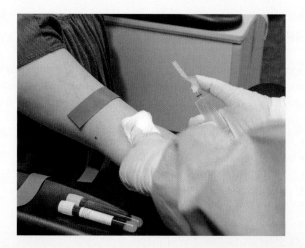

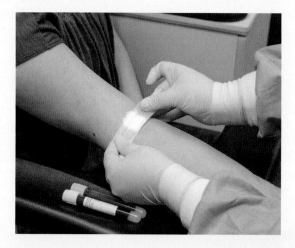

18. Apply pressure to the gauze or instruct the patient to do so. The patient may elevate the arm but should not bend it.

19. Label the tubes with the patient's name, the date, and the time, or apply the preprinted tube labels.

22. Disinfect the work area, dispose of any blood-contaminated materials (e.g., gauze) in the biohazard container, remove your gloves, and sanitize your hands.

23. Complete the laboratory requisition form and route the specimen to the proper place. Record the procedure in the patient's record.

(Figures from Warekois RS, Robinson R: Phlebotomy: worktext and procedures manual, ed 4, St. Louis, 2016, Saunders.)

successful. The first rule is to remain calm so that you can think clearly and can systematically determine the possible cause of the problem.

A hematoma is a large, painful, bruised area at the puncture site caused by blood leaking into the tissue, which causes the tissue around the puncture site to swell. The most common causes of hematoma formation

during the draw are excessive probing with the needle to locate a vein, failure to insert the needle far enough into the vein, and a needle that goes through the vein. A hematoma also can form after a draw if you fail to remove the tourniquet before removing the needle, fail to withdraw the vacuum tube before the needle is withdrawn, or fail to apply adequate pressure on the puncture site, or if the elbow is bent while pressure is applied. If a hematoma forms, discontinue the procedure stat, apply pressure to the area for a minimum of 3 minutes, and then apply an ice pack to the area. Notify the physician and observe the site to determine whether the bleeding has stopped. Depending on the facility's policy, an incident report may have to be completed and recorded in the patient's record.

Fainting, or syncope, can have serious consequences, and the patient care technician must always be prepared. Securing the patient in a blood collection chair prevents bodily injury if the person faints. Constant conversation with the patient during the procedure can help identify an impending episode, as can observing the patient's face and breathing rate.

Fainting

According to CLSI, the procedure for a fainting patient or one who is nonresponsive is as follows:

- If the patient begins to faint, quickly remove the tourniquet and needle from the arm and immediately dispose of the unit in a sharps container to prevent an accidental exposure.
- Notify staff members for assistance.
- Lay the patient flat or lower the head if the patient is sitting.
- Loosen tight clothing.
- Do not use ammonia inhalants/capsules because these are associated with adverse effects and are no longer recommended.
- Apply a cold compress or washcloth to the patient's forehead and back of the neck.

- Stay with the patient until recovery is complete.
- Document the incident according to facility policies.
- When the patient regains consciousness, he or she must remain in the facility for at least 15 minutes and should not operate a vehicle for at least 30 minutes.

Nerve damage can be a consequence of venipuncture, although an unlikely one. Preventive measures include avoiding the basilic vein and refraining from blind probing if the vein is missed.

Table 24.4 lists some probable solutions to complications. As a general rule, it is wise to limit yourself to two attempts to obtain blood from any one patient. If you fail on the second attempt, ask the patient whether he or she would prefer having someone else try, or whether it would be better to come back at another time. This maneuver lets the patient feel that he or she is in control of the situation. At one time or another, everyone is unsuccessful in obtaining a needed blood sample, so do not feel that you are a failure. Many facilities have policies in place which limit the number of times you may stick someone without success.

SPECIMEN RE-COLLECTION

Sometimes problems with a sample cannot be determined until the specimen is analyzed in the laboratory. Rejected specimens must be re-collected. The laboratory may reject a specimen for reasons that include the following:

- Unlabeled or mislabeled specimen
- Insufficient quantity
- Defective tube
- Incorrect tube used for the test ordered

Table 24.4	Managing Blood Draw Complications

Possible Complication	Strategies
Burned area	Choose another site, because these areas are prone to infection.
Convulsions	Stay calm. Remove the needle and quickly dispose of it in a sharps container, and then help guide the patient to the floor, protecting him or her from injury. Call for help.
Damaged or scarred veins or infected areas	Look for an alternative site; do not draw blood from scarred or infected areas.
Edema	Avoid the area; look for an alternative site.
Hematoma	Adjust the depth of the needle or remove the needle and apply pressure.
Intravenous (IV) therapy or blood transfusion sites	Blood samples should not be drawn from an arm that is also the site for IV infusion or blood transfusion because of the dilution factor.
Mastectomy	Do not draw blood from the side of the mastectomy, because mastectomy surgery causes lymphostasis, which may produce false results.
Nausea	Place a cold cloth on the patient's forehead, give the patient a basin in case of vomiting, and instruct him or her to take deep breaths. Alert the nurse.
No blood	Manipulate the needle slightly or remove the Vacutainer and perform the blood draw again using a syringe or butterfly setup.
Petechiae	Loosen the tourniquet, because this complication usually results from the tourniquet being in place for longer than 2 minutes.
Syncope	Position the patient's head between the knees (if in a sitting position). Check and record the patient's pulse, blood pressure, and respiration rate, and continue to observe the patient. Never leave the patient unattended.

- Hemolysis
- Clotted blood in an anticoagulated specimen
- Improper handling

Hemolysis is the major cause of specimen rejection. Because it cannot be detected until the blood cells separate from the plasma or serum, it is crucial to take steps to prevent red blood cell damage during collection. Hemolyzed serum or plasma appears rosy to bright red in color because of the release of hemoglobin from the cells. Some of the more routine tests that are adversely affected by hemolysis are chemistry tests for electrolytes (e.g., potassium, sodium), bilirubin, total protein, and numerous liver enzymes (e.g., alkaline phosphatase,

gamma glutamyl transferase). Table 24.5 reviews the major causes of hemolysis during collection.

CAPILLARY PUNCTURE

Capillaries are small blood vessels that connect small arterioles to small venules. A capillary, or dermal, puncture is an efficient means of collecting a blood specimen when only a small amount of blood is required, or when a patient's condition makes venipuncture difficult. Because the requisition will not indicate that the collection is to be made in this manner, you must be familiar with the advantages, limitations, and appropriate uses

Table 24.5	Major Causes of Hemolysis During Collection	
Cause of Hemolysis	**Explanation**	**Prevention**
Alcohol preparation	Transfer of alcohol into the specimen causes hemolysis.	Allow venipuncture site to dry completely.
Incorrect needle size	A high-gauge needle causes the blood to be forced through a small lumen with great force, shearing the cell membranes; a very-low-gauge needle allows a large amount of blood to suddenly enter the tube with great force, causing frothing.	Choose the correct needle for the job, aiming for a 19- to 23-gauge needle.
Loose connections on the vacuum tube assembly	If the connection between the needle holder and the double-pointed needle or the syringe and the needle is loose, air can enter the sample and cause frothing.	Ensure that all connections are tight before beginning the venipuncture.
Removing the needle from the vein with the tube intact	The remaining vacuum in the tube can cause air to be drawn forcefully into the tube, causing frothing.	Remove the final tube from the needle holder before withdrawing the needle from the patient's vein.
Underfilled tubes	Underfilling tubes lead to an improper blood/additive ratio. Certain additives in disproportionate amounts (e.g., sodium fluoride) can cause hemolysis.	Permit blood to flow into the tubes until no more movement can be seen.
Syringe collections	Pulling back forcibly on the plunger draws blood too quickly through the needle, shearing cell membranes; transferring blood into a vacuum tube further traumatizes red blood cells.	Pump the plunger several times before use to loosen it in the barrel. Use the smallest syringe possible. Pace the aspiration rate so that no more than 1 mL of air space is present at any time. Transfer blood into the vacuum tube immediately, preferably using a transfer device. *Never* push on the plunger when transferring to a vacuum tube. Angle the syringe so that the blood runs gently down the side of the tube, preventing the cells from hitting the bottom of the tube with force.
Mixing tubes too vigorously	All tubes except the red-topped tube must be mixed.	Gently invert tubes immediately after the draw. Anything other than gentle inversion (e.g., shaking) can hemolyze cells.
Temperature and transport problems	Trauma and temperature extremes can damage cells. Freezing results in ice crystals that puncture cell membranes.	Tubes should be transported in the upright position with as little trauma as possible. Temperature should be controlled—not too hot and too cold.
Separation of plasma or serum from red blood cells	Removing the serum or plasma from the cells minimizes the risk of contaminating the specimen with red blood cell contents.	Blood samples should be centrifuged, when applicable, as soon as possible and serum or plasma removed from the cells.
Prolonged tourniquet time	While the tourniquet restricts blood flow, interstitial fluid can leak into the veins and hemolyze red blood cells.	Adhere to the 1-minute rule for tourniquet application.
Poor collection; blood flowing too slowly into the tube	The needle lumen may be blocked because it is too close to the inner wall of the vein.	Withdraw the needle slightly to center it within the vein.

of this technique. Capillary puncture is warranted in the following situations:

- Older patients
- Pediatric patients (especially younger than age 2)
- Patients who require frequent glucose monitoring
- Patients with burns or scars in venipuncture sites
- Obese patients
- Patients receiving intravenous therapy
- Patients who have had a mastectomy
- Patients at risk for venous thrombosis
- Patients who are severely dehydrated
- Tests that require a small volume of blood

Because capillaries are bridges between arteries and veins, capillary blood is a mixture of the two. Small amounts of tissue fluid also are present in capillary blood, especially in the first drop. Analyte levels are usually the same in capillary and venous blood, with a few exceptions. Hemoglobin and glucose values are higher in capillary blood; potassium, calcium, and total protein are higher in venous blood.

Equipment

Skin Puncture Devices

The device used to perform a dermal puncture is the lancet, which delivers a quick puncture to a predetermined depth (Fig. 24.22). OSHA has directed that lancets must have retractable blades; they also must have locks that prevent accidental puncture after use and that prevent the device from being reused (Table 24.6). Skin puncture devices should always be discarded in a sharps container.

Collection Containers

Different types of collection devices and containers are available, and the ones used depend on the test to be performed (Fig. 24.23). Microcollection, or Microtainer®, tubes hold up to 750 L (0.75 mL) of blood and are available with a variety of anticoagulants and additives. The tops are color-coded in the same fashion as evacuated tubes. Blood is collected drop-wise into these tubes through a funnel-like device. Capillary tubes are another means of collecting blood from a dermal puncture. These are glass or plastic tubes that draw blood by

Table 24.6	Lancet Blade Recommendations	
Device Depth and Dimension	**Blood Volume**	**Application**
2.25-mm, 28-gauge needle	Single drop	Fingersticks
2.25-mm, 23-gauge needle	Single drop	Fingersticks, glucose test
1 × 1.5-mm blade	Low blood flow	Fingersticks, microhematocrit tube, or drop of blood for glucose or cholesterol test
1.5 × 1.5-mm blade	Medium blood flow	Fingersticks; to fill a single Microtainer tube
2 × 1.5-mm blade	High blood flow	Fingersticks; to fill multiple Microtainer tubes

(Modified from Becton, Dickinson and Company, at http://www.bd.com/vacutainer/faqs/#urine_faq)

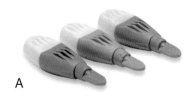

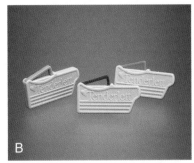

FIGURE 24.22 Dermal puncture devices. (A, Courtesy and © Becton, Dickinson and Company. IN Warekois RS, Robinson R: *Phlebotomy: worktext and procedures manual*, ed 4, St. Louis, 2016, Saunders. B, Courtesy Accriva Diagnostics.)

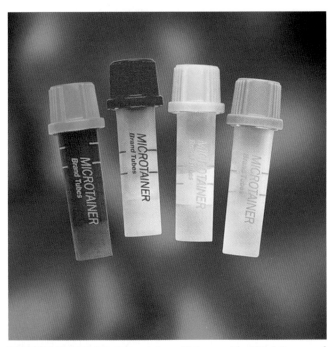

FIGURE 24.23 BD Microtainer Tubes with BD Microgard Closure. (Courtesy and © Becton, Dickinson and Company. IN Warekois RS, Robinson R: *Phlebotomy: worktext and procedures manual*, ed 4, St. Louis, 2016, Saunders.)

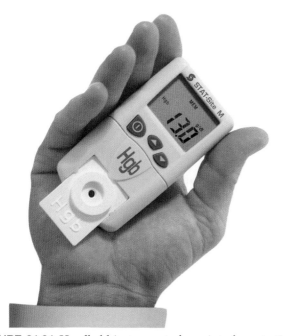

FIGURE 24.24 Handheld instruments for point-of-care testing. (Courtesy Stanbio Laboratory, Boerne, Texas. In Warekois RS, Robinson R: *Phlebotomy: worktext and procedures manual*, ed 4, St. Louis, 2016, Saunders.)

capillary action; that is, the blood fills into these narrow tubes without the need for suction. If the capillary tube is coated with the anticoagulant heparin, a red band will be seen at the top.

Manufacturers also provide various collection devices for obtaining small amounts of blood for "point-of-care" testing, such as for glucose, hemoglobin A_{1c}, troponin levels, and cholesterol (Fig. 24.24). The blood is pulled into the collecting device by capillary action after puncture, or it is dropped onto a reagent strip, which is inserted into the instrument to be analyzed.

Blood from a capillary puncture also can be deposited on paper cards. One such card, the Guthrie card, is used to test neonates for certain metabolic disorders, such as phenylketonuria (PKU). Blood is deposited into circles on biologically inactive filter paper and is sent to a referral laboratory for analysis within 24 hours of sampling. Each spot must be filled with capillary blood to soak through the paper. These cards typically dry before placing them in a mailing envelope. Federal postal regulations for the mailing of biohazardous material must be followed (Fig. 24.25).

Routine Capillary Puncture

Site Selection

In adults and children, the usual puncture site is the ring finger, but capillary blood can be obtained from the middle finger or heel (Fig. 24.26). The thumb usually is too callused, and the index finger has extra nerve endings that make the puncture more painful. The fifth

finger has too little tissue for a successful puncture. The puncture is made at the tip and slightly to the side of the finger. Be sure to puncture a fleshy area closer to the center of the finger to prevent damage to underlying bone. Avoid areas that are callused, scarred, burned, infected, cyanotic, or edematous.

For children younger than 1 year, dermal puncture is performed on the medial and lateral surfaces of the plantar surface (bottom) of the heel. Areas other than these are unsafe, and bone or nerve damage to an infant may occur. Blood flow from an infant's heel can be increased as much as sevenfold by applying a warm, moist towel (or other warming device) at a temperature no higher than 42° C (108° F) for 3 to 5 minutes. Never place bandages on the heel or anywhere on infants younger than age 2 because they may peel off and become a choking hazard.

Patient Preparation

Preparation for a capillary puncture is similar to that for venipuncture. Put on gloves and cleanse the finger well with an alcohol prep pad. If the patient's hands are dirty, ask the person to wash them before the procedure. If the patient's hands are cold, warm them in warm water and dry them thoroughly, or ask the person to rub or shake them vigorously.

In general, you must work very efficiently when performing a capillary puncture because blood flow stops quickly. Be sure to have your supplies organized and within easy reach. Grasp the finger firmly and apply gentle, intermittent pressure, but do not squeeze or "milk" it. Press the puncture device firmly against the skin and quickly depress the plunger.

Collecting the Specimen

After the dermis is punctured, it is important to wipe away the first drop of blood with sterile gauze. This drop contains tissue fluid that could interfere with test results. Fill the sampling containers according to the manufacturer's directions. Touch the container to the drop of blood as it is released from the puncture site, but do not touch the skin. If blood flow stops, wiping the site with sterile gauze may restart the flow. Be prepared for blood to contaminate your gloves or surfaces by having spare gloves, extra gauze pads, and disinfectant nearby. After the containers have been filled, ask the patient to apply pressure to the gauze you have placed over the puncture site if he or she is able. Seal containers as recommended by the manufacturer if necessary.

Specimen Handling

Capillary collection containers often are too small for a label to be applied. The most efficient way to transport

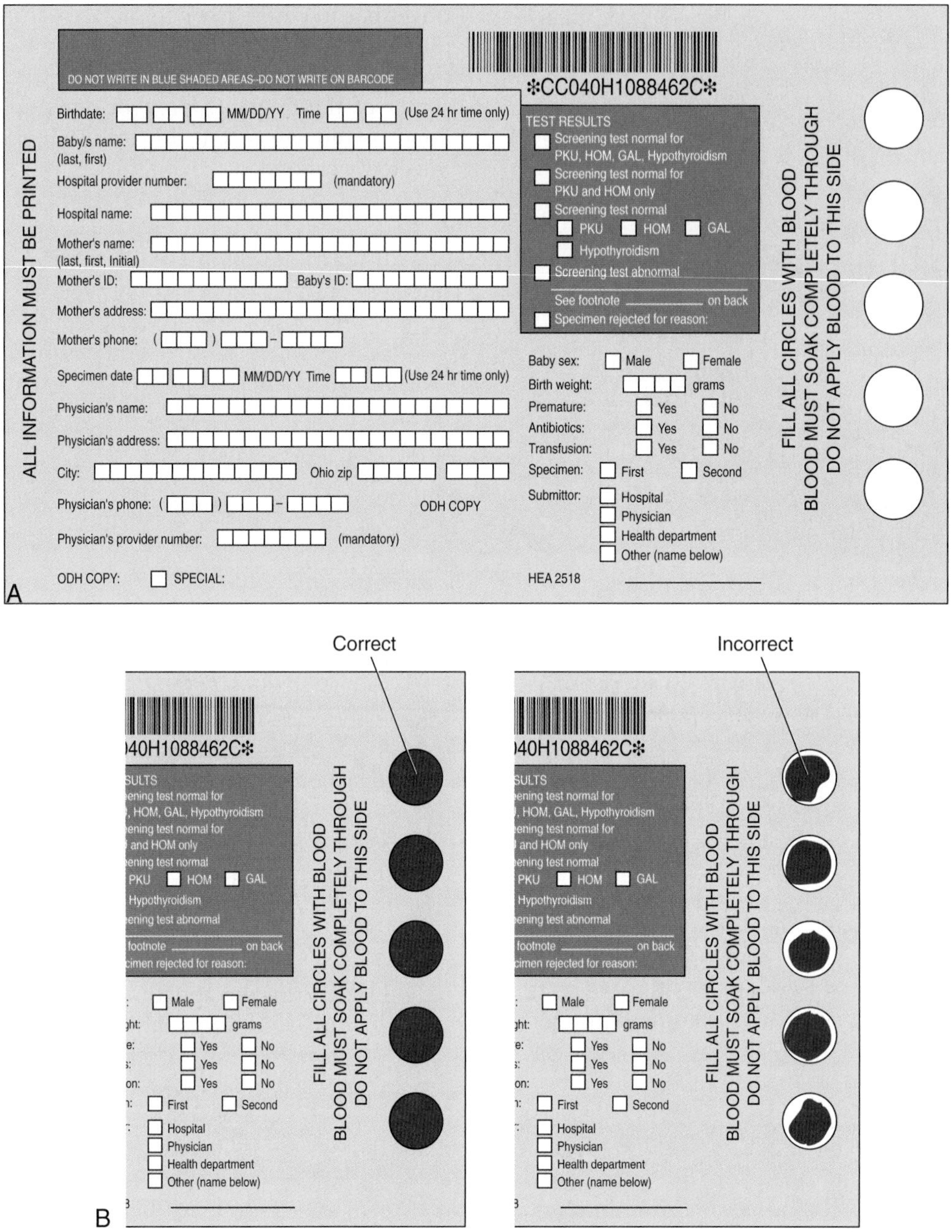

FIGURE 24.25 A, A Guthrie card used in neonatal screening. B, Correct and incorrect ways to fill in the circles. (Modified from Bonewit-West K: *Clinical procedures for medical assistants,* ed 7, Philadelphia, 2008, Saunders. IN Sommer SR, Warekois RS: *Phlebotomy: worktext and procedures manual*, Philadelphia, 2002, Saunders.)

capillary tubes is to remove the stopper from a red-topped tube, insert the capillary tubes, sealed-end down, replace the stopper, and label the tube. Micro-tainer tubes have plastic plugs that fit over the top. They may be placed in a labeled tube or in a labeled zipper-lock bag for transport. Always decontaminate collection containers before delivering them to the laboratory if blood was deposited on the surface during collection. The procedure for collecting capillary blood using a dermal procedure is outlined in Procedure 24.3.

PEDIATRIC PHLEBOTOMY

Obtaining blood from children and infants may be difficult and potentially hazardous. The procedure should be performed only by personnel trained in the techniques for pediatric phlebotomy. Successfully obtaining blood from children requires skill and an understanding of pediatric psychological development, as well as appropriate communication skills. The patient care technician must gain the child's confidence and often

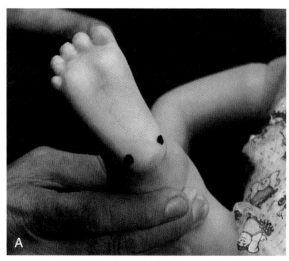
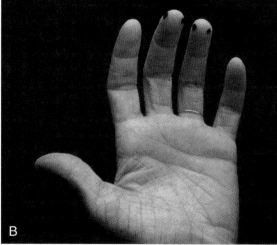

FIGURE 24.26 Capillary puncture sites on the heel and on the fingers. (From Proctor D, Adams A: *Kinn's the medical assistant: an applied learning approach*, ed 12, St. Louis, 2014.)

PROCEDURE 24.3

Collecting Capillary Blood Using Dermal Puncture

1. Read the requisition and gather all needed supplies on the basis of the physician's requisition.
2. Sanitize your hands. Put on nonsterile gloves.
3. Identify the patient and explain the procedure.
4. Select a puncture site depending on the patient's age and the sample to be obtained (side of middle or ring finger of nondominant hand, and medial or lateral curved surface of the heel for an infant).
5. Gently rub the finger along the sides.
6. Clean the site with alcohol, allow it to air-dry, or dry it with sterile gauze.

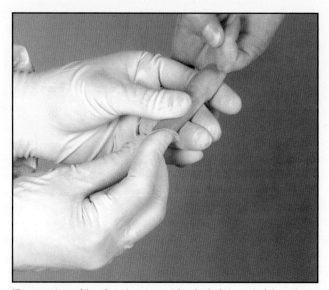

(Puncturing skin that is wet with alcohol is painful and can hemolyze the specimen.)

7. Grasp the patient's finger on the sides near the puncture site with your nondominant forefinger and thumb. Hold the lancet at a right angle to the patient's finger and make a rapid, deep puncture on the side of the patient's fingertip.

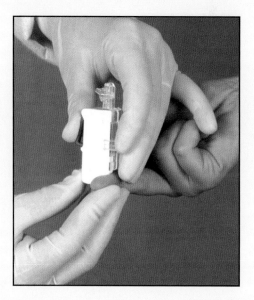

8. Dispose of the lancet in the sharps container. Wipe away the first drop of blood with clean, sterile gauze.

Continued

PROCEDURE 24.3

Collecting Capillary Blood Using Dermal Puncture—cont'd

9. Apply gentle pressure to cause the blood to flow freely.

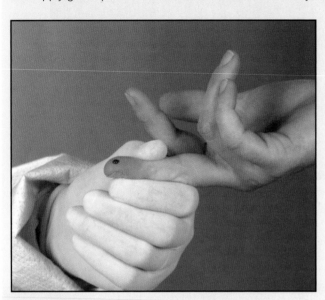

10. Collect blood samples.
    a. Express a large drop of blood, touch the end of the tube to the drop of blood (not the finger), fill the capillary tubes, place the finger over the blood-free end of the tube, and seal the other end of the tube by inserting it into the sealing clay. The tube should be approximately three quarters full before it is sealed.

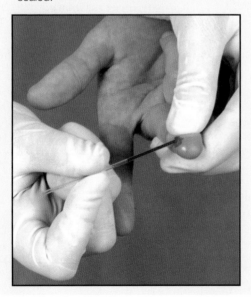

b. Wipe the finger with a clean, sterile gauze pad, express another large drop of blood, and fill a Microtainer. Do not touch the container to the finger. If more blood is needed, wipe the puncture with clean gauze and gently squeeze another drop. Cap the tube when the collection is complete.

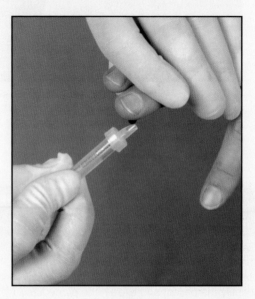

11. When collection is complete, apply pressure to the site with clean sterile gauze. The patient may be able to assist with this step.
12. Select an appropriate means of labeling the containers. Capillary tubes can be placed in a red-topped tube, which is subsequently labeled. Microtainers can be placed in zipper-lock bags that are subsequently labeled.
13. Check the patient for bleeding, clean the site if traces of blood are visible, and apply a nonallergenic bandage if indicated.
14. Dispose of used materials in the proper containers.
15. Disinfect the work area. Dispose of any blood-contaminated materials (e.g., gauze) in the biohazard container. Remove your gloves and sanitize your hands. *(To ensure infection control.)*
16. Record the procedure in the patient's record. *(A procedure is considered not done until it is recorded.)*

PROCEDURE 24.3

Collecting Capillary Blood Using Dermal Puncture—cont'd

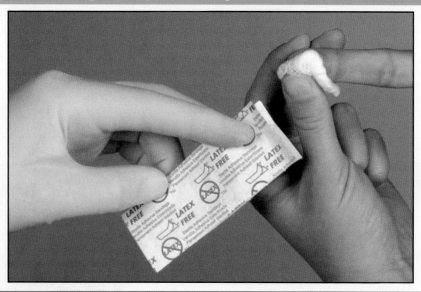

(Figures from Garrels M, Oatis C: Laboratory testing for ambulatory settings, *ed 3, St. Louis, 2015, Saunders.)*

that of the parent as well. Parents often ask to explain the tests being done and why. You should be very careful when divulging information; never tell the parents what disease or condition a specific blood test detects. Refer questions to the child's physician or to your nurse. A parent or guardian may or may not be an asset during the procedure. Ask the parent about the child's previous phlebotomy experiences and how cooperative the child is likely to be. Carefully determine whether the parent is comfortable with assisting in restraining an uncooperative child. Parental behavior greatly influences the child's behavior during the procedure. Children should never be restrained in a way that might cause physical injury. If the parent is unable or unwilling to assist with necessary restraint, always refer to the office or laboratory policy on restraints and procedural holds. Table 24.7 provides information on the typical fears and concerns of children during the procedure and suggested parental involvement.

Removing large amounts of blood, especially from premature infants, may result in anemia (Table 24.8). The amount of blood withdrawn must be recorded in the child's chart. Puncturing deep veins in children may result in cardiac arrest, hemorrhage, venous thrombosis, damage to surrounding tissues, or infection. In addition, the child could be harmed during forceful restraint. To prevent these problems, blood should be collected only by dermal puncture from children younger than age 2 unless the procedure warrants venous collection (lead levels or blood culture). Venipuncture on children younger than age 2 should be performed only by the

nurse or phlebotomist from the laboratory who is specially trained on young children.

When the patient care technician is required to perform pediatric phlebotomy, wearing a colorful smock, being truthful about the discomfort the child will feel, and providing tokens and praise for bravery go a long way toward allaying the child's fears. Topical anesthetics, such as ethyl chloride (EC) spray or amethocaine gel (Ametop®), may be used to reduce pain at the puncture site. In most cases a calm, professional person who understands the developmental needs of the child and relates to the child on that level can gain the acceptance necessary to perform a successful venipuncture or dermal puncture with a minimum of restraint and frustration.

Measuring Blood Glucose

Patients who have diabetes typically have to check their blood glucose levels at different times throughout the day. As a patient care technician, this may be a procedure you are asked to do, known as point-of-care testing. Point-of-care testing takes place at the bedside of the patient. This means that you can perform the test at the bedside and have a result within minutes. It does not typically require transporting a specimen to the laboratory.

The patient must monitor blood glucose levels with a blood glucose monitoring system periodically throughout the day to determine whether the levels are

Table 24.7	Childhood Behavior and Parental Involvement During Phlebotomy	

Age	Typical Mental State	Suggested Parental Involvement
Newborns (0–12 months)	Trust that adults will respond to their needs.	Parent should assist by cradling and comforting child.
Infants and toddlers (1–3 years)	Minimal fear of danger but fear of separation. Limited language and understanding of procedure.	Parent should assist by holding the child and providing emotional support.
Preschoolers (3–6 years)	Fearful of injury to body; still dependent on parent.	Parent may be present to provide emotional support and to assist in obtaining child's cooperation.
School-aged children (7–12 years)	Less dependent on parent and more willing to cooperate; fear of loss of self-control (crying).	Child may not want parent present.
Teenagers (13–18 years)	Fully engaged in the process; embarrassed to show fear and may show hostility to cover emotions.	Teen may not want parent present.

Table 24.8	General Guidelines for Pediatric Venipuncture

Weight (lb)	Limit During a Single Draw, mL
8–10	3.5
11–15	5
16–40	10
41–60	20
61–65	25
66–80	30

within the normal range. A glucometer is a hand-held device that measures the level of glucose in the blood, using capillary blood. The physician typically prescribes blood guclose testing in the morning before breakfast, before dinner, and possibly before lunch and at bedtime if the patient is having difficulty keeping blood plasma levels stabilized. An important responsibility of the patient care technician is to perform a blood guclose screening (Procedure 24.4).

Blood glucose monitoring systems are palm sized and use very small amounts of capillary blood from a site in the finger, forearm, upper arm, or abdomen. Many different types of blood glucose monitoring systems are available, but all display test results within seconds, and the results are stored in the memory function of the machine for future reference. The patient care technician should know that the accuracy of blood glucose results depends on following the instructions for the particular type of blood glucose monitoring system used by the patient. When performing outpatient blood guclose screening, the patient care technician must use the same machine the patient will use at home and must stress the importance of keeping a record of blood guclose readings to determine long-term serum glucose control. Patients should be encouraged to bring their glucometers with them to each office visit so that the physician can review glucose levels. When performing inpatient blood guclose testing, most facilities require that you use the hospital's blood glucose monitoring systems because they are tested for accuracy and often link to the patient's electronic health record (EHR).

Safe and effective blood glucose monitoring system use should include not only the steps for successfully

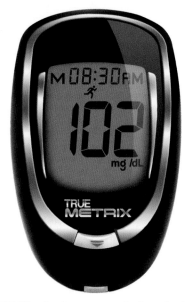

FIGURE 24.27 Blood glucose monitoring device (TrueTrack Smart System). (Courtesy Trividia Health, Fort Lauderdale, Fla.)

checking blood glucose levels but also quality-control mechanisms as suggested by the manufacturer of the device (Fig. 24.27). Some examples of quality controls include the following:

- Follow the manufacturer's intended use statement and instructions exactly.
- Perform the instrument maintenance specified by the manufacturer, including correct cleaning and storage of the instrument.
- Check the expiration dates on test strips and solutions and store these products correctly.
- Match and correctly enter the test strip code into the instrument before use.
- Notify the nurse if test results are out of range.

Patients with diabetes also need to find the best method of disposing of their syringes and lancets. Local pharmacies or hospitals may offer assistance with disposal of used sharps. If the patient does not have access to a sharps return program, a puncture-resistant container with an opening that can be easily and tightly sealed before disposal is a good choice.

PROCEDURE 24.4

Measuring Blood Glucose

1. Check the physician's order and collect the necessary equipment and supplies. Perform quality-control measures according to the manufacturer's guidelines and office policy.
2. Sanitize your hands and put on gloves.
3. Ask the patient to wash his or her hands in warm soapy water and then rinse them in warm water and dry them completely.
4. Check the patient's index and ring fingers and select the site for puncture.
5. Turn on the Accu-Chek® monitor by pressing the ON button.

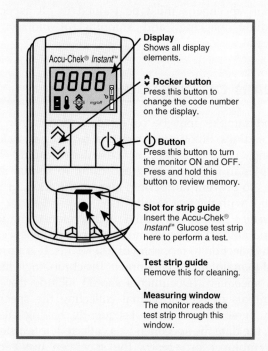

Display
Shows all display elements.

Rocker button
Press this button to change the code number on the display.

Button
Press this button to turn the monitor ON and OFF. Press and hold this button to review memory.

Slot for strip guide
Insert the Accu-Chek® Instant™ Glucose test strip here to perform a test.

Test strip guide
Remove this for cleaning.

Measuring window
The monitor reads the test strip through this window.

6. Ensure that the code number on the LED display matches the code number on the container of test strips.
7. Remove a test strip from the vial and immediately replace the vial cover.
8. Check the strip for discoloration by comparing the color of the round window on the back of the test strip with the designated "unused" color chart provided on the label of the test strip vial.
9. Do not touch the yellow test pad or round window on the back of the strip when handling the strip.
10. When the test strip symbol begins flashing in the lower right corner of the display screen, insert the test strip into the designated testing slot until it locks into place. If the test strip has been inserted correctly, the arrows

on the test strip will face up and point toward the monitor.

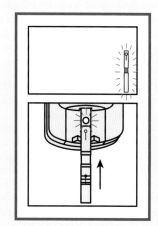

11. Cleanse the selected site on the patient's fingertip with the alcohol wipe and allow the finger to air-dry.
12. Perform the finger puncture and wipe away the first drop of blood.
13. Apply a large, hanging drop of blood to the center of the yellow testing pad.

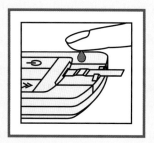

- Do not touch the pad with the patient's finger.
- Do not apply a second drop of blood.
- Do not smear the blood with your finger.
- Ensure that the yellow test pad is saturated with blood.

14. Give the patient a gauze square to hold securely over the puncture site.
15. The monitor automatically begins the measurement process as soon as it senses the drop of blood.
16. The test result will be shown in the display window in milligrams per deciliter (mg/dL).
17. Turn off the monitor by pressing the OFF button.
18. Discard all biohazardous waste in the proper waste containers.
19. Clean the glucometer according to the manufacturer's guidelines, disinfect the work area, remove your gloves and dispose of them properly, and sanitize your hands.
20. Record the test results in the patient's medical record.

(From Stepp CA, Woods MA: Laboratory procedures for medical office personnel, Philadelphia, 1998, WB Saunders.)

Regardless of the type of diabetes, for treatment to be successful, patients must play an active role in the management of their disease. The patient care technician should consistently encourage patients to be active participants in maintaining blood glucose levels within the normal range and constantly be on alert for possible complications from their disease. The ideal is to maintain blood plasma levels as close to the norm as possible to prevent complications. The American Diabetes Association recommends blood levels between 90 and 130 mg/dL before meals and below 180 mg/dL 2 hours after starting a meal, with a glycated (glycosylated) hemoglobin level (HbA$_{1c}$) below 7%.

Postcollection Specimen Handling

It has been said that the results of laboratory testing are only as good as the specimen sent for testing. Specimens handled improperly after collection may provide errors in the results and unnecessarily delay treatment for the patient. From the moment the specimen is collected, analytes in the blood begin to decay, and it is a race against time to provide results that accurately represent a patient's condition at the time of the blood collection. After collection, blood may need to be processed before the sample is sent to its final destination. For most samples, this involves separation of the plasma or serum from the red blood cells. If the tube contains no anticoagulant, blood begins to clot when it comes in contact with the glass tube. Plastic tubes require the addition of a clot activator; the SST speckle-topped tube has silica additives to accelerate clotting. "Clot" tubes should be allowed to sit upright in a rack for 30 to 60 minutes at room temperature while a solid clot forms. Tubes with clot accelerator should form a dense clot within 30 minutes. The presence of anticoagulants in the blood, such as warfarin (Coumadin) or heparin, may delay clotting. Once the clot has formed, every effort should be made to remove the clot from the serum within 2 hours.

Removal of the clot from the serum requires centrifugation. For the thixotropic gel to form the barrier between the clot and the serum, certain g-force, time, and temperature requirements must be met. A minimum g-force of 1000 g must be achieved by centrifugation; the gel must be at 25° C (77° F), and the tube must be centrifuged for 10 to 15 minutes. The serum does not have to be removed from the tube after centrifugation, because the gel has formed a barrier over the red blood cells. Once a tube with thixotropic gel has been centrifuged, it cannot be centrifuged again. The serum, however, can be decanted and centrifuged in another tube.

For tests that require plasma, the plasma should be removed from the cells as soon as possible. This can be accomplished with centrifugation followed by aspiration of the plasma and transfer to another tube using a disposable pipet. The green-gray marbled-topped tube, with lithium heparin anticoagulant, has a thixotropic gel which forms the necessary barrier when centrifuged as described previously. Certain blood tests, such as the complete blood count, require whole blood. It is wise to check the requirements of the laboratory that will perform the test as to how the specimen should be transported and stored. The College of American Pathologists recommends that whole blood for automated blood counts be refrigerated and tested within 72 hours.

Often specimens must be transported by courier to other facilities. The Hazardous Materials Shipping Regulations established by the Department of Transportation apply to the packaging or shipping of hazardous materials by ground transportation. Those who ship human specimens must be trained in all aspects of handling, packing, and shipping of biohazardous materials.

CHAIN OF CUSTODY

Blood samples may be collected as evidence in legal proceedings. Blood may be drawn for drug and alcohol testing, DNA analysis, or parentage testing. These samples must be handled according to special procedures to prevent tampering, misidentification, or interference with the test results.

Chain of custody is a legal term that refers to the ability to guarantee the identity and integrity of the specimen from collection to reporting of test results. It is a process used to maintain and document the chronologic history of a specimen. (Documents should include the name or initials of the individual collecting the specimen, each person or entity subsequently having custody of it, the date the specimen was collected or transferred, the employer or agency, the specimen number, the patient's or employee's name, and a brief description of the specimen.)

Collection kits are available that contain everything needed for the venipuncture, including the tube, the needle, the chain of custody forms and seals, the antiseptic, and even the tourniquet. Familiarize yourself with these kits before you are required to use them. You may be required to testify at a legal proceeding if you are involved in the collection or testing of a sample involved in a legal proceeding.

Patient Education

Patient care technicians who work as phlebotomists must maintain a professional attitude, yet remain sympathetic to the patient's fears and anxiety about being "stuck with a needle." Establishing an environment that encourages the person to relax can minimize the patient's pain and discomfort during the procedure.

Always remember to identify your patient and explain what you are going to do. Answer any questions the patient may have, and perform the procedure skillfully before anxiety has time to set in.

Provide as much explanation as needed to ease the patient's anxiety. Often the patient can help by identifying the site of the last successful blood draw. Follow the patient's suggestion in choosing the site for obtaining a blood specimen. When a patient is allowed to become an active participant in the procedure, he or she remains more relaxed, talkative, and confident in your expertise.

The atmosphere can change dramatically if the patient has had an unpleasant experience and associates pain and discomfort with venipuncture. Such a patient usually is ill at ease and apprehensive. In this case, you need to make every effort to perform the procedure quickly, efficiently, and effectively. Once the blood has been drawn and the patient has relaxed, you can help the patient develop a positive attitude.

If your patient has a history of syncope when blood is drawn, or if you suspect that the patient may faint during the procedure, have the person lie down. Assemble your equipment and alert the nurse before beginning the procedure. This type of professional care may help the patient get through the procedure without a traumatic effect.

Legal and Ethics Issues

Venipuncture and microcapillary blood collection are invasive procedures in which a sterile needle or a lancet is inserted through the skin. Because the skin is penetrated, drawing blood becomes a surgical procedure and is subject to the laws and regulations of surgery. When venipuncture is performed, the rules and regulations must be enforced with no deviations. Be sure to follow the procedures as written and to become familiar with the regulations and standards established by local and state agencies, as well as CLSI and OSHA. Not following policy and standards leave the patient care technician open to accusations of malpractice. Document any situations that arise in which observation of the standard of care comes into question. Notify your nurse any time there is a traumatic or difficult venipuncture.

On rare occasions, patients who have scarred veins as a result of intravenous drug use may ask to draw their own blood. You should never permit this and should always take precautions that your supplies are secure.

CHAPTER SUMMARY

Venipuncture requires a double-pointed safety needle, evacuated collection tubes, a needle holder or a syringe fitted with a safety needle, a tourniquet, an alcohol prep pad, gauze or cotton, a sterile bandage, latex gloves, and a biohazard disposal container. A tourniquet is used to prevent venous flow out of the site, which causes the veins to bulge. The tourniquet makes veins easier to locate and puncture. Tourniquets are applied snugly around the upper arm (or wrist for a hand draw) in a fashion that permits easy release. Leaving the tourniquet on a prolonged time results in hemoconcentration; applying the tourniquet too tightly results in unnecessary discomfort to the patient and the release of tissue fluid into the blood.

The various colors of vacuum tube stoppers indicate the contents of the tube. Certain additives are compatible with certain laboratory tests. The phlebotomist must be knowledgeable about blood tests and the types of tubes needed. Consulting literature provided by the manufacturer ensures the proper choice of a collection tube.

The venipuncture needle has a shaft with one end cut at an angle (bevel). The other end (the hub) attaches to the syringe or to a needle holder. The opening in the tip, the lumen, is measured in gauge numbers. Double-pointed needles are used for the evacuated tube method.

Needles with special adapters are used with disposable syringes. Lancets are used for dermal puncture.

Syringes are more commonly used for blood collection from elderly patients, whose veins tend to be more fragile; from children, whose veins tend to be small; and from obese patients, whose veins tend to be deep. Using a syringe allows a more controlled draw. Syringes commonly are used with winged infusion sets.

OSHA requires that all sharps used for phlebotomy should be engineered with safety devices, such as retractable needles, self-sheathing needles, and blunting devices. Needles should never be recapped, and in most cases they are not removed from the venipuncture unit. All sharps must be disposed of in an approved sharps container.

OSHA requires employers to have a postexposure plan in place for accidental sharps exposures. These plans generally include a means to cleanse the wound with an appropriate antiseptic cleanser; evaluation of the exposure to determine whether the employee is at risk for contracting HBV, HCV, or HIV, depending on the circumstance of the injury; gathering of information about the source of the blood involved; prophylactic care if necessary; confidential counseling for the injured; and follow-up on the exposure.

The median cephalic vein is the vein of choice for phlebotomy, but blood can be drawn from the cephalic vein and the median basilic vein. The basilic vein should not be used if possible. The dorsal vein on the hand may be used.

The middle two fingers (the lateral sides of each) generally are used for capillary puncture. In infants, the heel is the site of choice. The center of the heel must be avoided. Capillary blood can be collected in Microtainer devices, in capillary tubes, or on paper test cards. The Microtainer devices may contain anticoagulants and have stopper colors consistent with vacuum tubes.

Whole blood coagulates unless mixed with an anti-coagulant. The anticoagulant must be matched with the test so as not to interfere with the results. Whole blood is required for the complete blood count and differential. When clotted blood is centrifuged, the cells and the liquid separate; the liquid portion is the serum. Most chemistry and serology testing is performed on serum. When anticoagulated blood is centrifuged, the liquid that remains is plasma. Plasma may be used for coagulation studies and for blood glucose testing.

Blood cells can easily hemolyze, which alters test results; therefore serum or plasma should be separated from the cells as soon as possible after collection. This is done by centrifugation. Blood samples to be transported must be packaged securely and sent according to regulations set forth by governmental agencies.

Chain of custody is a legal term that refers to the ability to guarantee the identity and integrity of the specimen from collection to reporting of the test results. It is a process used to maintain and document the chronologic history of a specimen. Collection kits are available that contain everything needed for the venipuncture.

Case Scenario

Leah, a recent graduate of a patient care technician program, is a new employee at the Health Alliance Medical Clinic. The class on medical laboratory procedures was Leah's favorite in her program at the community college; in that class, she learned the principles of phlebotomy and performed several phlebotomy procedures both in the school's laboratory and at her externship site. Her employer has arranged for Leah to spend time with an experienced phlebotomist at the clinic so that she is prepared to perform phlebotomy duties in her new position. Nervous but excited, she begins her training.

Leah is in her second week at the clinic, and she is confident that she can perform phlebotomy on her own. Melissa has been a good mentor, and Leah has done quite a few successful "sticks" without any problems. Today, however, she is just having a bad day. Mr. Godfrey Lawrence has come to the clinic with numerous problems, and Dr. Gupta has ordered several blood tests. Mr. Lawrence is uncooperative when he sees that Leah must draw four tubes of blood. He angrily tells her that she cannot take that much blood out of him; she is a vampire and she will drain him. How should Leah deal with this problem?

Leah next must draw a sample from Ms. Danielle Rollins. Ms. Rollins indicates that she has a history of bruising after venipuncture, and sure enough, a hematoma begins to rise shortly after Leah inserts the needle. She then notices that Ms. Rollins has become pale and is perspiring. What should Leah do first? What other steps should Leah take? Can she still obtain the sample?

REVIEW QUESTIONS

1. Which of the following is the most common anti-septic used in routine venipuncture?
   a. Povidone-iodine solution
   b. Bleach
   c. Isopropyl alcohol
   d. Chlorhexidine gluconate

2. How many times may a needle be used before discarding it?
   a. 1
   b. 2
   c. 3
   d. No limit

3. Which of the following indicates the largest sized needle?
   a. 20 gauge
   b. 23 gauge
   c. 16 gauge
   d. 21 gauge

4. Which color-coded tube does not contain any additives?
   a. Red
   b. Yellow
   c. Lavender
   d. Green

5. The smaller the gauge number, the _____.
   a. Larger the lumen diameter
   b. Longer the needle
   c. Shorter the needle
   d. Smaller the lumen diameter

6. Upon entering the patient's room, you should
   a. Assemble your equipment
   b. Put on your gloves
   c. Introduce yourself
   d. Identify the patient

7. Which vein lies close to the brachial artery?
   a. Cephalic
   b. Median cubital
   c. Basilic
   d. Iliac

8. Tourniquets should be placed _____ inches above the venipuncture site.
   a. 1 to 2
   b. 2 to 3
   c. 3 to 4
   d. 4 to 5

9. The most common injury patients suffer from phlebotomy is _____.
   a. Hemoconcentration
   b. Occluded radial pulse
   c. Hematoma
   d. Nerve injury

10. During the venipuncture procedure, the tourniquet should stay on no longer than _____.
    a. 30 seconds
    b. 45 seconds
    c. 1 minute
    d. 2 minutes

Specimen Collecting and Testing

LEARNING OBJECTIVES

1. Understand the purpose of routine urinalysis.
2. Display sensitivity to patient rights and feelings when collecting specimens.
3. Explain the various means and methods used to collect urine specimens.
4. Instruct a patient in the collection of a 24-hour urine specimen.
5. Instruct a patient in the collection of a clean-catch midstream urine specimen.
6. Perform a complete urinalysis using a chemical reagent strip.
7. Describe methods for determining fertility and menopause using Clinical Laboratory Improvement Amendments (CLIA)–waived urine tests.
8. Discuss the steps in collecting a stool specimen.
9. Identify how to obtain a sputum specimen.
10. Discuss the legal and ethical responsibilities of the patient care technician who is assisting with specimen collection.

KEY TERMS

bilirubinuria The presence of bilirubin in the urine.

cytology The study of cells, including their formation, origin, structure, function, biochemical activities, and pathologic processes.

culture and sensitivity (C&S) A procedure performed in the microbiology laboratory in which a specimen is cultured on artificial media to detect bacterial or fungal growth, followed by appropriate screening for antibiotic sensitivity.

enzymatic reaction The reaction that occurs when a chemical or enzyme changes its composition or reacts due to the substance that just combined with the enzyme.

expectorate Eject mucus, sputum, or fluids from trachea and lungs by coughing or spitting.

filtrate The fluid that remains after a liquid is passed through a membranous filter.

metabolite The product of the metabolism of a substance, such as a drug.

mononuclear white blood cells Leukocytes with an unsegmented nucleus; monocytes and lymphocytes in particular.

phenylalanine An essential amino acid found in milk, eggs, and other foods.

polymorphonuclear white blood cells Leukocytes with a segmented nucleus; also known as polymorphonuclear neutrophils (PMNs) or segmented neutrophils.

renal thresholds Levels above which substances cannot be reabsorbed by the renal tubules and therefore are excreted in the urine.

sediment Insoluble material that settles to the bottom of a urine specimen.

The role of the patient care technician (PCT) has expanded to include collecting many different types of specimens. Allowing the PCT to do this can improve the care of the patient by freeing up the nurse to provide the care that only the nurse can provide. Allowing the PCT to collect the specimens while the nurse focuses on delivering the care plan for the patient allows everyone to work as a team. Specimen collection of urine, stool, and sputum will be covered in this chapter.

SPECIMEN COLLECTION

The PCT is often responsible for collecting specimens that have been ordered. Laboratory examination of specimens of urine, stool, and sputum provides important information about body functioning and contributes to the assessment of the patient's health status. Laboratory test results often help the physician or practitioner diagnose healthcare problems, provide information about the stage and activity of a disease process, and measure the response to therapy.

Patients often experience embarrassment or discomfort when giving a sample of body excretions or secretions. Most people believe that excretions should be handled discreetly; ensuring that the patient's privacy is maintained is helpful in keeping the patient comfortable during the sample collection. Anxiety is also brought on by how intrusive some collection procedures are, coupled with the fear of what the test results will reveal. Patients given a clear explanation about the purpose of the specimen and how it is to be obtained will be more cooperative in its collection. With proper instruction, many patients are able to obtain their own specimens of urine, stool, and sputum, thus minimizing embarrassment. Often the success of specimen collection depends on cooperation.

Guidelines for Specimen Collection

Laboratory tests are often expensive. The PCT can help prevent unnecessary costs by using the correct procedures for obtaining and processing specimens. When a patient has questions about laboratory tests, notify the nurse, who may consult the physician or laboratory.

It is the responsibility of the nurse to notify the prescribing healthcare provider when results of laboratory and diagnostic studies are returned. Never tell the patient the results of the specimens you help obtain. Each healthcare facility has its own policy and procedure manuals related to proper collection, processing, and results posting to the patient's chart.

A routine urinalysis (UA) is one of the more common laboratory examinations used in the diagnosis and treatment of disease. It is easily and quickly performed, and invasive techniques such as collecting with the use of a needle are generally not needed to collect the specimen. The results of a routine UA can reveal diseases of the bladder or kidneys; systemic metabolic or endocrine disorders, such as diabetes; and diseases of the liver, such as hepatitis or cirrhosis, or obstruction of the bile ducts. UA is routinely performed on all patients undergoing physical examination and on those entering the hospital for treatment.

PHYSIOLOGY OF URINE FORMATION

For centuries, abnormalities in the urine have been recognized as possible indicators of a disruption of homeostasis. One of the earliest known tests of urine involved pouring it on the ground to see whether it attracted insects. Such attraction indicated "honey urine," which was known to be excreted by people with skin eruptions. Today, urine is still checked for glucose as a means of detecting diabetes.

Historically, examination of the urine became a game for quacks and charlatans. Paintings from the Middle Ages show physicians peering into round-bottomed flasks of urine, claiming not only to be able to diagnose disease, but also to see into the future by simply looking at the fluid. These charlatans became known as "pisse prophets." During the twentieth century, UA became a practical laboratory procedure, and today urine is the most commonly analyzed body fluid in the clinical laboratory.

Urine is analyzed for several reasons—first to detect conditions such as diabetes, when patients may excrete glucose in the urine when they are experiencing hyperglycemia, or high blood glucose. The second reason is to detect conditions that involve the kidneys or the urinary tract, such as the presence of kidney stones or of a urinary tract infection. In addition, because chemicals are excreted through the kidneys, UA can be used to determine the effectiveness of medications and/or the possibility of urinary system side effects from prescribed drugs. Many medications are flushed out of the body by way of the urine. Finally, the urine can be observed for specific gravity to determine whether a person is adequately hydrated or not.

Anatomy of the Urinary Tract

It is important for the PCT to have a basic knowledge of kidney structure and urine formation to understand the results of a UA. The urinary tract consists of two kidneys, two ureters, one bladder, and one urethra. The functional unit of the kidney is the nephron. Each kidney has more than 1 million nephrons, and each nephron is composed of five distinct areas, each playing a role in urine formation (Fig. 25.1). Each nephron consists of a glomerulus, which acts in filtering, and a tubule, through which the filtrate passes. As the filtrate passes through,

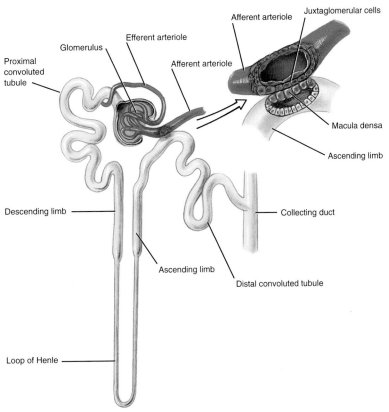

FIGURE 25.1 A nephron. (From Applegate EJ: *The anatomy and physiology learning system*, ed 4, Philadelphia, 2011, Saunders.)

various changes occur. Certain solutes are reabsorbed, and others are secreted into the kidney for eventual excretion. Nearly all of the water that passes through the glomeruli is reabsorbed.

The glomerulus is composed of a network of capillaries surrounded by a membrane called *Bowman's capsule.* The *afferent* arteriole carries blood from the renal artery into the glomerulus, where it then divides to form a capillary network. Where they reunite, the capillaries form the *efferent* arteriole, through which blood exits the glomerulus.

The tubular portion of the nephron is composed of the proximal convoluted tubule, the thin-walled segment, and the distal convoluted tubule. The thin-walled descending portion forms a loop known as the *loop of Henle.* Filtrate from several nephrons drains into a collecting tubule, several of which join to form a collecting duct. The collecting ducts join to form the papillary ducts, which empty at the tips of the papillae into the calyces. The filtrate then drains into the renal pelvis and is now called *urine.* Urine passes from the pelvis of the kidney down the ureter and into the bladder, where it remains until it is voided through the urethra.

Formation of Urine

The kidney selectively excretes (lets go of) or retains (holds on to) substances according to the body's needs and renal thresholds. Approximately 1200 mL of blood flows through the kidneys each minute. The blood enters the glomerulus through the afferent arteriole. The capillary walls of the glomerulus are highly permeable to water and to the low-molecular-weight solutes of the plasma, and they filter through into Bowman's capsule and then into the tubules. Many components of the filtrate, including glucose, water, and amino acids, are partially or completely reabsorbed by the capillaries surrounding the proximal tubules. More water is absorbed, and hydrogen and potassium ions are secreted in the distal tubules. Urine is concentrated in the system of collecting tubules and the loop of Henle. The kidneys convert nearly 180,000 mL of filtered plasma per day into a final urine volume of 750 to 2000 mL—approximately 1% of the filtered plasma volume. The largest component of urine is water; the solutes consist mostly of urea, chloride, sodium, potassium, phosphate, sulfate, creatinine, and uric acid.

COLLECTING A URINE SPECIMEN

Patient Sensitivity

The request for a urine specimen may create an embarrassing moment for the patient. The request should be made in private, such as after the patient's visitors leave.

The individual should be given detailed instructions so that he or she understands what is expected. Use good communication techniques to explain the details of the procedure to the patient and be observant for indications of confusion. If a language barrier exists, be creative but respectful of the patient's need to follow through correctly on the instructions for collection of the specimen.

Containers

The most important requirement for a collection container is cleanliness. Disposable, nonsterile, plastic, or coated paper containers are the most common and are available in many sizes with tight-fitting lids. If the sample is being sent to the laboratory for a culture, the specimen must be collected in a sterile container, and the patient must understand how to collect the specimen and how to handle the sterile specimen cup. Special pliable polyethylene bags with adhesive are used to collect urine from infants and children who are not toilet-trained. Collecting specimens from infants and children will be discussed later in this chapter. For specimens that must be collected over a specified period, large, wide-mouth plastic containers with screw-cap tops are used. Most routine UA testing, pregnancy testing, and tests for abnormal analytes are performed on urine collected in nonsterile containers.

As mentioned, when a urine culture is ordered, the specimen must be collected in a sterile container. Such containers are packaged with an intact paper seal over the cap and/or in sterile envelopes (Fig. 25.2). The label on all specimens must include the patient's name, the date and time of collection, and the type of specimen. Always put on gloves before handling filled specimen containers. Many healthcare facilities provide self-sticking labels that are placed on the patient's specimen. This creates a safer environment, ensuring that the urine is not mixed up with the specimens of other patients.

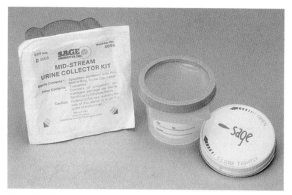

FIGURE 25.2 A sterile container for a midstream specimen. (From Proctor D, Adams A: *Kinn's The Medical Assistant: an applied learning approach*, ed 12, St. Louis, 2014, Saunders.)

Methods of Specimen Collection

Most analyses are performed on freshly voided urine collected in clean containers; this is called a *random specimen.* If the specimen is ordered to be collected when the patient arises in the morning, it is called a *first morning specimen.* These specimens are most concentrated and are best for nitrite and protein determination, bacterial culture, pregnancy testing, and microscopic examination. Two-hour postprandial urine specimens, collected 2 hours after a meal, are used in diabetes screening and for home diabetes testing programs. The 24-hour urine specimen is collected over 24 hours to provide a cumulative chemical analysis, such as hormone levels and creatinine clearance rates (a procedure for evaluating the glomerular filtration rate of the kidneys) (Procedure 25.1).

A second-voided specimen usually is collected to determine glucose levels; the first void of the morning is discarded, and the second void of the day is collected. For a catheterized specimen, the physician, the physician's assistant, or the nurse must insert a sterile catheter into the bladder to collect the specimen. A suprapubic specimen is collected with a needle inserted directly into the bladder. The PCT may *assist* with this type of collection; however, the PCT will not collect a suprapubic specimen.

The minimum volume of urine for a routine UA usually is 12 mL, but 50 mL is preferred. For any type of collection, it is important that the patient receives adequate verbal and/or written instructions. The easiest directions for the patient are to ask the person to fill the container halfway.

A clean-catch midstream specimen (CCMS) is ordered when the physician suspects a urinary tract infection and therefore orders a urine culture for examination of microorganisms. The clean-catch technique is used to remove microorganisms from the urinary meatus by thoroughly cleansing the area around the meatus and to flush out the distal portion of the urethra. The PCT needs to give complete, understandable instructions to the patient on the method of collection (Procedure 25.2). Failure to do so may mean that the patient will have to provide another specimen. For a urine culture, the urine is collected either by catheterization or by the clean-catch method in a sterile container.

Collecting a Urine Specimen From an Infant or Child

The easiest way to obtain a urine sample from a child older than 2 years who is toilet-trained is to give the parent the container and instructions ahead of time. Then, when the child appears at the office for the examination, the sample is available to be tested. If the sample is needed while the child is at the office, consult with

PROCEDURE 25.1

Collection of a 24-Hour Urine Specimen

1. Greet the patient by name.
2. Label the container with the patient's name and the current date, identify the specimen as a 24-hour urine specimen, and include your initials.
3. Explain the following instructions to adult patients or to the guardians of pediatric patients.
4. After explaining the following instructions, give the patient the specimen container with written instructions to confirm understanding.

Patient Instructions for Obtaining a 24-Hour Urine Specimen

1. Empty your bladder into the toilet in the morning without saving any of the specimen. Record the time you first emptied your bladder.
2. For the next 24 hours, each time you empty your bladder, the urine should be voided directly into the large specimen container.

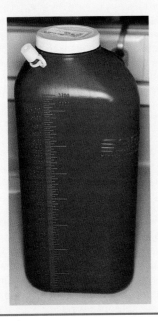

3. Put the lid back on the container after each urination and store the container in the refrigerator or in an ice chest throughout the 24 hours of the study.
4. If at any time you forget to empty your bladder into the specimen container, or if some urine is accidentally spilled, the test must be started all over again with an empty container and a newly recorded start time.
5. The last collection of urine should be done at the same time as the first specimen on the previous day so that exactly 24 hours of urine collection is completed. The collection ends with the first voided morning specimen that completes the 24-hour collection period.
6. As soon as possible after collection is completed, notify the nurse.
7. Document the details of the patient education intervention in the patient's record.

Processing a 24-Hour Urine Specimen

1. Ask the patient whether he or she collected all voided urine throughout the 24-hour period or whether any problems occurred during the collection process.
2. Complete the laboratory request form and prepare the specimen for transport.
3. Store the specimen in the refrigerator until it is picked up by the laboratory.
4. Document that the specimen was sent to the laboratory, including the type of test ordered, the date and time, and the type of specimen.

---

the parent for the best method to use. If the child is younger than 2 years, a pediatric urine collection device can be put on him or her to collect the sample (Fig. 25.3 and Procedure 25.3). This device is placed as soon as the order is received in to increase the chance of obtaining the needed sample soon. Once the device is in place, the child can be diapered to help hold it properly. Ensure that the adhesive sticks tightly so that the specimen collects in the device when the child urinates.

In some situations, the child may need to be catheterized to obtain the specimen. Pediatric catheterization kits contain all the supplies needed for this procedure. When preparing the kit for the nurse's or pediatrician's use, always remember that this is a sterile procedure. The pediatrician usually asks the parent to help with the

infant, whereas the PCT labels and prepares the specimen for the laboratory.

Handling and Transportation of a Specimen

Proper handling of specimens is essential. The chemical and cellular components of urine change if the urine is allowed to stand at room temperature (Table 25.1). Urine specimens should be kept refrigerated and should be processed within 1 hour of collection. If the specimen must be transported to a different laboratory, evacuated transport tubes are available; these contain preservatives and look much like blood collection tubes

1. Label the container and give the patient the supplies.

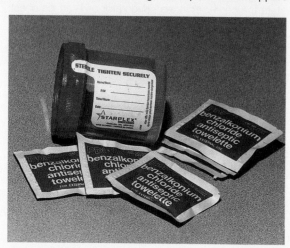

2. Explain the following instructions to adult patients or to the guardians of pediatric patients, being sensitive to privacy issues.

Obtaining a Clean-Catch Midstream Specimen (Female Patient)

1. Wash your hands and open the towelette packages for easy access.
2. Remove the lid from the specimen container, being careful not to touch the inside of the lid or the inside of the container. Place the lid, facing up, on a paper towel.
3. Remove your underclothing and sit on the toilet.
4. Expose the urinary meatus by spreading apart the labia with one hand.

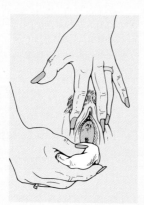

5. Cleanse each side of the urinary meatus with a front-to-back motion, from the pubis to the anus. Use a separate antiseptic wipe to cleanse each side of the meatus.
6. Cleanse directly across the meatus, front to back, using a third antiseptic wipe.

7. Hold the labia apart throughout this procedure.
8. Void a small amount of urine into the toilet.

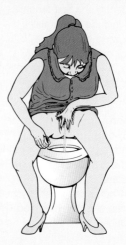

9. Move the specimen container into position and void the next portion of urine into it. Fill the container halfway. Remember that this is a sterile container. Do not put your fingers on the inside of the container.
10. Remove the cup and void the last amount of urine into the toilet. (This means that the first part and the last part of the urinary flow have been excluded from the specimen. Only the middle portion of the flow is included.)
11. Place the lid on the container, taking care not to touch the interior surface of the lid. Wipe in your usual manner, redress, and return the sterile specimen to the place designated by the medical facility.

Obtaining a Clean-Catch Midstream Specimen (Male Patients)

1. Wash your hands and expose the penis.
2. Retract the foreskin of the penis (if not circumcised).
3. Cleanse the area around the glans penis (meatus) and the urethral opening by washing each side of the glans with a separate antiseptic wipe.

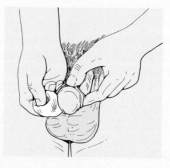

4. Cleanse directly across the urethral opening using a third antiseptic wipe.
5. Void a small amount of urine into the toilet or urinal.

PROCEDURE 25.2

Collection of a Clean-Catch Midstream Urine Specimen—cont'd

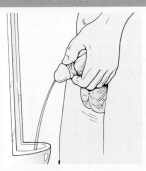

6. Collect the next portion of the urine in the sterile container, filling the container halfway without touching the inside of the container with the hands or the penis.

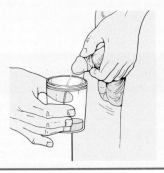

7. Void the last amount of urine into the toilet or urinal.
8. Place the lid on the container, taking care not to touch the interior surface of the lid. Wipe and redress.
9. Return the specimen to the designated area.

Processing a Clean-Catch Urine Specimen

1. Document the date, time, and collection type.
2. Process the specimen according to the physician's orders. Perform urinalysis in the office or prepare the specimen for transport to the laboratory.
   If it is to be sent to an outside laboratory, complete the following steps:
   - Ensure that the label is properly completed with patient information, date, time, and test ordered.
   - Place the specimen in a biohazard specimen bag.
   - Complete a laboratory requisition and place it in the outside pocket of the specimen bag.
   - Keep the specimen refrigerated until pickup.
   - Document that the specimen was sent.

PROCEDURE 25.3

Collecting a Urine Specimen From an Infant or Child

1. Assemble all needed supplies.
2. Sanitize your hands and put on gloves.
3. Ask the parent to remove the child's diaper or place the child in a supine position on the examination table and remove the diaper.
4. Cleanse the genitalia with antiseptic wipes.
5. *Male:* Cleanse the urinary meatus in a circular motion, starting directly on the meatus and working in an outward pattern. Repeat with a clean wipe. If the child has not been circumcised, gently retract the foreskin to expose the meatus; when you have completed the cleansing, return the foreskin to its natural position.
   Female: Hold the labia open with your nondominant hand; with your dominant hand, cleanse the inner labia, from the clitoris to the vaginal meatus, in a superior to inferior pattern. Discard the first wipe and repeat with a clean wipe, cleaning both sides of the inner labia.
6. Ensure that the area is dry. Unfold the collection device, remove the paper from the upper portion, place this portion over the mons pubis, and press it securely into place. Continue by removing the lower portion of the paper and securing this portion against the perineum (see Figure 25.3). Ensure that the device is attached smoothly and that you have not taped it to part of the infant's thigh.
7. Rediaper the infant or, if the parent is helping, have the parent rediaper the infant at this time. The diaper will help hold the bag in place.
8. Suggest that the parent give the child liquids, if allowed; check the bag for urine at frequent intervals.
9. When a noticeable amount of urine has collected in the bag, put on gloves, remove the device, cleanse the skin area where the device was attached, and rediaper the child.
10. Pour the urine carefully into the laboratory urine container and handle the sample in a routine manner.
11. Dispose of all used equipment in a biohazard waste container.
12. Remove your gloves, dispose of them in a biohazard container, and sanitize your hands.
13. Record the procedure in the patient's record.

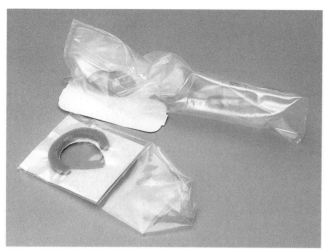

FIGURE 25.3 Urine collection devices. (From Proctor D, Adams A: *Kinn's The Medical Assistant: an applied learning approach,* ed 12, St. Louis, 2014, Saunders.)

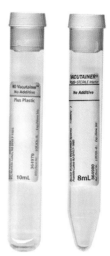

FIGURE 25.4 BD Vacutainer urine preservation tubes. (Courtesy Becton, Dickinson & Company, Franklin Lakes, New Jersey.)

Table 25.1	Changes in Urine at Room Temperature
Constituent	**Change**
Clarity	Becomes cloudy as crystals precipitate and bacteria multiply
Color	May change if pH becomes alkaline
pH	Becomes alkaline as bacteria form ammonia from urea
Glucose	Decreases as it is metabolized by bacteria
Ketones	Decrease because of evaporation
Bilirubin and urobilinogen	Undergo degradation in light
Blood	May hemolyze; false-positive results are possible because of bacterial peroxidase
Nitrite	May become positive as bacteria multiply and reduce nitrate
Casts	Lyse or dissolve in alkaline urine
Cells	Lyse or dissolve in alkaline urine
Bacteria	Multiply twofold approximately every 20 minutes
Yeasts	Multiply
Crystals	Precipitate as urine cools; may dissolve if pH changes

Box 25.1	Guidelines for Caring for a Urine Specimen Obtained at Home

- Do not put anything but your urine into the bottle.
- Do not pour out any liquid or powdered preservative from the container.
- If you accidentally spill some of the preservative on yourself, immediately wash with water and call the testing center or designated laboratory.
- Always keep the collection bottle cool. Refrigerate or keep the bottle in an ice-filled cooler or pail.
- Keep the cap on the container.

(Fig. 25.4). The vacuum in the tube allows for the delivery of 7 to 8 mL of urine, using a transfer straw or a urine collection cup with an integrated sampling device. Alternatively, the urine can be poured into the tube after the stopper is removed. The preservatives in the Becton Dickinson (BD) Vacutainer cherry red/yellow-stoppered tube—chlorhexidine, ethylparaben, and sodium propionate—prevent the overgrowth of bacteria and inhibit changes in the urine that can affect test results. Chemical reagent strip testing can be performed on preserved specimens; however, it should be performed within 72 hours. Tubes may be held at room temperature during this time.

A different preservative must be used for urine specimens slated for culture. The BD Vacutainer urine collection kit contains the preservatives sodium formate and boric acid to help preserve the level of bacteria present at the time of collection. This transport system should be used only for urine specimens that will be cultured. Results on the chemical reagent strip may be altered by these preservatives. Culture and sensitivity (C&S) testing should be performed within 72 hours. Tubes may be held at room temperature.

A laboratory request form must be completed for all specimens that will be transported to another site for analysis. Typical forms include the patient's name and the date, the type of UA ordered, the name of the physician requesting the examination, the appropriate code for the diagnosis that warranted the test, and a signature line for the physician to sign after he or she has reviewed the results. Specimens are sent to the laboratory in a plastic biohazard bag with zips closed and has an outside pocket where the laboratory request is placed (Box 25.1).

ROUTINE URINALYSIS

Physical Examination of the Urine

The first part of a complete UA is assessment of the physical properties of the urine and measurement of selected chemical constituents that are diagnostically important (Table 25.2).

Appearance

Color

Normal urine is a shade of yellow, ranging from pale straw to yellow to amber. The color depends on the concentration of the pigment urochrome and the amount of water in the specimen. A dilute specimen should be pale, and a more concentrated specimen should be a darker yellow. Variations in color may be caused by diet, medication, and disease. Abnormal colors may be related to pathologic or nonpathologic factors (Table 25.3).

Turbidity

Both normal and abnormal urine specimens may range in appearance from clear to very cloudy. Cloudiness may be caused by cells, bacteria, yeast, vaginal contaminants, or crystals. Often a urine specimen that was clear when voided becomes cloudy as it cools, as crystals form and precipitate.

Volume

The amount of urine is rarely measured in a random specimen. With a timed specimen, volume is measured by pouring the entire collection into a large, graduated cylinder. In general, it is not accurate enough to use the markings on the side of the collection container. Once the volume has been measured and recorded, a portion of well-mixed specimen, called an *aliquot*, is removed for testing. The remainder is discarded or stored, depending on the preference of the laboratory.

The normal volume of urine produced every 24 hours varies according to the age of the individual. Infants and children produce smaller volumes than adults. The normal adult volume is 750 to 2000 mL in 24 hours; the average amount is about 1500 mL. Excessive production of urine is called *polyuria*. This is common in diabetes and in certain kidney disorders. Oliguria is insufficient production of urine, which can be caused by dehydration, decreased fluid intake, shock, or renal disease. The absence of urine production, anuria, occurs in renal obstruction and renal failure.

Foam

Normally the presence of foam is not recorded, but careful observation of this property can be a significant clue to an abnormality. Foam is seen as small bubbles that persist for a long time after the specimen has been shaken; they must not be confused with any bubbles that rapidly disperse. White foam can indicate the

Table 25.2 Components of Macroscopic Urinalysis

Physical Properties	Chemical Properties
Color	Protein
Clarity	Glucose
Specific gravity	Ketones
Volume*	Bilirubin
Odor*	Blood
Foam*	Nitrite
	pH
	Urobilinogen
	Leukocyte esterase

*Not always assessed.

Table 25.3 Causes of Urine Colors

Color	Pathologic Cause	Nonpathologic Cause
Straw	Diabetes	Diuretics; high fluid intake (coffee, beer)
Amber	Dehydration	Excessive sweating; low fluid intake
Bright yellow		Carotene, vitamins
Red	Blood, porphyrins	Menstruation, beets, drugs, dyes
Orange-yellow	Bile, hepatitis	Pyridium (phenazopyridine hydrochloride), dyes, drugs
Greenish yellow	Bile, hepatitis	Senna, cascara, rhubarb
Reddish brown	Old blood, methemoglobin	
Brownish black	Methemoglobin, melanin	Levodopa
Salmon pink		Amorphous urates
White (milky)	Fats, pus	Amorphous phosphates
Blue-green	Biliverdin, infection with *Pseudomonas* organisms	Vitamin B, drugs, dyes

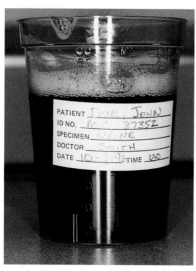

FIGURE 25.5 Dark amber urine with foam indicates possible increased protein and possible hematuria. (From Proctor D, Adams A: *Kinn's The Medical Assistant: an applied learning approach,* ed 12, St. Louis, 2014, Saunders.)

presence of increased protein (Fig. 25.5). Greenish yellow foam can mean bilirubinuria. Care should be taken in handling such urines, because the color of the foam may indicate that the patient has viral hepatitis.

Odor

As with foam, odor is not normally recorded but can be an important clue to metabolic disorders. Normal urine is said to be aromatic. Changes in the odor of urine may be caused by disease, the presence of bacteria, or diet. The odor of the urine of a patient with uncontrolled diabetes is described as fruity because of the presence of ketones, which are the products of fat metabolism. An ammonia or putrid smell in the urine can be caused by an infection or may be noted in urine that has been allowed to stand before it is tested. The bacteria break down the urea in the urine to form ammonia. Foods such as asparagus and garlic also can produce an abnormal odor in the urine. Urine from a child with phenylketonuria (PKU) is said to smell "mousy." PKU is a rare hereditary condition in which the amino acid phenylalanine is not properly metabolized, which can lead to severe mental retardation. Accumulation of phenylalanine in the blood and urine gives body fluids an odor like wet fur. (Blood sampling for PKU is discussed in Chapter 30.)

Specific Gravity

Specific gravity is the weight of a substance compared with the weight of an equal volume of distilled water. In UA, it is the rough measurement of the concentration, or amount, of substances dissolved in urine. The specific gravity of distilled water is 1.000. The normal specific gravity of urine ranges from 1.005 to 1.030, depending on the patient's fluid intake. Most samples fall between 1.010 and 1.025. The urine specific gravity indicates whether the kidneys are able to concentrate the urine and is one of the first indications of kidney disease. The presence of glucose, protein, or an x-ray contrast medium used in diagnostic studies also may increase the specific gravity of urine. To measure the specific gravity of urine, laboratories may use a urinometer, a refractometer, or a chemical reagent strip.

Waived Testing

All facilities in the United States that perform laboratory testing on human specimens for health assessment or the diagnosis, prevention, or treatment of disease are regulated by the Clinical Laboratory Improvement Amendments (CLIA) of 1988. Waived tests include test systems cleared by the U.S. Food and Drug Administration for home use and those tests approved for waiver under the CLIA criteria. Although CLIA requires that waived tests must be simple and have a low risk for errors in the results obtained, this does not mean that waived tests are completely error-proof. Errors can occur anywhere in the testing process, particularly when the manufacturer's instructions are not followed and when testing personnel are not familiar with all aspects of the test system.

Some waived tests have the potential for serious health impacts if performed incorrectly. For example, results from waived tests can be used to adjust medication dosages, such as prothrombin time testing in patients undergoing anticoagulant therapy and glucose monitoring in diabetics. In addition, erroneous results from diagnostic tests, such as those for human immunodeficiency virus (HIV) antibody, can have unintended consequences. To decrease the risk of erroneous results, the test needs to be performed correctly, by trained personnel and in an environment where good laboratory practices are followed (www.cdc.gov)

The reagent strip (dipstick) test is the method most commonly used and it is considered a CLIA-waived test. The pad on the strip contains a chemical that is sensitive to positively charged ions, such as sodium (Na^+) and potassium (K^+). The strip detects specific gravity in the range of 1.005 to 1.030.

Chemical Examination of Urine

Tests can be performed on urine to detect the presence of certain chemicals, which can provide valuable information to the physician. In certain situations, these chemical test results can be critical to the diagnosis.

Reagent strip testing is the most widely used technique for detecting chemicals in the urine (Procedure 25.4); these strips are available in a variety of types

PROCEDURE 25.4

Testing Urine With Chemical Reagent Strips

1. Sanitize your hands. Put on nonsterile gloves and eye protection.
2. Check the time of collection, the container, and the mode of preservation.
3. If the specimen has been refrigerated, allow it to warm to room temperature.
4. Check the reagent strip container for the expiration date.
5. Remove the reagent strip from the container. Hold it in your hand or place it on a clean paper towel. Recap the container tightly.
6. Compare nonreactive test pads with the negative color blocks on the color chart on the container.
7. Thoroughly mix the specimen by swirling.
8. Following the manufacturer's directions, note the time, dip the strip into the urine, and then remove it.

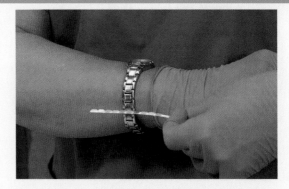

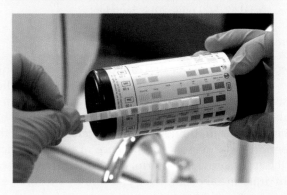

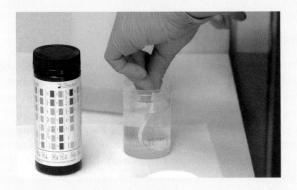

9. Quickly remove the excess urine from the strip by touching the side of the strip to a paper towel or to the side of the urine container.
10. Hold the strip horizontally. At the required time, compare the strip with the appropriate color chart on the reagent container. Document on the reagent strip flow sheet each result as it is read. Alternately, the strip can be placed on a paper towel.

11. Read the concentration by comparing the strip with the color chart on the side of the bottle.
12. Clean the work area, remove your gloves, and sanitize your hands. If a paper towel was used, dispose of it, the reagent strip, and your gloves in the biohazard container.
13. Document the results in the patient's record.

(Figures from Mosby's nursing video skills: basic intermediate & advanced skills, *ed 4, 2015, Elsevier.)*

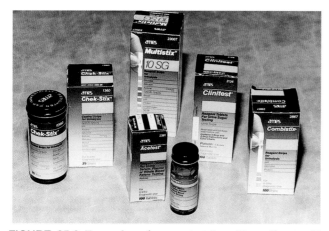

FIGURE 25.6 Examples of reagent strips. (From Proctor D, Adams A: *Kinn's The Medical Assistant: an applied learning approach,* ed 12, St. Louis, 2014, Saunders.)

(Fig. 25.6). In general, they are plastic strips to which one or more pads containing chemicals are attached. Tests are available for pH, specific gravity, vitamin C, leukocyte esterase, protein, ketones, glucose, blood, bilirubin, nitrite, urobilinogen, phenylketones, and other chemicals. The presence or absence of these chemicals in the urine provides information on the status of carbohydrate metabolism, liver and kidney function, and the patient's acid-base balance.

Reagent strips are designed to be used once and then discarded. The directions for each strip are included inside the package, and these instructions must be followed exactly if accurate results are to be obtained. A color comparison chart is provided on the label of the container. In addition to reagent strips, various tablet tests are available. Some facilities require color testing to ensure that their employees can notice color variations and differences. Those who are found to have a deficiency in determining color may be disqualified from a particular position, because of being unable to participate in this type of testing.

All strips and tablets must be kept in tightly closed containers in a cool, dry area and should be removed immediately before testing. To prevent contamination of the bottle, never touch a strip that has been exposed to urine against the color comparison chart. If both a UA and a C&S have been ordered for a specimen, the urine must be cultured before the UA is started, because introducing a reagent strip into the urine contaminates it.

pH

The pH is a measurement of the degree of acidity or alkalinity of the urine. A urine specimen with a pH of 7 is neutral. A value below 7 indicates acidity, and one above 7 indicates alkalinity. Normal, freshly voided urine may have a pH range of 5.5 to 8. The urinary pH

varies with an individual's metabolic status, diet, drug therapy, and disease. In the case of gross bacteriuria, the urine pH is alkaline as a result of bacterial conversion of urea to ammonia. Knowing the pH of the urine also assists in identification of crystals if they are found in the urine sediment.

Glucose

Glucose is filtered at the glomerulus, but under normal conditions most of it is reabsorbed in the tubules. The minute quantities normally present in the urine are not detected by reagent strips and tablets. Detectable glycosuria occurs whenever the renal tubules cannot reabsorb the filtered glucose load. A positive glucose finding is common in urine from patients with diabetes and may be the first indication of the disease. The reagent strip glucose testing method is based on an enzymatic reaction. It detects only glucose; in other words, it is specific for glucose.

Protein

Protein in the urine in detectable amounts is called *proteinuria* and is one of the first signs of renal disease. We normally excrete a small amount of protein every day; proteinuria may be light to heavy, constant, or sporadic. It may be affected by posture; in orthostatic proteinuria, protein is excreted only when the patient is in an upright position. In general, first morning specimens from these patients are negative, but protein is found in urine passed throughout the day. Proteinuria is a common finding in pregnancy. It also is almost always present after heavy exercise. The reagent strip is highly sensitive to urinary albumin and is less sensitive to hemoglobin, immunoglobulin, and mucoproteins.

Ketones

Ketones are the end product of fat metabolism in the body. Acetoacetate, acetone, and beta-hydroxybutyric acid are collectively called *ketone bodies,* or *ketones.* Ketonuria is common with starvation, low-carbohydrate diets, excessive vomiting, and diabetes mellitus. Because ketones evaporate at room temperature, urine should be tested immediately, or the specimen should be tightly covered and refrigerated. The reagent strip detects only acetoacetate. The Acetest, discussed later in this chapter, can be used to detect both acetone and acetoacetate.

Blood

The presence of blood in the urine may indicate infection or trauma to the urinary tract or bleeding in the kidneys. The blood test pad on the reagent strip reacts with three different blood constituents: intact red blood cells, hemoglobin from red blood cells, and myoglobin, a hemoglobin-like molecule that transports oxygen in muscle tissue.

Hematuria is the presence of intact red blood cells in urine. The color reaction on the reagent strip ranges from yellow through green to dark green when hematuria is present, revealing a speckled appearance. Hematuria can be caused by irritation of the ureters, bladder, or urethra. It also is a common finding in cystitis and in individuals passing kidney stones. A random specimen may contain blood from vaginal contamination if the woman is menstruating.

Hemoglobinuria is the presence of hemolyzed red blood cells. True hemoglobinuria is rare. It occurs as a result of intravascular red blood cell destruction and can be caused by transfusion reactions, malaria, drug reactions, snake bites, and severe burns.

Bilirubin and Urobilinogen

Bilirubin is a product of the breakdown of hemoglobin. Hemoglobin is released from old red blood cells and is gradually converted to bilirubin in the liver, and then further to urobilinogen in the intestines. Bilirubin is a bile pigment not normally found in urine. Its presence in urine is one of the first signs of liver disease or other disease in which the liver may be involved, such as infectious mononucleosis.

Bilirubinuria can occur even before jaundice or other symptoms of liver disease are evident. It is the result of liver cell damage or obstruction of the common bile duct by stones or neoplasms (tumors). Excessive bilirubin colors the urine yellow-brown to greenish orange. Because direct light causes decomposition of bilirubin, urine samples must be protected from light until testing is complete.

Urobilinogen normally is present in urine in small amounts. Increases are seen with increased red blood cell destruction and in liver disease. With total obstruction of the bile duct, no urobilinogen is formed in the intestines, none is reabsorbed into the circulation, and therefore none is present in the urine. Reagent strip methods cannot detect a decrease in urobilinogen.

Nitrite

Nitrite occurs in urine when bacteria break down nitrate, a common component of urine. A positive nitrite test result may indicate the presence of a urinary tract infection. However, not all bacteria are able to reduce nitrate to nitrite. Negative nitrite test results also can occur when bacteria are insufficient, or when the urine has not incubated in the bladder long enough for the reaction to occur. *Escherichia coli,* the organism that causes most urinary tract infections, reduces nitrate to nitrite. False-positive results can occur if a specimen is allowed to sit at room temperature and contaminating bacteria multiply. False-negative results may occur if the bacteria

further metabolize the nitrite they have produced to ammonia.

Leukocyte Esterase

Leukocytes (white blood cells) occur in urine with infections of the urinary tract. They also can be contaminants from the vagina. The leukocyte esterase test on reagent strips detects intact and lysed polymorphonuclear white blood cells. However, it does not detect mononuclear white blood cells, which occasionally are present during infection. The test does not react with the small numbers of white blood cells found in normal urine.

Limitations of Reagent Strip Testing

The reagent strip is a reliable method of chemical analysis of urine if used properly. The normal urine reference ranges for a reagent strip can be found in Table 25.4. Error can arise from a number of sources; for example, if the strip is soaked excessively in the specimen, chemicals in the pads may be diluted. If the strip is not held horizontally while read, colors from one pad may bleed onto another. Finally, certain chemicals, such as ascorbic acid, may affect the results of nitrite, glucose, bilirubin, and occult blood tests. Normal levels of vitamin C do not interfere, but if a person consumes large amounts of the vitamin, a special strip can be used to detect interfering levels of vitamin C. If an elevated level is found, the patient should be instructed to discontinue vitamin C intake for 24 hours and then another urine specimen should be collected for testing.

Quality Assurance and Quality Control in Urinalysis

The U.S. Food and Drug Administration (FDA) categorizes the chemical analysis of urine performed by an

Table 25.4	Normal Urine Reference Ranges for Reagent Strips
Reference	**Range**
Color	Pale yellow to straw
Clarity	Clear to slightly turbid
Specific gravity	1.001 to 1.035
pH	4.6 to 8
Protein (mg/dL)	NEG
Glucose (mg/dL)	NEG
Ketone (mg/dL)	NEG
Bilirubin (mg/dL)	NEG
Blood (mg/dL)	NEG
Nitrite (mg/dL)	NEG
Urobilinogen (Ehrlich units)	0.1 to 1
White blood cells	NEG

NEG = Negative

instrument or a reagent strip as a CLIA-waived test. The chemical analysis includes the reagent strip (dipstick) tests for bilirubin, glucose, hemoglobin or blood, ketones, leukocyte esterase, nitrite, pH, protein, specific gravity, and urobilinogen. To perform a microscopic UA procedure, a laboratory must be certified to perform moderate-complexity tests. Such a laboratory can also perform waived tests if it meets those qualifications.

A commercially available control strip should be used to determine the reliability of the reagent strip used in chemical analysis. One such control strip is the Chek-Stix® (Bayer, Tarrytown, NY). The plastic control strip has seven pads (Fig. 25.7), each of which contains synthetic ingredients that mimic human urine when reconstituted in water. After reconstitution, a reagent strip is immersed in the solution and the results are compared with a chart that accompanies the Chek-Stix. Both positive and negative Chek-Stix strips are available.

Quality control is as important in the microscopic examination as in the chemical analysis of urine. To ensure consistency, standardized, commercially available systems can be used, such as the KOVA® System (Hycor Biomedical, Garden Grove, CA) or the UriSystem™ (Fisher Scientific, Hampton, NH). These systems may include specially designed, graduated centrifuge tubes with devices or pipets that allow easy decanting of supernatant and retention of an exact amount of sediment. They also use specially designed plastic slides with wells or coverslips that accept only a given amount of sediment. Whatever system is used, the Clinical and Laboratory Standards Institute (CLSI) recommends the following:

- The urine volume should be 12 mL.
- The specimen should be centrifuged for 5 minutes at a relative centrifugal force of 400 g (i.e., 400 times normal gravity).
- A standardized slide should be used to view the sediment.
- A consistent reporting format should be used.

Additional Tests Performed on Urine

Clinitest®

The glucose test on the reagent strip detects only glucose, the most common sugar found in the urine. However, sugars other than glucose also can appear in the urine. Certain metabolic disorders can result in the excretion of sugars such as galactose, fructose, lactose, maltose, or pentoses. Galactosemia, a rare pathologic condition, is a congenital deficiency in the body's ability to metabolize galactose to glucose; galactosemia results in excretion of galactose in the urine. Seen in infants, it results in failure to thrive, vomiting, and diarrhea. If detected early, galactose can be eliminated from the diet, and the child develops normally. Lactose may be found in the urine of pregnant women or premature infants. In rare cases, urine may contain fructose or pentoses (e.g., xylose, arabinose) as a result of excessive consumption of honey or fruit. Maltose may be excreted in patients with diabetes. Of the many sugars, only the presence of glucose or galactose signifies a pathologic condition.

Acetest®

Acetest reagent tablets provide an alternative to strip testing when urine must be tested for the presence of ketones. Ketonuria results when the body metabolizes stored fat because of inadequate cellular uptake of carbohydrates. This is common with diabetes, starvation, and excessive vomiting. The Acetest tablet test (Bayer) is based on the same chemical reaction as the reagent strip test, but its advantage is that the tablet can be used with specimens other than urine, and it detects both acetone and acetoacetate.

Urine Pregnancy Testing

All pregnancy tests detect the presence of human chorionic gonadotropin (hCG), a hormone produced by the placenta and present in urine during pregnancy. After implantation of the fertilized egg in the uterus, the hCG levels in serum double every few days. This rapid rise occurs for approximately 7 weeks, and then the level begins to decline. Within 72 hours of delivery, the hormone disappears.

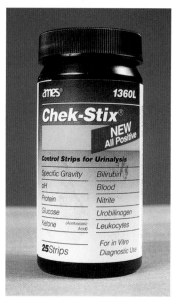

FIGURE 25.7 Chek-Stix control strips. (From Sorrentino SA, Remmert LN: *Mosby's essentials for nursing assistants*, ed 5, St. Louis, 2014, Mosby.)

The most common type of test for pregnancy is the lateral flow immunoassay test. Many brands are available for laboratory use and are also available over the counter. These tests can be sensitive enough to detect the presence of hCG as early as 1 week after implantation or 4 to 5 days before a missed menstrual period. The tests can be performed in as little as 5 minutes, and the results are easy to interpret—usually as easy as reading a color change. For the best results, the test should be performed on the first morning voided specimen. The test is based on reactions that occur between antibodies and antigens. Antibodies are proteins formed in response to antigens. When they come in contact, the antibody binds to the antigen, as long as the two are present in sufficient quantity and the antibody is specific for the antigen (e.g., as with a lock and key).

Ovulation Testing

CLIA-waived lateral flow urine tests are available to assist in the prediction of ovulation for women attempting to conceive either naturally or using artificial insemination. During the menstrual cycle, human luteinizing hormone (LH) remains at a relatively stable level. Approximately 14 days before menstruation, the body experiences the "LH surge"—a brief, rapid increase in LH. This surge triggers the release of the ovum from the ovary. Two to 3 days after the surge, the LH level returns to the base level. Conception is most likely to occur within 36 hours after the LH surge. The principle of this test is similar to that of the pregnancy test: the reservoir pad contains anti-LH antibodies conjugated to colloidal gold. A positive test result indicates a urine LH level of 20 mIU/mL or higher. Testing usually is performed for 5 consecutive days in the middle of the cycle. Once the surge is detected, ovulation can be expected within 2 to 3 days.

Menopause Testing

A woman is said to have reached menopause when menstruation, or the monthly cycle, has not occurred for at least 12 months. The time before menopause, called *perimenopause*, can last for years, bringing with it uncomfortable symptoms such as irregular periods, hot flashes, vaginal dryness, or sleep problems. Some of this may be because of an increase in follicle-stimulating hormone (FSH). Levels of FSH, which is produced by the pituitary gland, increase temporarily each month to stimulate the ovaries. When a woman enters menopause, the ovaries stop producing eggs, and the levels of FSH rise. CLIA-waived lateral flow tests detect FSH in the urine. A positive test result indicates that a woman may be in a stage of menopause; a negative test result, along with symptoms of menopause, may indicate that a woman is in perimenopause. The qualitative lateral flow test should never be used to direct a woman to stop using birth control methods if she does not want to conceive, because pregnancy is still possible during perimenopause.

URINE TOXICOLOGY

Toxicology is the study of poisonous substances and their effects on the body. The clinical laboratory performs testing on body fluids and tissues to monitor the use of therapeutic drugs such as digoxin (a cardiac medication) or to detect poisoning by herbicides, metals, animal toxins, and poisonous gases (e.g., carbon monoxide).

Laboratory testing for illegal drugs or alcohol also is performed, most commonly as an employment, insurance, or legal requirement (Table 25.5). Although serum (blood) tests are more accurate for determining current impairment or the time of ingestion, urine is the specimen of choice for most routine screening procedures. For routine screening, a random specimen usually is collected. Often, safeguards are used to ensure that a specimen is fresh and is truly from the patient. Water may be temporarily unavailable in the restroom, bluing agents may be added to the toilets, a container with a temperature-sensitive strip may be provided, and someone may accompany the patient into the restroom. In some cases, a strict chain of custody is required. The substance for which the test is performed or its metabolite often remains in urine much longer than the impairment or intoxication lasts. This is one reason that urine screening is favored over serum or blood screening.

As a PCT, you may be responsible for collecting specimens for toxicology tests and for performing certain tests. Rapid drug screening devices are about the size and shape of a credit card (Fig. 25.8). The device is dipped into a urine sample, or urine is directly applied to the device. The results are read according to the manufacturer's instructions in just minutes. "Negative" results indicate that none of the targeted drugs were

Table 25.5	Commonly Abused Drugs and Body Retention Times
Drug	**Retention Time**
Alcohol	2 to 10 hours
Amphetamine	24 to 48 hours
Methamphetamine	3 to 5+ days
Barbiturates	
Phenobarbital	2 to 6 days
Secobarbital	24 hours
Cocaine, cocaine metabolites	12 hours to 3 days
Opiates, heroin, morphine	3 to 4 days
Phencyclidine (PCP)	3 to 7+ days
Marijuana (tetrahydrocannabinol metabolites)	2 days to 11 weeks

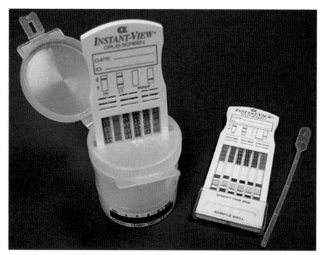

FIGURE 25.8 Instant-View Drug Test. (Courtesy Alfa Scientific, Poway, California.)

detected in the urine sample at specified cutoff levels; "inconclusive" results indicate that the device reacted with something in the urine and confirmation testing is required.

The Instant-View Multi-Drug Screen™ (Alfa Scientific, Poway, CA) urine test is a lateral flow chromatographic immunoassay that tests for urine metabolites of a variety of drugs, including amphetamines, barbiturates, benzodiazepines, cocaine, morphine, methadone, phencyclidine (PCP), tricyclics, marijuana, Ecstasy, and methamphetamines. Available in cartridges that test from two to six drugs, the test is a competitive binding immunoassay in which drug and drug metabolites in a urine sample compete with immobilized drug conjugate for limited labeled antibody binding sites. By using antibodies specific to different drug classes, the test permits independent, simultaneous detection of up to six drugs from a single sample in 5 minutes.

Drug testing has legal ramifications. Therefore additional testing often is necessary to ensure that samples have not been adulterated. Adulteration is the intentional manipulation of a urine sample to allow someone to falsely pass a drug screening test. It may involve using urine from another person or an animal, diluting the sample with water, or adding substances such as bleach, vinegar, eye drops, baking soda, drain openers, soft drinks, or hydrogen peroxide. Urine collection cups with built-in thermometer panels often are used to ensure that urine has been freshly voided from the bladder. A temperature of 32° C to 38° C (90° F to 100° F) within 4 minutes of collection is expected. Test strips that detect human immunoglobulins (antibodies) in urine can determine whether the specimen is human in origin and if it is naturally dilute or has been diluted. Human immunoglobulin G (IgG) is exclusive to humans and is always found at certain levels in urine, even if it is dilute. The addition of chemicals to the urine will prevent the reaction on the test strip.

Each step from collection of the specimen to reporting of test results to the patient must be strictly monitored. Requirements include sealed specimen containers; supervised laboratory analysis throughout the process; and authorized signatures at each step.

Alcohol Testing

Alcohol testing is not performed on urine, but CLIA-waived tests are available to detect alcohol using saliva. Saliva-based tests have a high degree of correlation to blood alcohol analysis. The saliva alcohol test manufactured by STC Technologies (Bethlehem, PA) uses a Dacron swab saturated with saliva to detect ethanol. The test is used primarily for workplace testing, including the federally mandated testing of transportation workers, but also in private company "drug-free workplace" programs and by emergency departments.

FEDERAL DRUG TESTING CUSTODY AND CONTROL FORM

SPECIMEN ID NO.   **1234567**   LAB ACCESSION NO.

OMB No. 0930-0158

STEP 1: COMPLETED BY COLLECTOR OR EMPLOYER REPRESENTATIVE

A. Employer Name, Address, I.D. No.

B. MRO Name, Address, Phone and Fax No.

C. Donor SSN or Employee I.D. No. _____

D. Reason for Test: ☐ Pre-employment ☐ Random ☐ Reasonable Suspicion/Cause ☐ Post Accident ☐ Return to Duty ☐ Follow-up ☐ Other (specify)_____

E. Drug Tests to be Performed: ☐ THC, COC, PCP, OPI, AMP ☐ THC & COC Only ☐ Other (specify)_____

F. Collection Site Address:

Collector Phone No. _____

Collector Fax No. _____

STEP 2: COMPLETED BY COLLECTOR

Read specimen temperature within 4 minutes. Is temperature between 90° and 100° F? ☐ Yes ☐ No, Enter Remark

Specimen Collection: ☐ Split ☐ Single ☐ None Provided (Enter Remark) ☐ Observed (Enter Remark)

REMARKS

STEP 3: Collector affixes bottle seal(s) to bottle(s). Collector dates seal(s). Donor initials seal(s). Donor completes STEP 5 on Copy 2 (MRO Copy)

STEP 4: CHAIN OF CUSTODY - INITIATED BY COLLECTOR AND COMPLETED BY LABORATORY

I certify that the specimen given to me by the donor identified in the certification section on Copy 2 of this form was collected, labeled, sealed and released to the Delivery Service noted in accordance with applicable Federal requirements.

X _____   Signature of Collector   Time of Collection   AM PM

_____ (PRINT) Collector's Name (First, MI, Last)   Date (Mo./Day/Yr.)

SPECIMEN BOTTLE(S) RELEASED TO:

Name of Delivery Service Transferring Specimen to Lab

RECEIVED AT LAB:

X _____   Signature of Accessioner

_____ (PRINT) Accessioner's Name (First, MI, Last)   Date (Mo./Day/Yr.)

Primary Specimen Bottle Seal Intact ☐ Yes ☐ No, Enter Remark Below

SPECIMEN BOTTLE(S) RELEASED TO:

STEP 5a: PRIMARY SPECIMEN TEST RESULTS - COMPLETED BY PRIMARY LABORATORY

☐ NEGATIVE   ☐ POSITIVE for: ☐ MARIJUANA METABOLITE ☐ CODEINE ☐ AMPHETAMINE ☐ ADULTERATED
☐ DILUTE   ☐ COCAINE METABOLITE ☐ MORPHINE ☐ METHAMPHETAMINE ☐ SUBSTITUTED
☐ REJECTED FOR TESTING ☐ PCP ☐ 6-ACETYLMORPHINE ☐ INVALID RESULT

REMARKS _____

TEST LAB (if different from above) _____

I certify that the specimen identified on this form was examined upon receipt, handled using chain of custody procedures, analyzed, and reported in accordance with applicable Federal requirements.

X _____   Signature of Certifying Scientist   _____ (PRINT) Certifying Scientist's Name (First, MI, Last)   Date (Mo./Day/Yr.)

STEP 5b: SPLIT SPECIMEN TEST RESULTS - (IF TESTED) COMPLETED BY SECONDARY LABORATORY

Laboratory Name

Laboratory Address

☐ RECONFIRMED ☐ FAILED TO RECONFIRM - REASON_____

I certify that the split specimen identified on this form was examined upon receipt, handled using chain of custody procedures, analyzed, and reported in accordance with applicable Federal requirements.

X _____   Signature of Certifying Scientist   _____ (PRINT) Certifying Scientist's Name (First, MI, Last)   Date (Mo./Day/Yr.)

PRESS HARD - YOU ARE MAKING MULTIPLE COPIES

PEEL   **1234567** A   SPECIMEN ID NO.   PLACE OVER CAP   **1234567** SPECIMEN BOTTLE SEAL   Date (Mo. Day Yr.)   Donor's Initials

PEEL   **1234567** B (SPLIT)   SPECIMEN ID NO.   PLACE OVER CAP   **1234567** SPECIMEN BOTTLE SEAL   Date (Mo. Day Yr.)   Donor's Initials

COPY 1 - LABORATORY

0000-0000-0225

Drug Form Part 1
Face Inks: 000 BLK / 000 RED
Date: 05/09/00
Not To Use For Colormatch
Follow PMS Guide For Colors

FIGURE 25.9 First page of a five-page Federal Drug Testing Custody and Control form. (From Proctor D, Adams A: *Kinn's The Medical Assistant: an applied learning approach,* ed 12, St. Louis, 2014, Saunders.).

Collecting a Stool Specimen

Stool specimens are collected and examined for a variety of reasons, including the following: to determine the presence of infection or blood; to observe the amount, color, and consistency of the stool; to determine the presence of fats; or to identify parasites, ova, and bacteria. The PCT collects the feces, labels the specimen appropriately, and sends the specimen and the laboratory request to the laboratory. When stool is to be examined for parasites, it must be taken immediately to the laboratory in order for parasites to be examined under the microscope while they are alive. It is also possible to collect a stool specimen from a colostomy or an ileostomy.

The PCT should inform the patient that a stool specimen is needed; it is then essential to carry out collection in a manner that will not cause stress or make the patient feel hurried or embarrassed. Supplies should be arranged if the patient is to collect the stool. When a stool specimen is to be obtained, the specimen hat should be placed toward the back of the toilet or commode. When a urine specimen is to be obtained, the specimen hat should be placed toward the front. If both urine and stool specimens are to be collected, two specimen hats are used: one placed at the front and one placed toward the back of the toilet or commode. A bedpan may be used to collect a stool specimen if the patient is cautioned not to void in the bedpan, which would compromise the stool specimen. The PCT must understand why the stool specimen is being collected in order to correctly choose the appropriate supplies. If the stool specimen is for ova and parasites, an appropriate container with a special solution must be obtained (Procedure 25.5).

PROCEDURE 25.5

Collecting a Stool Specimen

1. Refer to the healthcare provider's order.
2. Assemble supplies.
3. Introduce self.
4. Identify patient.
5. Explain procedure to patient; ensure that the patient understands what is expected.
6. Perform hand hygiene and don nonsterile gloves according to agency policy and guidelines from the CDC and OSHA.
7. Assist patient to bathroom when necessary.
8. Ask patient to defecate into commode, specimen device, or bedpan, preventing urine from entering specimen.

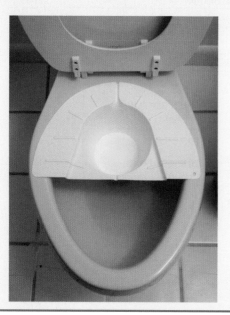

9. Transfer stool to specimen cup with use of a tongue blade, and close the lid securely.

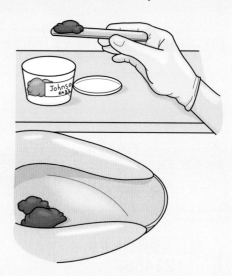

10. Remove gloves, discard them in proper receptacle, and perform hand hygiene.
11. Attach requisition slip, enclose specimen in a biohazard bag, label the bag, and send specimen to laboratory (it is necessary to take specimens for ova and parasites to the laboratory stat; it is acceptable to keep other stool specimens at room temperature).
12. Assist patient to bed.
13. Document procedure and observations.

CDC, Centers for Disease Control and Prevention; *OSHA*, Occupational Safety and Health Administration; *PPE*, personal protective equipment. *(Step 8 and 9 figures from Sorrentino SA, Remmert LN: Mosby's essentials for nursing assistants, ed 5, St. Louis, 2014, Mosby.)*

Collecting a Sputum Specimen

Sputum is secretion from the lungs. It contains mucus, cellular debris, microorganisms, or some combination of these, and it sometimes contains blood or pus. A sputum specimen must be obtained from deep in the bronchial tree. Expectoration of throat and mouth secretions is not to be used as a sputum specimen because saliva with food particles does not produce desired results. Early morning is the best time to collect a sputum specimen because the patient has not yet cleared the respiratory passages. Many tests are possible to perform on sputum, such as culture (a laboratory test involving cultivation of microorganisms or cells in a special growth medium) and sensitivity (a laboratory method of determining the effectiveness of antibiotics, usually performed in conjunction with culture); cytologic analysis (cytology is the study of cells, including their formation, origin, structure, function, biochemical activities, and pathologic processes); and examination and testing for acid-fast bacillus (the organism responsible for tuberculosis of the lung).

Collecting a Sputum Specimen by Expectoration

Some patients are able to expectorate (eject mucus, sputum, or fluids from trachea and lungs by coughing or spitting) a sputum specimen. Closed-method collection containers, such as a Lukens specimen container, protect the PCT from contamination with body fluids. The PCT should explain the procedure and prepare the patient for the test. Instructions should be given to the patient the night before the test to drink extra fluids, which will help loosen secretions and make expectoration for the specimen easier. The PCT should instruct the patient that it is not possible to use saliva as a specimen. Saliva is clear, whereas sputum is thick, sometimes colored, and tenacious (sticky) and requires the ability to initiate a deep cough, to raise the mucus (Procedure 25.6).

Injury & Illness Prevention Box 25.1

- When handling a sputum collection, wear gloves.
- If you are assisting the patient with the collection, it is best to wear gloves and a mask to protect yourself from the respiratory mucus splashing in your face.
- Anytime there is suspected respiratory infection, wear a mask when assisting with a sputum collection.

Patient Education

Frequently a PCT is called upon to explain collection techniques to the patient. Patients want to do the

---

PROCEDURE 25.6

Collecting a Sputum Specimen by Expectoration

1. Refer to the healthcare provider's order.
2. Assemble supplies.
3. Introduce self.
4. Identify patient.
5. Explain procedure.
6. Perform hand hygiene and don nonsterile gloves according to agency policy and guidelines from the CDC and OSHA.
7. Position patient in Fowler's position.
8. Instruct patient to take three breaths and force cough into sterile container.
9. Label specimen container.
10. Enclose specimen in biohazard bag and attach laboratory requisition. Immediately send specimen to laboratory. If any sputum is present on outside of container, wash it off with disinfectant.
11. Remove gloves, discard them in proper receptacle, and perform hand hygiene.
12. Document procedure and observations.

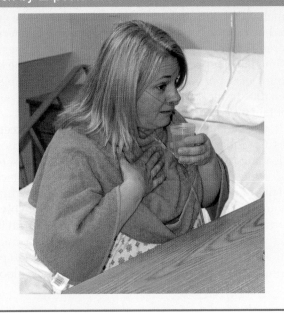

CDC, Centers for Disease Control and Prevention; OSHA, Occupational Safety and Health Administration.

procedure correctly but often lack the knowledge of urinary terminology and are embarrassed to or do not know how to ask questions regarding cleaning of the genital area. When explaining a urinary collection procedure, use pictures and words that the patient will understand. As you explain the procedure in terms that the patient knows, he or she will feel comfortable telling you or asking you pertinent details that may have a definite impact on treatment of the problem. Providing the patient with a clearly written instruction sheet is also helpful. The instruction sheet should be personalized with his or her name, the time to begin collection or testing (if applicable), what supplies should be used, and a phone number to call if questions arise.

LEGAL AND ETHICAL ISSUES

Similar to all other procedures, the test is only as valid as the specimen and the procedure performed on that specimen. You are responsible for that when you instruct the patient and when you perform the test.

You have the responsibility for properly collecting specimens and accurately testing them. In addition, you are responsible for strict adherence to protocol when collecting and testing specimens when legal ramifications are associated with the test results. Patient confidentiality is paramount when drug testing is performed, as is rigid conformation to all established rules and regulations.

CHAPTER SUMMARY

Routine UA is performed primarily as a screening test to detect metabolic and physiologic disorders. Urine is easily obtained, making it an ideal specimen for testing. Urine is analyzed for detection of extrinsic and intrinsic pathologic conditions. Urine is formed through a filtration mechanism in the kidney via the nephrons. As the filtrate passes through the tubules, various changes occur. Urine is stored in the bladder and is voided through the urethra.

Requesting a urine specimen from a patient may be an embarrassing moment for the patient. The request should be made in private, and the patient should be given explicit instructions so that he or she understands what is expected. Some urine collections, such as the 2-hour postprandial specimen, must be timed around meals or fasts. Routine UA requires no special preparation, whereas a CCMS requires cleansing of the external genitalia. Only urine that will be cultured must be collected in a sterile container. Urine to be sent to a referral laboratory may require the addition of preservatives.

Timed urine specimens are collected to determine the amount of a particular analyte in the urine during a given time frame. Proper patient instruction is necessary to obtain an acceptable specimen.

Proper patient instruction is necessary for an acceptable CCMS. Both men and women are given instructions in cleaning the external genitalia to prevent contamination of the urine. Urine must be collected in a sterile container and refrigerated if it cannot be tested within 1 hour. Physical examination of the urine involves determination of the color, turbidity, and specific gravity. Odor and foam color may be noted. The chemical examination of urine involves determination of the pH level and the levels of glucose, protein, ketones, blood,

bilirubin, urobilinogen, and nitrite, as well as specific gravity and leukocyte esterase, with the use of a reagent strip.

Pregnancy tests detect hCG, a hormone produced by the placenta. Anti-hCG antibodies embedded in test cartridges bind to hCG and initiate color changes in test areas. Urine moves through lateral flow devices by capillary action. Fertility can be assessed using lateral flow tests that detect LH, a hormone that increases in concentration in the urine shortly before ovulation. Menopause can be assessed using lateral flow tests that detect FSH, which increases as menopause approaches.

Laboratory tests are only as valid as the specimen and the procedure performed on that specimen. The PCT is responsible for ongoing education to maintain standards and skills in use of certain laboratory equipment. Patient confidentiality is paramount when drug testing is performed.

Case Scenario

Dr. Hill has ordered a UA on the specimen from Mr. Parks, a UA and pregnancy test on the specimen from Mrs. Carpenter, and a UA and C&S on the specimen from Ms. Hillman. After reviewing the requisitions and entering the patient information into the daily logbook, Rosa notes that Mrs. Carpenter's specimen was collected at 6 AM— 3 hours ago. Is this acceptable? Explain your answer. Rosa also notes that the specimen collected in the sterile container from Ms. Hillman is marked "CCMS." Why is this important?

REVIEW QUESTIONS

1. The normal color of urine is _____.
   a. Pale straw yellow
   b. Brown
   c. Red
   d. Orange

2. The presence of greenish yellow foam may mean that the patient has _____.
   a. Cancer
   b. Hepatitis
   c. Diabetes
   d. Heart disease

3. What is the minimum amount of urine required for a routine urinalysis?
   a. 5 mL
   b. 10 mL
   c. 12 mL
   d. 15 mL

4. When does the 24-hour urine specimen begin?
   a. At a specific time
   b. When the patient wakes up in the morning
   c. Before the patient goes to bed
   d. Once the patient voids and discards the urine

5. What should the patient use to collect his or her stool to be sent to the laboratory?
   a. A urine collection bag
   b. Nothing; the patient should use the toilet to catch the stool.
   c. A specimen hat
   d. A Foley catheter

Surgery and Immobility

Care of the Surgical Patient

LEARNING OBJECTIVES

1. Define the concepts of aseptic technique.
2. Explain the differences among sanitization, disinfection, and sterilization.
3. Explain the types and uses of sterilization indicators.
4. Perform a skin prep for surgery.
5. Properly apply sequential compression devices and elastic stockings.
6. Discuss the legal and ethics concerns regarding surgical asepsis and infection control.

KEY TERMS

asepsis The condition of being free from infection

infection Invasion of body tissues by microorganisms, which then proliferate and damage tissues

sterilization Complete destruction of all forms of microbial life

surgical asepsis The complete destruction of organisms on instruments or equipment that will enter the patient's body

Asepsis is the condition of being free of infection or infectious material. *Medical asepsis* is the destruction of organisms after they leave the body, or the state of being free from disease-causing organisms. The principles of medical asepsis are put in place by a healthcare facility to prevent reinfection of a patient and cross-infection of another patient or ourselves. To prevent cross-contamination, potential microorganisms and pathogens must be isolated by following standard blood and body fluid precautions and by disinfecting or sterilizing objects as soon as possible after they become contaminated. Medical asepsis is the process of either reducing the number of pathogens or destroying them; this creates an environment that is clean but not sterile (free of microorganisms).

Surgical asepsis is the complete destruction of organisms on instruments or equipment that will potentially enter the patient's body. This technique is mandatory for any procedure that invades the body's skin or tissues, such as surgery. Everything that comes in contact with the patient must be sterile, including surgical gowns, drapes, and instruments, in addition to the gloved hands of the surgeon and surgical assistants. Anytime the skin or a mucous membrane is punctured or pierced, as in venipunctures or injections, aseptic techniques must be practiced. Urinary catheterizations, biopsies, and dressing changes on open wounds are performed using sterile technique.

Sometimes the patient care technician (PCT) will be asked to remove dirty instruments for cleaning and sterilization after surgical procedures. Careful attention must be given to sterilizing all items at all times. Frequent checking and rechecking of procedures helps ensure that invasive procedures are effective and are performed without any "breaks" in technique. Single-use, disposable items offer the best method of infection control, and they are being used more frequently in medical offices and hospitals. However, when disposable equipment is used, the PCT must know the specific disposal guidelines for contaminated instruments and supplies.

STERILIZATION

Before an instrument or piece of equipment can be used in a surgical procedure, it first must be sanitized, then disinfected, and finally sterilized to remove all forms of microorganisms.

Instruments and other items used in surgery, childbirth, examinations, or treatments must be carefully cleaned before proceeding with the steps of disinfection or sterilization. *Sanitization* is the cleansing process that reduces the number of microorganisms to a safe level as dictated by public health and infection control guidelines. This cleansing process removes debris such as blood and other body fluids from instruments or equipment. Blood and debris (also known as "bioburden") must be removed so that, later in the process, disinfection with chemicals or sterilization with steam, heat, or gases can penetrate to all the instrument's surfaces. The sanitization procedure should be completed immediately after the instruments are used. If this is not possible, rinse the used items under cold water immediately after the surgical procedure and place them in a low-sudsing, rust-inhibiting, enzyme-containing, detergent solution. Never allow blood or other substances that can coagulate to dry on an instrument. Leaving dry blood or other substances can cause "pitting" of the metal finishing and ruin the instrument.

The PCT should always wear gloves while performing sanitization (thick utility gloves if the instruments have sharp or pointed edges) to prevent possible personal contamination with potentially infectious body fluids that may be present on the articles being cleaned. When you are ready to sanitize instruments, drain off the soak solution and rinse each instrument in cold, running water. Separate the sharp instruments from the others, because metal instruments may damage the cutting edges, and sharp instruments may damage the other instruments or injure you. Clean all sharp instruments at one time, when you can concentrate on preventing injury to yourself. Open all hinges and scrub serrations and ratchets with a small scrub brush or toothbrush. Rinse the instruments in hot water and then check them carefully for proper working order before they are disinfected or sterilized. The items should be hand-dried with a towel to prevent spotting.

Disinfection is the process of killing pathogenic organisms or of rendering them inactive. However, it is not always effective against spores, the tubercle bacilli, and certain viruses. Disinfectant chemicals may kill microbes within a short time but are usually very hard on instruments. Some chemicals, such as Cidex®, are effective enough to kill all organisms, but the usual immersion time for these sterilants is 10 hours or longer. Many types of disinfecting agents are available and have varying degrees of effectiveness. It is important to follow the manufacturer's guidelines on the proper use of each product and also to understand the product's advantages and disadvantages and the possible sources of error.

To ensure proper sterilization for surgical aseptic procedures, an area (usually a utility room) should be set aside in each office for just this purpose. The area should be divided into two sections, one dirty and one clean. The dirty section is used for receiving contaminated instruments and other materials at the conclusion of surgical procedures. This area should have a sink, receiving basins, proper cleaning agents, brushes, utility gloves, autoclave wrapping paper or cloth, autoclave envelopes and tape, sterilizer indicators, and disposable gloves. Designated biohazardous waste containers with red bags are needed to safely discard gloves and other contaminated disposable products worn when handling contaminated items. Personal protective equipment (PPE) for autoclave procedures includes the following:

- Heat-resistant autoclave gloves for loading and unloading
- Fluid-resistant gloves to prevent contact with contaminants
- A laboratory coat or impervious gown, if needed, to protect against splashes
- A face shield and/or goggles if a splash hazard exists

The clean section of the utility room should be reserved for receiving the sterile items after they have been removed from the sterilizer. Clear, clean plastic bags in which to store sterile packs may be kept in the clean area. Both areas should be spotlessly clean and well organized. Sterilization can be achieved by moist heat in an autoclave, by gas, or with chemicals. Most medical offices use the autoclave method.

Autoclave

Steam under pressure in the autoclave (Fig. 26.1) is the best method of sterilization, because it kills all pathogens and spores. Pressurized steam is fast, convenient, and dependable. The pressure allows for heat higher than the boiling point, and when combined with moisture, these two factors create a very effective mechanism for killing all microorganisms. When steam is admitted into the autoclave chamber, it simultaneously heats and wets the object, coagulating the proteins present in all living organisms. When the cycle is complete and the chamber has cooled, the steam condenses and explodes the cells of microorganisms, thus destroying them. To be effective, the steam moisture must come in contact with all surfaces being sterilized. Steam under pressure is capable of much faster penetration of fabrics and textiles than dry heat, but its use has definite limitations if the proper techniques are not followed.

The recommended temperature for sterilization in an autoclave is 121° to 123° C (250° to 255° F). Unwrapped items should be sterilized for 20 minutes, small wrapped items for 30 minutes, and large or tightly wrapped items for 40 minutes. Processing time starts *after* the autoclave reaches normal operating conditions of 121° C (250° F) and 15 pounds per square inch (psi) pressure.

The three basic autoclave cycles are as follows:

- *Gravity ("fast exhaust") cycle:* This cycle is used to sterilize stainless steel instruments, glassware, and so on. The autoclave fills with steam and is held at a set temperature for a set period. When the cycle is complete, a valve opens and the chamber rapidly returns to atmospheric pressure. Drying time may be added to the end of the cycle.
- *Liquid ("slow exhaust") cycle:* This cycle is used to prevent sterilized liquids from boiling. Steam is exhausted slowly at the end of the cycle, allowing the liquids to cool.
- *Prevacuum cycle:* This cycle is used for porous materials. The chamber is partially evacuated before the introduction of steam for greater steam penetration; this is not available on all machines.

Incorrect operation of an autoclave may result in superheated steam. If steam is brought to extremely high temperature, it is literally dried out, and the advantage of a higher heat is diminished. Wet steam is another cause of incomplete sterilization. Wet steam results from failing to preheat the chamber, which causes excessive condensation in the interior of the chamber. Condensation is necessary, but too much prevents the sterilization process from being completed properly. It can be compared with taking a hot shower in a cold bathroom, which results in heavily steamed mirrors, walls, and towels. If packs become too saturated to dry during the drying cycle, the packs pick up and absorb bacteria from the air or any surface on which they are placed after removal from the autoclave. Placing cold instruments in a hot chamber also increases condensation. Other causes of wet steam include opening the door too wide at the end of the cycle or allowing a rush of cold air into the chamber. Overfilling the water reservoir may produce this same effect.

The main cause of incomplete sterilization in the autoclave is the presence of residual air. Without the complete elimination of air, an adequately high temperature to sterilize the contents within the autoclave's chamber cannot be reached. Air and steam do not mix. Because air is heavier than steam, it pools wherever possible. One tenth of 1% (0.1%) residual air trapped around an instrument prevents complete sterilization. This is especially dangerous in older autoclaves that do not have a chamber thermometer separate from the

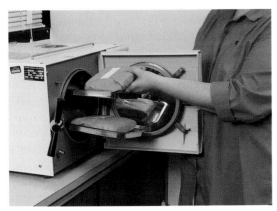

FIGURE 26.1 Steam autoclave. (From Bonewit-West K: *Clinical procedures for medical assistants*, ed 7, Philadelphia, 2008, Saunders.)

pressure gauge. Adequate chamber pressure does not guarantee a proper chamber temperature.

Sterilization Indicators

Sterilization is achieved only when steam reaches the optimum temperature for a designated duration and has penetrated to the center of the articles. Sterilization indicators must be used routinely to determine whether all microorganisms have been destroyed. The two basic types of sterilization indicators are chemical indicators (autoclave tape) and biologic indicators (bacterial spore strips).

Chemical Sterilization Indicators

Autoclave tape, a commonly used sterilization indicator, contains a chemical dye that changes color when exposed to steam. The tape is not an absolute indication that the proper sterilization time, temperature, and steam have been maintained; it merely indicates that a high temperature was reached while the article was in the autoclave. The strip must completely change color (colors vary by manufacturer) or reveal the word "autoclaved" to ensure effective operation. The main function of autoclave tape, besides holding the wrapping material together or closing a sterilization bag, is to verify that the package has been autoclaved.

Biologic Sterilization Indicators

The facility should have a policy for how frequently the autoclave is tested using biologic methods. One type, a spore strip indicator, contains a temperature-sensitive dye that changes color when the proper combination of steam, temperature, and time has been achieved. An indicator strip should be placed in the center of the largest pack that typically would be autoclaved in the facility to determine the accuracy of the autoclave and autoclave procedures. Test indicator kits are available that use ampules of *Bacillus stearothermophilus*, which is destroyed at 121° C (250° F). On completion of the cycle, the ampule is sent to the laboratory for analysis of any type of microbial growth, which would indicate that the autoclave is not sterilizing properly.

Autoclave Unloading Guidelines

When the autoclave's sterilization cycle is complete, release the pressure according to the manufacturer's guidelines. Once the pressure gauge reads "0," stand back from the door and, with heat-resistant gloves, open the door approximately ¼ inch. Allow the load to dry for at least 15 minutes (this time varies according to the type of autoclave and the size of the load). Capillary attraction is the action that draws moisture through the surface of materials. Packs can act like a sponge,

attracting outside moisture and microorganisms. Touching a wet pack allows microorganisms on your hands to penetrate the wrappings, making the contents of the pack nonsterile. Dry, wrapped packs may be removed with clean, dry hands, but it is safer to wear heat-resistant gloves to reduce the possibility of burns from the hot instruments inside the packs. If possible, allow all packs to cool in the autoclave with the door open. Place the packs on a dry, dust-free surface inside an enclosed cupboard or drawer for storage. Do not place the packs on cold surfaces, because hot packs may cause condensation, and moisture will contaminate the contents.

Guidelines for unloading an autoclave include the following:

- Stand behind the door when opening it to prevent accidental steam burns.
- Slowly open the door only a crack, allowing the items to cool for 15 to 20 minutes before removing them.
- If for any reason the integrity of the sterilization process is in question, the load should be considered contaminated and autoclaved again. Reasons for concern include the following:
  - Any load that fails to convert a sterilization indicator strip
  - Any load processed after a biologic test indicates that the autoclave is not working properly

Shelf Life of Sterilized Packs

Sterilized instruments should be stored in a manner that preserves the integrity of the packaging material. Storage practices can be either date related or event related. Although some facilities continue to date every sterilized package and use shelf-life practices (first in, first out), other facilities have switched to event-related practices. This approach recognizes that the product should remain sterile until some event causes the item to become contaminated (e.g., a package becomes torn or wet). The quality of the packaging material, the conditions under which items are stored and transported, and the amount that they are handled all affect the chances that the package and its contents will remain sterile. All packages containing sterile items should be inspected before use to verify barrier integrity and dryness. Any package that is wet, torn, dropped on the floor, or damaged in any way should not be used. The instruments should be recleaned, packaged in new wrap, and sterilized again (www.cdc.gov).

Even for event-related packaging, the date of sterilization should be placed on the package. If multiple sterilizers are used in the facility, the sterilizer used should also be indicated on the outside of the packaging material. This information can facilitate retrieval of processed items in the event of a sterilization failure (www.cdc.gov).

In general, muslin and autoclave paper packs are considered sterile for up to 28 days from the date of sterilization. Polypropylene autoclave bags are sterile for up to 6 months from the sterilization date. All sterile packs should be stored on dry, dust-free, covered shelves or in drawers. Fabric wrappers must be inspected for holes and laundered after each use. A damaged pack or a broken seal renders the package nonsterile; spills of any fluid onto a package also contaminate it. When a pack is no longer sterile for any reason, including the expiration date, the contents must be reprocessed as if the pack had been used for surgery. The contents must be sanitized, disinfected, wrapped, and sterilized as usual.

SURGICAL PROCEDURES

Common surgical procedures that are routinely performed with the PCT's assistance may include suturing, cyst removal, incision and drainage (I&D) of abscesses, and collection of biopsy specimens. The PCT may need to be knowledgeable about preparing the patient and the room, assisting the physician with the surgery, and applying a dressing and bandage after the procedure is finished.

Each surgical procedure requires appropriate skin preparation and draping with a *fenestrated* drape, also called an *eye sheet*. This is a surgical drape with an opening in the center. The size of the opening depends on the size of the surgical field. The opening is placed directly over the surgical site after the site has been suitably prepared (or "prepped," as it is called in healthcare practice). A minor surgery tray is opened, and a sterile field is created on an instrument stand.

After numbing the area with a local anesthetic, the physician opens the skin with an incision. If a cyst is being removed, the physician cuts around it and usually tries to "deliver" it from the wound intact. If the procedure is an I&D, foul matter will start oozing from the wound immediately after the skin is incised. The wound is drained completely and flushed with copious amounts of sterile saline solution. A drain may be placed in the wound and left for several days. If the procedure is a biopsy, a small amount of tissue is removed and placed in a specimen container with preservative. The specimen container must be carefully labeled with the appropriate patient information, the date, and specifics about the specimen type and location. It then is sent to the laboratory, where it is examined microscopically for changes or abnormalities.

Electrosurgery

Electrosurgery is also known as *electrocautery*. An electrosurgical unit (ESU) uses high-frequency current to cut through tissue and coagulate blood vessels. A small probe with an electric current running through it is used to *cauterize* (burn or destroy) the tissue. When the electric current comes in contact with tissue and blood cells, they are vaporized, producing carbon and steam. This process seals blood vessels, minimizing cellular oozing and bleeding. Electrosurgery may be used to destroy granulations and small polyps.

The necessary components are the ESU's power source, the grounding cable and pad, and the active electrode (a pencil-like instrument with a tip and cord). Tips are disposable and are used according to the type of procedure performed. The two most commonly used tips are the needle and flat designs.

Holding the pencil-like instrument, the surgeon touches the tissue with the tip and activates the electric current with a switch on the instrument or a foot pedal. The electric current is delivered to the tissues, and tissue is vaporized at the site of contact. Operating room fires represent a potentially life-threatening hazard and are triggered by the ESU pencil. Carbon dioxide is a fire suppressant and is a routinely used medical gas. Each facility should have fire safety plans in place within the operating room in the event a fire should occur from use of electrosurgical instruments.

Injury & Illness Prevention Box 26.1

Important Tips About the Grounding Pad

- Carefully inspect the pad, cable, and skin before the procedure.
- Place the pad close to the operative site.
- The pad must be tight against the patient's skin.
- Apply the pad to a fleshy area, such as the thigh.
- Do not place the pad over a bony area.
- Do not place the pad over body hair.
- Do not place the pad over metal implants or a pacemaker.
- Carefully inspect the pad site on the skin after the procedure.

ASSISTING WITH SURGICAL PROCEDURES

Surgery performed in a medical office or outpatient center is restricted to the management of minor problems and injuries. The PCT is expected to assist with preparing the patient and setting up the sterile field. The following procedures must be used without exception when assisting with minor surgery. Individual facilities may have specific guidelines for some of these procedures; however, the theory behind sterile technique is universal, regardless of where you work.

Preparation of the Patient

Whether minor surgery is performed because of an unplanned accident or is a planned, elective procedure, the patient needs both psychological and physical support. A patient facing a surgical procedure may be concerned about pain, disfigurement, and a possible diagnosis of cancer. An injured patient may feel anxious about medical bills or possible loss of employment. Because surgery is a frightening experience, the PCT must take the time, both preoperatively and at the time of surgery, to help the patient deal with fears and anxieties. The best way to help is to ensure that the patient understands the details of the procedure, that all questions are answered by the physician or nurse, and that the patient has the opportunity to talk about the procedure and voice any concerns.

Questions should be answered directly, but you should answer only the questions that are within your scope of knowledge and the policies of the hospital. Notify the nurse if the patient has questions that have been unanswered. What may seem to be a minor or unimportant question to you may be a very frightening concern to the patient. The minor surgery room can be intimidating, so unless the patient is sedated, try to make conversation with him or her while you prepare for the physician's arrival.

Preoperative preparation may include blood and urine tests, completion of a consent form, and gathering of the current history concerning any recent illnesses, medications, and allergies. Patient preparations before surgery may include a skin prep, cleansing enemas, food intake restrictions, special bathing, and administration of a sedative medication. On the day of surgery, the patient is instructed to empty the bladder and undress and gown as requested. The vital signs are recorded in preparation for the procedure.

Positioning

Have the patients remove their clothes so that they will expose the surgical site completely. If a patient gown is being worn, have the patient remove all underclothes, including the woman's bra. Underwire bras especially can cause burns from use of the ESU. Clothing may also act as a tourniquet or may make applying a proper dressing or bandage difficult if it is left on the body during a surgical procedure. In addition, the patient's clothing may be stained by the skin prep solution or may interfere with adequate site preparation.

The patient needs to be positioned as comfortable as possible for the procedure. An uncomfortable position can be held for only a limited time, and the patient may have to move, perhaps in the middle of a procedure, if you have not ensured his or her comfort from the beginning. The nurse will typically inform you what position the patient needs to be placed in for the procedure. If the patient has an open wound that will need rinsing during the procedure, wear nonsterile gloves to assist the patient into position. If there is active and profuse bleeding, an impermeable gown and gloves should be worn. If there is danger of blood and body fluid contamination to your face or eyes, wear goggles, a mask, or a face shield.

Skin Preparation

The human skin is a reservoir of bacteria, but it cannot be sterilized without the risk of damaging cells and tissues. The goal of adequate skin preparation for a surgical procedure is to reduce the number of microorganisms so that transference of harmful organisms at the incision site is limited. Cleansing the patient's skin before surgery with surgical soap and an antiseptic and clipping the hair from the area if needed is called a *skin prep* (Procedure 26.1). Sometimes the patient may be instructed to repeatedly cleanse the surgical area with bacteriostatic or antiseptic soap several days before the surgery. Disposable skin prep trays and razors are commonly used in the hospital setting. The hair is clipped more than shaved, to prevent injury to the skin from cuts and nicks. Sometimes an electrical razor is used, which has been shown to limit the number of nicks to the skin, which result in a break in the skin's integrity, or protective layer.

PROCEDURE 26.1
The Surgical Skin Prep

1. Sanitize your hands.
2. Instruct the patient in the skin preparation procedure, ensuring that the person understands the procedure and the rationale for it.
3. Ask the patient to remove any clothing that might interfere with exposure of the site and provide a gown if needed.
4. Assist the patient into the proper position for site exposure. Provide a drape if necessary to protect the patient's privacy.
5. Expose the site. Use a light if necessary.
6. Put on gloves and open the skin prep pack.
7. Add the antiseptic soap to the two bowls.
8. Start at the incision site and begin washing with the antiseptic soap on a gauze sponge in a circular motion, moving from the center to the edges of the area to be scrubbed.

PROCEDURE 26.1

The Surgical Skin Prep—cont'd

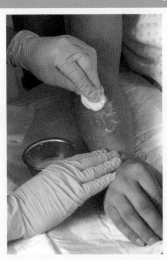

14. Rinse the area with a sterile normal saline solution.

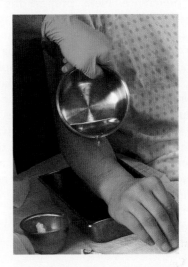

9. After one complete wipe, discard the sponge and begin again with a new sponge soaked in the antiseptic solution.
10. When you return to the incision site for the next circular sweep, you must use clean material.
11. Repeat the process, using sufficient friction for 5 minutes (or follow facility policy for the duration required for a particular prep).
12. If hair is present, the area may need to be clipped. Hold the skin taut and shave in the direction of growth. Take care to prevent injury to yourself or your patient. Immediately after completion, dispose of the razor in the sharps container.

15. Dry the area, using the same circular technique with dry sponges. The area may be dried by blotting with a sterile towel.
16. Paint on the antiseptic with the cotton-tipped applicators or gauze sponges, using the same circular technique and never returning to an area that has already been painted.

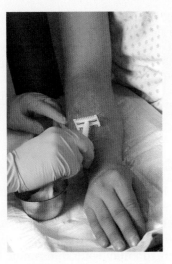

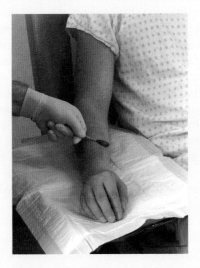

13. After shaving, scrub the skin a second time.

17. Place a sterile drape and/or towel over the area.
18. Answer all the patient's questions to relieve anxiety about the upcoming surgical procedure.
19. Document completion of the skin prep in the patient's chart.

Preparation of the Room

If you are to assist in a minor surgical procedure, ask the nurse which materials are needed according to the physician's preference. Next, prepare the room and gather the supplies to be used. Sterile supplies are opened just before the procedure. Opened materials that have been exposed longer than 1 hour, usually because of a delay, are considered nonsterile. Supplies should not be placed where they can be knocked over or dropped. Wrapped sterile supplies that have fallen to the floor must not be used. Once supplies have been opened, the sterile field should be covered with a sterile drape, and a team member should stay in the room to monitor them. Ensure that the patient and family members understand that they should not approach or touch the sterile field.

Sterile Technique

Accurately performing surgical aseptic technique involves a degree of coordination with the hands that can come only with practice. It requires a great deal of concentration and planning of all movements and procedural steps. The procedures covered in this chapter are for minor surgery, but they are the same techniques used during major surgery. To develop a sound knowledge of sterility and sterile technique, use the following memory aid: *Everything sterile is white and everything that is not sterile is black. There is no gray!* Sterile surfaces must *never* come in contact with nonsterile surfaces. If this occurs, the sterile surface immediately is considered contaminated or nonsterile. Absolute honesty is essential for maintaining sterile techniques. When a sterile surface comes in contact with a nonsterile item, this is called a "break" in sterility or a "break" in the sterile field. During any procedure, everything must stop at this point and the "break" must be corrected immediately—which usually means that the PCT must start over again at the very beginning of the procedure. Any break could lead to serious wound contamination, postoperative infection, and even death. Medical asepsis directly affects the health and well-being of the patient and the healthcare team, and must be practiced without fail.

Sterile Field

A sterile field is any sterile surface on which sterile items are placed. In the office, a sterile field most often is set up on a small metal table. In surgery, a sterile field is created by draping sterile towels (either disposable or from autoclaved packs) over a stand or table. The surgical site on the patient's skin is prepared and then draped with sterile towels or drapes so that it also becomes a sterile field.

Hands and hair are two of the greatest sources of contamination when a sterile field is set up. With practice, you will learn to know what may be touched with your hands and what must be touched only with sterile gloved hands. Hair that falls freely over the shoulders and forward gives off a cloud of bacteria with every movement. It must always be secured back and up, not touching the shoulders.

Rules for Maintaining a Sterile Field

- Talking should be kept to a minimum because air currents carry bacteria.
- Sterile team members should always face one another.
- Always keep the sterile field in your view. If you turn your back on a sterile field or lose sight of it, it is considered contaminated.
- Nonsterile persons or items should never cross over the sterile field.
- Tables are sterile only at table level; anything that falls below the edge of the Mayo tray is considered contaminated. A 1-inch border surrounding the tray is considered contaminated, so anything placed on the tray within that 1-inch border is contaminated.
- Consider a sterile barrier contaminated if it has been wet, cut, or torn.
- Packages placed on a clean surface are contaminated on the outside, but the inside of the sterilized package may be used as a sterile field.
- Keep sterile gloved hands above waist level at all times; do not let hands drop below the waist.
- Never remove and then replace any item in the field (e.g., using sterile forceps to cleanse a wound), or the field is contaminated.
- The inside of a sterile package remains so if the package is peeled open properly; it should be opened the entire way, and the contents then tossed onto the field without crossing over the sterile area.
- If a sterile package has fallen to the floor, it must be discarded.
- *If you are in doubt about the sterility of anything, consider it contaminated.*

Specimen Collection

If a specimen is collected during a procedure, it is placed in a sterile glass or basin. You may be asked to deliver the specimen to the laboratory. Do not remove the specimen from the sterile field until the physician gives the order. The surgeon may want to examine the specimen again during the surgery. After the procedure is complete, place the specimen in an appropriate container, label it, and send it to the laboratory for analysis.

Completing the Surgical Procedure

At the conclusion of the procedure, the physician will close the wound with staples, sutures, or a glue-like substance known as Dermabond™. The techniques and methods of tissue closure vary greatly; all of them cannot be described or illustrated here.

After the skin closure, the wound site is cleansed with wet (using sterile, normal saline solution) and sterile dry sponges by the surgeon or the nurse. Care must be taken not to disturb the wound edges or sutures. Next, a sterile dressing is placed over the incision, and a bandage is applied to support the dressing.

Postoperative Responsibilities

After caring for the patient, the PCT may need to clean up the room; this should be done by following *standard precautions*. Wear disposable gloves until all contaminated materials have been properly removed and handled. Place disposable equipment and supplies in biohazardous waste containers and/or sharps containers. The room should be checked for any blood spills or other contamination and disinfected appropriately. After completing this process, remove the contaminated gloves and sanitize your hands.

Use clean gloves to disinfect the room, including the table, stand, side and back tables, any other equipment in the room, and the floor. Used instruments must be sanitized, disinfected, and resterilized for future use.

Postoperative Instructions and Care

The patient should be given time to rest after the surgery. If a sedative was administered, ensure that the patient does not get out of bed on his or her own the first time. Be sure to assist the patient to the bathroom to ensure that he or she can safely walk. If the patient has been given a topical or local anesthetic, the nurse will explain to the patient that the anesthesia effect will wear off and that some discomfort may be felt at the operative site.

Injury & Illness Prevention Box 26.2

- Anytime a patient has had sedation or anesthesia for a surgical procedure, the patient should have assistance with ambulation the first time.
- Be prepared for the person to fall when he or she goes to get up out of the bed.
- Know where your call lights are so that you can initiate an emergency response system if the patient were to fall.
- Falls have better outcomes if the PCT anticipates it ahead of time and care plan for a safe landing of the patient.

Postoperative care extends for the total recovery period, not just for the time of immediate care after the procedure. Many instructions will be given to the patient in writing. They should be simple in style and easily understood by both the patient and caregivers. These instructions can be preprinted forms for each type of surgery, or a general form with checked boxes for particular postoperative instructions that apply specifically to the individual patient.

Dressings

A dressing is a sterile covering placed over a wound for the purposes of the following:

- Protecting the wound from injury and contamination
- Maintaining constant pressure to minimize bleeding and swelling
- Holding the wound edges together
- Absorbing drainage and secretions

A dressing usually consists of a strip of lubricated mesh gauze, a nonstick Telfa™ pad, or a clear dressing placed over a sutured wound. Gauze sponges may be placed over nonadhering material, depending on the physician's preference. Body cavities or wounds that need to remain open for a time are dressed with long, thin packing material that often is impregnated with an antiseptic or a lubricant; this sometimes is called *packing*. A good dressing must be effective and comfortable and must remain in place. If the dressing covers a hairless area, it may be anchored with tape, but no tape should touch the wound.

Frequently, small, clean lacerations may be closed with Steri-Strips™ (Fig. 26.2). These strips reduce the chance of infection and do not leave suture scars. Steri-Strips are used on areas of the body that are protected from movement and stress. They often are used on the face. Because they are a suture replacement, only the physician should place them on a fresh wound. However, if they are applied after suture removal to provide

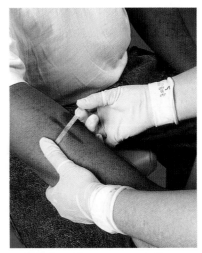

FIGURE 26.2 Steri-Strips on a wound. (From Bonewit-West K: *Clinical procedures for medical assistants*, ed 7, St. Louis, 2008, WB Saunders.)

further support for healing tissues, the nurse may apply them. They fall off once the wound heals.

Bandages

Bandages hold dressings in place and also help maintain even pressure, support the affected part, and help protect the wound from injury and contamination. Bandages can be gauze, cloth, or elastic cloth rolls and are bound by clips, tape, or ties. Dressings and bandages frequently appear easy and simple to apply; however, special skill is required to use different types of bandaging techniques (see Chapter 28). Bandages that are too loose fall off; those that are too tight may compromise circulation and further harm the patient.

Plain roller gauze is seldom used. It is difficult to handle, has no elasticity, and tends to bind. It also tends to slip, because it does not adhere to itself. Wrinkled crepe-type roller bandages (e.g., Coban™) are preferred, because they easily conform to various shapes of the body and adhere to themselves (Fig. 26.3). If the bandage is to cover a wound, it should always be applied over a sterile dressing.

Plain elastic cloth (e.g., Ace™) bandages or elastic roller cloth with adhesive backing makes flexible, secure covers. When an Ace elastic roller bandage is applied as a pressure bandage, especially to the lower limbs, it is essential to keep the bandage consistent in spacing and tension to ensure even pressure. Even, gentle pressure stimulates circulation and healing. Uneven pressure causes constriction points that can create pressure sores, ulcers, or edema.

POSTOPERATIVE CARE

Preventing Thrombus Formation

After a surgical procedure, patients may be at risk of clot formation in their lower extremities, especially if they are on bedrest for an extended duration. One way to decrease the risk of a clot formation, otherwise known as a deep vein thrombosis, is with the use of elastic stockings or sequential compression devices (SCDs). SCDs are sleeves or stockings made of fabric or plastic that are wrapped around the legs and secured with Velcro® (Procedure 26.2). Once they are applied, connect the sleeves to a pump that inflates and deflates the stocking around the leg. Typically, the inflation cycle lasts 10 to 15 seconds, and the deflation lasts for 45 to 60 seconds. Use of the SCDs decreases the amount of blood remaining in the veins and instead promotes the blood to return to the heart for reoxygenation. SCDs are most effective if begun as soon after a surgical procedure as possible.

Elastic stockings (also called antiembolitic stockings) also help to promote venous return and prevent formation of blood clots in the lower extremities (Procedure 26.3). These are specially fitted stockings that are ordered according to the patient's size of calf, thigh, and leg. You may be asked to measure these areas of the patient's lower extremities in order to obtain the correct size stockings. These are normally very tight fitting and should be removed once per shift.

Delegation and Documentation Box 26.1

The skill of applying SCDs can be delegated to the PCT. The nurse is responsible for assessing circulation in the extremities. The PCT should notify the following to the nurse:
- If patient complains of pain in leg
- If discoloration develops in extremities

The nurse can delegate the skill of applying antiembolitic elastic stockings to the PCT. Before delegation, instruct the PCT to inform the following to the nurse:
- If patient complains of leg pain or leg swelling
- If patient has any skin irritation

Also instruct the PCT to direct the patient to do the following:
- To avoid activities that promote venous stasis (e.g., crossing legs, wearing garters)
- To elevate legs while sitting and before applying stockings to improve venous return
- Not to massage legs
- To avoid wrinkles in stocking

Legal and Ethics Issues

Personal discipline for maintaining an awareness of the surgical field is the primary concern in surgical asepsis. Often the PCT is alone when setting up the room for a surgical procedure; if contamination occurs, no one may know except the PCT. It is the PCT's responsibility to

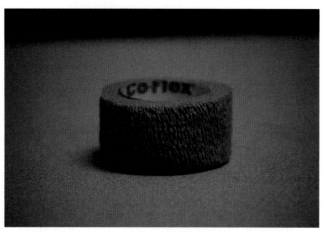
FIGURE 26.3 Koban latex-free self-adhesive wrap.

PROCEDURE 26.2

Applying Sequential Compression Devices

1. Receive the request from the nurse to apply sequential compression stockings.
2. Perform hand hygiene.
3. The nurse may ask you to obtain baseline data about status of circulation such as the lower extremity pulses.
4. Identify patient using two identifiers (i.e., name and birth date or name and account number, according to agency policy). Ask patient to state name.
5. Perform hand hygiene. Provide hygiene to patient's lower extremities as needed.
6. Assemble and prepare equipment.
7. Arrange sequential compression device (SCD) sleeve under patient's leg according to leg position indicated on inner lining of sleeve.

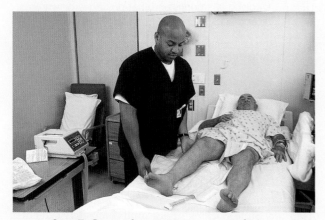

Step 7: Correct leg position on inner lining.

a. Back of patient's ankle should line up with ankle on inner lining of sleeve.
b. Position back of the knee with popliteal opening.

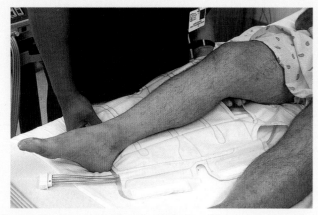

Step 8: Position back of patient's knee with popliteal opening.

8. Wrap SCD sleeve securely around patient's leg.
9. Verify fit of SCD sleeves by placing two fingers between patient's leg and sleeve.

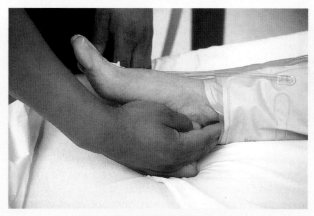

Step 9: Check fit of SCD sleeve.

10. Attach connector of SCD sleeve to plug on mechanical unit. Arrow on compressor lines up with arrow on plug from mechanical unit (See illustration above Step 10).

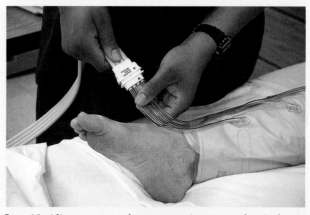

Step 10: Align arrows when connecting to mechanical unit.

11. Turn mechanical unit on. Green light indicates that unit is functioning.
12. Observe functioning of unit for one complete cycle.
13. Reposition patient for comfort and perform hand hygiene.
14. Remove compression stockings at least once per shift.
15. Document the procedure.

(Figures from Potter PA, Perry AG: Fundamentals of nursing: concepts, process, and practice, *ed 9, St. Louis, 2017, Elsevier.)*

PROCEDURE 26.3

Applying Antiembolitic Elastic Stockings

1. Identify patient using two identifiers (i.e., name and birth date or name and account number, according to agency policy).
2. Observe for signs, symptoms, and condition of patient skin that contraindicate use of antiembolitic elastic stockings. Signs and symptoms include the following:
   a. Dermatitis or open skin lesion
   b. Recent skin graft
   c. Decreased circulation in lower extremities as evidenced by cyanotic (blue) or cool extremities
   Notify the nurse if any of these is present.
3. Assess and document condition of patient's skin and circulation to leg and foot (i.e., presence of popliteal and pedal pulses, edema, and discoloration of skin; temperature; lesions; or abrasions).
4. Use tape measure to measure patient's legs to determine proper stocking size.
5. Explain procedure and reasons for applying stockings.
6. Perform hand hygiene. Provide hygiene to patient's lower extremities as needed.
7. Position patient in supine position.
8. Apply elastic stockings as follows:
   a. Turn elastic stocking inside out up to heel. Place one hand into stocking, holding heel. Pull top of stocking with other hand inside out over foot of stocking.
   b. Place patient's toes into foot of elastic stocking, ensuring that stocking is smooth.

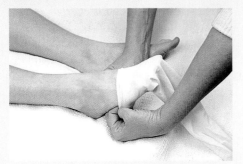

Step 10b: Place toes into foot of stocking.

   c. Slide remaining portion of stocking over patient's foot, ensuring that toes are covered. Make sure that foot fits into toe and heel position of stocking.

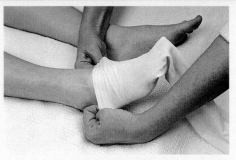

Step 10c: Slide heel of stocking over foot.

   d. Slide top of stocking up over patient's calf until stocking is completely extended. Be sure that stocking is smooth and that no ridges or wrinkles are present, particularly behind knee.

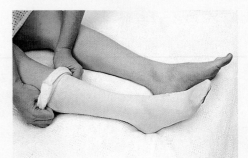

Step 10d: Slide stocking up leg until completely extended.

   e. Instruct patient not to roll stockings partially down.
9. Reposition patient for comfort and perform hand hygiene.
10. Remove stockings at least once per shift.
11. Inspect stockings for wrinkles or constriction.
12. Inspect elastic stockings to determine that there are no wrinkles, rolls, or binding.
13. Observe circulatory status of lower extremities. Observe color, temperature, and condition of skin. Palpate pedal pulses.
14. Observe patient's response to wearing antiembolitic elastic stockings.
15. Document the procedure.

(Figures from Potter PA, Perry AG: Fundamentals of nursing: concepts, process, and practice, ed 9, St. Louis, 2017, Elsevier.)

begin the procedure again with clean or sterile supplies if it is possible that contamination occurred. The PCT's main responsibilities include carrying out sanitization, disinfection, and sterilization procedures with precision and with total effectiveness. There is no room for compromise.

Patients should have absolute assurance that they are being taken care of in an aseptic atmosphere and under the most stringent aseptic conditions. Absolute honesty on the part of the PCT builds self-respect and contributes to professional achievement and satisfaction. Never take short cuts.

CHAPTER SUMMARY

Medical asepsis is the process of reducing the number of pathogens or destroying all pathogens; surgical asepsis is the complete destruction of all organisms on instruments or equipment that will enter the patient's body. Using proper surgical aseptic technique is the primary means of preventing postoperative infections in surgical patients. Everyone on the healthcare team is responsible for preventing and correcting breaks in technique.

Sanitization is the cleaning of instruments and the environment to reduce the number of pathogens. *Disinfection* is the destruction of pathogens by physical or chemical means. *Sterilization* is the destruction of all microorganisms.

Typical minor surgical procedures include I&D of a cyst; electrosurgery, which uses high-frequency current to cut through tissue and coagulate blood vessels; laser surgery, which uses tiny light beams to safely treat specific tissues with minimal damage to surrounding tissues and to limit scar formation; microsurgery, which involves the use of an operating microscope to perform delicate surgical procedures; endoscopic procedures, which use a fiberoptic instrument with a miniature camera mounted on a flexible tube to examine the area within an organ or cavity and which are named according to the organs or areas they explore; and cryosurgery, which is the use of extreme cold to destroy tissues such as warts and skin lesions.

The PCT may be responsible for preparing the patient for surgery; assisting with positioning of the patient; performing skin preparation if ordered; and preparing the room for the procedure.

Sterile surfaces must never come in contact with nonsterile surfaces. If this occurs, the sterile surface immediately is considered contaminated. The rules for maintaining a sterile field include keeping talking to a minimum; maintaining sight of the sterile field; and never crossing over the sterile field. Anything that falls below the edge of the stand and within a 1-inch border surrounding the tray is considered contaminated. A sterile barrier that is wet, cut, or torn is contaminated. Sterile gloved hands must be kept above waist level at all times. An item is never removed from and then again put into the field. A sterile package should be opened the entire way and the contents tossed onto the field without crossing over the sterile area. If a sterile package falls to the floor, it must be discarded. If any doubt exists about sterility, the field must be considered contaminated and the process must start all over again.

Case Scenario

Melissa works as a PCT in the labor and delivery suite. She is responsible for assisting with the setup of the Cesarean section operating room once deliveries have occurred there in preparation for the next patient. Melissa has taken great care to set up the room under strict surgical asepsis. As she walks by the room about 15 minutes later, she notices that someone from her unit has entered the surgical suite without putting the appropriate gown and gloves on. What should Melissa do, knowing that the sterile sense of the room has been broken? It is one of her peers, and she does not want to make her mad, so she is afraid to say anything about it. The friend was only in the room for a minute or so, grabbing a pen she had left in the room during the earlier surgery.

REVIEW QUESTIONS

1. The PCT has just put elastic stockings on a patient after surgery. The family asks what the purpose of these stocking is. How should the PCT respond? The stockings help to _____.
   a. Prevent varicose veins
   b. Prevent muscular fatigue
   c. Ensure joint mobility
   d. Promote venous return to the heart

2. The recommended temperature for sterilization in an autoclave is _____.
   a. 110° to 115° C
   b. 115° to 118° C
   c. 118° to 121° C
   d. 121° to 123° C

3. What are two of the greatest sources of contamination when setting up a sterile field?
   a. Floor and walls
   b. Hands and hair
   c. Socks and shoes
   d. Nose and mouth

4. Where should the grounding pad be placed on the patient for electrosurgery?
   a. Over bony prominences
   b. As far away from the incision as possible
   c. On a fleshy area, such as the thigh
   d. In the patient's armpit area, over their hair

5. Which type of precautions is required for surgical procedures?
   a. Handwashing
   b. Surgical asepsis
   c. Medical asepsis
   d. Contact precautions

Heat and Cold Applications

LEARNING OBJECTIVES

1. Identify reasons for using heat and cold applications.
2. Discuss heat and cold therapy and procedures for each.
3. Differentiate between the benefits of heat versus cold applications.
4. Discuss safety precautions to take when applying heat or cold to the skin.

KEY TERMS

ice collar A bag or pack that is filled with ice that can be wrapped around a part of the body
vasoconstriction Narrowing of the blood vessels
vasodilation Dilation of the blood vessels

HEAT AND COLD THERAPY

Patients who have experienced injury to some part of the body often benefit from the use of heat or cold therapy, or both. The heat or cold can be either dry or moist, depending on the injury, or need, and on the healthcare provider's order. Because the application of heat or cold affects the blood circulating throughout the body, it is the responsibility of the healthcare team to ensure patient safety during this therapy. The body's reaction to heat therapy can include a rapid pulse, faintness, or difficulty breathing, and the reaction to cold therapy includes shivering. Therefore it is important to monitor the patient closely during the administration of heat or cold therapy. The nurse must be able to evaluate the skin integrity of the body part being treated and determine the patient's ability to perceive temperature variations to the body part affected. The nurse will delegate to the patient care technician (PCT) when it is appropriate to use heat and/or cold therapy.

The body can generally adapt well to temperatures between 59° F (15° C) and 113° F (45° C). Typically, patients exposed to temperatures below 59° F (15° C) experience numbness followed by pain, and when exposed to temperatures above 113° F (45° C), patients experience pain and burning. Initially, healthy patients are able to sense these temperature changes, but within a short time, the patient's skin adapts to the temperature, and the patient no longer feels sensations of warmth or coolness. This wide range of being able to adapt to temperature, along with a decreased sensitivity to temperature extremes, creates the risk of injury. It becomes very important to identify patients at greatest risk for developing injuries related to heat and cold applications.

Injury & Illness Prevention Box 27.1

- Older adults and young children are more sensitive to cold.
- Remain with the patient for the first 5 minutes of treatment to evaluate subjective response.
- If the patient response to the therapy is poor, discontinue the therapy and notify the nurse.
- Evaluate skin every 2 to 3 minutes after first 10 minutes of therapy.
- Older adults and young children frequently require more covering for warmth.

Local Effects of Heat and Cold

Heat applications are generally used to provide comfort and to speed healing. Patients with musculoskeletal discomfort, such as joint or back pain, may benefit from application of heat to the area. Cold is normally used to decrease swelling and to reduce pain. Cold is often used for sprains, fractures, and nosebleeds or after some surgical procedures, such as tonsillectomies.

Effects of Heat Application Within the Body

Heat produces vasodilation (dilation of the blood vessels). Vasodilation causes increased blood flow to the area of the body being treated; as a consequence, blood flow to the rest of the body decreases, which can potentially result in increased pulse, dizziness, and shortness of breath as the body works to get blood to those other areas of the body while the majority is being pushed to the area of heat. In addition, more nutrients are brought to the area, which produces an increase in metabolism and tissue growth. In situations in which infection is involved, the application of heat brings more antibodies and white blood cells (leukocytes) to the area to fight infection and speed healing. If heat applications are left in place for more than 1 hour, a heat-conserving mechanism sets in, and vessels begin to constrict, which decreases blood flow to that area. Extended heat application may also cause damage to epithelial cells and produce erythema (redness), tenderness, and blistering. The healthcare provider's order should include frequency and duration of heat therapy, and it may even specify a temperature. The nurse should provide this information to you as the PCT.

Systemic Effects of Cold Application

Exposure of the skin to cold results in vasoconstriction (narrowing of blood vessels). Vasoconstriction decreases blood flow to the area; as a consequence, blood flow to the other organs and tissues increases, which causes the body to shiver in an attempt to produce heat. If the cold application is left in place for too long, or if the temperature is too low, the cold interferes with adequate circulation to the area, and the tissue involved is damaged. Such damage to the skin is often accompanied by a burning type of pain. If exposure to extreme cold continues for an extensive period, the skin could freeze and die, as in frostbite. Again, the healthcare provider's order or facility policy should be followed to prevent complications. The nurse should share this information with the PCT.

Patient Safety

To prevent injuries related to heat or cold application, it is important to know the patient's ability to be able to tell difference in heat and cold temperature variations before application. It is also important for the nurse to check for any contraindications to therapy or intolerance to heat or cold before applying either therapy. The nurse should share this information with you as the PCT before asking you to apply heat or cold to the patient.

Contraindications to heat therapy include any bleeding, because vasodilation increases bleeding; inflammation, which sometimes worsens as a result of the vasodilation; and cardiovascular problems, because heat applied to large areas of the body has the potential to interrupt blood flow to vital organs.

Cold therapy should not be used if edema has already occurred. The cold decreases circulation to the area and prolongs the reduction of the edema. Anyone with impaired circulation or an acute injury in which nerve damage is suspected should not receive cold therapy, because cold decreases blood supply further and increases complications. Also, cold tends to increase shivering, which results in a significant increase in body temperature; therefore patients with an already increased temperature may suffer complications from cold therapy.

Patients who have an altered level of consciousness or are disoriented should be observed frequently during heat or cold application because they are at increased risk of injury from either type of application because of their inability to communicate adequately. In addition, ensure that the equipment being used for heat and cold applications is in proper working order. Equipment must be checked for leaks, and electrical equipment must be inspected for damaged cords or wires before use. It is also necessary to check for even distribution of temperature of the equipment because uneven temperature distribution may suggest that the equipment is not functioning properly. By ensuring that both the patient and the equipment are appropriately prepared before application of heat or cold therapy, the PCT is able to determine the effectiveness of therapy and identify any complications after the application of heat or cold.

Hot, Moist Compresses

When hot, moist compresses are ordered, the solution is heated to the appropriate temperature, gauze or cloth is dipped in the solution, and the damp gauze or cloth is then applied to the designated area. If a wound is open, sterile technique and sterile gauze must be used. Hot, moist compresses increase circulation to the affected area and decrease edema.

To maintain the temperature of a compress, it may be necessary to change the compress frequently or wrap the compress in an aquathermia pad (K-pad), a waterproof heating pad, a piece of plastic, or a dry towel. Moist heat is a better conductor of heat than is dry heat; therefore it may be necessary to lower the temperature settings for moist heat. Because moist heat causes evaporation of heat from the skin, it is important to cover the patient with a blanket and minimize drafts in the room to keep the patient warm, especially for elderly patients (Procedure 27.1).

Delegation and Documentation Box 27.1

Heat and Cold Therapy

In some states, the task of applying moist heat, or warm, moist compresses, may be delegated to the PCT under the supervision of the nurse. When this task is delegated to the PCT, keep in mind that the nurse is responsible for evaluating the condition of the patient's skin and preventing injury to the patient. The nurse should remind the PCT to observe the following guidelines:
- Maintain proper temperature of heat or cold applications.
- Maintain application only for the prescribed duration.
- Check patient's skin for excessive redness and pain during application and to report any such adverse reactions to the nurse.
- Report to the nurse when the treatment is complete so that the nurse has the opportunity to evaluate the patient's response.

The task of applying cold therapy to intact skin may also be delegated to the PCT. Again, the nurse must evaluate the condition of the patient's skin and protect the patient from harm.

Injury & Illness Prevention Box 27.2

Home Applications of Heat and Cold

Heat Applications
- Do not apply heat immediately after an injury; heat will increase bleeding and edema.
- A washcloth or towel soaked in hot or warm water can be used as a moist compress in emergency situations.
- Never put washcloths or linen in the microwave because this may cause a fire.
- Check electrical cords on lamps and heating pads if they are to be used for heat therapy.
- Instruct patient not to lie on heating pads; the heat cannot disperse appropriately and may cause burns.
- Never use the high setting on heating pads.
- Instruct patients not to sleep with a heating pad on; this may increase the risk for burns.
- Use a cloth or towel between the heating device and the skin to prevent burns and skin damage.

Cold Applications
- Keeping gel packs in the freezer at home makes at-home cold treatments easy.
- Instruct patients never to use cold packs designed for use in freezer chests for food or beverages on the skin.
- Suggest using a bucket filled with ice and water to immerse foot, hand, or elbow. Use a bath thermometer to test temperature.
- Freeze water in a plastic foam cup, and use it to treat a sprain or strain. Peel off the rim of the cup to or below the level of the ice, and apply ice in a circular motion.
- A bag of frozen vegetables conforms readily to a body part needing cold therapy for a brief time.
- Put ice and water in a zipper-locked bag to quickly make an ice bag for home use.
- Use a cloth or towel between the cooling device and skin to prevent skin damage.

PROCEDURE 27.1

Applying Heat Applications

1. Sanitize your hands.
2. Explain the procedure to the patient and answer any questions.
3. Ask the patient to remove all jewelry from the area to be treated.
4. Place one or two towel layers over the area to be treated.
5. Apply the commercial moist heat packs.
6. Cover with the remaining portion of the towel (see figure).
7. Advise the patient to leave the heat pack in place no longer than 20 to 30 minutes, off for the same amount of time, and then repeat if needed.
8. Record the procedure in the patient's medical record.

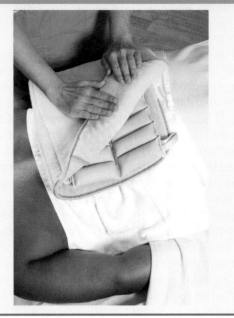

(Figure from Salvo S: Massage therapy: principles and practice, ed 5, St. Louis, 2016, Elsevier.)

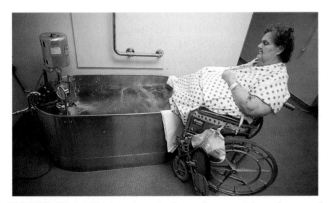

FIGURE 27.1 Whirlpool moist heat therapy. Note the towel placed over the edge of the tub beneath the patient's legs to prevent injury and promote comfort. (From Elkin MK, Perry AG, Potter PA: *Nursing interventions and clinical skills,* ed 4, St. Louis, 2008, Mosby.)

Warm Soaks

Warm soaks are accomplished by soaking a body part in a warm solution or wrapping a body part in dressings that have been saturated with a warm solution. A whirlpool treatment may also be used to apply a warm soak (Fig. 27.1). Warm soaks increase circulation to the affected area, reduce edema, help with removing the dead skin from wounds, and relax muscles, and can be used to apply a medicated solution to large areas.

To administer a warm soak, the PCT heats the solution to 105° to 110° F (40.5° to 43° C) and then immerses the patient's affected body part in the solution. Waterproof pads are placed under the container, and the container is covered with towels or waterproof pads to minimize heat loss. The solution usually retains the desired temperature for approximately 10 minutes; it is necessary afterward to add more of the heated solution to maintain a constant temperature. To prevent injury to the body part, it is removed from the water while the heated solution is added. Upon completion of the soak, the body part is dried completely.

Another form of warm soak is a paraffin bath. A paraffin bath consists of a warmed mixture of heated paraffin wax and mineral oil (Fig. 27.2). Patients with painful arthritis or other joint discomforts of the hands and feet may benefit from these baths. In many institutions, physical therapists administer the paraffin bath, but there are now appliances available for home use. It is important to instruct patients not to allow the bath temperature to exceed 128° to 130° F (53.3° to 54.5° C), to prevent burns and skin damage.

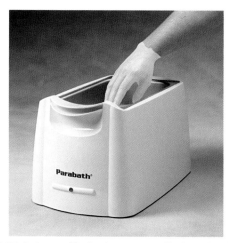

FIGURE 27.2 A paraffin bath is especially helpful for relieving pain in patients with arthritis. The hand is dipped in warm paraffin, which is left on for about 30 minutes and then peeled off. (From Proctor D, Adams A: *Kinn's the patient care technician*, ed 12, St. Louis, 2014, Saunders.)

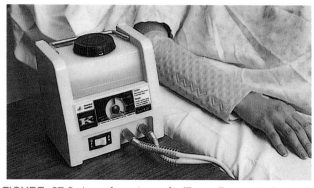

FIGURE 27.3 Aquathermia pad. (From Perry A, Potter P, Ostendorf W: *Nursing interventions and clinical skills*, ed 6, St. Louis, 2016, Mosby.)

Aquathermia (Water-Flow) Pads (K-Pads)

In healthcare institutions, the aquathermia pad, also known as a *water-flow pad* or *K-pad* (Fig. 27.3), is used as a source of moist or dry heat application in lieu of conventional heating pads. Aquathermia pads, which are waterproof, tend to be safer than heating pads because a precise temperature is set by inserting a plastic key into the temperature regulator, or the temperature is preset before use. In aquathermia pads, distilled water is circulated through internal channels in the pad via hoses connected to an electrical unit that houses a heating element and motor.

The recommended temperature setting for the aquathermia pad is between 105° and 110° F (40.5° and 43° C). To ensure proper functioning and safety of the unit and even distribution of water circulation, ensure that the tubing is kept even with the unit and is secured in place. As the water reservoir runs low, the unit is filled with distilled water rather than tap water to prevent mineral deposits from forming in the unit.

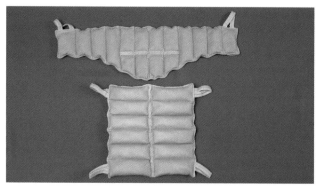

FIGURE 27.4 Commercial hot packs made of canvas that contain a silicone gel. (From Proctor D, Adams A: *Kinn's the patient care technician*, ed 12, St. Louis, 2014, Saunders.)

As with all heat or cold applications, a thin towel or pillowcase is placed next to the patient's skin so that the pad is not in direct contact with the patient. The pad may be secured with tape, ties, or gauze rolls. An aquathermia pad must never be secured with safety pins because those may cause the pad to leak. In addition, patients should not be allowed to lie on the pad because this prevents even heat distribution, and burns may occur. Applications typically last for 20 to 30 minutes. Some healthcare providers may order the application to be applied for longer periods, depending on the reason and the patient's condition. No matter how long the application is on, it is always important to check the patient's skin periodically during the application for any signs of burning.

Dry Heat Application

Warm, dry heat can be applied with commercially available disposable hot packs (Fig. 27.4), electric heating pads, or hot water bottles. With the commercially prepared hot packs, the heat is released when the chemicals contained in the pack are mixed by squeezing, kneading, or breaking the internal container according to package directions.

Hot water bottles are not recommended in acute care facilities, but they may be used in the home setting. If they are used in the home, it is essential to instruct the patient to practice extreme caution to prevent burns.

Heating pads are also frequently used in the home setting but are not recommended for use in acute care or long-term care facilities. Heating pads contain an electrical coil surrounded by a waterproof pad covered by cotton or flannel fabric. The temperature regulation for these units is limited to the choice of low, medium, and high settings instead of exact temperatures. Safety precautions include teaching the patient to avoid lying on the pad, to avoid using the high setting, and to avoid securing the pad with a safety pin, which may cause an electrical shock.

PROCEDURE 27.2

Applying Cold Applications

1. Sanitize your hands.
2. Explain the procedure to the patient and answer any questions.
3. Check the bag for leaks.
4. Fill the bag with small cubes or chips of ice until it is about two thirds full.

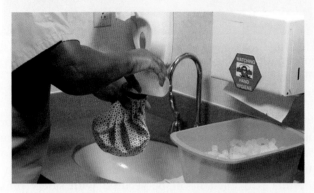

5. Push down on the top of the bag to expel excess air and put on the cap or seal the plastic bag.
6. Dry the outside of the bag and cover it with one or two towel layers.
7. Help the patient position the ice bag on the injured area.

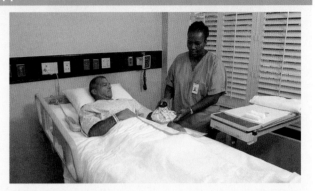

8. Advise the patient to leave the ice bag in place for about 20 to 30 minutes or until the area feels numb, whichever comes first. *(Leaving the ice in place for more than 20 to 30 minutes may cause tissue damage.)*
9. Check the skin for color, feeling, and pain. *(If the treated area becomes very painful, remains numb, or is pale or cyanotic, the ice bag should be removed and the nurse notified.)*
10. Record the procedure in the patient's medical record.

(Figures from Mosby's nursing assistant video skills 4.0, *St. Louis, 2015, Elsevier.)*

Cold, Moist, and Dry Compresses

Cold compresses are typically used to treat inflammation and prevent edema. They can be either clean or sterile and are usually applied for 20 minutes at 59° F (15° C). The procedure for application of cold compresses is similar to that used for warm compresses (Procedure 27.2). A thin towel or cloth should be applied between the skin and the compress, and the healthcare provider orders frequency and duration of treatment.

Commercially prepared disposable cold packs work like disposable hot packs. They are packaged in various sizes and shapes and permit dry cold application. The nurse is responsible for evaluating the patient for signs of complications from cold therapy, including erythema, burning sensation, numbness, mottling, extreme paleness, and cyanosis. The nurse also needs to teach the patient the normal progression of sensations experienced during cold therapy; first cold, then pain relief followed by burning skin pain, and finally numbness. Ensure to apply towels (sterile towels over an injured area) between the cold application and the skin (Fig. 27.5). To prevent frostnip (a mild form of frostbite) or frostbite, remove the cold pack or compress after 20 minutes, and inspect the skin for signs of complications.

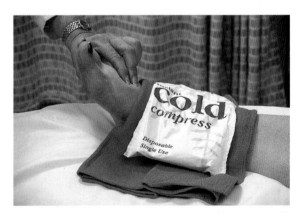

FIGURE 27.5 Commercial cold pack used for therapy. (From Perry A, Potter P, Ostendorf W: *Nursing interventions and clinical skills,* ed 6, St. Louis, 2016, Mosby.)

Ice Bags or Collars

Ice bags or ice collars can be used to reduce edema formation and bleeding and provide a numbing effect to areas of bleeding and bruising formation, as well as for patients who have undergone dental surgery or those with muscle strain. When these devices are used, the PCT must ensure that there are no leaks by filling the device with water before use. The device is filled two thirds full of crushed ice. This allows the device to mold well to the body part, and it does not apply too much pressure on the area being treated. Excess air must be expelled from the device before the cap is secured because conduction of cold is interrupted by excess air in the device. Excess moisture should be dried from the device, and the device is covered with flannel material, a towel, or a pillowcase. The ice pack or collar is applied according to the healthcare provider's order or facility policy. The nurse should provide you with this information before you apply the ice collar or compress.

CHAPTER SUMMARY

Heat and cold applications can be beneficial in both providing comfort, and decreasing inflammation in a patient. The PCT may be asked to apply either heat or cold applications to the patient. Safety is your most important concern when applying either heat or cold, as either one can cause problems and further injury to the patient if left in place for too long. Be sure to follow your agency's policy and your nurse's direction in applying either heat or cold.

Case Scenario

Kaiwan is helping a 56-year-old patient with rheumatoid arthritis who is receiving a paraffin bath treatment for both hands. He did not check the temperature before having the patient put her hands in the bath, and when she puts her hands in, she immediately pulls them out and complains that it is too hot. How should Kaiwan handle this situation? What should he say to the patient? What steps should he take to prevent this from occurring with another patient?

REVIEW QUESTIONS

1. To administer a warm soak, the water temperature should be between what range?
   a. 100° to 105°F
   b. 105° to 110°F
   c. 110° to 115°F
   d. 115° to 120°F

2. Washclothes may be warmed using which method?
   a. Microwave
   b. Boiling water from stove
   c. Heating over a fire
   d. Soaked in hot water

3. An aquathermia pad is used for what type of application?
   a. Moist heat
   b. Moist cold
   c. Dry cold
   d. Ice pack

4. What should be placed between the patient's skin and an ice pack?
   a. Paper towel
   b. Bath blanket
   c. Thin towel
   d. Nothing

5. For what duration should cold compresses be applied to the skin before removing?
   a. 10 minutes
   b. 20 minutes
   c. 30 minutes
   d. 60 minutes

Care of Wounds and Pressure Ulcers

LEARNING OBJECTIVES

1. Discuss the body's response during each stage of wound healing.
2. Discuss the role of nutrition in wound healing.
3. Identify common complications of wound healing.
4. Differentiate between healing by primary intention and healing by secondary intention.
5. Discuss the factors that impair wound healing and the interventions for each type of wound.
6. Describe the purposes of and precautions taken when applying bandages and binders.
7. Identify interventions for the prevention and treatment of pressure ulcers.

KEY TERMS

bandage A strip or roll of cloth or other material that can be wound around a part of the body in a variety of ways for multiple purposes

binder A bandage that is made of large pieces of material to fit a specific body part

dehiscence Rupture of the wound at the incisional line

drainage The removal of fluids from a body cavity, wound, or other source of discharge by one or more methods

epithelialization The formation of new cells during wound healing

eschar A piece of dead tissue that is cast off from the surface of the skin, particularly after a burn injury, but also seen in an ulcer

exudate Fluid, cells, or other substances that have been slowly exuded, or discharged, from cells or blood through small pores or breaks in cell membranes

granulation A sign of healing; soft, pink, fleshy projections that consist of capillaries surrounded by fibrous collagen

incision A cut produced surgically by a sharp instrument that creates an opening into an organ or space in the body

macerated The softening and breaking down of skin resulting from prolonged exposure to moisture

primary intention Wound healing that occurs when wound edges are close together and little tissue is lost, such as those made surgically

puncture A stab wound for a drainage system

purulent Producing or containing pus

sanguineous Composed of or pertaining to blood

secondary intention Wound healing that occurs when a wound must granulate during healing, occurs when skin edges are not close together (approximated) or when pus has formed

serosanguineous Thin and red, composed of serum and blood

serous Thin and watery, composed of the serum portion of blood

tertiary intention A type of wound healing where the practitioner leaves a contaminated wound open and closes it later, after the infection is controlled, by suturing two layers of granulation tissue together in the wound

T-tube A drainage tube into the duct to maintain a free flow of bile

wound Any injury to the body's tissues that involves a break in the skin

The term wound refers to any injury to the body's tissues that involves a break in the skin. Injury results in either an open or a closed wound. This break in the integrity of the skin results in a potential compromise to the individual's protective barriers against outside pathogens, or germs. Prompt assessment and interventions to reduce the potentially negative impact of the breakdown in the skin's protective mechanism are important. Stressors experienced by the individual affect how well the wound heals. Healing is affected by age, nutritional status, physical well-being, and medication therapies. Social factors, including smoking, can impair wound healing. Chronic illnesses, including diabetes, cancer, and heart disease, slow the body's ability to heal. Stress and strain (nausea, vomiting, abdominal distention, coughing, respiratory efforts) place tension against a surgical incision, especially an abdominal incision. During this postoperative phase, the abdominal muscles contract and cause intraabdominal pressure; if the incisional area is weak, dehiscence (or a breaking through of the incision) is possible. Other factors that have the capacity to affect wound healing include preoperative skin preparation, type of surgical procedure, environment within the operating room, and postoperative wound care.

WOUND CLASSIFICATION

Wound classifications are determined based on a series of factors that include cause, the severity of injury, how contaminated the wound may be, and size. An understanding of what caused the wound is very important to determine the proper treatment plan.

In planned surgery, the surgeon makes a wound by incision (a cut produced surgically by a sharp instrument that creates an opening into an organ or space in the body) or puncture (stab wound for a drainage system); the surgical wound is usually closed or managed (e.g., a drain inserted, a stoma created) in the final stage of the procedure. A traumatic injury (e.g., from a knife stabbing) and unplanned or emergency surgeries is very different, because the practitioner brings wound edges together to aid healing. Unless a "dirty surgery" is performed (e.g., a perforated bowel, ruptured appendix where bowel contents are spilled into the abdominal cavity), a surgical incision is cleaner and easier to repair than a traumatic wound.

WOUND HEALING

The healing process begins immediately after an injury and sometimes continues for a year or longer. Although the healing process follows the same pattern, the type of wound and tissue, the wound's severity, and the overall condition of the patient influence the overall process. Wound healing follows four phases: hemostasis, inflammatory phase, reconstruction, and maturation.

Phases of Wound Healing

Hemostasis (termination of bleeding) begins as soon as the injury occurs. As blood platelets adhere to the walls of the injured vessel, a clot begins to form. Fibrin in the clot begins to hold the wound together, and bleeding subsides.

During the *inflammatory phase*, there is an initial increase in the flow of blood elements (antibodies, electrolytes, plasma proteins) and water out of the blood vessel into the vascular space. This process causes the cardinal signs and symptoms of inflammation: erythema (redness), heat, edema (swelling), pain, and tissue dysfunction. Leukocytes appear and begin to engulf bacteria, fungi, viruses, and toxic proteins. If an infection is not present, the number of leukocytes decreases. During the inflammatory phase, cells in the injured tissue spread out, divide, and form new cells. Slowly, blood clots dissolve and the wound fills; the sides of the wound usually meet in 24 to 48 hours. As the inflammatory phase ends, new cells and capillaries fill in the wound from the underlying tissue to the skin surface. This process seals the wound and protects it from contamination.

Collagen formation occurs during the *reconstruction phase*. This phase begins on the third or fourth day after injury and lasts for 2 to 3 weeks. Fibroblasts produce collagen, a glue-like protein substance that adds tensile strength to the wound and the tissue. Collagen formation increases rapidly between postoperative days 5 and 25. During this phase, the wound takes on the appearance of an irregular, raised, purplish, immature scar. Wound dehiscence, or rupture of the wound at the incisional line, most frequently occurs during the reconstruction phase.

Approximately 3 weeks after surgery, fibroblasts begin to exit the wound. The wound continues to gain strength, although healed wounds rarely return to the strength the tissue had before surgery. Although tissue heals at varying speeds, internal wounds (stomach, colon) regain strength faster than skin wounds. Occasionally, a *keloid*, which is an overgrowth of collagenous scar tissue at the site of a wound, forms during this *maturation phase*. The keloid's color ranges from red to pink to white. This new tissue is elevated, rounded, and firm. African Americans, dark-complexioned whites, and young women have the highest incidence of keloid formation.

Process of Wound Healing

The process of wound healing occurs by primary intention (primary union), secondary intention (granulation),

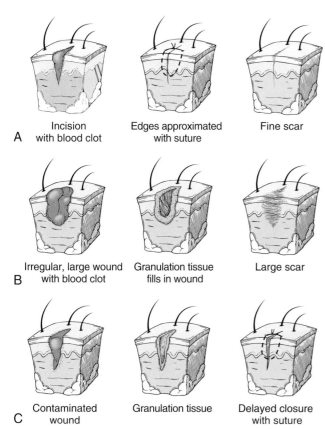

FIGURE 28.1 Types of wound healing. **A,** Primary intention. **B,** Secondary intention. **C,** Tertiary intention. (From Lewis SL, Dirksen SR, Heitkemper MM, et al: *Medical-surgical nursing: assessment and management of clinical problems,* ed 9, St. Louis, 2014, Mosby.)

In healing by tertiary intention (delayed primary intention), the practitioner leaves a contaminated wound open and closes it later, after the infection is controlled, by suturing two layers of granulation tissue together in the wound. This type of healing also occurs when a primary wound becomes infected, is opened, is allowed to granulate, and is then sutured. Tertiary intention healing results in a larger and deeper scar than does healing by either primary or secondary intention.

These stages provide a model for acute (as opposed to chronic), or quicker, wound healing. An important concept in wound healing is that the stages of wound healing, although progressive, do not necessarily occur in a particular order. Some normally healing wounds are in all three stages of wound healing simultaneously.

Factors That Affect Wound Healing

To promote healing, the patient should be encouraged to drink plenty of fluids and to eat a balanced diet. Protein is necessary in wound healing, so that new cells are formed. If the patient is not able to tolerate food or fluids, the patient might need to be fed via a tube or an IV. Patients who are unable to tolerate large meals or solid foods may need to eat small, frequent meals. Supplementation may be needed. Foods rich in protein, vitamins A and C, and zinc assist in wound repair. Sources of protein include meats, peanut butter, and legumes. Dark leafy vegetables and yellow or orange fruits and vegetables provide vitamin A. Strawberries, tomatoes, spinach, and cruciferous vegetables, including broccoli, cauliflower, and cabbage, are rich sources of vitamin C. Zinc may be obtained from fortified cereals, red meat, and seafood. Offer fluids, when tolerated, on an hourly basis. Unless your nurse states otherwise, encourage an intake of 2000 to 2400 mL in 24 hours. As the patient progresses from clear to full liquids, provide fluids the patient enjoys. Until the patient's hydration level is stable (usually 48 to 72 hours), monitor the patient's intake and output (I&O).

Assist the patient to achieve a balance between rest as a means to facilitate healing and activity to decrease pooling of blood in the veins. The location and size of the incision influence the patient's movements. Care should be taken to avoid strain on the suture line. When the patient is on bedrest, provide instruction about the best means to move in bed, moving one body section at a time—head, chest, hips, and legs. To sit up, the patient should roll to the side and, with the elbow as a lever, push to a sitting position; this reduces the stress placed on the incision. If coughing occurs, apply a pillow, rolled bath blanket, or the palms of the hands to the incisional area to lessen intraabdominal pressure; this technique is called *splinting.* Limiting of visitors may sometimes be necessary if the patient tires too easily.

or tertiary (third) intention (Fig. 28.1). Wounds in which skin edges are close together and little tissue is lost, such as those made surgically, heal by primary intention; minimal scarring results. Primary intention healing begins during the inflammatory phase of healing; in surgery, this is usually during closure of the wound.

Healing by secondary intention, when a wound must granulate during healing, occurs when skin edges are not close together (approximated) or when pus has formed. Some wounds develop a purulent (producing or containing pus) exudate (fluid, cells, or other substances that have been slowly exuded, or discharged, from cells or blood through small pores or breaks in cell membranes) when injured or diseased tissue dies. In this case, the surgeon creates an opening for its release through a drainage system or by packing the wound with gauze. Slowly, the necrotized (dead) tissue decomposes and escapes, and the cavity begins to fill with granulation tissue, or soft, pink, fleshy projections that consist of capillaries surrounded by fibrous collagen. The amount of granulation tissue necessary to fill the wound depends on the wound's size; scarring is greater in a large wound.

Preexisting conditions, such as malnourishment, and chronic diseases (arthritis, diabetes mellitus, hypertension) add stress to the recovering body and necessitate ongoing monitoring.

SURGICAL WOUND

The selection of the site for the surgical wound (intentional incision) is based on the tissue and the organs involved, the nature of the injury or disease process, the presence of inflammation or infection, and the strength of the site. If a surgical procedure calls for a drainage system, the positioning of the drain also influences the placement of the incision. The surgeon's goal is to enter the cavity involved and repair the injured or diseased area as quickly and with the least trauma possible. To facilitate the surgery, patients are often placed in positions that add stress to the tissue. Pain after surgery results from strained muscles and ligaments, as well as from the surgical procedure itself, and sometimes caused by how the patient was positioned during the procedure.

Many options are available to the surgeon for closing the surgical incision. Common closures are sutures, staples, adhesive skin closure strips, butterfly strips, and transparent sprays and films. A binder or bandage helps support the incision and/or secures dressings, making use of adhesive materials unnecessary in some cases. A protective dressing is often used to cover the surgical wound for the first 24 hours. It is removed the day after surgery by the surgeon.

Table 28.1	Types of Wound Drainage
Type	**Appearance**
A. Serous 	Clear, watery plasma
B. Purulent 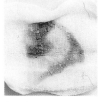	Thick, yellow, green, tan, or brown
C. Serosanguineous	Pale, red, watery: mixture of serous and sanguineous
D. Sanguineous 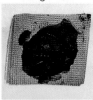	Bright red: indicates active bleeding

(From Lewis SL: Medical-surgical nursing: assessment and management of clinical problems, *ed 8, St. Louis, 2011, Mosby.)*

Delegation and Documentation Box 28.1

- The first dressing on a postoperative patient is always removed by the surgeon, unless otherwise directed.
- Never remove a dressing from a postoperative patient until the nurse directs you to do so.
- Always save any dressing that has drainage that seems excessive or is in a color you are unfamiliar with. Show it to your nurse.

After surgery, the nurse will inspect the dressing hourly during the first 4 hours after the procedure. Then, the nurse will inspect dressings every 2 to 4 hours for the first 24 hours. On the day of surgery, most wounds produce either sanguineous (composed of or pertaining to blood) or serosanguineous (thin and red, composed of serum and blood) exudate. Later, as the exudate subsides, it becomes serous (thin and watery, composed of the serum portion of blood) (Table 28.1). Because pressure to wounds slows bleeding, the general practice is to keep surgical wounds covered with a gauze dressing. To prevent undetected hemorrhaging, the nurse must inspect both the dressing or incisional area and the area under the patient. Exudate follows the flow of gravity; therefore depending on the contour of the body, the dressing sometimes remains dry even though blood or exudate is flowing away, under the body.

Injury & Illness Prevention Box 28.1

- You may be asked to observe a patient's dressing when you are in the room.
- If you ever note blood on the underpad of a patient, notify the nurse at once. Blood flows in a downward direction because of gravity. If the patient has excessive blood under his or her buttocks, the wound may be bleeding excessively.

CARE OF THE INCISION

Surgical wounds, because they are created under aseptic conditions, generally heal well and quickly. For prevention of trauma until new skin growth occurs, and for

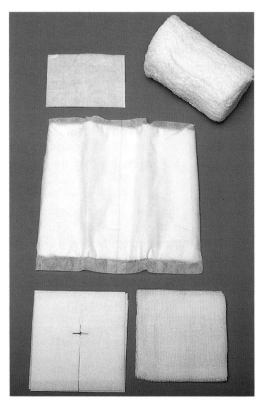

FIGURE 28.2 Types of dressings. *Top to bottom:* Telfa, rolled gauze, ABD, flat gauze 4 × 4, and drain dressing. (From Perry AG, Potter PA: *Clinical nursing skills & techniques,* ed 8, St. Louis, 2014, Mosby.)

keeping bleeding and exposure to bacteria to a minimum, the wound is usually covered at least initially by a dressing. Dressings over closed wounds are usually removed by the second or third day.

Incision coverings take the form of gauze, semiocclusive, or occlusive dressings (Fig. 28.2). Gauze dressings permit air to reach the wound; semiocclusive dressings permit oxygen but not air impurities to pass; and occlusive dressings permit neither air nor oxygen to pass. Occlusive and semiocclusive dressings are thought to promote healing by keeping wounds moist (yet sterile) so that epithelial cells are able to slide more easily over the surface of the wound during epithelialization. Tape, ties, bandages, or cloth binders may sometimes be used to secure a dressing over a wound site. The selection depends on the wound size, the location, the presence of drainage, the frequency of dressing changes, and the patient's level of activity. Montgomery straps, which remain in place around the wound while permitting the dressing over the wound to be changed, are one possibility; they reduce the need for frequent removal and reapplication of tape, which can cause considerable skin irritation (Box 28.1). If an occlusive dressing is used, place tape strips on all sides of the dressing. Otherwise, place the tape strips several inches apart to make the wound accessible to atmospheric oxygen.

Box 28.1   How to Make Montgomery Straps

Use of Montgomery straps to secure dressings helps prevent tape irritation of skin when dressings require frequent changing. If ready-made Montgomery straps are not available, follow these steps to make them:

1. Cut four to six strips of 2- to 3-inch-wide (5 to 7.6 cm) hypoallergenic tape of sufficient length to allow the tape to extend about 6 inches beyond the wound on each side. *(The length of the tape depends on the patient's size and the type and amount of dressing.)*
2. Fold each strip 2 to 3 inches back on itself (sticky sides together) to form a nonadhesive tab. Then, cut a small hole in the folded tab's center, close to its top edge. Make as many pairs of straps as you need to snugly secure the dressing.
3. Clean the patient's skin to prevent irritation. After the skin dries, apply skin protectant. Then, apply the sticky side of each tape to a skin barrier sheet composed of opaque hydrocolloidal or nonhydrocolloidal materials, and apply the sheet directly to the skin near the dressing. Thread a separate piece of gauze tie, umbilical tape, or twill tape (about 12 inches [30.5 cm]) through each pair of holes in the straps, and fasten each tie similar to shoelace. Do not stress the surrounding skin by securing the ties too tightly.
4. Repeat this procedure according to the number of Montgomery straps needed.
5. Replace Montgomery straps whenever they become soiled (every 2 to 3 days). If skin maceration occurs, place new tape about 1 inch (2.5 cm) away from any irritation.

(Adapted from Springhouse: Handbook of nursing procedures, *Philadelphia, 2001, Lippincott Williams & Wilkins.)*

The surgeon may leave sutured, clean wounds undressed after surgery or may use loose dressings. These methods allow oxygen in the air to circulate above the wound, aiding in the healing process. In many cases, if a dressing has been used for closed wounds, it is removed within 24 hours after surgery to allow air circulation. Within 24 hours, enough fibrin has usually been produced at the wound site to stop the entry of microorganisms. In most cases, the surgeon does the initial dressing change.

A dry dressing (as opposed to wet-to-dry, or semiocclusive or occlusive dressings) is often the choice for management of a wound with little drainage, such as abrasions and nondraining postoperative incisions. In addition to keeping initial bleeding to a minimum, the dressing protects the wound from injury, prevents introduction of bacteria, reduces discomfort, and speeds healing. A dry dressing also prevents deeper tissues from drying out by keeping the wound surface moist

1. Healthcare-associated infections are a continual threat to patients, especially the patient after surgery.
2. Virulence of the bacterial contamination and resistance of the patient are two major factors in determining whether a wound becomes infected.
3. Because wound infections usually have an incubation period of 4 to 6 days, some patients are discharged before problems are noted.
4. Exudate and drainage are signs of healing, but accurate assessments sometimes provide signals of potential complications of wound healing.

(www.woundsource.com is a helpful resource). The dry dressing should not rub against the wound. If a dry dressing adheres to a wound, moisten the dressing with sterile normal saline solution or sterile water before removing the gauze. Moistening the dressing in this manner decreases the dressing sticking to the wound and reduces the risk of further trauma to the wound.

Dressing removal may be stressful to the patient. Provide instruction about what will be experienced during the procedure. If the dressing removal is anticipated to be painful, the nurse will usually provide analgesic at least 30 minutes before exposing a wound.

Follow sterile technique whenever handling the wound or the dressing. *Asepsis* (absence of germs) not only protects the patient care technician (PCT) from wound drainage but also decreases the introduction of *pathogenic* (capable of producing disease) organisms into the wound. Use of sterile asepsis lessens the chance of the patient acquiring a healthcare-associated infection (Box 28.2). Use standard precautions when handling body secretions. Good hand hygiene technique and the use of sterile aseptic procedures are essential when providing surgical wound care. Wear a gown, mask, and protective goggles if soiling or splashing of wound exudate is anticipated.

Transparent Dressings

Thin, self-adhesive transparent film dressings (e.g., OpSite™, Tegaderm™) belong in the semiocclusive or occlusive categories. As a synthetic permeable (capable of allowing the passage of fluids or substances in solution) membrane, this type of dressing acts as a temporary second skin. It has several advantages. It adheres to undamaged skin to contain exudate and minimize wound contamination. It also serves as a barrier to external fluids and bacteria yet still allows the wound to breathe. It promotes a moist environment that speeds epithelial cell growth. This dressing type allows for wound assessment without removal of the protective film. Underlying tissue is protected against disruption caused by dressing removal. Film-type dressings are beneficial when dressing sites over joints—allowing for a greater range of motion when the patient moves. Transparent dressings are available with and without adhesive borders. These dressings can stay in place up to 7 days if complete occlusion is maintained. They are unable to absorb large amounts of wound drainage. Monitoring is needed to ensure that the surrounding skin does not become macerated (Jones et al., 2006).

For best results, these dressings are used on clean, debrided wounds that are not actively bleeding. The film is ideal for small, skin-surface wounds and as a dressing over an intravenous catheter site. Nonadhesive transparent dressings fall off as the wound heals. Saline solution can be used to moisten dressings that may be adhering or stuck to the wound bed. Showering and bathing are permitted with the healthcare provider's approval.

EXUDATE AND DRAINAGE

Exudate is fluid, cells, or other substances that have slowly leaked from cells or blood vessels through small pores or breaks in cell membrane. Drainage is the removal of fluids from a body cavity, wound, or other source of discharge by one or more methods; it may occur passively on its own or with mechanical assistance (see the following section on drainage systems).

Exudate and drainage are described as serous, sanguineous, or serosanguineous. Serous exudate or drainage is a clear, watery fluid that has been separated from its solid elements (e.g., the exudate from a blister). Serous fluid has the characteristics of serum. Serum is the clear, thin, sticky fluid portion of blood that remains after coagulation. In contrast, sanguineous exudate or drainage is fluid that contains blood. Thus serosanguineous exudate or drainage is thin and red (usually described as pink) because it is composed of both serum and blood. If the tissue is infected, exudate or drainage is likely to be purulent or brown-green. Exudate or drainage from specific organs has its own particular color (e.g., bile from the liver and gallbladder is green or green-brown).

The type and the amount of exudate or drainage produced depend on the tissue and organs involved. The nurse will treat exudate or drainage in quantities greater than 300 mL in the first 24 hours as abnormal. If you are collecting data on output and note an increase in wound drainage, report it to the nurse immediately. When patients first ambulate, a slight increase of exudate or drainage sometimes occurs. If sanguineous exudate or drainage continues, small blood vessels may possibly be oozing.

Not all surgical wounds drain. If exudate or drainage does occur, accurate assessments are vital. The following exudate and drainage characteristics are important to note and chart: color, amount, consistency (thick or thin), and odor. If the exudate or drainage has a pungent or strong odor, infection is likely. Exudate most likely is contained either in a drainage system or on a dressing. If a dressing is used, you can monitor the amount of exudate or drainage (such as from a Penrose drain) by weighing the soiled dressing (1 g of exudate or drainage equals 1 mL). This may be a task delegated to you by the nurse. Until the surgeon orders a dressing change, never remove the soiled dressings; only reinforce them.

Drainage Systems

Frequently, surgical procedures are performed to remove or repair organs that lie within the body (e.g., gallbladder removal). In these cases, something is needed to assist gravity in removal of drainage from the cavity. If a gastrectomy is performed with an upper abdominal midline incision, fluid collects and remains at the surgical site. To help with drainage, the surgeon makes a secondary incision, or stab wound, close to the surgical incision. The site for the stab wound is planned deliberately. The surgeon's intent is to drain exudate or drainage away from the incision, not toward it. If the exudate enters the surgical incision, contamination and infection are likely to follow.

Several methods are available to facilitate the flow of exudate away from the wound site. *Closed drainage* is a system of tubing and other apparatus attached to the body to remove fluid in an airtight circuit that prevents environmental contaminants from entering the wound or cavity. *Open drainage* passes through an open-ended tube into a receptacle or out onto the dressing. *Suction drainage* uses a pump or other mechanical device to help extract a fluid.

Gentle suction is needed in some surgeries to help gravity move the exudate. A drainage system is chosen to fit the area to be drained and according to the type of exudate and amount of drainage expected. A rubber or plastic drain is sometimes used to remove exudate from the wound and deposit it out through the skin onto a dressing (open drainage system); sometimes it is positioned through the surgical incision or stab wound. The Penrose drain commonly serves this purpose. When it is inserted, a sterile safety pin is placed through the drain to keep it from sliding into the wound. When the surgeon wants a gentle vacuum, a closed drainage system is possible to use. The portable vacuum container (e.g., Hemovac®) is an expandable unit connected by tubes to the drainage site. As the unit expands and creates gentle suction, exudate collects in the drainage receptacle. The Jackson-Pratt evacuator is another type of closed drainage system that uses a bulb to provide the needed vacuum (Figs. 28.3 and 28.4).

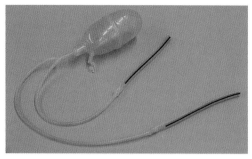

FIGURE 28.3 Jackson-Pratt drains have wide, flat areas that have to be brought through the stab wound with great force. (From Elkin MK, Perry AG, Potter PA: *Nursing interventions and clinical skills,* ed 4, St. Louis, 2008, Mosby.)

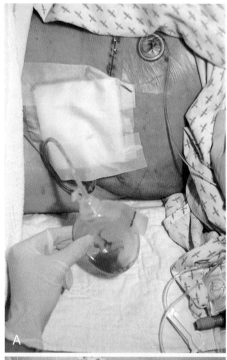
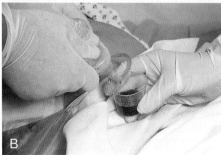

FIGURE 28.4 Jackson-Pratt drainage device. **A,** Drainage tubes and reservoir. **B,** Emptying drainage reservoir. (From Perry AG, Potter PA: *Clinical nursing skills and techniques,* ed 8, St. Louis, 2014, Mosby.)

T-Tube Drainage System

After surgical removal of the gallbladder (an open cholecystectomy), the bile duct is often inflamed and edematous. The healthcare provider frequently inserts a drainage tube into the duct to maintain a free flow of

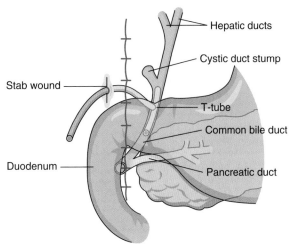

FIGURE 28.5 T-tube. (From Beare PG, Myers JL: *Adult health nursing,* ed 3, St. Louis, 1998, Mosby.)

bile until edema subsides. This tube is called a T-tube. The long end of the T-tube exits through the abdominal incision or through a separate surgical wound (Fig. 28.5). The tube drains by gravity into a closed drainage system. The collection bag is emptied and measured every shift or as necessary.

BANDAGES AND BINDERS

A bandage is a strip or roll of cloth or other material that can be wound around a part of the body in a variety of ways for multiple purposes. Bandages are available in rolls of various widths and materials, including gauze, elasticized knit, elastic webbing, flannel, and muslin. Gauze bandages are lightweight and inexpensive, mold easily around contours of the body, and permit air circulation that helps prevent skin maceration (the softening and breaking down of skin from prolonged exposure to moisture). Elastic bandages fit well to body parts but also can be used to place pressure over a body part. Flannel and muslin bandages are thicker than gauze and thus stronger for supporting or applying pressure. A flannel bandage also insulates to provide warmth.

A binder is a bandage that is made of large pieces of material to fit a specific body part (e.g., an abdominal binder or a breast binder). Most binders are made of elastic, cotton, muslin, or flannel.

Correctly applied bandages and binders do not cause injury to underlying and nearby body parts or create discomfort for the patient (Procedures 28.1 and 28.2; Table 28.2). For example, a chest binder must not be so tight as to restrict chest wall expansion.

After a bandage is applied, document and immediately report changes in circulation, skin integrity, comfort level, and body function, such as ventilation

Check institutional policy and the state's nurse practice act regarding which wound care interventions can be delegated to unlicensed assistive personnel (UAP), such as the PCT. In some states, aspects of wound care such as dressing change are permitted to be delegated. Possibly this includes the changing of dry dressings with use of clean technique for chronic wounds. In this situation, instruct staff on what to report when a wound is cleansed. The PCT must also know how to use clean technique to avoid cross contamination. All wound assessment—the care of acute new wounds and those that require sterile technique for dressing changes—generally remains within the domain of professional nursing practice. The assessment of the wound requires the critical thinking and knowledge application unique to a nurse even when the dressing change is delegated to others.

The procedure of applying a transparent dressing can be delegated to a PCT.

Assessment of wound drainage and maintenance of drains and the drainage system require the critical thinking and knowledge application unique to a nurse. Delegation to a UAP is often appropriate for emptying a closed drainage container, measuring the amount of drainage, and reporting the amount on the patient's I&O record.

The procedure of suture removal requires the critical thinking and knowledge application unique to the nurse. For this procedure, delegation is inappropriate.

The procedure of applying a binder (abdominal or breast) can be delegated to the PCT. However, it is the responsibility of the nurse to assess the patient's ability to breathe deeply, cough effectively, and move independently before and after binder application. The nurse is also responsible for assessing the patient's skin for irritation or abrasion, the underlying wound, and patient's level of comfort.

or movement. When applying a bandage, it is acceptable to loosen or readjust it as necessary. Obtain the direction from the nurse before loosening or removing a bandage the healthcare provider applied. Explain to the patient that any bandage or binder by definition feels relatively firm or tight. Assess any bandage carefully to be sure that it is properly applied and replace soiled bandages. Like a damp dressing, a bandage or binder is a potential harbor for microorganisms (Box 28.3).

Pressure Ulcers

Prevention and treatment of skin breakdown is one of the highest priorities of care. Prevention is the ultimate goal, but when this is not possible, good care can result in (1) healing of the broken skin without complications;

Text continued on p. 517

PROCEDURE 28.1

Applying a Bandage

Steps to remember before performing the procedure are as follows:

1. Refer to the medical record, care plan, or Kardex for special interventions.
2. Provide an introduction to the patient; include name and title or role.
3. Identify patients by checking armband and requesting that patients state their name.
4. Explain the procedure and the reason for the procedure in terms the patient is able to understand; give the patient time to ask questions. Advise the patient of any potential unpleasantness that will be experienced.
5. Perform hand hygiene and don clean gloves according to agency policy and guidelines from the Centers for Disease Control and Prevention (CDC) and the Occupational Safety and Health Administration (OSHA).
6. Assemble equipment and complete necessary charges.
7. Prepare patient for intervention:
   - Close door or pull privacy curtain.
   - Raise bed to comfortable working height; lower side rail on side nearest you.
   - Position and drape patient as necessary.
8. Ensure that skin and dressing are clean and dry.
9. Separate any adjacent skin surfaces.
10. Align part to be bandaged, providing slight flexion as appropriate and not contraindicated.
11. Apply bandage from distal to proximal part.
12. Apply bandage with even distribution of pressure.
    a. For the circular bandage, see Table 28.2.
    b. For the spiral bandage, see Table 28.2.
    c. For the spiral-reverse bandage, see Table 28.2.
    d. For the recurrent (stump) bandage, see Table 28.2.
    e. For the figure-of-8 bandage, see Table 28.2.
    f. Secure first bandage before applying additional rolls. Apply additional rolls without leaving any uncovered areas.
13. Assess tension of bandage and circulation of extremity.
14. During the procedure: Promote patient involvement as possible.
15. Assess patient's tolerance, being alert for signs and symptoms of discomfort and fatigue. Inability to tolerate a procedure is described in the nursing notes.
16. Completion of procedure: Assist patient to a position of comfort and place needed items within easy reach. Be certain patient has a means to call for assistance and knows how to use it.
17. Raise the side rails and lower the bed to the lowest position.
18. Remove gloves and all protective barriers, such as gown, goggles, and masks, if worn. Store or remove and dispose of soiled supplies and equipment according to agency policy and guidelines from the CDC and the OSHA.
19. Perform hand hygiene after patient contact and after removing gloves.
20. Document patient's response, expected or unexpected outcomes, and patient teaching. Specific notes for documentation are included in each procedure.
21. Report any unexpected outcomes immediately to the nurse. Specific notes for reporting are included in each procedure.

PROCEDURE 28.2

Applying a Binder, Arm Sling, and T-Binder

Steps to remember before performing the procedure are as follows:

1. Refer to the medical record, care plan, or Kardex for special interventions.
2. Provide an introduction to the patient; include name and title or role.
3. Identify patients by checking armband and requesting that patients state their name.
4. Explain the procedure and the reason for the procedure in terms the patient is able to understand; give the patient time to ask questions. Advise the patient of any potential unpleasantness that will be experienced.
5. Perform hand hygiene and don clean gloves according to agency policy and guidelines from the Centers for Disease Control and Prevention (CDC) and the Occupational Safety and Health Administration (OSHA).
6. Assemble equipment.
7. Prepare patient for intervention:
   - Close door or pull privacy curtain.
   - Raise bed to comfortable working height; lower side rail on side nearest you.
   - Position and drape patient as necessary.
8. Change dressing if appropriate; cleanse skin if needed.
9. Separate skin surfaces or pad bony prominences.
10. Apply binder.
    a. Triangular binder (sling)
       (1) Have patient flex arm at approximately 80-degree angle, depending on purpose of binder.

Continued

PROCEDURE 28.2

Applying a Binder, Arm Sling, and T-Binder—cont'd

(2) Place end of triangular binder over shoulder of the uninjured side, anterior to posterior.

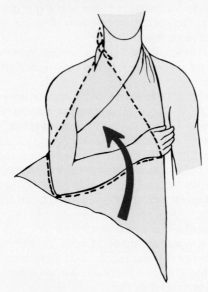

(3) Grasp other end of binder and bring it up and over injured arm to shoulder of injured arm.

(4) Use square knot to tie two ends together at lateral area of neck on uninjured side.

(5) Support wrist well with binder; do not allow it to extend over end of binder.

(6) Fold third triangle end neatly around elbow and secure with safety pins.

b. T-binder
(1) Using appropriate binder, place the waistband smoothly under patient's waist; patient should be positioned lying supine; tails should be under patient.

(2) Secure two ends of waistband together with safety pin.

(3) Single tail: bring the tail up between legs to secure dressing in place. Two tails: bring tails up one on each side of penis or large dressing.

(4) Bring tails under and over waistband; secure with safety pins.

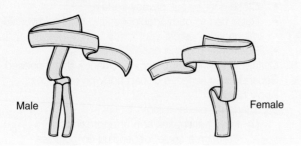

Male   Female

c. Elastic abdominal binder (see illustration)
(1) Center binder smoothly under appropriate part of patient.

(2) Close binder: pull one end of binder over center of patient's abdomen while maintaining tension on that end of binder; pull opposite end of binder over center and secure with Velcro closure tabs, metal fasteners, or horizontally placed safety pins.

(3) Observe patient's respiratory status.

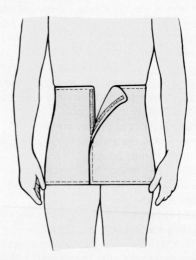

d. For postsurgical application of abdominal binders, proceed upward from bottom (except for a patient after cesarean delivery) to minimize pull on the suture line.

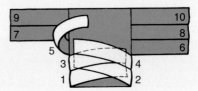

11. Note comfort level of patient. Smooth out binder to prevent wrinkles. Adjust binder as necessary.

12. During the procedure: Promote patient involvement as possible.

13. Assess patient's tolerance, being alert for signs and symptoms of discomfort and fatigue. Inability to tolerate a procedure is described in the nursing notes.

14. Completion of procedure: Assist patient to a position of comfort and place needed items within easy reach. Be certain that patient has a means to call for assistance and knows how to use it.

15. Raise the side rails and lower the bed to the lowest position.

16. Remove gloves and all protective barriers, such as gown, goggles, and masks, if worn. Store or remove and dispose of soiled supplies and equipment according to agency policy and guidelines from the CDC and OSHA.
17. Perform hand hygiene after patient contact and after removing gloves.
18. Document patient's response, expected or unexpected outcomes, and patient teaching. Specific notes for documentation are included in each procedure.

19. Report any unexpected outcomes immediately to the nurse. Specific notes for reporting are included in each procedure.
20. Document the following:
    - Time of application
    - Type of binder
    - Patient's response

(Figures from Potter PA, Perry AG: Fundamentals of nursing: concepts, process, and practice, *ed 9, St. Louis, 2017, Mosby.)*

Table 28.2   Basic Bandage Turns

Basic Bandage Turns	Use
Circular 1. Unroll 3 to 4 inches of bandage from back of roll. 2. Place flat bandage surface on anterior surface of portion of body to be covered and hold end in place with thumb of nondominant hand. 3. Continue rolling bandage around same area until two overlapping layers of bandage cover part. Remove excess bandage roll. 4. Secure end of bandage with safety pin or clip if it is attached to end of bandage. If end of bandage has raw edge, fold 0.5 to 1 inch under before securing bandage. Gauze bandage is possible to secure with strip of adhesive tape.	Circular turns are used to cover small body regions such as a digit or wrist and are used to anchor bandaging materials. 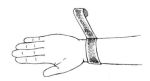
Spiral 1. Anchor bandage at distal end of body part with two circular turns (note steps 1 through 3, Circular). 2. Advance bandage on ascending angle, overlapping each preceding turn by half to two thirds the width of bandage roll until proximal border of area is covered. 3. Secure end of bandage.	Used to cover cylindrical body parts where contour of part does not vary significantly in size (e.g., slender wrist and forearm). 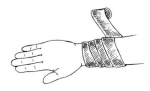
Spiral-Reverse 1. Anchor bandage at distal border of area to be covered (use one to three circular turns). 2. Advance bandage on ascending angle of approximately 30 degrees. 3. Halfway through each turn, fold bandage toward you and continue around part in downward stroke. 4. Continue advancing bandage as in steps 2 and 3 until desired proximal point is reached. Secure bandage.	Used to cover inverted cone-shaped body parts such as calf or thigh. 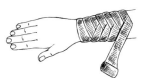

Continued

| Table 28.2 | Basic Bandage Turns—cont'd |

Basic Bandage Turns

Use

Figure-of-8

1. Anchor bandage at center of joint (see steps 1 through 3, Circular).
2. Ascend obliquely around upper half of circular turn above joint followed by turn that descends obliquely below joint.
3. Continue in same manner, overlapping half of previous turn until desired immobilization is attained.
4. Be certain to cover the joint with bandage to prevent fluid shift to those tissues and subsequent impaired circulation.
5. Secure end of bandage.

Used to cover joints and provide immobilization. Outer surface of fabric is against skin during ascending application of bandage. Each reverse turn places alternate side of bandage toward skin.

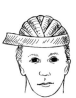

Recurrent

1. Anchor bandage with two circular turns (see steps 1 through 3, Circular) at proximal ends of body part to be covered.
2. Make reverse turn at center front, and advance fabric over distal end of the body part to center back, forming covering perpendicular to first circular turns.
3. Make reverse turn at back and bring bandage forward, overlapping one half of perpendicular bandage on one side. Make reverse turn at front and overlap opposite side of center, continuing on to back. Repeat these steps, overlapping each previous strip of bandage until entire area is covered.
4. Anchor bandage with two circular turns.
5. Secure end of bandage.

Provides caplike coverage for scalp or amputation stump.

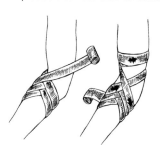

| Box 28.3 | Guidelines for Applying a Bandage or Binder |

1. Position body part to be bandaged in comfortable position of normal anatomic alignment. Bandages cause restriction in movement. Immobilization in position of normal functioning reduces risk of deformity or injury.
2. Prevent friction between and against skin surfaces by applying gauze or cotton padding. Skin surfaces in contact with each other (e.g., between toes, under breasts) are likely to rub against each other and cause abrasion or chafing. Bandages over body prominences often rub against skin and cause impairment of skin integrity.
3. Apply bandages securely to prevent slippage during movement. Friction between bandage and skin can cause impairment of skin integrity.
4. When bandaging extremities, apply bandage first at the distal end and progress toward the trunk (heart).
5. Gradual application of pressure from the distal toward the proximal portion of the extremity promotes venous return and keeps the risk of edema or circulatory impairment to a minimum.
6. Apply bandages firmly, with equal tension exerted over each turn or layer. Avoid excess overlapping of bandage layers. (*Approximately one third to one half of previous layer should be covered by successive*

layers.) Proper application prevents unequal pressure distribution over bandaged body part. Localized pressure causes circulatory impairment.
7. Position pins, knots, or ties away from wound or sensitive skin areas. These materials potentially exert localized pressure and cause irritation.
8. Remove and reapply an elastic bandage at least once every 8 hours unless otherwise directed by healthcare provider.
9. Remove elastic bandage whenever necessary to readjust wrinkles, looseness, or tightness; because of patient discomfort; or when you note signs and symptoms of nerve or vascular impairment.
10. Apply bandages to the lower extremities before the patient sits or stands (i.e., with patient lying down).
11. Use increasingly wider bandages as size of area to be covered increases.
12. Use adhesive tape rather than loose clips or pins to fasten bandages on small child or infant. Safety pins are more effective than clips and do not fall out of bandage. Many facilities prefer tape for safety and maintenance of skin integrity.
13. Patients with tubes or drains who have binders need frequent assessment to ensure patency of tubes for drainage.

(2) a decrease in the patient's pain; (3) a decrease in length of stay in the facility if a discharge is planned; and (4) a decrease in the cost of ongoing care.

Approximately 2.5 million hospitalized patients have pressure ulcers develop each year despite national guidelines regarding their prevention and treatment. Of these 2.5 million patients, 60,000 die of complications, and the financial cost incurred from treating patients with pressure ulcers is estimated at $9 to $11 billion each year (AHRQ, 2011).

To encourage acute care facilities to become more aggressive in the prevention of pressure ulcer development, as of October 2008, the Centers for Medicare and Medicaid stopped covering the costs of treatment of pressure ulcers that develop during the patient's hospitalization, which means that if a patient gets a pressure ulcer while they are hospitalized, there will not be payment for the hospital's costs associated with the treatment of the pressure ulcer. The goal is to prevent patients from experiencing the pain, loss of function, complications such as infection, prolonged hospital stays, and the increased costs associated with the development of pressure ulcers (Medscape, 2008).

Pressure ulcers occur when pressure on the skin causes the blood vessels in an area to collapse. The flow of blood and fluid to the cells is delayed, resulting in ischemia, or lack of oxygen and nutrients, to the cells. When the external pressure against the skin is greater than the pressure in the capillary bed (network of capillaries), blood flow decreases to the adjacent tissue. If the pressure continues without relief for more than 2 hours, cells in the involved layers of skin tend to undergo necrosis (death of tissue). Pressure is usually most severe over bony prominences (e.g., sacrum, scapulae, ears, elbows, heels, inner and outer malleoli, inner and outer knees, back of head, trochanteric areas of the hips, and heels).

In addition to unrelieved pressure, two mechanical factors play a common role in the development of pressure ulcers. The first is *shearing force.* This occurs when the tissue layers of skin slide on each other, causing subcutaneous blood vessels to kink or stretch and resulting in an interruption of blood flow to the skin (see Chapter 18).

The second mechanical factor is *friction.* The rubbing of skin against another surface produces friction, which may remove layers of tissue. This might occur when moving patients in bed by sliding them across the bed linen, when improperly lifting patients, and when improperly placing bedpans.

The appearance of pressure ulcers is a major sign of impaired skin integrity. A patient who stays in one position without relief of pressure, especially over bony prominences, is at risk for development of a pressure ulcer. Patients especially at risk are chronically ill, debilitated, older, disabled, or incontinent and those with spinal cord injuries, limited mobility, circulatory impairment, or poor overall nutrition.

Those who are incontinent are at risk because continual contact of the skin with urine and feces often causes chemical irritation, which frequently leads to impaired skin integrity. Nutritional factors play a role both for those who are overweight and those who are underweight. Obesity increases the risk because fat tissue has less vascularity and resilience, and the added bulk and weight increase the pressure on bony prominences. Obesity also causes increased skin-on-skin contact, especially in skin folds. Underweight increases the risk because of a lack of cushion over the bones and muscles and lack of nutrition to the skin cells. In addition, any condition that results in a decreased supply of oxygen and nutrients to the cells, such as anemia, atherosclerosis, or edema (swelling), increases the risk of skin impairment because the cells are not adequately nourished. Patients who are at increased risk for any reason need careful ongoing assessment and a plan of care aimed at preventing skin impairment.

Delegation and Documentation Box 28.3

Although assessment for the presence of skin impairment is a nursing responsibility and is not to be delegated, UAPs such as the PCT, provide hygienic care in many settings. Therefore be knowledgeable in the following areas:

- Report any changes in the patient's skin condition, such as redness, irritation, dryness, maceration, or discomfort to the nurse at once.
- Provide care to prevent the patient from exposure to body fluids such as urine, feces, wound drainage, and gastric secretions.
- Observe bony prominences (e.g., sacrum, scapulae, ears, elbows, heels, inner and outer malleoli, inner and outer knees, back of head, ischial tuberosities, trochanteric areas of the hips, and heels) for any signs of redness, irritation, or skin breakdown.
- Observe and prevent any areas of pressure from external devices such as oxygen tubing, nasogastric tubing, casts, braces, urinary catheter tubing, or drainage tubing.
- Provide perineal care as needed and observe the area for any signs of skin breakdown. Apply protective barrier creams as allowed by facility policy.

Definition and Staging

The definition of a pressure ulcer was revised by the National Pressure Ulcer Advisory Panel (NPUAP) in 2007, when the staging system of pressure ulcers was expanded from four to six categories. The two new categories include unstageable/unclassified and suspected deep tissue injury. The NPUAP defines a pressure ulcer as a localized injury to the skin or underlying tissue, usually over a bony prominence, caused by pressure with shear or friction. The following sections describe the revised stages of pressure ulcer development. Additional information regarding pressure ulcers can be found at www.npuap.org.

The nurse must assess any reports taken from the PCT regarding potential or actual skin integrity issues. If reddened areas are found, the nurse should assess the area by noting any blanching of the area (by gently pressing on the reddened area with a gloved finger; if the area does not blanch when pressure is applied, injury to the tissue is likely). This finding is documented and reported to the healthcare provider. If actual skin impairment has already occurred, the nurse must measure and document the area according to facility protocol and report the findings to the healthcare provider.

Stage I

A stage I pressure ulcer is a localized area of skin, typically over a bony prominence, that is intact with non-blanchable redness. Skin with darker tones may not have visible blanching, but its color is likely to differ from the surrounding area. The wound characteristics vary; areas may be painful, firm, soft, warm, or cool compared with adjacent tissue. This stage is typically difficult to detect in patients with dark skin tones.

Stage II

A stage II pressure ulcer involves partial-thickness loss of dermis. It appears as a shallow open ulcer, usually shiny or dry, with a red-pink wound bed without slough or bruising (bruising raises the suspicion of deep tissue injury). Some stage II ulcers manifest as intact or open (ruptured) serum-filled blisters. Do not use the term *stage II* to describe skin tears, tape burns, perineal dermatitis, maceration, or excoriation.

Stage III

A stage III pressure ulcer involves full-thickness tissue loss in which subcutaneous fat is sometimes visible, but bone, tendon, and muscle are not exposed. If slough is present, it does not obscure the depth of tissue loss. Possible features are undermining and tunneling. The depth of a stage III pressure ulcer varies depending on its anatomic location. On the bridge of the nose, the ear, the occiput, and the malleolus, which lack subcutaneous tissue, these ulcers are shallow. Extremely deep stage III pressure ulcers do develop in areas with significant layers of deep adipose tissue.

Stage IV

A stage IV pressure ulcer involves full-thickness tissue loss with exposed bone, tendon, or muscle. Sometimes slough or eschar is present on some parts of the wound bed. The ulcer often includes undermining or tunneling. As with stage III pressure ulcers, stage IV pressure ulcers vary in depth depending on their location. Because these ulcers extend into muscle and supporting structures, the patient is at risk for osteomyelitis.

Unstageable/Unclassified

An unstageable pressure ulcer involves full-thickness tissue loss, a wound base covered by slough (yellow, tan, gray, green, or brown), and eschar in the wound bed that usually is tan, brown, or black. The true depth and stage of the ulcer cannot be determined until the base of the wound has been exposed. Stable eschar on the heels provides a natural biologic cover; do not remove it.

Suspected Deep Tissue Injury

During this stage, the wound appears as a localized purple or maroon area of discolored intact skin or a blood-filled blister. This is caused by underlying soft tissue damage from pressure or shear. Characteristics of the area range from painful, firm, mushy, boggy, or warm to cool compared with adjacent tissue. In patients with dark skin tones, deep tissue injury is sometimes difficult to detect but often starts with a thin blister over a dark wound bed. The wound sometimes becomes covered with thin eschar. Even with prompt treatment, some wounds develop quickly, exposing additional layers of tissue.

Interventions

Interventions for patients with pressure ulcers include ongoing assessment and evaluation of improvement. Assessment data include the size and the depth of the ulcer (see Chapter 18), the presence of any undermining, the amount and the color of any exudate, the presence of pain or odor, and the appearance of the exposed tissue. Healing is a long-term process. Interventions are determined according to the stage of the ulcer (Boxes 28.4 and 28.5).

Box 28.4   General Guidelines for Care of Pressure Ulcers

- Never massage reddened areas (risk of further skin breakdown). Massage over bony prominences is no longer recommended. *(Massage results in decreased blood flow and tissue damage in some patients.)*
- Nutritional support, which promotes healthy tissue repair, is likely to be as important as local wound care for the patient.
- Observe the patient's hydration. If it is inadequate or if signs of dehydration (decreased skin turgor and recessed eyes) are present, carefully observe the patient's intake and output (I&O) and monitor fluid replacement therapy as ordered.
- Turn patients who are on complete bed rest or unable to reposition themselves every 2 hours. It is important to avoid the full lateral position, which results in direct pressure on the trochanteric region. The 30-degree lateral-incline position is preferable (see Box 28.5).
- Reposition chair-bound patients every hour. If chair-bound patients are able to shift their weight, teach them to do so every 15 minutes.
- Place patients who are at risk for skin impairment on a pressure-relieving mattress or chair cushion. Doughnut

types of cushions are not advisable because they sometimes cause a congestion of blood to the area, resulting in edema and decreased blood flow to the area. Placement of a rolled bath blanket under the distal extremity helps prevent pressure ulcers on the heel by "floating" the heel (raises the heel off the bed) (see Chapter 18).
- Other pressure-relieving devices to try are therapeutic beds and mattresses. Examples of pressure-relieving beds are low-air-loss beds and oscillating support surface beds. In addition, there are the alternating air mattress and the water mattress.
- Many kinds of topical agents to facilitate healing are available to apply to the wound and edges of the wound. Take care to evaluate the effectiveness of any product used on the ulcer. The nurse will administer these topical healing medications. The nurse should use with caution any products that have the capacity to damage fragile skin and prevent epithelialization (formation of new cells), such as hydrogen peroxide or alcohol.

Box 28.5   Moving Dependent Patient to 30-Degree Lateral (Side-Lying) Position

This move removes pressure from bony prominences of the entire back, but especially the greater trochanters. *(If patient is able to move freely, a side-lying position with upper and lower shoulders aligned is acceptable.)*

Procedure

1. Lower the head of the bed as much as patient can tolerate, keeping head of bed below 30-degree angle. Lower side rail.
2. Using a pull sheet, move patient to the side of the bed opposite the one toward which the patient will be turned. Raise side rail. Go to opposite side of the bed and lower side rail.
3. Assist patient to raise arm nearest you above head, adjusting pillow if needed.
4. Grasp patient's shoulder and hip, and assist patient to roll toward you onto side.

5. Flex both of the patient's knees after the turn, and support upper leg from knee to foot with a pillow or folded blanket.
6. Ease lower shoulder forward, and bring upper shoulder back slightly. Assess patient's comfort.
7. Support upper arm with pillows so that arm is level with shoulder.
8. Optional: Place pillow behind and under patient's back so that it is tucked smoothly against back.
9. Make certain that patient's back is straight without evidence of twisting. Adjust as needed for comfort.
10. Pressure points to assess include the ear, the shoulder, the anterior iliac spine, the trochanter, the lateral side of the knee, the malleolus, and the foot.

CHAPTER SUMMARY

Wounds are described as open or closed. Care of the open wound is determined by the extent of the wound. Maintenance of sterile technique is essential when providing care for an open wound.

After a bandage or binder is applied, document and immediately report changes in circulation, skin integrity, comfort level, and body function, such as ventilation or mobility.

Remove dressings gently to prevent further injury to the wound. Dispose of used dressings appropriately to prevent cross contamination.

Major types of wound exudate are serous, purulent, and sanguineous. The main complications of wound healing are hemorrhage, infection, and dehiscence. Physical stress from vomiting, coughing, or sudden muscular contraction has potential to cause separation of wound edges or dehiscence. Apply bandages and binders in a manner that does not impair circulation or irritate the skin. The best treatment for pressure ulcers is with prevention. Once a pressure ulcer is present on the skin, it is difficult to treat and takes a long time to heal. There are several devices, such as cushions and pillows, that can be used to help position the patient in an ideal position that prevents excess pressure on bony prominences.

Case Scenario

Melissa is working in an outpatient urgent care setting as a PCT. She applied a figure-of-8 elastic bandage to the hand and wrist of a patient who came into the urgent care after a sports injury. She immediately sent the patient home after applying the bandage. She did not document the procedure in the patient's medical record at the time because the urgent care was so backed up with patients to be seen. Discuss all of your concerns regarding this situation. In what ways were safe patient practices ignored? What would be the worst-case scenario for the outcome of this situation? How can this potentially serious situation be corrected after the fact?

REVIEW QUESTIONS

1. Which of the following statements is correct in regard to the use of an abdominal binder?
   a. It replaces the need for underlying dressings.
   b. It should be kept loose for patient comfort.
   c. The patient has to be sitting or standing when it is applied.
   d. The patient must have adequate ventilatory capacity.

2. Which of the following phrases best describes serous drainage?
   a. Fresh bleeding
   b. Thick and yellow
   c. Clear, watery plasma
   d. Beige to brown and foul smelling

3. The healthcare provider has ordered an abdominal binder placed around a surgical patient with a new abdominal wound. What is the likely indication for this intervention?
   a. Collection of wound drainage
   b. Reduction of abdominal swelling
   c. Reduction of stress on the abdominal incision
   d. Stimulation of peristalsis from direct pressure

4. What can be done to reduce surgical wound infection?
   a. Adhering to the principles of hand hygiene
   b. Cleansing the incision from the least contaminated to the most contaminated area
   c. Leaving the incision open to the air
   d. Changing the dressing using sterile technique

5. Which wound drain is classified as providing gravity-assisted drainage?
   a. Jackson-Pratt
   b. Hemovac
   c. Penrose
   d. Wound VAC system

Rehabilitative and Restorative Care

LEARNING OBJECTIVES

1. Identify patients who would benefit from rehabilitation services.
2. Discuss the goals of rehabilitation therapies and restorative care.
3. Describe the interdisciplinary rehabilitation team concept and the function of each team member.
4. Discuss the role of the patient care technician in the specialized practice of rehabilitation.
5. Recognize the importance and significance of family-centered care in rehabilitation.
6. Discuss two major disabling conditions.
7. Recognize polytrauma as a difficult challenge for rehabilitation.
8. Describe the goals of pediatric and gerontologic rehabilitation nursing care.

KEY TERMS

chronic illness An irreversible lifelong disease state or impairment for which disease management programs may offer supportive care, function, and prevention of further disability

Commission on Accreditation of Rehabilitation Facilities A nonprofit, private, international standard-setting, and accreditation body whose mission is to promote and advocate the delivery of quality rehabilitation

comprehensive rehabilitation plan A plan that encourages the patient to reach individual goals through the services provided in the rehabilitation setting

disability Any restriction in or lack of ability to perform an activity in the manner or within the range considered normal as the result of impairment

family-centered care A philosophy that recognizes the important role of the family in the lives of children with disabilities or other chronic conditions

functional limitation Any loss of ability to perform tasks or activities of daily living

gerontologic rehabilitation nursing A specialty practice that focuses on the unique requirements of older adult rehabilitation patients

handicap A physical, mental, or emotional impairment or disability that interferes with a person's normal functioning

impairment Any loss or abnormality of psychological, physical, or anatomic structure or function

interdisciplinary rehabilitation team A team that collaborates to identify individuals' goals and features a combination of expanded problem-solving beyond the boundaries of the individual disciplines, together with discipline-specific work toward goal attainment

multidisciplinary rehabilitation team A rehabilitation team that develops discipline-specific goals, clear boundaries between disciplines, and outcomes that are the sum of each discipline's efforts

pediatric rehabilitation nursing Care that provides a continuum of care so that affected children can become contributing members of society and function at their maximal potential

physiatrist Physicians specializing in physical medicine or rehabilitation

posttraumatic stress disorder (PTSD) A psychological reaction to the experience of trauma outside the normal range of human experience

spinal cord injury (SCI) Any injury in which the spinal cord undergoes compression by fracture or displacement of vertebrae by bleeding or by edema

transdisciplinary rehabilitation team A rehabilitation team that participates in cross-training of their staff to minimize any duplication of effort toward individual goal attainment

traumatic brain injury (TBI) A type of injury to the brain that can result in temporary or permanent damage

Rehabilitative and restorative care attempts to help patients regain any function they may have lost, as well as keep any function they have without losing more. The goals include improving one's self-esteem, dignity, independence, and level of functioning. In rehabilitative care, every aspect of the patient's needs and care are assessed and addressed. Rehabilitation has the potential to be used for all major areas of illness or injury that may cause disability (Smeltzer et al., 2010). Restorative care is the care the healthcare team provides every day that assists patients in their rehabilitation.

Rehabilitation is defined in several ways. For the purposes of this chapter, rehabilitation is a process of delivering good patient care that results in positive outcomes for the patient, delivered by a team of highly trained professionals with the goal of restoring the patient to the fullest physical, mental, social, vocational, and economic capacity of which he or she is capable. Rehabilitation is the process of regaining strength or adjusting to a new set of needs by finding new ways to do the things previously done (Medline Plus, 2013). The underlying philosophy of rehabilitation is to focus on abilities rather than disabilities, to continually make the most of the abilities that remain intact. This means focusing on the positive rather than the negative—focusing on what patients can do versus what they cannot do. The individual, the family, and the support system are the focus of all rehabilitation efforts. Quality rehabilitation will result in the person continually striving to reach his or her highest potential of living independently, or without the help of others, in today's complex world.

NEED FOR REHABILITATION

Rehabilitation is required and valuable in a variety of circumstances. What requires the need for rehabilitation may include one or more of the following:

- Impairment: Any loss or abnormality of psychological, physical, or anatomic structure or function.
- Disability: Any restriction in or lack of ability to perform an activity in the manner or within the

range considered normal as the result of impairment. According to the World Health Organization (Zheng et al., 2011), disability includes loss of the ability to function physically or psychologically in normal activities in work, school, home, or community or social activities.

- Handicap: A physical, mental, or emotional impairment or disability that interferes with a person's normal functioning ("Handicap," n.d.). A given disability may be a handicap for one person but not for another individual.
- Functional limitation: Any loss of ability to perform tasks or activities of daily living (ADLs).
- Chronic illness: An irreversible lifelong disease state or impairment for which disease management programs may offer supportive care, function, and prevention of further disability (PubMed Health, 2007).

It is important to recognize the differences and uniqueness between these terms. In rehabilitation, the individual is recognized to have a disability, and the focus is on the individual rather than on the disability. Thus the rehabilitation team works with individuals who have disabilities, rather than "the disabled."

CHRONIC ILLNESS AND DISABILITY

Although managing chronic illness and disability is one of the biggest healthcare problems facing developed countries, the U.S. healthcare system still has some work to do to provide optimal care for the individuals who need it. The emphasis on acute care continues even though the largest group of healthcare consumers (people who seek healthcare) consists of people with chronic illnesses. In 2012, nearly 50% of Americans were found to have a chronic illness or disability, and the associated medical costs account for 86% of all healthcare expenses (Centers for Disease Control and Prevention, National Center for Chronic Disease Prevention and Health Promotion, 2013). This means that a large portion of money spent on healthcare is for those who have chronic illnesses. The U.S. Department of Health and Human Services (U.S. DHHS) developed a way to manage chronic illness, to improve the quality of life for people with disabilities, and to focus toward health promotion and disease prevention, titled *Healthy People 2020* (U.S. DHHS, 2013). The set of objectives outlines health goals, starting with identifying people with disabilities and reducing the difficulty in accessing needed care (Box 29.1). It takes everyone, including healthcare consumers and the healthcare team, to accomplish these goals.

Healthcare providers must learn to recognize the special needs of the person with a chronic illness or disability and to organize, plan, and provide care to meet these needs. To appreciate the need for a specific, unique approach to planning and providing care for individuals with chronic illnesses and disabling conditions, providers first need to understand the concepts of chronicity and disability.

CHRONIC ILLNESSES

Unlike acute illnesses, which usually come on fast and are limited to that illness, chronic illnesses have the potential to be abrupt or come on gradually and, by definition, last for an extended and unknown period. Patients affected by a chronic illness are still able to function but often with some limitation because of the chronic illness.

SCOPE OF INDIVIDUALS REQUIRING REHABILITATION

Rehabilitation is a bridge for the patient, closing the gap between uselessness and usefulness, between hopelessness and hopefulness, and between sadness and happiness. Many conditions that require rehabilitation can occur at different points in one's life. Living longer in

the United States can mean retiring and enjoying the so-called golden years but also includes a strong chance of acquiring one or more chronic, disabling conditions. Chronic illnesses and the physiologic changes of aging increase the likelihood of physical limitations and disability for older people. Although many families continue to care for older people with disabling conditions in their homes, many also live in nursing homes. Whether an older patient is in the acute stage of an illness or injury or in the community, rehabilitation services are built around helping the patient to maintain functional abilities, ensuring their safety, promoting effective coping, preventing complications, and modifying the environment for maximal independence.

A disability has a number of potential effects on both the patient and the family, including behavioral and emotional changes and changes in roles, body image, self-concept, and family dynamics.

GOALS OF REHABILITATION

Rehabilitation is a goal-oriented (outcome-oriented) process. These goals are personal, and the rehabilitation team individualizes them to meet the holistic needs of each patient served. To determine goals, a collaborative goal-setting process includes the members of the rehabilitation team, with the patient and the family at the center of the process.

It is appropriate to include the following criteria in all rehabilitation goals:

- The goals maximize the quality of life of the patient.
- The goals address the patient's specific needs.
- The goals assist the patient with adjusting to an altered lifestyle.
- The goals are directed toward promoting wellness and minimizing complications.
- The goals assist the patient in attaining the highest degree of function and self-sufficiency possible.
- The goals assist the patient with home and community reentry.

All rehabilitation efforts must be outcome-focused and comprehensive, and must include an educational process.

CORNERSTONES OF REHABILITATION

Rehabilitation involves several important aspects of care in helping the patient meet agreed-upon goals. The following are important factors to keep in mind while helping the patient to reach these goals:

- *Focus on the individual:* All efforts of rehabilitation are centered on the patient's goals and objectives. When the patient sets or holds goals that are not realistic, the team works with the patient in reshaping expectations.

- *Community reentry:* Rehabilitation is considered successful if the patient is able to reenter the community through participation in social, vocational, and recreational activities.
- *Independence:* The goals of rehabilitation focus on promoting and maintaining the patient's physical and emotional independence.
- *Functional ability:* Progress in rehabilitation is measured in terms of functional outcomes.
- *Team approach:* Rehabilitation goals are achieved through the work of the rehabilitation team members, including the patient and the family.
- *Quality of life:* Goals focus on improving the quality of life (how good the patient's life is), rather than increasing the quantity of life (number of days the patient is to live).
- *Prevention and wellness:* Because many problems that require rehabilitation are long-lasting, rehabilitation goals focus on preventing complications and maximizing function.
- *Change process:* Patients who experience a disabling condition or chronic illness experience the change process, as do their families. There are many changes that occur when someone experiences a disability. The rehabilitation team is responsible for directing the change in as positive a manner as possible. Sometimes mind over matter can make the most difference in how the patient responds to the new disability or chronic illness.
- *Adaptation:* Although patients with disabilities do not always accept their disability, learning to adapt to the circumstances created by the limits of their abilities is a positive method of coping.
- *Patient and family education:* Knowledge and skills are essential components of the rehabilitation program. Patients with substantial disability have potential to obtain a degree of independence through patient education, which enables them to direct their own care.

COMPREHENSIVE REHABILITATION PLAN

The more comprehensive the rehabilitation program is, the better the chances the patient will be able to function at a higher level. According to the Commission on Accreditation of Rehabilitation Facilities (a nonprofit, private, international standard-setting, and accreditation body whose mission is to promote and advocate the delivery of quality rehabilitation), it is necessary to initiate an overall individualized comprehensive rehabilitation plan of care within 24 hours of the patient's hospital admission and have it ready for review and revision by the rehabilitation team within 3 days of the

admission. The results of the interdisciplinary admission assessment provide the basis for developing the plan. The patient's individual goals incorporating the unique strengths, needs, abilities, and preferences are the underlying basis of the plan. This plan reflects the environment where the patient will go upon hospital discharge. The goals must be measurable, must be described in functional or behavioral terms (what the patient will do or how he or she will function), and must have associated time frames for achievement, and the responsible team member or members must be listed.

All clinicians treating the patient use this comprehensive plan of care. Your role as the patient care technician (PCT) is to support the patient's rehabilitation plan during his or her time of your care. Evaluation conferences and family conferences take place regularly. You will more than likely not take part in these evaluation conferences, but may be asked questions by the nurse as to how the patient is doing with his or her ADLs. The active participation of the patient and family is an integral part of planning and implementing the discharge process.

REHABILITATION TEAM

Because no one discipline offers the knowledge and expertise necessary to provide all the components of the rehabilitation program, the rehabilitation team is composed of people from multiple disciplines. It may include a physician, a nurse practitioner, a physiatrist (physicians specializing in physical medicine or rehabilitation) (American Association of Physiatrists, 2013), a physical/occupational/speech therapist, a recreational therapist, a psychologist, a spiritual adviser, and a social worker, and it always includes the patient and patient's family. The team coordinates the comprehensive rehabilitation program for each patient in an individualized manner (Table 29.1 and Fig. 29.1).

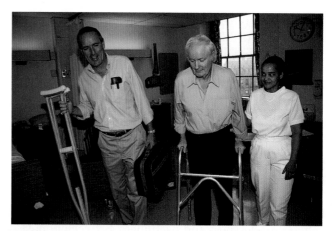

FIGURE 29.1 A nurse and a physical therapist, members of the rehabilitation team, helping a patient with ambulation. (From Leahy JM, Kizilay PE: *Foundations of nursing practice: a nursing process approach*, Philadelphia, 1998, Saunders.)

Table 29.1	Rehabilitation Team	
Member	**Role**	**Actions**
Patient	Key member	Participates in goal setting
		Takes control of own life
Physiatrist	Rehabilitation physician	Is team leader and coordinator of program
Rehabilitation RN	Coordinator, educator	Provides support
		Educates patient and family concerning rehabilitation process
		Promotes independence
Rehabilitation LPN/LVN	Care provider; patient's advocate	Provides support
		Reinforces education to the patient and family concerning the rehabilitation process
		Assists in treatment plan and implementation
Physical therapist	Designing exercise program	Provides therapy
		Assesses patient's needs
		Provides training
Occupational therapist	Assessing independent living needs	Recommends equipment modifications
		Adapts equipment
Speech-language pathologist	Performing assessment of communication and swallowing abilities Designing rehabilitation communication program	Helps patient regain communication skills
		Teaches patient
Therapeutic recreation therapist	Recreation planner	Plans leisure activities
		Promotes patient's interest in activities
Clinical psychologist	Emotional evaluator	Assesses patient's position on the mental health continuum
		Promotes patient's independence by maximizing active participation
		Assists patient in developing realistic positive attitudes
Chaplain	Spiritual consultant	Provides spiritual support and guidance
Vocational rehabilitation counselor	Vocational planner	Helps patient obtain training for new or current employment

LPN/LVN, Licensed practical nurse or licensed vocational nurse; *RN*, registered nurse.

Models of Team Functioning

There are three primary models of rehabilitation team functioning. One model, primarily of service in the past, is the multidisciplinary rehabilitation team. Characteristics of this model are discipline-specific goals, clear boundaries between disciplines, and outcomes that are the sum of each discipline's efforts. Effective communication is the key to success for this type of team.

The type of team most commonly used today in rehabilitation hospitals is the interdisciplinary rehabilitation team. This type of team collaborates to identify individuals' goals and features a combination of expanded problem-solving beyond the boundaries of the individual disciplines, together with discipline-specific work toward goal attainment.

A third type of team is the transdisciplinary rehabilitation team. What characterizes this model is the blurring of boundaries between disciplines, as well as cross-training and flexibility to minimize any duplication of effort toward individual goal attainment. The roles of each member are not necessarily unique to that particular staff member; rather, each person is trained in providing the care regardless of the role he or she serves.

Major strengths of the team methods of care delivery are that they are well established, promote good communication and collaboration among disciplines, address comprehensive aspects of care, energize staff, and view the patient holistically. Each of the models provides a structure for rehabilitation, and it is still necessary to integrate services to ensure a comprehensive, appropriate experience. The PCT may play an active role in the rehabilitation of the team depending on the setting and type of facility.

Rehabilitation Nurse

The rehabilitation nurse with diverse expertise in various roles and work settings plays a vital, unique role on this team. Rehabilitation nurses are with the patient on a 24-hour basis. Because of this constant exposure, nurses can note small changes. It is necessary for rehabilitation nurses to have broad knowledge of the pathophysiology of a wide range of medical-surgical conditions and highly specialized knowledge and skills regarding rehabilitation.

In addition to a set of specialized knowledge and skills, rehabilitation nursing requires an attitude of believing that one can achieve progress toward a goal rather than focusing strictly on one's limitations. In rehabilitation, the work is predicated on the belief that individuals with functional disabilities or chronic illnesses have an intrinsic worth that transcends the disability or illness. William Barclay put it this way:

One of the highest of human duties is the duty of encouragement. … It is easy to laugh at men's ideals; it is easy to pour cold water on their enthusiasm; it is easy to discourage others. The world is full of discouragers. … We have a duty to encourage one another. Many a time a word of praise or thanks has kept a man on his feet. Blessed is the man who speaks such a word.

Rehabilitation nurses are obliged to offer encouragement regularly. The role of a rehabilitation nurse is to put the individual in charge of his or her own care rather than taking charge.

The Association of Rehabilitation Nurses (2014) gives the following definition related to rehabilitation nursing:

Rehabilitation nursing is the diagnosis and treatment of human responses of individuals and groups to actual or potential health problems relative to altered functional ability and lifestyle. The goal of rehabilitation nursing is to assist the individual who has a disability and/or chronic illness in restoring, maintaining, and promoting his or her maximal health. This includes preventing chronic illness and disability.

Specialized training is necessary to become an effective team member. Many facilities have specific units that are dedicated for rehabilitation. The care you provide on this unit may be very different from the care you would provide on an acute-care, medical/surgical type of unit.

Rehabilitation is practiced in a variety of settings across the continuum of care: primary care clinics, home health agencies, outpatient services, hospitals and rehabilitation facilities, skilled nursing facilities, subacute or transitional care facilities, residential facilities, day care agencies, insurance companies, and private companies.

The focus in rehabilitation is on enabling the patient to move from a totally dependent state to a level of independence. Extensive family and patient education, modern adaptive equipment, numerous community integration activities, specialized programs, and professional, effective team therapies all combine to help patients learn to make the most of their lives.

Basic rehabilitation can be used whether the patient is suffering from arthritis, multiple sclerosis, mental illness, brain attack or stroke, spinal cord injury (SCI), burn, or traumatic brain injury (TBI). The PCT's responsibility is to apply appropriate concepts and techniques throughout the continuum of care. All basic care measures are essential; these include position changes and maintaining body alignment, which prevent skeletal and muscular deformities (contractures) and pressure ulcers.

Rehabilitation is a challenge that requires knowledge, teamwork, coordination, planning, and patience. To care for people with disabilities, it is important for rehabilitation professionals to learn and stay informed of current knowledge and techniques.

Assessment

The nurse begins to develop a plan of care for the patient by assessing the ability of the patient to perform ADLs in a safe manner; this assessment helps the nurse determine the patient's level of independence. This assessment is best performed through observation of the patient completing different basic tasks, such as ambulation and bathing. Observation of the abilities or disabilities of the patient provides information on which to base the plan of care. Additional areas to observe include ability of the patient to dress himself or herself, including fastening clothing, and self-feeding ability, including holding of the utensils and chewing and swallowing food and liquids. The PCT will assist the patient in carrying out these tasks according to the patient's ability to do so.

FAMILY AND FAMILY-CENTERED CARE

Family-centered care is a philosophy that recognizes the important role of the family in the lives of patients with disabilities or other chronic conditions. It is a philosophy in which healthcare providers strive to support families in their natural caregiving roles by building on the family's unique strengths as individuals. This means that the healthcare team promotes normal patterns of living at home and in the community, and families and professionals are viewed as equals in a partnership striving for excellence at all levels of healthcare. The ability and willingness of healthcare providers to share knowledge of health resources with families, encouraging them to act as supporters for themselves and their family members, is an important part of family-centered care.

Collaboration and communication between family and professional is essential for providing appropriate and optimal care.

It is a process that will differ according to variations in situations, families, cultures, healthcare settings, and providers. Family-centered care requires learning new ways of relating to and working with families, in rehabilitation and throughout the continuum of care.

CROSS-CULTURAL REHABILITATION

Society is in a state of transformation. Many countries are experiencing considerable shifts across an increasingly wide range of ethnic identification, religions, material reality, beliefs, and behaviors, all leading to rich diversity and cultural complexity. At the same time, health professionals, including rehabilitation teams, are becoming much more aware of the need to become culturally knowledgeable in order to be effective in their interaction with patients.

Rehabilitation team members must engage in genuine collaboration with patients and colleagues, including community-level workers and those trained in other disciplines, in order to obtain the best possible functional outcome for the patient. Disability exists in all societies, but the definition and significance of disability in an individual culture depends on that culture's values. Attitudes also vary toward individuals with a disability; toward concepts of rehabilitation; toward the sociocultural, biologic, and economic implications of disability; and toward policy affecting individuals with a disability.

Cultural competence includes recognizing and including—at all levels—the importance of culture, the assessment of diverse populations with varying cultural differences, and the adaptation of services to meet culturally unique needs (Cultural Competency Advisory Group, 2009).

The following describes a culturally competent healthcare team member:

- Has the capacity for cultural assessment of one's own cultural values and beliefs
- Provides healthcare that is sensitive to the culture and values of the patient
- Is conscious of the dynamics of difference between the cultural groups
- Adapts to diversity in race, color, ethnicity, national origin, immigration status, religion, age, gender, sexual orientation, political beliefs, social and economic status, education, occupation, spirituality, and any other differences (Cultural Competency Advisory Group, 2009).

ISSUES IN REHABILITATION

In rehabilitation, sometimes there are issues that affect the delivery of care. The issues involved include but are not limited to the following:

- *Quality of life versus quantity of life:* Rehabilitation focuses on continually improving the quality of the person's life, not merely maintaining life itself for more days or years.
- *Care versus cure:* Because of the suddenness and catastrophic effect of many conditions that necessitate rehabilitation, it is necessary to consider the care of the individual in relation to the cure of the condition. Many conditions are irreversible; therefore the focus

of care is on adapting and accepting an altered life rather than resolving an illness.
- *High cost of interdisciplinary care versus long-term care:* Rehabilitation is expensive, mainly because the care is delivered by a team of highly trained professionals. Studies of resource allocation have shown that starting rehabilitation early saves thousands of dollars and increases the chance that the patient will be able to live independently and return to the workforce, thereby eliminating the expense of a caregiver or residential long-term care (Lipshutz et al., 2012; American Physical Therapy Association, 2014). In some cases, the success of rehabilitation is viewed as a person's return to productive employment; in other cases, a disability means that two people become unemployed: the individual with the disability and the caregiver. Rehabilitation in this scenario can be successful, and the savings still considerable, if the individual with the disability becomes independent enough to not require a caregiver even though he or she remains unable to return to work.

CHRONIC CONDITIONS REQUIRING REHABILITATION THERAPY

Cardiac Rehabilitation

Many patients who have experienced a cardiac event, such as a myocardial infarction (heart attack) or cardiac surgery, require rehabilitation in order to return to normal activities (Rosdahl and Kowalski, 2012). A cardiac rehabilitation program is designed to meet the needs of the patient through exercise, education about heart-healthy living, and counseling in stress reduction in an effort to reduce modifiable risk factors associated with cardiac disease and to prevent future hospitalizations (National Heart, Lung, and Blood Institute, 2013). The rehabilitation team evaluates baseline levels of physical fitness and develops an individualized program. The focus is also on improving the patient's emotional adaptation to the cardiac condition and related limitations.

Pulmonary Rehabilitation

Patients with chronic breathing problems, such as chronic obstructive pulmonary disease (COPD), and those who require or have just recently undergone lung surgery may benefit from pulmonary rehabilitation. This type of rehabilitation includes an exercise program; counseling regarding diet and nutrition; education regarding the lung disease process; and management, energy conservation techniques, and breathing strategies (National Heart, Lung, and Blood Institute, 2010). The program may be located in the hospital or offered on an outpatient basis in the community. Home-based

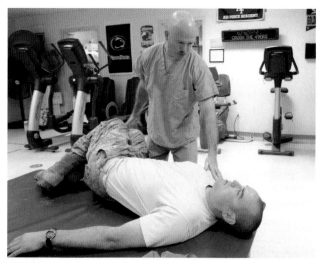

FIGURE 29.2 Wounded army veteran receiving rehabilitative nursing care. (U.S. Army photo by Spc. Cody Barber/Released.)

services are common. Healthcare team members involved in pulmonary rehabilitation include physicians, nurses, respiratory therapists, physical and occupational therapists, dietitians, and nutritionists. Social services may also be represented (National Heart, Lung, and Blood Institute, 2010).

Polytrauma and Rehabilitation Nursing

Soldiers wounded in the war or in conflict, including those in Iraq and Afghanistan, brought about challenges to today's healthcare system. These soldiers experience multiple traumas, a phenomenon known as polytrauma–blast-related injury (PT/BRI), as a result of explosions. Rehabilitative nurses in the military and in the Veterans Administration have responded to these challenges (Fig. 29.2).

Blast-related injuries are categorized as primary, secondary, tertiary, or quaternary (miscellaneous) (Pennardt, 2011). Air-filled cavities in the body (ears, lungs, and gastrointestinal tract) and organs covered with fluid (brain and spinal cord) are most likely to suffer from compression damage from high-explosive blasts. These injuries are considered primary blast-related injuries (Pennardt, 2011). Injuries from airborne debris, bomb fragments, and shrapnel embedded in any body part are considered secondary blast-related injuries. Any injury sustained from being thrown as the result of an explosive shock wave or dynamic overpressure is a tertiary blast-related injury; examples include broken bones and traumatic head and spinal cord injuries. Inhalation of and exposure to toxic chemicals, traumatic amputations of limbs, and burns are examples of quaternary injuries (Nelson, 2008).

In an effort to deal more effectively with PT/BRI, medical treatment for these soldiers is focusing on postacute care with the goal of reducing disabilities associated with these injuries (Rosenfeld and Ford, 2013). The rehabilitation teams for soldiers who have experienced PT/BRI gear their care toward discovering and treating additional injuries that were not detected during the postacute phase, as well as treating those originally identified injuries (Rosenfeld and Ford, 2013). The earlier the injuries are identified, the more successful treatment outcomes are and the lower the costs incurred during treatment are (Rosenfeld and Ford, 2013).

It is important to understand, identify, and treat PT/BRIs in order to avoid focusing care solely on the more visible injuries. Identification of this newly identified group of injuries allows successful treatment of a variety of conditions, ranging from concussions that cause cognitive and vestibular deficits to posttraumatic stress disorder (Rosenfeld and Ford, 2013).

Posttraumatic Stress Disorder

Posttraumatic stress disorder (PTSD) is defined as a psychological reaction to the experience of trauma outside the normal range of human experience (Mayo Clinic, 2011). Studies indicate that an estimated 7.7 million Americans are affected by PTSD (National Institute of Mental Health, n.d.).

The American Psychiatric Association first identified PTSD in 1980. Before 1980, the field described soldiers who experienced the symptoms now known as PTSD as suffering from "shell shock" or "war neurosis" (Glass, 1969), and many people believed that affected soldiers were making up the symptoms in order to avoid being involved in further combat (Clark, 1997). After the Vietnam War, PTSD received acceptance as a psychiatric diagnosis, and other forms of trauma, such as rape and natural disasters, were also identified as causes of PTSD (American Psychiatric Association, 1980).

Events such as the September 11, 2001, terrorist attacks in the United States, Operation Iraqi Freedom, and Hurricane Katrina have again brought attention to PTSD in survivors. However, the veracity of the disorder still raises doubt among some family members and healthcare providers. PTSD diagnosis is dependent on the identification of a traumatic event—a historical event such as a hurricane, a tornado, or a bombing—that is different from a painful stressor, such as a personal event (Mayo Clinic, 2011).

There are effective treatments for PTSD, intense therapy and use of medications being the most common forms. Studies have shown that a combination of cognitive and prolonged-exposure therapy (brain training) is the most effective in treating the disorder, sometimes with the aid of medications such as antidepressants (National Center for PTSD, 2013).

For the PCT on the rehabilitation team, it is important to be aware that other psychological conditions often go along with PTSD. The PCT plays a critical supportive role during rehabilitation in assisting the patient to adapt or regain control over the symptoms of PTSD (Rehabilitation Institute of Chicago, 2013). Through early assessment of PTSD symptoms and the use of therapeutic communication, PCTs are able to assist patients in achieving the goal of treatment. Therapeutic communication techniques include listening, normalizing responses, and working to develop trust in the healthcare team member–patient relationship. PCTs should also be aware of their own reactions, emotions, and communication skills when caring for trauma victims. If the PCT is feeling overwhelmed, he or she may need to consult with a mental healthcare provider.

DISABILITY

The Americans with Disabilities Act became law in 1990. This landmark legislation provides protection against discrimination for people with disabilities. Universally accepted, the Americans with Disabilities Act defines an individual as disabled if he or she has a physical or mental impairment that substantially limits one or more major life activities, has a record of such an impairment, or is regarded as having such an impairment.

As is the case with chronic illness, it is important to recognize that having a disability is just one of many changes of the normal human experience. It is crucial to develop a level of awareness to avoid labeling groups of people in ways that risks giving them care that is less than the best.

People with disabilities are not defined by their illness or their disability. They are complex individuals with unique combinations of skills, and you must identify them as such. The basis for planning care that promotes health and positively affects the quality of life is a holistic, person-first approach in which the shared experience of being human, along with the uniqueness of the individual, is honored and the strengths, as well as impairments, are recognized.

Furthermore, providers are called on to offer interventions that address the need of people with chronic illnesses or disabilities to develop personally within the context of that illness or disability.

The following sections concern two of the major conditions for which dedicated rehabilitation efforts are necessary.

Spinal Cord Injuries

A spinal cord injury (SCI) is any injury in which the spinal cord undergoes compression by fracture or displacement of vertebrae, by bleeding, or by edema. Injury at each level has its unique characteristics, but in general, the higher the injury point is, the greater is the loss of function. The body parts and the functions located above the injury point continue to operate as they should. Injury to the spinal cord is irreversible in that the cord is unable to repair itself. Spinal function is sometimes present below the level of the lesion. In general, however, the effects of an injured spinal cord include paralysis, loss of normal bowel and bladder function, and loss of sensation (Fig. 29.3). Terminology associated with SCI includes, but is not limited to, the following:

- *Complete injury:* No motor or sensory function below the level of injury
- *Incomplete injury:* Some or all motor or sensory function below the level of injury
- *Quadriplegia:* Damage to the cervical spine or the neck that involves weakness or paralysis in all four extremities
- *Paraplegia:* Damage below the cervical area that involves weakness or paralysis in the trunk and lower extremities
- *Paresis:* A slight paralysis, incomplete loss of muscular power, or weakness of a limb

SCIs are categorized as follows:

- *Cervical cord injury:* Level of injury is at the cervical spine (C2 to C7) and involves paralysis of all extremities and trunk, respiratory failure, bladder and bowel disturbance, bradycardia, perspiration, elevated temperature, and headache.
- *Thoracic cord injury:* Level of injury is at the thoracic spine (T1 to T12) and involves paralysis of lower extremities. Initially after the injury, muscles are flaccid (weak, soft, flabby, lacking normal muscle tone) and later become spastic (having spasms or other uncontrolled contractions of the skeletal muscles). Other potential symptoms are paralysis of bladder, bowel, and sphincters; pain in chest or back; abdominal distention; and loss of sexual function.
- *Lumbar cord injury:* Level of injury is at the lumbar spine (L1 to L2) with paralysis of lower extremities, bladder, and rectum and loss of sexual function.

SCIs occur mainly as a result of traumatic accidents, and the individuals paralyzed are primarily young men. Because of improved emergency and medical care techniques, typical patients are more likely to survive the injury. Most of these patients are young enough that they have the potential to work. Injury level and the extent of damage to the spinal cord largely determine functional disabilities. Functional limitations occur in nearly every aspect of an individual's life after an SCI.

The effect of SCI on the individual remains one of the most compelling challenges in the field of rehabilitation. Patients with SCI often require considerable motivation and reeducation to regain a satisfying quality of life and to ensure community reintegration. Crucial for rehabilitation is the effort of an interdisciplinary team whose

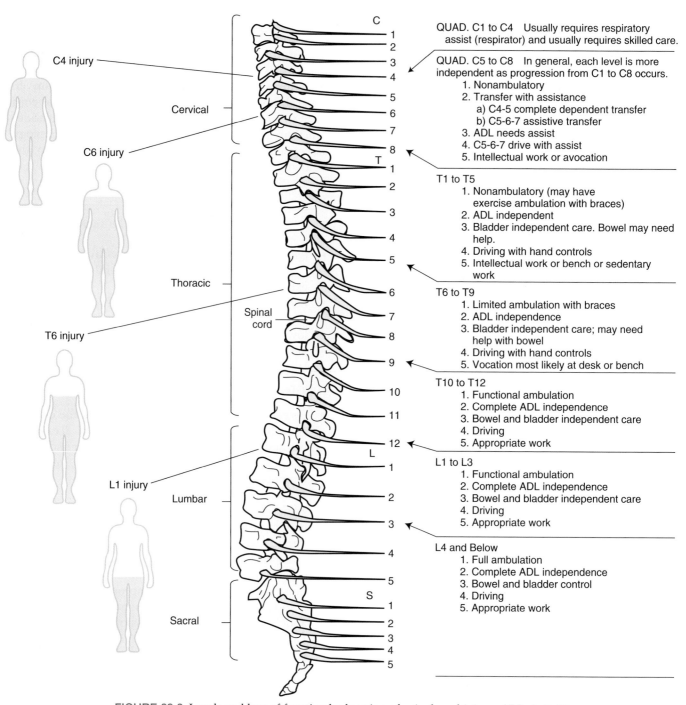

C4 injury

C6 injury

T6 injury

L1 injury

Cervical

Thoracic

Spinal
cord

Lumbar

Sacral

C
1
2
3
4
5
6
7
8
T
1
2
3
4
5
6
7
8
9
10
11
12
L
1
2
3
4
5
S
1
2
3
4
5

QUAD. C1 to C4   Usually requires respiratory
assist (respirator) and usually requires skilled care.

QUAD. C5 to C8   In general, each level is more
independent as progression from C1 to C8 occurs.
1. Nonambulatory
2. Transfer with assistance
   a) C4-5 complete dependent transfer
   b) C5-6-7 assistive transfer
3. ADL needs assist
4. C5-6-7 drive with assist
5. Intellectual work or avocation

T1 to T5
1. Nonambulatory (may have
   exercise ambulation with braces)
2. ADL independent
3. Bladder independent care. Bowel may need
   help.
4. Driving with hand controls
5. Intellectual work or bench or sedentary
   work

T6 to T9
1. Limited ambulation with braces
2. ADL independence
3. Bladder independent care; may need
   help with bowel
4. Driving with hand controls
5. Vocation most likely at desk or bench

T10 to T12
1. Functional ambulation
2. Complete ADL independence
3. Bowel and bladder independent care
4. Driving
5. Appropriate work

L1 to L3
1. Functional ambulation
2. Complete ADL independence
3. Bowel and bladder independent care
4. Driving
5. Appropriate work

L4 and Below
1. Full ambulation
2. Complete ADL independence
3. Bowel and bladder control
4. Driving
5. Appropriate work

FIGURE 29.3 Levels and loss of function by location of spinal cord injury. *ADL,* Activities of daily living. (From Cooper K, Gosnell K: *Foundations of nursing,* ed 7, St. Louis, 2015, Mosby.)

members work together to meet the specific needs of both the patient and the family.

Traumatic Brain Injuries

Every year an estimated 2 million Americans suffer from traumatic brain injury (TBI), ranging in nature from mild concussion to the more devastating kind that renders injured people comatose for the remainder of

their life. Although some people are fortunate enough to return to their previous functioning level shortly after their injury, statistics related to TBI are rather depressing. Of the 75,000 to 100,000 people who die each year from TBI, many are children and young adults. Of the individuals who do survive, 500,000 receive injuries severe enough to necessitate hospitalization, and 90,000 of the injuries result in severe and permanent disability (www.cdc.gov). Most brain-related disabilities, including physical, cognitive, and psychosocial difficulties, necessitate at least 5 to 10 years of difficult and painful rehabilitation; many affected patients require lifelong treatment and attention. When these statistics expand to include families of individuals with brain injuries, the number of people whose lives are forever altered by TBI rises to staggering proportions.

The primary goal of the rehabilitation professional treating the survivor of brain injury is to restore the patient to the highest possible level of independent functioning.

Head injuries are classified as either penetrating or closed-head injuries. In penetrating injuries, an object lacerates the scalp, fractures the skull, and injures the soft tissue in its path, thus destroying nerve cells. In a closed-head injury, some application of force causes the brain to collide with an inner surface of the skull. There is often violent twisting action, which causes the upper section of the brain to rotate while the lower end remains securely anchored in a stationary, or still position. This results in widespread damage throughout the brain. Brain injuries are also possible as a result of other traumas (e.g., electrocution, drug overdose).

Brain injuries are classified as *mild, moderate, severe,* or *catastrophic*. Brief or no loss of consciousness characterizes mild brain injury, which is the majority of head injuries. Neurologic examination findings are often normal. Postconcussive syndrome sometimes persists for months, years, or indefinitely. Signs and symptoms include fatigue, headache, vertigo, lethargy, irritability, personality changes, cognitive deficits, decreased information processing speed, and difficulties with memory, understanding, learning, and perception. These symptoms can lead to feelings of incompetence, guilt, and frustration. Family members also may become impatient and frustrated at times.

Moderate brain injuries are characterized by a period of unconsciousness ranging from 1 to 24 hours. Cognitive skills—including planning, sequencing, judgment, reasoning, and computation skills—are usually impaired. In general, some psychosocial problems also occur, such as self-centeredness, denial, mood swings, agitation, depression, lethargy, sexual dysfunction, emotional lability, low tolerance for frustration, poor judgment, and behavioral outbursts.

Patients with severe brain injuries experience unconsciousness or posttrauma amnesia for longer than 8 days. Cognitive, psychosocial, and behavioral disabilities result.

In catastrophic brain injury, a defining characteristic is a coma lasting several months or longer. Affected individuals sometimes appear to be awake. However, they generally never regain significant, meaningful communication with their environment.

A patient with TBI commonly observes inconsistent performance, anger, and frustration. However, ineffective problem-solving strategies can usually be changed. Cognitive limitations to rehabilitative recovery include problems in thinking and reasoning (impaired memory), impaired concentration and attention, and impaired informational processing speed. Psychosocially, the patient appears to lack initiative; however, this is a normal consequence of a head injury. Egocentric (self-centered) behavior is often noted in brain-injured individuals, as is depression. In general, the more the memory improves, the more the patient becomes depressed. Abstinence from alcohol is a primary injunction for any patient with a brain injury because alcohol increases the chance of abnormal electrical impulse and seizure activity.

Continuous and honest involvement of the family, as both a victim of the injury and an equal participant in the rehabilitation process, is crucial for successfully rehabilitating a patient with TBI. Rehabilitation professionals must be available and honest when reporting to families. Equal communication with all family members is important, as is encouraging the family to become involved in counseling and education. Family members should be reminded to be aware of each other's needs and interests. The nurse should assist them to become involved in a support group and inform them of available community resources.

Regardless of personality types, any disability, particularly a TBI, is a crisis that threatens many aspects of the patient's and family's life: job income, pleasures, family, community ties, health, and life itself. The fears are real.

PEDIATRIC REHABILITATION NURSING

Pediatric rehabilitation nursing is a specialty practice area that also continues to expand within the field of rehabilitation. The field of pediatric rehabilitation has undergone marked development since the early 1900s. The number of children with chronic disabling conditions has increased as a result of improved rates of survival from illnesses and injuries that once were fatal.

Since the 1990s, the field has evolved from a mere combination of pediatrics and rehabilitation into a true specialty committed to the care of children with disabilities or other chronic conditions and their families. PCTs who work with nurses in this field, in a collaborative relationship with the interdisciplinary team, provide a continuum of care so that affected children can become contributing members of society and function at their maximal potential. Infants, children, and adolescents with a variety of disabling conditions receive specialized care from hospital to home, from clinic to school. Physical, emotional, social, cultural, educational, developmental, and spiritual dimensions are all subjects of consideration in a holistic approach to care. The goal is to cherish and foster the unique qualities of each child.

The primary difference between rehabilitation of children and rehabilitation of adults is the developmental potential of each child. Children will continue to grow and develop, even though they have a disability. Children and adolescents can receive an injury resulting in disability at any age, with very different consequences for the patient's future, depending on the age and developmental level at which the trauma occurred. Children who are born with genetic disorders, who are premature, or whose fetal development is affected by maternal disease, injury, or substance abuse require services focused on habilitation rather than rehabilitation. Whereas *rehabilitation* refers to the relearning of skills or behaviors lost as a result of disease or injury, *habilitation* refers to the process of acquiring skills and behaviors by an individual whose development has been affected by disease or other disabling conditions since birth or very early childhood.

In summary, the pediatric PCT who works in rehabilitation units has the power to have a very positive influence on the lives of children with disabilities and chronic conditions, as well as on their families. By helping to transition from hospital to home and community and by offering support to families, the PCT provides assistance in meeting identified needs. By following the individualized plan of care that incorporates the values and beliefs supported in rehabilitation, the PCT has the opportunity to affect the quality of the child's life for the better and to facilitate the child's interactions with family and friends within the community.

Delegation and Documentation Box 29.1

- Although the nurse is responsible for developing the plan of care for the pediatric patient, you are an active member of carrying out the plan of care.
- Involve the entire family when providing care to the child, under the direction and delegation of the nurse.
- Documenting the child's age and developmental level is important in caring for children because they will continue to develop despite their disability.

GERONTOLOGIC REHABILITATION NURSING

Gerontologic rehabilitation nursing is a specialty practice that focuses on the unique requirements of older adult rehabilitation patients. Because the needs of older adults differ from those of the rest of the population, the knowledge and skill needed to provide quality patient care needs special attention. Gerontologic rehabilitation nurses are knowledgeable both about techniques of caring for the aged and about rehabilitation concepts and principles. This unique type of nursing combines knowledge of both the aging process and rehabilitation practice in the specialized task of caring for older adults with a disability or long-term health problem.

A primary goal in gerontologic rehabilitation nursing is the assistance of older adult patients in achieving their personal optimal level of health and well-being through holistic care in a therapeutic environment. This goal is similar to that of general rehabilitation nursing but with a special focus on the geriatric population, considering their special needs, roles, and social relationships, and the potential physical limitations that are possible as a result of the aging process. As a PCT, your role in providing gerontologic rehabilitation involves following the plan of care developed by the nurse and other members of the healthcare team.

Gerontologic rehabilitation nurses strive not only to provide rehabilitative care but also to teach prevention. Thus gerontologic rehabilitation nurses have an opportunity to function within primary, secondary, and tertiary levels of care, with the universal goal of helping older adult patients to achieve optimal wellness and self-care.

Injury & Illness Prevention Box 29.1

- It is important to encourage use of any functional abilities the older adult may still have.
- Failure to use certain muscles and limbs because of injury could result in the inability for them to function over time.
- Involve older adults in their care as much as possible to encourage independence and discourage depression from lack of involvement.

CHAPTER SUMMARY

Rehabilitation nursing is a career with several key mandates and rewards. This type of responsibility should be taken seriously because it can significantly affect the future of patients with disabilities. Rehabilitation nurses facilitate the change from resistance to openness, turning inertia into action. The focus must be maintained on the assets and the successes of people who have disabilities.

Ralph Waldo Emerson (1803–1882) summed it up succinctly when he wrote, "It is one of the most beautiful compensations of this life that no man can sincerely try to help another without helping himself."

Rehabilitation is the process of maximizing an individual's capabilities or resources to foster optimal independent functioning.

The patient is the most important team member and must be involved in planning the programs and learning in detail about the disabilities, the ways of accomplishing the goals, and the options available. Rehabilitation aims toward preventing complications of disease or trauma and toward maintaining or restoring function. Basic rehabilitation is possible regardless of cause of disability. The rehabilitation team individualizes care by developing a goal-directed, comprehensive care plan for each patient.

A disability has a number of potential effects on both the patient and the family, including behavioral and emotional changes and changes in roles, body image, self-concept, and family dynamics. Holistic interventions are used to assist the patient in attaining an optimal level of functioning and well-being. The focus of all rehabilitation is on the patient's abilities, not on his or her disabilities.

Case Scenario

A 70-year-old patient has suffered a traumatic brain injury from falling out of a tree. He is alert and able to assist with the ADLs, though he appears to be mad and not willing to take part in his care. Specifically, he tells you to leave him alone and that he just wants to die. How would you handle this situation? Is it important for him to take part in his ADLs, or should you complete them for him? What are ways you can involve him in his care while respecting his desires for privacy?

REVIEW QUESTIONS

1. An 11-year-old boy has had a head injury from being struck in the skull by a baseball bat. When he awakens in the hospital 3 weeks later, how would his head injury be classified?
   a. Mild brain injury
   b. Moderate brain injury
   c. Severe brain injury
   d. Catastrophic brain injury

2. What term is the PCT referring to that describes a disadvantage for a person that results from an impairment or a disability and limits that person's fulfillment of his or her normal roles?
   a. Disability
   b. Impairment
   c. Handicap
   d. Inconvenience

3. What is known as any loss of ability to perform tasks or activities of daily living?
   a. Functional limitation
   b. Disability
   c. Handicap
   d. Inconvenience

4. What is the focus of rehabilitation?
   a. Curing the disease
   b. Preventing any complications
   c. Promoting a sense of dependence
   d. Promoting a high level of functioning

5. Damage to the cervical spine or the neck that involves weakness or paralysis in all four extremities is known as what?
   a. Paraplegia
   b. Hemiplegia
   c. Quadriplegia
   d. Paresis

Special Care Concerns and Settings

Care of Women and Children

1. Explain the anatomy and physiology of the female reproductive system.
2. Summarize the process of pregnancy and parturition.
3. Identify normal findings and common variations observed in the newborn.
4. Outline the patient care technician's role in gynecologic and reproductive examinations.
5. Discuss the legal and ethical implications in a gynecology or obstetrical setting.
6. Outline the patient care technician's role in a pediatric examination.
7. Obtain accurate vital signs and plot pediatric growth patterns.
8. Describe the characteristics and needs of the adolescent patient.

acrocyanosis When the hands and feet of a newborn may appear slightly blue because of poor peripheral circulation.

Bartholin's cyst When a Bartholin's gland, which lubricates the vagina, becomes blocked and is inflamed; it can be the size of a pea or as large as an egg.

circumcision Surgical removal of the foreskin from the penis.

clitoris A small, elongated erectile body above the urinary meatus at the superior point of the labia minora.

coitus Sexual union between male and female; also called intercourse.

colostrum A thin, yellow, milky fluid secreted by the mammary glands a few days before and after delivery.

dilation The opening of the cervix through the process of labor, measured as 0 to 10 cm dilated.

effacement The thinning of the cervix during labor, measured in percentages from 0% to 100% effaced.

fundus The curved, top portion of the uterus; the fundal height used as a measurement of fetal growth and estimated gestation.

human chorionic gonadotropin (HCG) A hormone secreted by the placenta that is found in the urine of pregnant females.

lactation Function of secreting milk or period during which milk is secreted.

lanugo Downy, fine hair characteristic of the fetus between 20 weeks of gestation and birth.

lochia Bloody vaginal discharge after a delivery that consists of blood, tissue, and mucus.

lochia alba Vaginal drainage that is slightly yellow to white.

lochia serosa Vaginal discharge that is pink to brown in color.

meconium The newborn's initial stools that are odorless, black-green, and sticky.

mons pubis The fat pad that covers the symphysis pubis.

multiparous Pertaining to women who have had two or more pregnancies.

parturition The act or process of giving birth to a child.

prolactin A hormone secreted by the anterior pituitary gland that is responsible for stimulating milk production in the mammary alveolar cells.

puerperium The period of time from when the woman delivers the placenta until the reproductive organs return to approximately the nonpregnant size and position, about 3 to 6 weeks.

umbilical cord The lifeline connecting the mother to the baby; it is whitish blue-gray with three vessels (one vein and two arteries) and contains a gelatinous tissue called Wharton jelly.

vernix caseosa A yellowish white, cream cheese–like substance that covers a newborn.

vulva The external female genitalia, which begins at the mons pubis and terminates at the anus.

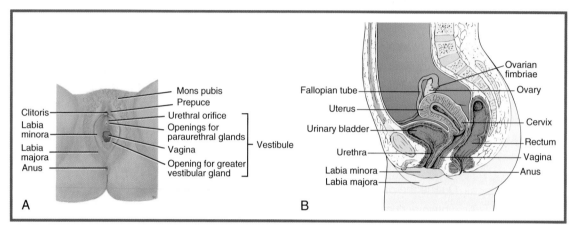

FIGURE 30.1 A, Female external genitalia. B, Normal female reproductive system. (A, from Applegate EJ: *The anatomy and physiology learning system,* ed 4, Philadelphia, 2011, Saunders; B, from Frazier MS, Drzymkowski JA: *Essentials of human diseases and conditions,* ed 6, St. Louis, 2016, Saunders.)

The branch of medicine that deals with pregnancy, labor, and the postnatal period is known as *obstetrics,* and the branch of medicine that deals with diseases of the genital tract in women is called *gynecology.* Frequently, a physician practices both specialties and is known as an *OB/GYN physician.* Assessment of the female reproductive system is an important part of healthcare. Patients often are hesitant and uncomfortable about talking about sexual matters, so they wait until symptoms are intolerable or disease is advanced before seeking medical care. The patient care technician must be aware of the patient's emotional state and must give support when needed.

ANATOMY AND PHYSIOLOGY

Female Reproductive System

The female reproductive system includes both internal and external organs. The internal organs are located in the pelvis and cannot be seen without special instruments, such as a vaginal speculum or a laparoscope. The external organs can be seen during the physical examination.

The primary parts of the female reproductive system are the vulva, vagina, uterus, fallopian tubes, and ovaries (Fig. 30.1). The vulva includes the clitoris, the urethral meatus, and the vaginal orifice. These structures are covered by two sets of lips of tissue. The inner set, the *labia minora,* is a thin layer of skin that extends from the top of the clitoris to the base of the vaginal opening. The external set, the *labia majora,* and the mons pubis are covered with hair in the adult.

The vagina connects the internal and external organs. This tubelike structure is constructed to receive the penis during coitus. It is lubricated by a mucous membrane lining, and its walls are made up of overlapping tissue in the form of rugae, which allows the vagina to expand during the birth of an infant. At the distal end of the vagina is the cervix, often called the *neck of the uterus,* which is approximately 1 to 1½ inches long. The uterus is an upside-down, pear-shaped muscular organ, and its sole purpose is to house and nourish the fetus from implantation shortly after conception until parturition. The uterine walls have three layers. The inner layer, the endometrium, is rich in blood and changes in consistency during the menstrual cycle. The middle layer, the myometrium, is the powerful muscular layer that contracts to make the birth of a baby possible. The outer layer, the perimetrium, protects the structure and attaches to ligaments that support and hold the uterus in place (Fig. 30.2).

On both sides of the fundus of the uterus are the fallopian tubes, also called the *oviducts.* These tubes extend from the uterus to the ovaries but do not attach

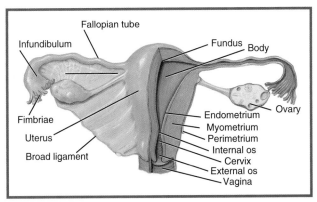

FIGURE 30.2 Uterus and fallopian tubes. (Modified from Applegate EJ: *The anatomy and physiology learning system,* ed 4, Philadelphia, 2011, Saunders.)

to the ovaries. The distal end of the tube opens freely into the abdominopelvic cavity and acts as a passageway for the ovum to the uterus and for the sperm as they search for the ovum. At the distal end of the fallopian tubes are fingerlike projections, called *fimbriae,* which move in a wavelike pattern to draw the released ovum into the fallopian tube.

The ovaries are almond-shaped organs that produce and release the egg (ovum) and excrete the hormones necessary for the development of secondary sexual characteristics and the maintenance of a pregnancy. The ovaries secrete the hormones progesterone and estrogen, which regulate reproductive function. For pregnancy to occur, the vagina must receive the sperm from the male; the sperm move up through the opening in the cervix (the cervical os), through the uterus, and into the fallopian tubes. As many as 200 million to 600 million sperm can be deposited, and about 100,000 survive the acidic environment of the vagina to swim toward the egg.

Fertilization occurs when one sperm cell penetrates and fertilizes an egg. Fertilization usually takes place in the distal third of the fallopian tube. The tiny fertilized ovum, now called a *zygote,* moves by peristalsis and the massaging motion of the cilia that line the fallopian tube into the uterus and implants itself into the uterine wall. After implantation, the placenta forms; this structure supplies the new life with all the nourishment needed for development. Once pregnancy begins, the serum levels of human chorionic gonadotropin (HCG) rise, and the hormone spills into the woman's urine, where it can be detected with a pregnancy test.

Breast Tissue

Mammary tissue develops from the increased estrogen secretion that occurs during puberty. In the center of each breast is a nipple surrounded by a pigmented region called the *areola.* Inside the breast are 15 to 20 lobes and their subunits—the lobules of glandular tissue

that are separated by connective support tissue and surrounded by adipose tissue. The amount and distribution of adipose tissue determine the size and shape of the breast (Fig. 30.3). Breast tissue also contains mammary glands, modified sweat glands that become the organs of milk production, and a system of ducts for delivery of milk to the nipple. Mammary ducts respond to elevated levels of estrogen and progesterone produced during the menstrual cycle by increasing in size, resulting in premenstrual fullness and tenderness of the breasts.

Four hormones control the mammary glands: *Estrogen* is responsible for the increase in size; *progesterone* stimulates the development of the duct system; *prolactin* stimulates the production of milk; and *oxytocin* causes the ejection of milk from the glands.

Menstruation

When a girl enters puberty, one of the many changes that occur is *menarche,* or the beginning of the menstrual cycle. Menstruation is a normal body process that occurs in every female. It is the physiologic means by which the body rids itself of the thickened endometrial wall that develops during the average 28-day cycle. The menstrual cycle involves a series of events controlled by hormones from the pituitary gland and the ovaries.

PREGNANCY

Anatomy and Physiology

Fertilization usually takes place in the distal third of the fallopian tube when one sperm cell penetrates and fertilizes an egg, which is then called a *zygote.* The zygote, which is made up of 23 chromosomes from the ovum and 23 chromosomes from the sperm, forms the first complete cell. This cell begins to grow and multiply immediately. The zygote travels down the fallopian tube and reaches the uterus in 5 to 6 days, implanting in the uterine endometrium. Enzymes are secreted by the zygote to aid the implantation process.

After implantation, the placenta forms within the uterine wall. It is derived from maternal endometrial tissue and from the chorion, the outermost membrane that surrounds the developing zygote. The amnion, the innermost layer of the membranes, holds the fetus suspended in an amniotic cavity surrounded by a fluid called *amniotic fluid.* The amnion and the fluid sometimes are called the "bag of water." In about 25% of pregnancies, breaking of the amniotic sac signals the onset of labor.

Within 2 weeks of fertilization, the zygote has undergone mitosis and is well established in the uterus. The next stage of development is the embryonic period, which includes the third to twelfth weeks of pregnancy

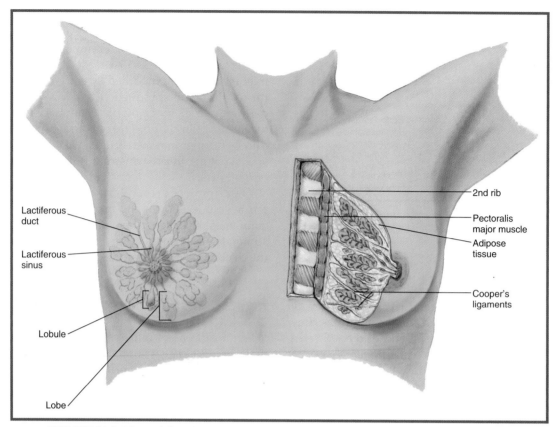

FIGURE 30.3 Normal female breast. (From Jarvis C: *Physical examination and health assessment*, ed 4, Philadelphia, 2004, Saunders.)

(the first trimester). The embryonic period is a crucial time for the developing fetus, because this is when all tissues and organs develop. During the second and third trimesters, the embryo becomes a fetus; this is when cells develop and begin their primary functions, organs mature, and the fetus gains weight and grows in length.

Throughout the pregnancy, maternal and fetal blood never mix. Nutrients and oxygen diffuse from the mother's blood across the placental membrane into the blood vessels of the fetus's umbilical cord. Carbon dioxide and waste materials pass from the umbilical cord, through the placenta, and into the mother's circulatory system for excretion.

The placenta also acts as a gland by producing HCG and progesterone to maintain the pregnancy. Low levels of progesterone can lead to spontaneous abortion in pregnant women and menstrual irregularities in non-pregnant women. The average gestation is calculated at 9 calendar months, 10 lunar months, or 266 to 280 days. As previously mentioned, it is divided into three trimesters.

First Trimester

The first trimester is the period from the beginning of the last monthly period (LMP) through the fourteenth week. It is a time of multiple physical and psychological changes for the woman and a crucial time for fetal organ development. It is essential that the pregnant woman understands the importance of a nutritious diet and of avoiding potential agents that could cause harm to the developing fetus. The woman may complain of breast tenderness, constipation, headaches, urinary frequency, and nausea and vomiting. Rest, relaxation exercises, plenty of fluids, regular exercise, and small, frequent meals help relieve these discomforts. During this time, the obstetrician obtains a complete health history of the patient, including family, medical, menstrual, and obstetric histories. The obstetric history includes the number of times the patient has been pregnant (gravida) and the number of times she has given birth to a live infant (para).

A series of blood tests also is performed during the initial prenatal visit. In follow-up prenatal visits, the patient care technician may be asked to collect a urine specimen for urinalysis, weigh the patient, and measure the blood pressure. The mother should gain approximately 10 to 12 lb in the first half of pregnancy and another 15 to 17 lb during the second half. Experts believe that a healthy weight gain is somewhere between 25 and 35 lb. The baby's heart tones can be picked up through a specialized method, called *Doppler ultrasound*, somewhere between 9 and 12 weeks of pregnancy. Once recorded, the fetal heart rate is assessed at each subsequent visit. The nurse or healthcare provider is responsible for obtaining the fetal heart rate.

Prenatal blood and laboratory tests include the following:

- Hematocrit and hemoglobin levels to check for anemia
- Blood type and Rh with antibody screening for possible Rh incompatibility
- Rubella titer to determine whether the mother is immune to German measles; rubella infection during pregnancy can cause multiple birth defects, including deafness, vision disorders, and mental retardation
- Syphilis screening; if the result is positive, antibiotic treatment is initiated to protect the fetus from congenital syphilis
- Hepatitis B screening, because this virus can be passed to the fetus in utero
- HIV screening is suggested; if the result is positive, treatment of the mother greatly reduces the risk of transmission to the fetus
- Pap smear to check for abnormal cervical cells
- Gonorrhea and chlamydia cultures to prevent infection of the baby at birth
- Urinalysis to detect protein, white blood cells, or glucose
- Group B streptococcus culture of the lower vagina for strep B infection, performed between the thirty-second and thirty-sixth weeks; if the result is positive, the mother is treated with antibiotics to prevent fetal exposure during vaginal birth
- Fetal nonstress test (NST) to evaluate the fetal heart rate; the mother is attached to a fetal monitor, with the goal of seeing accelerations in the fetal heart rate with movement (this is performed by the nurse)

Second Trimester

The second trimester extends from the fifteenth through the twenty-eighth week after the LMP. The uterus has enlarged to above the umbilicus, and the patient feels the first fetal movements, called *quickening*. In addition to the basic health history and physical examination, assessment is performed by abdominal palpation and fetal heart monitoring. The height of the fundus may be measured in centimeters from the symphysis pubis to the fundus. At each office visit, a urine sample is screened with a dipstick to detect protein or glucose, and the woman's blood pressure is monitored for signs of hypertension. The patient care technician may be responsible for performing these tasks at each prenatal visit. The mother may complain of backache, dizziness, leukorrhea, and leg cramps from the increasing size of the uterus.

Third Trimester

The third trimester begins at the twenty-eighth week and lasts until delivery. This period is marked by rapid fetal growth, with the baby gaining close to 1 lb per week. The patient continues to be closely monitored. Childbirth preparation classes usually begin during this time. The patient experiences noticeable breast enlargement and may have an occasional discharge from the nipples of the clear, sticky fluid colostrum. The pregnant woman may complain of uterine cramping (Braxton-Hicks contractions), heartburn, edema, and frequent urination. Lightening, the dropping of the fetus into the pelvis, may occur a few weeks before birth, especially in primigravidas (women in their first pregnancy).

Assisting With the Examination

The female reproductive system examination is probably the most emotionally charged medical experience the average woman undergoes. Even women with relatively sophisticated attitudes toward their bodies and sexuality may be embarrassed by the casual, impersonal approach of the medical team during this procedure. Many women fear the physician's findings. Anxieties and fears are best handled through explanations and by showing a genuine interest in the patient's concerns.

If the physician is male, a female assistant should be present during the examination; this could be the patient care technician. The only exception to this rule is when the patient requests that the assistant leave the room; if this is done, the request is noted on the patient's medical record. The patient care technician is responsible for supporting the patient, nurse, and the physician during the procedure. The physician will sometimes ask for certain instruments that you may need to be familiar with if you work on a labor & delivery unit. In preparation for the examination, the patient should empty her bladder, completely disrobe, and put on an examination gown.

Pelvic Examination

The patient care technician should remain in the examination room to provide reassurance to the patient and as legal protection for a male physician while the patient's vaginal and perineal areas are examined. Furthermore, the lithotomy position is awkward to assume without assistance and may be embarrassing to the patient. Never place the patient in the lithotomy position until the physician or midwife is ready to begin the examination. When you assist the patient into the lithotomy position, always keep her totally covered.

You should stand at the patient's side so that you can observe the patient, yet still be able to move quickly if needed by the physician. First, the physician inspects the external genitalia and palpates the perineal body. The patient may be asked to bear down to show any muscular weaknesses that may be the result of lacerations of the perineal body during a previous childbirth. A third-degree laceration may have involved the rectal sphincter and may cause rectal incontinence.

Next, sometimes the physician or midwife will need to obtain a Pap specimen. They will use the vaginal speculum, without lubrication, for examination of the cervix and the vaginal canal and for obtaining the Pap specimen. The speculum should be prewarmed with warm water. Have the patient take some deep breaths to help relax the abdominal muscles. The normal cervix points posteriorly and has smooth, pink, squamous epithelium. Abnormalities most frequently seen are ulcerations (erosions), Bartholin's cysts, and cervical polyps. Because erosions cannot be palpated, inspection is the only method of detecting them. Healed lacerations from childbirth are common in a multiparous patient. Pregnancy increases the size of the cervix, and hormone deficiency causes it to atrophy. The vaginal wall is reddish pink and has a corrugated appearance from the overlapping tissue (rugae) lining. Vaginal infections change the appearance of the vaginal mucosa. After the Pap specimen has been obtained, you may be responsible for labeling the specimen and preparing it for transport to the cytology laboratory. Be sure to follow laboratory instructions during the preparation to avoid having to repeat the examination.

Postexamination Duties

When the examination is finished, help the patient into a sitting position and into the dressing room if needed. Following the Standard Precautions established by the Occupational Safety and Health Administration (OSHA), remove the examination equipment and supplies while the patient is repositioned in the bed (Box 30.1). Offer a clean set of linens if there is any discharge noted on the bed.

Box 30.1	Safety Alert: Instrument Use and Care

Instruments that come in contact with a patient, including vaginal speculums, should be sanitized, disinfected, and sterilized before they are used for another patient. If the instrument does not penetrate tissue, it can be stored under clean or medically aseptic conditions. Some physicians prefer to use disposable speculums for routine pelvic examinations. Instruments that penetrate tissue (e.g., uterine biopsy punch, uterine tenaculum, cervical dilators and sounds) must be sterilized and stored and handled under sterile conditions.

Parturition

Labor is the physiologic process by which the uterus expels the fetus and the placenta (Fig. 30.4). To be born vaginally, the baby must drop down into the pelvic floor, and the cervix must efface (thin out) and dilate (open up). Effacement is the thinning of the cervix from its prelabor length of 1 to 1½ inches to a completely thin tissue (Fig. 30.4A). This occurs when uterine contractions pull cervical tissue upward as labor progresses so that the bottom uterine segment (the cervix) becomes thinner and the top uterine segment (the fundus) becomes thicker. Effacement is measured as a percentage; the cervix is said to be 0% to 100% effaced. Dilation (sometimes called *dilatation*) is the opening of the cervix, which allows the infant to pass out of the uterus and into the vaginal birth canal. Dilation is measured in centimeters, which are estimated during vaginal examinations by manual palpation. Labor is divided into three stages:

- Stage I—from the onset of labor through complete dilation and effacement of the cervix (Fig. 30.4B). During this time, uterine contractions become longer, stronger, and closer together until complete dilation and effacement occur and pushing begins. Stage I is divided into early active (up to 3 cm dilation and 80% to 100% effaced), active (4 to 7 cm dilation and completion of effacement), and transition (8 to 10 cm dilation). The average length of time for primigravidas in stage I is 9 to 11 hours.
- Stage II—from complete dilation and effacement of the cervix through the birth of the fetus (Fig. 30.4C). This is the pushing stage, which lasts approximately 1 hour for primigravidas.
- Stage III—from the birth of the fetus through expulsion of the placenta (Fig. 30.4D). This occurs approximately 20 minutes after the birth of the baby.

The postpartum period, also called the puerperium, lasts from the time the woman delivers the placenta until the reproductive organs return to approximately the nonpregnant size and position. The puerperium lasts about 3 to 6 weeks and consists of two stages. The immediate postpartum period, which lasts up to 6 hours after delivery, is sometimes called the *fourth stage of labor*, or the recovery stage. The new mother needs emotional support and close assessment after giving birth. This is a time for close observation and assessment to ensure that no problems occur. The later postpartum stage follows the stage of recovery and lasts until about 6 weeks after delivery.

During the postpartum period, the mother's body makes rapid physiologic adaptations. The anatomic and physiologic changes that took place over 9 months begin a reversal within 6 short weeks. Many psychological changes also occur as the woman and her family adjust to expansion of the family.

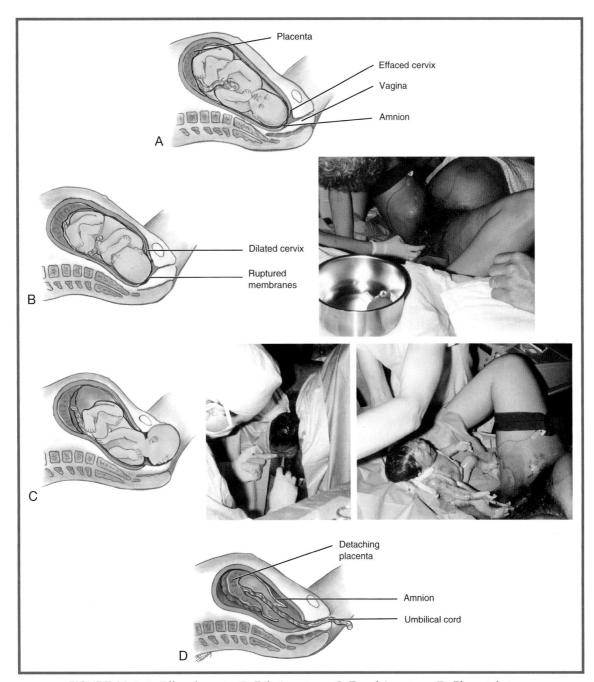

FIGURE 30.4 **A,** Effaced cervix. **B,** Dilation stage. **C,** Expulsion stage. **D,** Placental stage. (From Applegate EJ: *The anatomy and physiology learning system,* ed 4, Philadelphia, 2011, Saunders.)

ANATOMIC AND PHYSIOLOGIC CHANGES OF THE MOTHER

Reproductive Organs

Uterus

After the birth of the baby and the delivery of the placenta, the uterus contracts in response to *oxytocin* (a hormone produced by the posterior pituitary gland that stimulates uterine contractions and release of milk in the mammary glands [let-down reflex]). This contraction compresses blood vessels at the site where the placenta separated from the uterine wall. This site, an area 3 to 4 inches (8 to 10 cm) in diameter, has open venous sinuses. If the uterus does not contract adequately, the woman may lose too much blood. The placental site heals through exfoliation, in which necrotic tissue is sloughed from the uterine lining, leaving a fresh layer of endometrial tissue free from scars. This process is necessary for successive pregnancies to occur.

Immediately after delivery, the uterine fundus is about midway between the umbilicus and the symphysis pubis

Table 30.1	Lochia and Nonlochia Bleeding
Lochia	**Nonlochia Bleeding**
Lochia usually trickles from the vaginal opening. The steady flow is greater as the uterus contracts.	If the blood discharge spurts from the vagina, cervical or vaginal tears may exist in addition to the normal lochia.
A gush of lochia may result as the uterus is massaged. If it is dark in color, it has been pooled in the relaxed vagina, and the amount soon lessens to a trickle of bright red lochia (in the early puerperium).	If the amount of bleeding continues to be excessive and bright red, a tear may be the source.

or slightly higher. It weighs approximately 2 lb (907 g). During the first 12 hours after birth, it rises to the level of the umbilicus at midline. In the following 24 to 48 hours, the uterus begins a gradual descent. It moves approximately one fingerbreadth per day; within a week, it is barely palpable at the level of the symphysis pubis and weighs 1 lb (453 g). Within 6 to 8 weeks, the uterus again is a pelvic organ, approximately the nonpregnant size of 2 oz (57 g) and no longer palpable.

After delivery, the uterine lining is shed. This bloody discharge is termed lochia. It consists of blood, tissue, and mucus. As the uterine lining is shed, the necrotic tissue, blood, and mucus leave the body through the vagina. Lochia has a fleshy odor similar to that of menstrual discharge. For the first day or two after delivery, the lochia is made up mostly of blood, which results in a bright red drainage called *lochia rubra*. Some small clots may be passed during this phase. As the placental site heals, the discharge thins and becomes pink to brown; this is called lochia serosa. After the seventh day, the drainage is slightly yellow to white and is called lochia alba. This drainage continues for another 10 days to 2 weeks. If fragments of the placenta are retained in the uterus, the uterus is not able to contract and seal blood vessels adequately, which can result in excessive blood loss and may necessitate surgical intervention (Table 30.1).

Cervix, Vagina, and Perineum

The cervix appears edematous, with bruising. The external cervical os has a ragged, slit-like appearance instead of a round shape as seen in the nulliparous woman. The vaginal walls are thin and dry, with an absence of rugae. Vaginal mucus production returns with the return of estrogen production. Rugae reappear in 4 weeks.

Bruising and edema of the perineum is common. The episiotomy (if present) should be free of erythema, with the edges well approximated and without discharge. It should heal in 2 to 3 weeks. Sutures that are used are

absorbed by the woman's body. Lacerations of the perineum are classified from first to fourth degree, depending on depth of involvement. The repaired laceration should also have well-approximated edges and no drainage. Healing time depends on laceration depth. Return of these areas to the nonpregnant state should be complete in 6 to 8 weeks.

Most acute injuries and lacerations of the perineum, the vagina, the uterus, and their support tissues occur during childbirth. Ideally, injuries are repaired at the time of delivery, which facilitates healing, limits residual damage, and reduces the incidence of infection. Future gynecologic problems with female organs may be attributed to childbirth.

The tendency to get lacerations varies with each woman; in some women, the soft tissue may be less distensible. Heredity may be a factor in this. For example, the tissue of light-skinned women, especially those with reddish hair, does not heal as well as that of darker-skinned women.

Breasts

Breast changes begin early in pregnancy. Increased amounts of estrogen stimulate enlargement of breast size by increasing adipose tissue and fluid retention. Estrogen also stimulates the growth of the milk ducts to prepare for lactation (function of secreting milk or period during which milk is secreted).

The first secretion produced by the breast is colostrum. This precursor to milk is thin, watery, and slightly yellow. It is rich in protein, calories, antibodies, and lymphocytes. Colostrum production begins in the second trimester. Expectant mothers begin to leak colostrum in the later weeks of the third trimester. Its production continues for about 2 days after delivery, when true milk production begins.

Lactation is a combination of hormonal, neurologic, and psychological responses. After delivery, estrogen and progesterone levels diminish rapidly. As they drop, the level of prolactin increases. Prolactin, a hormone secreted by the anterior pituitary gland, is responsible for stimulating milk production in the mammary alveolar cells. Stimulation of the nipples, particularly by the infant's sucking, causes the release of oxytocin from the posterior pituitary gland. Oxytocin stimulates contraction of the mammary ducts, and milk is ejected from the breast. This cycle is called the *let-down reflex*.

TRANSFER FROM THE RECOVERY AREA

After the initial recovery period of 1 to 2 hours, the woman may be transferred to a postpartum room in the same or another nursing unit. In labor, delivery, recovery, postpartum (LDRP) room settings, the nurse who provided care during the recovery period usually continues to care for the woman. In the labor, delivery, recovery (LDR) room or a traditional setting, the woman is transferred to a separate unit where the postpartum nursing staff provide her care. In some settings, the baby remains with the mother wherever she goes. In other facilities, the baby is taken to the nursery for several hours of observation during the mother's initial recovery period.

The move to another area of the maternity unit requires the patient care technician to prepare a room for the postpartum patient. The type of bed that will need to be prepared is an open bed, and sometimes a surgical bed. If the patient has had an epidural that has created a numbing effect on the patient's legs, she will not be able to walk to her room and may arrive by stretcher. In this case, a surgical bed would need to be prepared for the patient. For the patient who has not had any anesthesia, the patient will more than likely arrive by wheelchair. In this case, an open bed may be prepared.

Childbearing practices and rituals of other cultures may be different from standard practices associated with bonding in the Anglo-American culture. For example, Chinese families traditionally use extended family members to care for the newborn so that the mother can rest and recover, especially after a cesarean birth. In some cultures, women do not initiate breastfeeding until their breast milk comes in. In other cultures, families do not name their babies until after the confinement month. The amount of eye contact also varies among cultures.

Become knowledgeable about the childbearing beliefs and practices of diverse cultural and ethnic groups. Because individual cultural variations exist within groups, clarify with the patient and family members or friends what cultural norms the patient follows. Incorrect judgments may be made about mother-infant bonding if you do not practice culturally sensitive care.

Postpartum Care

Recovery Stage

After the time and energy involved in labor and delivery, the mother is often hungry. Most women do not have dietary restrictions after vaginal childbirth. After a cesarean section, women often have restrictions that limit oral intake to ice or liquids for the first day with a gradual reintroduction to the diet. Fluids are important during the recovery phase to replace the fluids and blood lost during delivery; offer a variety of fluids such as water and juices. When a general anesthetic has been used, such as during a cesarean delivery, verify with the nurse before giving solid food, as many patients are on a clear liquids diet until the return of bowel sounds or the presence of flatus or a bowel movement.

If the woman used mouth-breathing techniques during labor such as Lamaze, she may have dry mucous membranes, cracked lips, and noticeable breath odor. Good oral hygiene relieves these symptoms and reduces discomfort. A complete sponge bath or a shower with assistance enhances well-being and comfort by removing perspiration and other waste products from the skin. The patient care technician may be asked to assist with this.

Hygiene

During the postpartum stage, excessive perspiration is normal. The lochia has a characteristic musty odor. It should not have a foul or decaying smell. Encourage regular bathing (showers are preferred) to minimize odors and promote comfort. Most women are permitted to be up as tolerated within hours of giving birth, but they may experience vertigo as a result of vascular shifts related to the heat of the shower. If this occurs while the woman is standing in the shower, she may experience syncope and injure herself. When the newly delivered woman takes a shower for the first time, provide for safety by instructing her on use of the emergency call signal and the length of shower time recommended, and provide a chair in the shower room. Also, check the patient frequently during her first shower to verify she is safe. Tub baths are not recommended until after the postpartum examination at 6 weeks so that no water that has been contaminated with body wastes enters the vaginal canal or uterus until healing is completed. Also, if in an LDRP unit, the patient will need a linen change after the recovery phase. This typically takes place when the patient gets up to void for the first time after delivery. Always include an underpad on the bed of a postpartum patient because of the continued bleeding that may occur after delivery.

Sitz baths may be used to reduce discomfort and promote healing of the perineum. Vasodilation from the warm water helps reduce edema and speed tissue repair. Instruct the patient about water temperature and length of time. As with a shower, vascular changes may occur; check on the patient regularly to promote safety. Proper cleaning of equipment must take place between patients if community facilities are used (Fig. 30.5). Today, most facilities use a personal, portable sitz bath that the patient can take home at discharge.

If the woman has delivered via cesarean section, she has an abdominal incision with sutures or staples. Traditionally, the patient has a dressing covering the incision the day of surgery. This is usually removed the next day by the surgeon. The incision likely is left open to the air. Those patients with staples closing their wounds have them removed in approximately 3 days. Adhesive strips may be applied after their removal and remain on for the next 5 to 7 days. Care should be taken so that

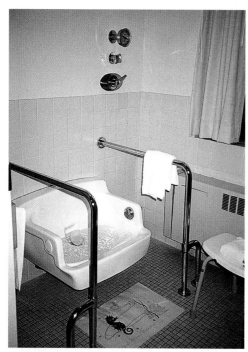

FIGURE 30.5 Sitz bath for perineal care. (From Perry AG, Potter PA, Elkin MK: *Nursing interventions and clinical skills,* ed 4, St. Louis, 2008, Mosby.)

clothing does not irritate the incision. The patient may shower with the incision that contains sutures or staples. Wounds with adhesive strips need to be protected from the direct flow of water during a shower.

Elimination

Recovery Stage

Diuresis and diaphoresis are common immediately after delivery. If the woman received IV fluids, urinary output may be increased. Encourage voiding because a full bladder may interfere with complete contraction of the uterus, potentially causing hemorrhage.

The initial voiding should occur within 4 to 6 hours after delivery. Tissue edema from the delivery may cause difficulty with voiding. In addition, some women may have reduced sensitivity and are unaware that the bladder is full. Some agencies have a policy to assess voiding three times in measurable amounts of 300 mL or more after delivery to determine urinary elimination. Try measures to stimulate voiding. If the patient is unsuccessful voiding a sufficient quantity, catheterization may be necessary. If repeated catheterization is needed, a Foley catheter may be inserted. An indwelling catheter is routinely inserted before cesarean delivery and may remain in place for 1 or 2 days after delivery. The patient care technician may be asked to insert a catheter (refer to Chapter 21).

MAINTENANCE OF SAFETY

Activity and Exercise

Recovery Stage

Monitor vital signs every 15 minutes for the first hour and then hourly for the next 4 hours during the recovery stage (Table 30.2).

Delegation and Documentation Box 30.1

- The nurse may delegate recovery vital signs to the patient care technician after the nurse has performed a baseline assessment.
- Be sure to record the vital signs accurately and immediately after taking them. *Do not* record all of the vital signs on a notepad for documenting later.
- Recovery vital signs are recorded every 15 minutes for the first hour; if any component is abnormal, notify the nurse at once, as this may signify that the patient is bleeding excessively.

Ensure that the mother is settled comfortably in bed. A patient who has just given birth may need to remain in bed for a time to allow her body systems to adjust to fluid volume changes. Early ambulation is key in the prevention of complications. The rapid decrease in intraabdominal pressure after birth results in a dilation of the blood vessels that supply the intestines (known as splanchnic engorgement), which causes blood to pool in the viscera. This contributes to orthostatic hypotension; when a woman who has recently given birth stands up, she may faint or feel lightheaded.

Instruct the patient to use her call bell to summon help before she attempts to get out of bed. Assess her color, pulse, and level of consciousness (LOC) in response to conversation and then assist her in ambulating to the bathroom. Once the woman has reached the bathroom, remain close with frequent inquiries as to her well-being. Have a wheelchair available in the room or just outside in case the woman is too weak to walk back to bed. Encourage her to rest after the ambulation so that she can regain her strength.

The patient who received conduction anesthesia (epidural block) is kept in bed until she can fully move, feels sensation in her legs, and has blood pressure and pulse within normal limits. Assess her ability to communicate, her LOC, and her vital signs for stability (within normal limits) before allowing her to get out of bed; the nurse will notify you when the patient is allowed out of bed. The patient should wear slippers when ambulating to prevent slipping or sliding.

The patient who has received analgesics needs to be observed closely until she is fully recovered from the medication (i.e., vital signs are stable within her normal range and she is fully awake).

Table 30.2	Vital Signs and Blood Pressure After Delivery

Normal Findings	Deviations From Normal Findings and Probable Causes
Temperature During first 24 hr, temperature may rise to 100.4°F (38°C) as a result of dehydrating effects of labor. After 24 hr, the woman should be afebrile.	A diagnosis of puerperal sepsis is suggested if a rise in maternal temperature to 100.4°F (38°C) is noted after the first 24 hr after delivery and recurs or persists for 2 days. Other possibilities are mastitis, endometritis, urinary tract infection, and other systemic infections.
Pulse Bradycardia is common for the first 6 to 8 days after delivery. It is caused by increased cardiac output and stroke volume. The pulse returns to nonpregnant levels by 3 mo after delivery. A pulse rate between 50 and 70 bpm is considered normal.	A rapid pulse rate or one that is increasing may indicate hypovolemia as a result of hemorrhage.
Respirations Respirations should fall to within the woman's normal predelivery range.	Hypoventilation may follow an unusually high subarachnoid (spinal) block.
Blood Pressure Blood pressure is altered slightly, if at all. Orthostatic hypotension, as indicated by feelings of vertigo or syncope immediately after standing up, can develop in the first 48 hr as a result of the splanchnic engorgement (the excessive filling or pooling of blood within the visceral vasculature after removal of pressure from the abdomen) that may occur after delivery.	Low or falling blood pressure may reflect hypovolemia as a result of hemorrhage. However, it is a late sign, and other symptoms of hemorrhage usually alert the staff. An increased reading may result from excessive use of vasopressor or oxytocic medications. Because gestational hypertension can persist into or begin in the postpartum period, routinely evaluate blood pressure. If a woman reports headache, rule out hypertension as a cause before administering analgesics. If the blood pressure is elevated, confine the woman to bed and notify the physician.

During the first 24 hours after giving birth, the woman's temperature may be slightly elevated if she is dehydrated. Elevations noted after the first 24 hours may signal the onset of an infection, and temperatures higher than 100.4°F (38°C) are significant and should be reported. Many women feel chilled after giving birth and appreciate an extra blanket or one that has been warmed. Sometimes a beverage such as hot tea or warm milk provides comfort. Tell the patient this chilling is a normal reaction to the stress of labor.

Slight bradycardia, 50 to 70 bpm, is sometimes observed and is not considered abnormal if the other vital signs are within normal limits. Tachycardia may also occur in response to increased blood loss or physical exertion.

Blood pressure may be slightly elevated from exertion, from excitement, and possibly from the oxytocic medications. If the blood pressure is consistently elevated, or if the patient also reports headache or visual disturbances, complications related to gestational hypertension could be occurring. These often persist even after delivery. Notify the physician immediately. A decrease in blood pressure could be caused by altered intraabdominal pressure or hemorrhage. Watch changes closely and report them.

Later Postpartum Stage

Vital signs normally stabilize within the first 2 hours after delivery; report immediately any abnormality to the nurse. If vital signs have not stabilized within this time, the nurse may have you continue to monitor them every 15 minutes to 1 hour and report significant changes.

A temperature of 100.4°F (38°C) or higher on 2 successive days during the first 10 days after delivery (not including the first 24 hours) is considered indicative of puerperal infection. Closely monitor any signs and symptoms of infection during the postpartum stage. Use good aseptic technique when caring for the postpartum patient.

The flow of lochia may increase suddenly when the patient gets out of bed; secretions that pooled in the vagina drain out of the body when she stands. Once the lochia has changed to *serosa* or *alba*, excessive exercise or activity may result in the lochia changing back to *rubra*. This is a sign to slow down and increase activity gradually.

CHARACTERISTICS OF THE NEWBORN

Body Size and Shape

The newborn's head is disproportionately large for the body. The abdomen is prominent, with a smaller chest and narrow hips. The body is usually held in a moderately flexed position. A wide variation of size is seen in healthy newborns. The average newborn weighs 7 lb, 8 oz (3400 g) and is approximately 20 inches (50 cm) long. Charts are available for plotting height and weight. The head circumference averages 13 to 14 inches (33 to 35.5 cm) and is generally about 1 inch (2.5 cm) larger than the chest circumference, which averages 12 to 13 inches (30.5 to 33 cm). The nurse may ask the patient care technician to assist with obtaining the head measurements. A paper tape measure is used.

Vital Signs

Respiratory rate averages from 30 to 60 breaths/min with brief periods of apnea. Breathing is more noticeable in the stomach and should be effortless, without evidence of respiratory distress. Rate and rhythm vary with activity. Pulse rate averages 120 to 160 bpm, with higher and lower variations depending on activity.

The heartbeat should have a regular rate and rhythm. Auscultate the apical beat between the fourth and fifth intercostal spaces. This is best done when the infant is asleep. The blood pressure averages 60 to 80/40 to 50 mm Hg and should be approximately the same in all four extremities. If the nurse asks the patient care technician to perform blood pressure measurements, it is important to obtain a blood pressure using all four extremities so that any variation can be assessed to rule out any heart defects. A drop in systolic blood pressure (about 15 mm Hg) in the first hour after birth is common. Crying and moving usually cause increases in systolic blood pressure. The axillary temperature of the newborn should be between 97.6° and 98.6°F (36.4° and 37°C), with stabilization of temperature occurring within 8 to 10 hours after birth.

Skin

The infant's skin can exhibit a wide range of rashes and color changes (Box 30.2). Most are not significant and disappear within a few days.

Color

The white newborn is usually pink to slightly reddish in appearance. The black newborn may appear pinkish or yellowish brown. Newborns of Spanish descent may have an olive tint or a slight yellow cast to the skin. Newborns of Asian descent may be a rosy or yellowish tan. The color of Native American newborns depends on the tribe and can vary from a light pink to a dark, reddish brown. By the second or third day, the skin turns to its more natural tone and is drier and flakier. The ruddiness results from normally elevated red blood cell concentration.

The hands and feet may appear slightly blue; this is called acrocyanosis and is caused by poor peripheral circulation. Acrocyanosis can last for 7 to 10 days. It is most commonly observed when the infant becomes cold. Mottling, a lacy pattern with dilated vessels on pale skin, is also common.

> **Box 30.2**   **Common Skin Observations in the Newborn**
>
> - *Milia* are small white spots usually seen on the nose and chin. They are a result of occluded sebaceous glands and disappear spontaneously within a few weeks.
> - *Newborn rash*, or erythema toxicum neonatorum, is an elevated, hive-like rash that may result in small white vesicles. It is not contagious and, like milia, disappears without treatment.
> - *Telangiectatic nevi*, "stork bites," are flat pink or red marks often seen on the eyelids, nose, or nape of the neck. These are dilated capillaries that become more vivid when the infant cries. They are not significant to the health of the infant and disappear at 1 to 2 years of age.
> - *Mongolian spots* are areas of increased pigmentation. The lumbar dorsal area is the most common location. The area may appear bluish black. These are most often seen in darker-skinned people.
> - *Nevus flammeus*, port-wine stain, is a reddish purple discoloration often seen on the face. This is a capillary angioma below the epidermis. Unfortunately, these do not disappear spontaneously. Medical techniques have been developed that reduce or remove port-wine birthmarks.
> - *Strawberry birthmarks*, nevus vasculosus, are capillary hemangiomas. These may continue to increase in size for several months. They normally then begin to shrink spontaneously and usually disappear early in childhood.

The newborn's hemoglobin and hematocrit levels frequently are elevated; hemoglobin may range from 14 to 24 g/dL, and hematocrit from 44% to 64%. These elevated levels are needed by the fetus to assist with oxygen transport. After delivery, the neonate does not require these same levels.

As the infant's body begins to manage this elevation and cells are broken down, jaundice results. *Jaundice*, a yellow discoloration caused by deposits of bile pigments, is first detected over bony prominences on the face and the mucous membranes. Normally occurring jaundice results approximately 48 hours after birth and is termed *physiologic jaundice*. It gradually disappears by the seventh to tenth day. Jaundice that occurs sooner than 48 hours after birth is termed *pathologic jaundice*. This type of jaundice is not normal and may be the result of a maternal-fetal blood incompatibility. Further assessment of jaundice is necessary. The physician may order laboratory and diagnostic tests to determine the nature of the problem and begin treatment to prevent complications.

Appearance

At birth, the skin is covered with a yellowish white, cream cheese–like substance called vernix caseosa. This substance protects the infant's skin from the amniotic fluid. When the vernix caseosa is removed, the skin may appear dry and may crack, flake, and peel. Another common finding is lanugo (downy, fine hair characteristic of the fetus between 20 weeks of gestation and birth); lanugo is most noticeable over the shoulders, forehead, and cheeks, but it is found on nearly all parts of the body, except the palms, soles, and scalp.

Umbilical Cord

The umbilical cord is whitish blue-gray with three vessels (one vein and two arteries) and contains a gelatinous tissue called Wharton jelly. Inspect the cord for the number of vessels because a two-vessel cord may indicate congenital anomalies. In Fig. 30.6, note the cord stump in *A* and the cord stump in *B* (triple dye gives it the purplish color).

Providing Cord Care

The cord clamp must be securely fastened with no skin caught in it. Purulent drainage or redness or edema at the base indicates infection. The cord becomes brownish black within 2 or 3 days and falls off in about 10 to 14 days. If there is any bleeding noted from the cord, notify the nurse at once.

Care of the cord varies in different agencies. It may be treated with a bactericidal substance, such as triple-dye solution (see Fig. 30.6B), antibiotic ointment, or alcohol, three times a day or allowed to dry naturally. None of the treatments commonly used is better at keeping the cord clean and dry than the others. When soiled, the cord should be cleaned with water. This natural treatment of cords may shorten the time to cord separation and does not lead to increased infections. The diaper is folded below the cord to keep the cord dry and free from contamination with urine.

The nurse may ask the patient care technician to remove the cord clamp about 24 hours after birth if the end of the cord is dry (Fig. 30.7). Although the base of the cord is still moist, it does not bleed if the end is dry and crisp.

Hypothermia

Maintenance of body temperature is a major concern in the care of newborns. Prolonged exposure to a cold environment can result in increased oxygen consumption and depleted fat reserves. Newborns have a relatively large surface area and a limited amount of protective adipose (fat) tissue. They lose heat through radiation, evaporation, conduction, and convection. Be aware of this and take precautions to reduce the losses (Table 30.3).

Right after delivery, a heat lamp will be used to keep the newborn warm. This is often called a warmer or

Table 30.3	Precautions to Minimize Heat Loss in Infants
Types of Heat Loss	**Nursing Interventions to Prevent Heat Loss**
Radiation: Loss that occurs when heat transfers from the body to cooler surfaces and objects not in contact with the body	Keep body well wrapped to prevent radiant loss. Work quickly to avoid excessive time with skin exposed. Use radiant warmer to minimize loss. Locate crib away from outside wall.
Evaporation: Loss when water is converted into a vapor	Dry infant thoroughly after delivery and promptly when bathing.
Conduction: Loss of heat to a cooler surface via direct skin contact	Pad surfaces under infant, including tables and scales. Warm other equipment, such as stethoscopes, before use.
Convection: Loss of heat to cooler air currents	Reduce drafts from open doors, windows, or air conditioning; wrap newborn to protect from cold.

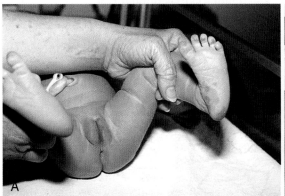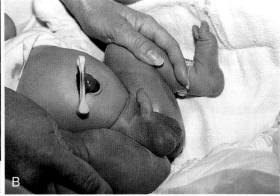

FIGURE 30.6 External genitalia. A, Genitalia in female term infant. Note mucoid vaginal discharge. B, Genitalia in male infant. Uncircumcised penis. Rugae cover scrotum, indicating term gestation. Cord has been swabbed with ethylene blue to prevent infection. (A, Courtesy Marjorie Pyle, RNC, LifeCircle, Costa Mesa, California, in Lowdermilk DL, Perry SE, Cashion K, et al.: *Maternity and women's health care,* ed 11, St. Louis, 2016, Mosby. B, Courtesy Marjorie Pyle, RNC, LifeCircle, Costa Mesa, California, in Lowdermilk DL, Perry SE, Cashion K, et al.: *Maternity and women's health care,* ed 10, St. Louis, 2012, Mosby.)

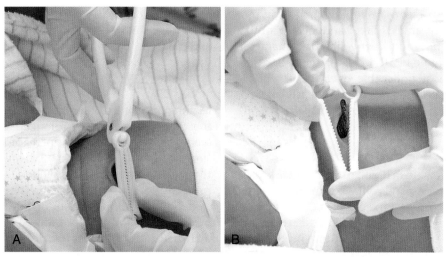

FIGURE 30.7 The cord clamp is removed when the end of the cord is dry and crisp. The clamp is cut (A) and separated (B). Note: No triple dye was used; the diaper is folded down away from the cord area. (From McKinney ES, James SR, Murray SS, et al.: *Maternal-child nursing,* ed 4, Philadelphia, 2013, Saunders.)

stabilette. Monitor temperature with a skin sensor or thermometer. Most facilities use the axillary route because it is considered safest. The normal axillary temperature is 97.6° to 98.6° F (36.4° to 37° C). Mercury thermometers are rarely used in healthcare settings today, although they may still be used in the home.

The First Bath

The patient care technician may be asked to give the newborn the first bath. Some facilities allow bathing the newborn in the patient's room to allow the parents to bond with the newborn. Other facilities require the newborn be taken to the nursery for the first bath. Bathing of the neonate take place after the body temperature has stabilized. The frequency and type of baths depend on facility policies. Bathing serves a number of purposes: complete cleansing, observation of the infant's condition, comfort, and parent-child bonding.

Gather all bathing articles and the infant's change of clothing before bathing. The room temperature should be 75° F (24° C), and the bathing area should be free of drafts to prevent heat loss. The bath water should be approximately 100° F (38° C). Heat loss in the infant is greater than heat loss in the adult because of the relatively large ratio of the skin surface to body mass in the newborn. To conserve the infant's energy, control heat loss by bathing the infant quickly, padding cold surfaces, exposing only a portion of the body at a time, and thoroughly drying the infant. Until the initial bath is completed, wear gloves when handling the newborn.

The Centers for Disease Control and Prevention (CDC) regulations related to standard precautions against human immunodeficiency virus and other bloodborne pathogens have increased the use of soap solutions for bathing newborn infants. Use a nonmedicated mild soap

for the initial bath. Shampoo the hair and use a brush or a comb to remove dried blood and vernix caseosa. Careful drying reduces the heat lost during bathing. The order of the bath is essentially the same as for an adult, beginning with the eyes, the face, and the head and ending with the anal region. Do not vigorously remove vernix caseosa (the white material that looks like cold cream) because it is attached to the upper, protective layer of the skin. Vernix caseosa may be left on for 48 hours; if it persists beyond that time, wash if off gently. Some nurses advocate massaging the vernix caseosa gently into the skin. To date, no studies have confirmed the benefits or disadvantages of this technique.

Reassess the temperature 30 minutes after completion of the bath.

After the initial bath, washing with warm water is sufficient for the first week. Full submersion into a tub of water should not be done until the cord has fallen off. The infant's skin is thin and delicate. The infant's fragile skin can be injured by vigorous cleansing. Daily bathing is not needed; however, the perineal area should be carefully washed with nonmedicated mild soap and warm water and carefully dried with each diaper change. Parents may make personal decisions about the brand and type of cleaning agents used. Recommendations are that oils and scented products should be avoided. After the bath, talc or baby powder should not be used because it may cause aspiration if too close to the nose and mouth.

Circumcision refers to the surgical removal of the foreskin. Many parents elect to have the procedure performed on their newborn infant (http://www .acog.org/Patients/FAQs/Newborn-Circumcision). In the United States, 64% of newborns are circumcised in the first days after birth (http://www.childrenshospital .org/conditions-and-treatments/treatments/circum cision). Regional differences are found with the procedure. Rates of circumcision are highest in the southern and midwestern states and lowest in the west. The reasons parents opt to have their sons circumcised are varied. Some parents choose circumcision to follow "family tradition," and others out of concern for their son's reproductive health. The Jewish faith promotes the circumcision of infant boys. Jewish families who follow the time-honored ritual of their faith opt to have the circumcision performed 7 days after birth. The procedure is performed in a religious ceremony by a religious figure (Goodman, 1999). The American Academy of Pediatrics (AAP) reported in 1999 that acknowledged health benefits were associated with circumcision but that these benefits were not significant enough to warrant a recommendation to mandate this procedure for all male infants. In 2012, the AAP again reaffirmed this position (American Academy of Pediatrics, 2012). The AAP further states that pain medicine should be used if a circumcision is performed; a consent form for both is required.

If circumcision is performed, the area should be kept clean. Sterile petroleum gauze is usually applied to the penis after circumcision and is left in place for 24 hours; it is replaced if it becomes dislodged prematurely.

Wash the penis gently at diaper changes to remove urine and feces, and reapply fresh sterile petroleum gauze. Do not attempt to remove the dried yellow exudate that forms in 24 hours and persists for 2 to 3 days; this is part of the normal healing process. Some practitioners may recommend the use of cloth diapers during the first week to promote healing. Loose diapering is necessary. These infants usually are fussy for about 2 to 3 hours and may refuse a feeding.

Injury & Illness Prevention Box 30.1

- If any bleeding is noted around the circumcision site, notify the nurse at once.
- A newborn can hemorrhage from the site of a circumcision.
- Bleeding from a circumcision site may be the first time the healthcare team would know whether the patient had any bleeding disorders.

Newborn Elimination

The newborn should void within 24 hours of delivery. The average newborn voids small amounts of poorly concentrated urine; it is normally clear and odorless. Occasionally, a small pink or brownish discharge may be observed as a result of uric acid crystals that were formed in the bladder in utero. As fluid intake increases and kidney function improves, urination becomes more frequent and assumes the normal color.

Bowel elimination should occur within 24 hours of birth. The newborn's initial stools are odorless, black-green, and sticky. This is called meconium and is made up of vernix, strands of lanugo, mucus, and other substances from the amniotic fluid. Occasionally, the first stool is encased in mucus and called a *meconium plug.* Once the infant begins to take nourishment, the stool changes. Transitional stools, which occur on about the second day, tend to be greenish and loose. These are seen until about the fourth day, when the milk stool is seen. Breastfed babies tend to pass stool frequently, sometimes with every feeding. The stool is pale yellow and sweet smelling. Small curds may be observed. Babies who are bottle fed tend to have fewer stools, usually two or three per day after the first 2 weeks. These are bright yellow and pasty in consistency; the odor may be slightly stronger than that of breastfed babies. This type of stool continues until solid food is introduced. Very watery stools, green stools (after the transition), or stools expelled with force may indicate gastrointestinal irritation or infection and should be reported promptly (Fig. 30.8). Newborns can lose a great deal of fluid rapidly and become dehydrated (see Box 30.3 for stooling patterns of newborns). (Note that newborns normally give the impression of straining with a stool because their muscles are underdeveloped. This can cause parents undue concern if they are not advised about it. The straining subsides as growth and maturity continue.)

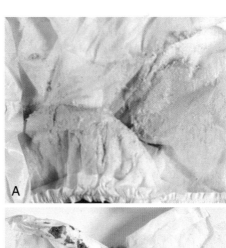

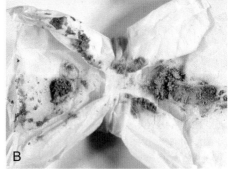

FIGURE 30.8 Infant stool. A, Breastfed. B, Formula fed. (From Zitelli BJ, McIntire SC, Nowalk AJ: *Zitelli and Davis' atlas of pediatric physical diagnosis,* ed 6, St. Louis, 2012, Saunders.)

Box 30.3	Change in Stooling of Newborns

Meconium
- Infant's first stool is composed of amniotic fluid and its constituents, intestinal secretions, shed mucosal cells, and possibly blood (ingested maternal blood or minor bleeding of alimentary tract vessels).
- Passage of meconium should occur within the first 24 to 48 hours, although it may be delayed up to 7 days in very-low-birth-weight infants.
- Colostrum has a laxative effect that aids the infant to expel the meconium.

Transitional Stools
- Transitional stools usually appear by the third day after initiation of feeding.
- They are greenish brown to yellowish brown, thin, and less sticky than meconium; they may contain some milk curds.

Milk Stool
- Milk stools usually appear by the fourth day.
- In *breastfed* infants, stools are yellow to golden, are pasty in consistency, and have an odor similar to that of sour milk.
- In *formula-fed* infants, stools are pale yellow to light brown, are firmer in consistency, and have a more offensive odor.

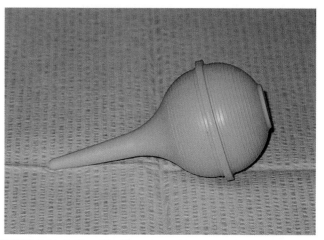

FIGURE 30.9　Nasal bulb syringe. (From Proctor D, Adams A: *Kinn's The Medical Assistant: an applied learning approach*, ed 12, St. Louis, 2014, Saunders.)

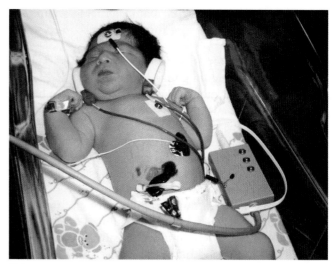

FIGURE 30.10　Hearing screening test. (Courtesy Dee Lowdermilk, Chapel Hill, NC. IN Lowdermilk D, et al.: *Maternity & women's health care*, ed 10, St. Louis, 2012, Mosby.)

Airway Clearance

Maintenance of a clear airway is critical. Many newborns need suctioning to remove mucus from the nose and mouth. Newborns are obligate (necessary or required) nose breathers; they must be able to breathe through the nose while suckling. Therefore the nasal passageway must be kept open and free from mucus. A small bulb syringe is commonly used. Squeeze it before insertion and then gently release it to suction secretions. For the first few days, a bulb syringe should always be kept with the newborn, particularly during feeding (Fig. 30.9).

Newborn Hearing Screenings

The AAP recommends universal screening of newborn hearing before discharge since studies have indicated that the incidence of hearing loss is as high as 2 to 4 per 1000 normal newborns (http://emedicine.medscape .com/article/836646-overview). The patient care technician may administer this noninvasive hearing screening in the newborn nursery. It involves placement of electrodes on different areas of the scalp and shoulder. Newborns should be in a passive quiet state, which means that they should not be active with movement,

nor should they be crying. This will help ensure that accurate results are obtained (Fig. 30.10).

Legal Implications

The patient care technician may be in the position to recognize and provide assistance to women who are being mistreated. Battered women seldom come forward and tell healthcare workers they are being abused. If the patient reports such problems to the patient care technician, or if an abusive situation is suspected, do not hesitate to report this information to the physician. The American Medical Association (AMA) has developed guidelines to help caregivers recognize victims of abuse.

- *Know what to look for:* Suspicious findings include multiple injuries at different sites, especially areas that normally are covered by clothing. Also, the patient may be frightened, anxious, and passive and may have a history of "accidents."

- *Know what to ask when obtaining a patient history:* Even patients who show no signs of abuse should be asked whether they have ever been in an abusive relationship; if verbal arguments ever become physical; if their partner acts differently when drinking or using drugs; and if their partner is overprotective and jealous.
- *Know what to say and do:* A battered woman suffers both physical and emotional abuse. She may begin to believe that she deserves to be mistreated, and she needs unconditional and nonjudgmental emotional support from the healthcare worker. She needs to be treated with warmth and respect and encouraged to develop a plan of action to deal with the next violent episode. Suggestions include having immediate access to important documents, keys, money, transportation, the address of a safe house, and phone numbers for the police and local domestic violence hotline if available. The National Domestic Violence Hotline can be reached at 1-800-799-SAFE (7233). It provides 24-hour help for victims seeking local shelters.

THE PEDIATRIC PATIENT

An infant's first physical assessment comes at the time of delivery, when the pediatrician assesses the newborn's ability to thrive outside the uterus. The Apgar score is a system for evaluating the infant's physical condition at 1 and 5 minutes after birth (Table 30.4). Developed by pediatrician Virginia Apgar, the scoring system evaluates the following: *a*ppearance (color); *p*ulse (heart rate); *g*rimace (reflex; response to stimuli); *a*ctivity (muscle tone); and *r*espiration (breathing). These parameters are each rated 0, 1, or 2. The maximum total score is 10.

Infants with low scores require immediate medical attention.

Well-Child Visits

The frequency of well-child visits, or how often a newborn visits the physician, varies with the physician and the community. It may follow this pattern: 2 weeks, 4 weeks, 8 weeks, 4 months, 6 months, 12 months, 18 months, 2 years, 5 years, 10 years, and 15 years. These visits focus on maintaining the child's health through basic system examinations, immunizations, and upgrading of the child's medical history record (Box 30.4).

The decision on whether the child is to be seen alone or with the parent depends on the pediatrician and the child's age. Often the child looks to the parent for approval before answering or performing a skill; for this reason, the physician may want to assess the child alone. If this is the case, explain to the parent that the physician wants to evaluate the child's independent abilities and that as soon as testing is complete, the physician will explain the results of the tests.

The medical history is an essential guide to the pediatric examination. With an infant, the physician depends on the caregiver for the history, but as the child gets older, some history may be obtained from the child and clarified or amplified by the parent. Close observation also gives the physician considerable information.

Sick-Child Visits

Sick-child visits occur whenever needed, usually on short notice. For this reason, most pediatric offices keep open appointments in the schedule to accommodate calls for sick-child visits. The length and frequency of this type of visit depends entirely on the child and the illness. The patient care technician who works in a pediatrician's office or on a pediatric unit frequently is the first point of contact for a sick child and his or her caregiver.

Table 30.4	Apgar Scoring System*		
	ASSIGNED SCORE		
Clinical Sign	0	1	2
Heart rate	Absent	100	100
Respiratory effort	Absent	Slow and irregular	Good and crying
Muscle tone	Limp	Some flexion of the arms and legs	Active movement
Reflex irritability	No response	Grimace	Coughing and sneezing
Color	Blue and pale	Body pink and extremities blue	Pink all over

*, http://www.acog.org/Resources-And-Publications/Committee-Opinions/Committee-on-Obstetric-Practice/The-Apgar-Score

Box 30.4	Lead Paint Exposure

Children are especially vulnerable to lead levels in their environment. High blood lead levels can result in serious brain injury, including seizures, coma, and death; lower levels can cause learning problems, stunted growth, and behavior disorders. Lead-based paint in homes and on imported toys and chronic exposure to lead-contaminated dust are the most common causes of lead exposure. The Centers for Disease Control and Prevention (CDC) recommends a screening blood lead test for all children between 1 and 2 years of age. This screening may be done using a capillary blood sample (see Chapter 24) and may be delegated to the patient care technician.

THE PATIENT CARE TECHNICIAN'S ROLE IN PEDIATRIC PROCEDURES

The patient care technician is responsible for assisting the pediatrician with examinations; upgrading patient histories; performing ordered screening tests, such as vision, hearing, urinalysis, and hemoglobin checks; measuring and weighing children as needed; and providing patient and caregiver support. A patient care technician must develop a relationship with the pediatric patient that encourages cooperation and compliance with tests and treatment plans. If the child becomes upset, everything you need to do to the child during that time will be done under stress for them, and the chance for them struggling with trusting you in the future will be greater. When entering the room of pediatric patients, it is best to address them on their eye level rather than looking down at them. Pediatric staff typically wear brightly colored uniforms, sometimes with friendly patterns, as a way to encourage trust with the pediatric patient.

Interacting with children requires special techniques, depending on the child's age. A calm, unhurried manner is essential to gaining cooperation. The tone of voice should be gentle but confident. Using a firm, direct approach about expected behavior is important in gaining the cooperation of older children. Offering sincere praise for the child during the examination or procedures helps ease anxiety and builds self-esteem. If the child is having an unusually difficult time, try to discover the reason. If he or she has had a bad medical experience in the past, the child may be afraid of what might happen. Each step should be explained in a language the child (as well as parent) can understand. Children younger than 2 years feel better when the parent holds them or remains very close. Preschool children enjoy playing, so making a game out of the situation is helpful (Fig. 30.11). Whatever the child's age,

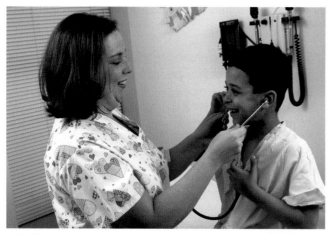

FIGURE 30.11 Making a game out of a procedure. (From Proctor D, Adams A: *Kinn's The Medical Assistant: an applied learning approach*, ed 12, St. Louis, 2014, Saunders.)

the patient care technician should be sensitive to his or her individual needs and should adapt the examination and procedures as much as possible to meet those needs.

The sequence of the physician's examination or nurse's assessment varies and frequently is adapted based on the child's cooperation. The pediatrician or nurse probably will leave procedures and tests that are likely to cause the most objections until the end of the examination. The physician or nurse is constantly evaluating the child's growth and development. A child's alertness and responses tell the physician or nurse a considerable amount. With infants and young children of preschool age, the parent is closely questioned about the child's eating, sleeping, and elimination habits. A school-aged child usually is a little more cooperative during an examination and can answer most questions without parental assistance. Adolescent patients should be given the option of not having parents present during an examination. This may permit teenagers to respond more honestly about lifestyle factors and also protects their privacy.

Measurement

Examination of the child includes measurement of the circumference of the infant's head to determine normal growth and development (see Chapter 15). The size of the child's head reflects the growth of the brain. Brain growth is 50% complete by 1 year of age, 75% by age 3, and 90% by age 6. Routine head measurement is recommended in children until 36 months of age and in older children whose head size is not within norms. It is important to discover any congenital problem as early as possible so that appropriate treatment can be started.

The patient care technician should record the child's length or height, weight, and head circumference on growth charts so that the physician can compare the child's measurement statistics with national standards. Growth charts consist of a series of percentile curves that illustrate the distribution of selected body measurements.

The current version of the CDC's growth records consists of 16 charts (8 for boys and 8 for girls) (Figs. 30.12 and 30.13). These charts represent revisions of the 14 previous charts and also the introduction of BMI-for-age charts for boys and for girls aged 2 to 20 years. The BMI is the recommended method of determining whether children or adults are overweight or obese. The BMI growth charts can be used beginning at 2 years of age, when height can be measured accurately.

Assisting With the Examination

Vital signs are measured first (Table 30.5). Depending on the child's age and level of cooperation, the temperature

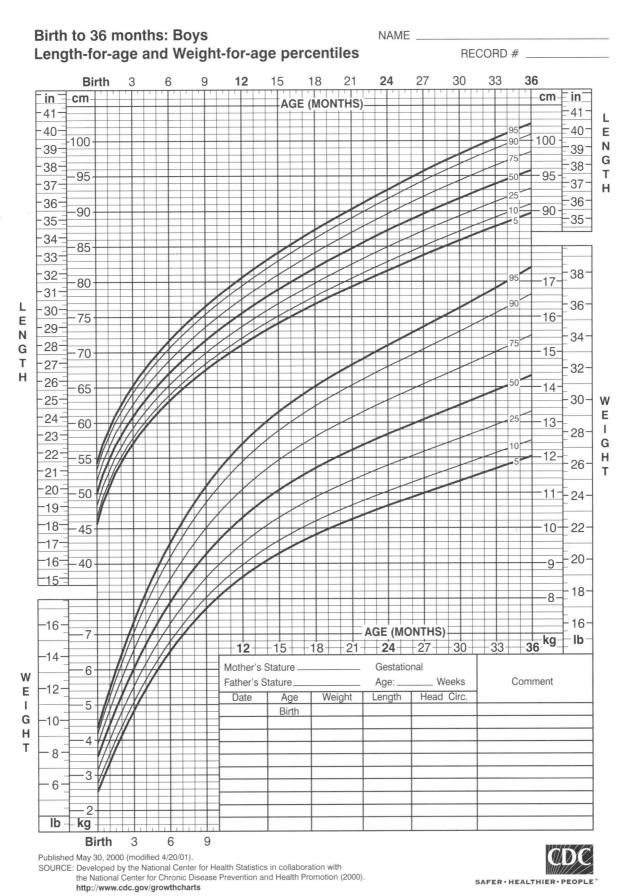

Birth to 36 months: Boys
Length-for-age and Weight-for-age percentiles

NAME _____

RECORD # _____

Published May 30, 2000 (modified 4/20/01).
SOURCE: Developed by the National Center for Health Statistics in collaboration with
    the National Center for Chronic Disease Prevention and Health Promotion (2000).
    http://www.cdc.gov/growthcharts

CDC
SAFER · HEALTHIER · PEOPLE™

FIGURE 30.12 Growth chart: males (birth to 36 months). (Developed by the National Center for Health Statistics in collaboration with the National Center for Chronic Disease Prevention and Health Promotion (2000). http://www.cdc.gov/growthcharts)

2 to 20 years: Girls
Stature-for-age and Weight-for-age percentiles

NAME _____

RECORD # _____

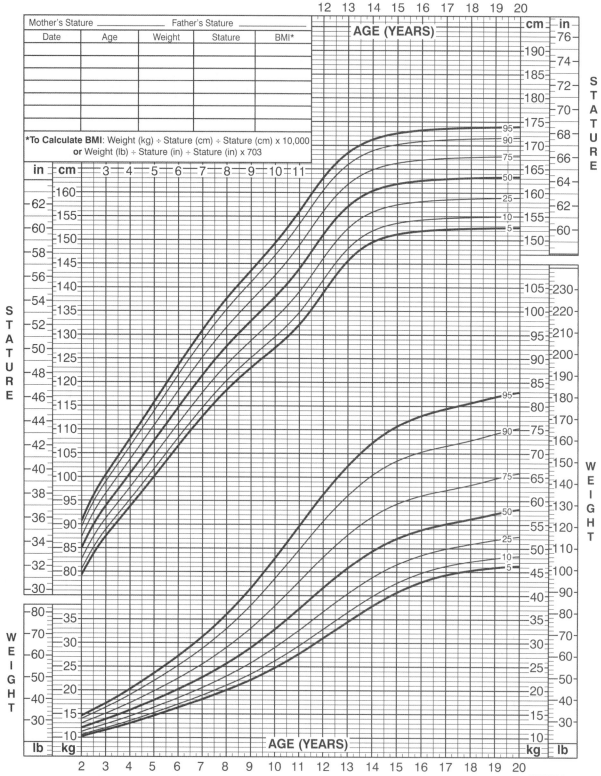

Published May 30, 2000 (modified 11/21/00).
SOURCE: Developed by the National Center for Health Statistics in collaboration with
the National Center for Chronic Disease Prevention and Health Promotion (2000).
http://www.cdc.gov/growthcharts

FIGURE 30.13 Growth chart: females (2 to 20 years). (Developed by the National Center for Health Statistics in collaboration with the National Center for Chronic Disease Prevention and Health Promotion (2000). http://www.cdc.gov/growthcharts)

Table 30.5	Reference Ranges for Pediatric Vital Signs
Vital Sign	**Reference Range**
Temperature	
Oral	98.6°F (37°C)
Aural	100.4°F (38°C)
Axillary	97.6°F (36.4°C)
Pulse	
Newborn	100 to 180 beats per minute
3 mo–2 yr	80 to 150 beats per minute
2 to 10 yr	65 to 130 beats per minute
Respirations	
Newborn	30 to 50 breaths per minute
1 to 3 yr	25 to 30 breaths per minute
4 to 6 yr	23 to 25 breaths per minute
7+ yr	16 to 20 breaths per minute
Blood Pressure	
Newborn	Systolic 90 mm Hg; diastolic 70 mm Hg
1 to 5 yr	Systolic 100 mm Hg; diastolic 70 mm Hg
6 to 12 yr	Systolic 120 mm Hg; diastolic 84 mm Hg
13+ yr	Systolic, 100 mm Hg + age; diastolic, 30 to 40 mm Hg less

may be obtained by the axillary, oral, rectal, tympanic, or temporal method. The rectal and temporal methods are considered most accurate in infants; however, the temporal method is easiest, quickest, and less invasive. It is important to remember that the younger the child, the more immature the ability to regulate body heat. Therefore the temperature of an infant may fluctuate easily and rapidly. The child's pulse rate is affected similar to that of an adult; it can increase as a result of activity, anxiety, illness, and environmental temperature. If the child is younger than 2 years, the pulse is measured apically by placing the stethoscope on the left side of the chest medial to the nipple. Always count the beats for 1 full minute for accuracy.

An alternative method of obtaining the pulse of a very young child is to use the brachial artery in the upper arm. After age 2 years, the child's pulse may be taken at the radial pulse site. Anticipate a pulse rate higher than that of an adult; the younger the child, the faster the pulse. The respiratory rate is easily obtained in a child because the chest can be readily observed. Expect the rate to be increased according to the child's age (the younger the child, the faster the normal respiratory rate) and health. The ratio of four pulse beats to one respiration should remain constant in a healthy child.

Blood pressure measurements are not included in most pediatric examinations. However, if the child has a heart or kidney defect, a blood pressure reading may be ordered. The cuff must be the appropriate width to obtain an accurate reading, and the bell of the stethoscope must be small enough to seal over the site. It is best to use a pediatric stethoscope with a pediatric bell when obtaining an infant's pressure. Blood pressure readings in a young child are lower than those in an adult.

To prevent a small child or infant from rolling the head from side to side during the physician's examination, stand at the head of the table and support the child's head between your hands. An infant needs not be draped, but privacy is important to an older child. Sincere respect and friendly conversation at the child's level accomplishes a great deal. Always be patient with children. Ensure that they understand what is expected. Always involve the parents or caregivers as much as possible.

INJURY PREVENTION

Unintentional injuries are the leading cause of death and disability in children in the United States. Injuries cause more childhood deaths than all diseases combined. The primary causes of childhood injuries are motor vehicle accidents, drowning, burns, falls, poisoning, aspiration with airway obstruction, and firearm accidents. Childhood injuries are linked to the child's growth and development level and usually are preventable. Young children are totally dependent on caregivers to keep them safe, so constant supervision and a childproof environment are essential for this age group. Older children need to be aware of health hazards and should be encouraged to protect themselves from injury (e.g., use bike helmets, protective padding when skateboarding, and seat belts). The highest incidence of accidental injuries is seen in children under age 9 years (http://www.cdc.gov/safechild/child_injury_data.html). Patient care technicians should always be sure that the patient care environment is safe for pediatric patients. This may include ensuring that all electric outlets are plugged, any equipment with cords is kept out of reach of children, and side rails are always up and engaged.

THE ADOLESCENT PATIENT

The adolescent patient may present the greatest challenge to health education and disease management. Adolescence begins with the onset of puberty, a time when the child's reproductive system matures, and is marked by rapid changes in the endocrine and musculoskeletal systems. The adolescent undergoes rapid growth spurts and the development of secondary sexual characteristics.

Health examinations for patients in this age group should include screening for height and weight; gathering details about diet and exercise routines; screening for sexually transmitted infections (STIs), and for sexually active female adolescents, a Pap test, especially to screen for infection with human papillomavirus (HPV); reviewing the vaccination history and administration of boosters as indicated; and assessing for high-risk behaviors, such as substance abuse and sexual behavior.

Some health problems most frequently seen in adolescent patients include eating disorders (anorexia nervosa and bulimia nervosa), obesity, and injury-related problems. Accidents are the leading cause of death and injury in adolescence, and suicide is the third leading cause of death. All healthcare personnel should be on the alert for indicators of suicide, including the following:

- Signs of depression, such as headaches, abdominal discomfort, anorexia, fatigue, aggressiveness, drug or alcohol abuse, and sexual promiscuity
- Verbal statements that hint at the adolescent's intention to commit suicide; talking about dying
- Actions such as giving away prized objects, withdrawing from social groups, sudden changes in normal behavior patterns, or writing a suicide note

CHILD ABUSE

The Child Abuse Prevention and Treatment Act states that all threats to a child's physical and/or mental welfare must be reported. This means that every teacher, healthcare worker, and social worker—in fact, every citizen—who suspects that a child is being neglected or abused must report this to the proper authority. The agency must record the report, and after three similar reports, the agency must investigate.

When suspected abuse is reported, the individual must provide his or her name; however, this is considered confidential information and is not given to the child's parent or guardian, nor is it given to the investigating officer. The individual making the report also is protected under the law from any liability for reporting suspicions of child abuse.

If the patient care technician suspects that a child is a victim of abuse, he or she should notify the nurse immediately. In most states, the patient care technician and the nurse can make separate reports to the authorities. However, state laws vary, so state and local reporting protocols should be outlined in the office procedures manual. See Box 30.5 for signs of child abuse.

Injury & Illness Prevention Box 30.2

- Children should cover their mouth with a disposable tissue when they cough and should blow the nose with disposable tissues.
- A tissue should be used only once and then immediately thrown away.
- Children should not be allowed to share toys they have put in their mouth.
- After a child has discarded a toy that was in the mouth, it should be placed in a bin for dirty toys that is out of reach of others. Wash and disinfect these toys before allowing children to play with them again.
- Ensure that all children and adults follow good hand-washing practices.

Legal and Ethical Issues

In the United States, children are considered persons who are growing and developing physically, emotionally, and mentally. Our laws view children as a distinct group, and laws and customs have been established that deal with the protection of children's rights.

Box 30.5   Signs of Child Abuse

Obvious Signs
- Previously filed reports of physical or sexual abuse of the child
- Documented abuse of other family members
- Different stories between parents and child on how an accident happened
- Stories of incidents and injuries that are suspicious
- Injuries blamed on other family members
- Repeated visits to the emergency department for injuries

Examination Findings
- Trauma to the nervous system
- Internal abdominal pain
- Discolorations/bruising on the buttocks, back, and abdomen
- Elbow, wrist, and shoulder dislocations

Changes in Behavior
- Too eager to please the parent
- Overly passive and too compliant
- Aggressive and demanding
- Parenting the parent (role reversal)
- Delays in the normal growth and development patterns
- Erratic school attendance

Physical Indicators
- Poor hygiene
- Malnutrition
- Obvious dental neglect
- Neglected well-baby procedures (e.g., immunizations)

CHAPTER SUMMARY

The female reproductive system is made up of the external genitalia and the internal organs, including the vagina; the cervix, which must dilate and efface for vaginal birth of a child; the uterus; the fallopian tubes; and the ovaries, which mature and produce ova.

Pregnancy occurs when the ovum and the sperm meet in the fallopian tube and a zygote is formed. The zygote implants in the uterine wall, and the placenta begins to form, which provides hormonal support for the pregnancy. The fetus is surrounded by an amniotic sac and floats in amniotic fluid. Oxygen and nutrients for the fetus pass through the placenta to the umbilical cord. The embryonic period ends at 12 weeks; by then, all tissues and organs have developed. During the remainder of the pregnancy, the organs mature and begin to function, and the fetus grows. Pregnancy is divided into three trimesters. The first trimester is a crucial time for fetal organ development; the second trimester brings quickening and many physiologic changes in the mother; during the third trimester, the fetal organ systems mature. The three stages of labor are dilation and effacement of the cervix, birth, and expulsion of the placenta.

The patient care technician prepares the patient for the examination, equips the room, ensures that supplies are available and properly prepared, positions and drapes the patient as needed, assists with the Pap smear or any other procedures, and provides support and understanding for the patient.

Confidentiality is crucial in dealing with obstetric and gynecologic disorders. Only healthcare professionals directly involved in the patient's care should know the purpose of the patient's visit, diagnosis, or treatment. The patient care technician may be in the position to recognize and provide assistance to women who are being mistreated. If the patient reports such problems to the patient care technician, or if an abusive situation is suspected, do not hesitate to report this information to the nurse.

The patient care technician assists the physician and/or nurse with the pediatric physical assessment; performs ordered screening tests such as vision, hearing, urinalysis, and hemoglobin checks; measures height and weight as needed; documents accurately; and provides support to patients and caregivers. Vital signs vary in children because of their growing physical and developmental systems.

Adolescents are going through extreme physical and emotional changes, and an extra measure of patience and understanding is required to establish therapeutic interactions. Ensuring their privacy and giving them the option of being assessed without their parents are important factors in establishing truth with an adolescent.

Case Scenario

You are assisting with opening a new pediatric unit in the hospital where you work as a patient care technician. Your unit manager has asked you to help ensure that all patient rooms are considered safe for the patients, regardless of their age. Considering all ages of children, what precautions would you take to make a patient room safe and why? Name the areas you would observe within a room for potential safety hazards for children. What could you do to take a potential safety hazard and make it safe?

REVIEW QUESTIONS

1. The average pregnancy lasts how long?
   a. 150 days
   b. 200 days
   c. 250 days
   d. 280 days

2. The umbilical cord typically falls off at what age?
   a. 2 to 3 days
   b. 5 to 7 days
   c. 10 to 14 days
   d. 1 month

3. What is the normal axillary temperature for a newborn?
   a. 97.6° to 98.6° F
   b. 97.5° to 98.0° F
   c. 98.0° to 98.6° F
   d. 98.0° to 99.0° F

4. Turning the fan off just before the delivery of a newborn will help prevent heat loss through which mechanism?
   a. Evaporation
   b. Conduction
   c. Convection
   d. Radiation

5. Drying newborns off with towels when they are born will help prevent which type of heat loss?
   a. Evaporation
   b. Conduction
   c. Convection
   d. Conduction

6. What act states that all threats to a child's physical or emotional well-being must be reported?
   a. Health Insurance Privacy & Portability Act
   b. Child Abuse Prevention and Treatment Act
   c. Patient's Bill of Rights
   d. Affordable Care Act

7. What is the leading cause of death and disability in children in the United States?
   a. Car accidents
   b. Cancer
   c. Unintentional injuries
   d. Fires

8. At what age can a radial pulse be taken from a pediatric patient?
   a. 6 months
   b. 1 year
   c. 18 months
   d. 3 years

Caring for the Older Adult

LEARNING OBJECTIVES

1. Discuss the impact of a growing aging population on society.
2. Identify the stereotypes and myths associated with aging.
3. Explain the changes in the anatomy and physiology of the body systems caused by aging.
4. Summarize the major diseases and disorders faced by older patients.
5. Describe various screening tools for dementia, depression, and malnutrition.
6. Explain the effect of aging on sleep.
7. Differentiate among independent, assisted, and skilled nursing facilities.
8. Summarize the role of the patient care technician in caring for aging patients.
9. Determine the principles of effective communication with older adults.
10. Identify legal and ethical issues associated with aging patients.

KEY TERMS

collagen The protein that forms the inelastic fibers of tendons, ligaments, and fascia
elastin An essential part of elastic connective tissue; when moist, it is flexible and elastic
lacrimation The secretion or discharge of tears
presbycusis A decreased ability to hear high frequencies and to discriminate sounds
presbyopia A difficulty in being able to focus on detailed objects close at hand
tinnitus A ringing or buzzing in the ears

According to the Administration on Aging, an agency of the U.S. Department of Health and Human Services, the aging population, those age 65 years or older, numbered 44.7 million in 2013. By 2030 almost 1 of every 5 Americans (about 72 million people) will be 65 years or older. The fastest growing segment of the U.S. population is those age 85 years or older.

The average life expectancy of an individual who reaches age 65 years is an additional 18.7 years (20 years for women, 17.1 years for men). A child born in 2010 has a projected life expectancy of 80.8 years, more than 30 years longer than a child born in 1900. Older women outnumber older men; 22.9 million women are older than age 65 years, as are 17.4 million men. About 30% of older people who live outside of institutions live alone; half of women over age 75 years live alone. More than half a million grandparents over the age of 65 years are the primary caregivers for their grandchildren who live with them. Most older people have at least one chronic medical condition, and many have multiple conditions. Hypertension, arthritis, heart disease, cancer, and diabetes are the health problems most commonly seen in the elderly, and a significant number also suffer from strokes, asthma, emphysema, and chronic bronchitis.

What does all this mean to those who have chosen careers in healthcare? As the aging population expands, it will affect all parts of society. One area in particular will be the individual's need to use health services in places such as physicians' offices, hospitals, and long-term-care facilities. To provide better services to the aging patient, the patient care technician should understand the aging process, which includes the physical and sensory changes with which older people must cope. This knowledge enables patient care technicians to recognize the special needs of the aged and to develop therapeutic management and communication skills that can help them effectively care for the older patient.

Aging is a complex physical, psychologic, and social process. Old age is not an illness but a normal life process that people experience in different ways. Lack of exercise, poor nutrition, substance abuse, continual stress, and air pollutants all are factors that cause a person to show the effects of aging decades earlier than someone who has practiced healthy living habits.

As people age, changes occur in their physical appearance and abilities, along with sensory changes in vision, hearing, taste, and smell. These changes do not occur at the same time in everyone; however, changes in the areas of their senses can have a huge effect on the person's ability to interact with his or her environment (Box 31.1).

CHANGES IN ANATOMY AND PHYSIOLOGY

The aging process brings about changes in all of the body's systems. Table 31.1 summarizes these changes and what can be done to encourage healthy aging.

Box 31.1   Stereotypes and Myths About Aging

- *Most aging people will develop dementia.* Dementia is not part of the normal aging process. However, the older the person, the greater the risk of dementia. About 6% of those aged above 65 years and 40% of those aged above 85 years are diagnosed with significant memory and disorientation issues.
- *Disease is a normal and an unavoidable part of the aging process.* Recent research verifies that people who have established healthy lifestyles as they age remain healthy well into their older years. Aging people are more likely to have health issues, but it does not mean that all persons aged above 65 years will have diseases.
- *Older workers are less productive than younger ones.* Older people who have a strong work ethic will continue to have a strong work ethic. It may take aging people longer to learn new material, but they continue to be capable of learning and applying new knowledge.
- *Most older people end up in long-term care facilities.* At any given time, approximately 5% of the aging population lives in long-term care facilities; 80% of aging individuals live alone with or without a partner.
- *Most aging people have no interest in or capacity for sexual relations.* Sexual interest does not change significantly with age; a decrease in sexual activity is usually related to the loss of a partner.
- *Deciding to make healthier choices to decrease the presence of diseases will do no good.* It is never too late to benefit from healthy lifestyle choices.

Cardiovascular System

Cardiovascular disease is the most frequent cause of illness and disability in the aging population, and congestive heart failure is the most common reason for hospitalization. Age-related changes occur in the cardiovascular system, but disease and lifestyle habits such as lack of exercise, poor diet, and stress contribute to these changes. Heart disease is ranked as the leading cause of death among men and women; therefore proper management of cardiovascular disease can help maintain the health of an aging population and reduce mortality rates.

Aging causes the walls of the veins to weaken and stretch. This damages the valves, especially in the veins of the legs, where the walls of the veins require more pressure in order to bring the blood back to the heart against the force of gravity. As a result, swelling and varicose veins of the lower legs are common in the elderly, increasing the risk of the formation of thrombi, or blood clots, in the deep veins, or deep vein thrombosis (DVT).

Arteriosclerosis is considered part of the aging process. The vessel walls thicken and become less elastic

Table 31.1	System Changes With Aging and Measures to Promote Health	
Body System	Age-Related Changes	Health Promotion
Cardiovascular system	Arteriosclerosis and atherosclerotic plaque buildup reduces blood flow to major organs; 50% of the aging population has hypertension; CVD is the number one killer of women and men in their 60s.	Regular exercise; weight control; diet rich in fruits, vegetables, and whole grains; cholesterol, blood glucose monitoring
Central nervous system	Brain shrinks by 10% between 30 and 90 years of age; takes longer to learn new material; attention span and language remain the same; signs and symptoms may be caused by depression, vascular disease, and drug reactions.	Aerobic exercise to increase blood flow to CNS; maintaining mental activities (e.g., reading, interacting with others)
Endocrine system	After age 50 years, women have a sharp decline in estrogen; men have a more gradual decline in testosterone.	Possible hormone replacement therapy or natural soy supplements
Gastrointestinal system	Decline in gastric juices and enzymes by age 60 years; decreased peristalsis with increased constipation; some nutrients are not absorbed as well.	High-fiber diet and adequate fluid intake; regular exercise to prevent constipation
Musculoskeletal system	Muscle mass decreases; tendency to gain weight; gradual loss of bone density; deterioration of joint cartilage	Strength training to increase muscle mass; stretching to remain limber; exercise; vitamin D and calcium supplements
Pulmonary system	At age 55 years the lungs become less elastic and the chest wall gradually stiffens, making oxygenation more difficult.	Regular aerobic exercise; quit smoking
Sensory organs	Hearing is intact through the mid-50s but declines by 25% by age 80 years; oral problems are common; skin thins and loses elasticity; presbyopia after age 40 years; cataracts common after age 60 years	Avoid exposure to loud noise; use of hearing aids; good dental hygiene; prevention of sun damage to the skin; annual eye examinations; diet rich in dark green, leafy vegetables to prevent cataracts and macular degeneration
Urinary system	Kidneys become less efficient; bladder muscles weaken; one third of seniors experience incontinence; prostate enlargement is common.	Pelvic exercises, drugs, or surgery for incontinence; annual PSA with digital rectal examination monitoring for men
Sexuality	Men: Impotence is not a symptom of normal aging; men over age 50 years may have some altered function. Women: Menopause causes vaginal narrowing and dryness, resulting in painful intercourse.	Men: Maintenance of cardiovascular health with exercise, weight control, no smoking, diabetes management Women: Use of vaginal lubricants or estrogen cream

CNS, Central nervous system; CVD, cardiovascular disease; PSA, prostate-specific antigen.

as a result of the calcification and buildup of connective tissue. In addition, the artery's ability to dilate and contract diminishes. To maintain an adequate blood supply throughout the body, the heart must work harder to overcome the resistance caused by stiffened vessels. Older adults have a higher incidence of orthostatic hypotension, which is a drop in blood pressure when the person stands or changes positions. The alteration in blood pressure from sitting to standing must drop more than 20 mm Hg in the systolic pressure or more than 10 mm Hg in the diastolic pressure when the position is changed in order to be orthostatic hypotension. This significant decrease is typically caused by a drop in the volume of circulating blood. The nurse may have the patient care technician take orthostatic blood pressures as part of the routine intake protocol for aging patients. This involves taking multiple blood pressures while the patient is in various positions, such as standing, sitting, and lying down.

Endocrine System

Hormonal changes that occur with aging are related to a general decrease in hormone production combined with changes in how the body's tissues receive the

hormones. The most common endocrine system disorder seen in aging patients is diabetes mellitus (DM) type 2. As a person ages, insulin production by the beta cells in the pancreas decreases and insulin resistance at the tissue level increases. According to the National Institutes of Health, more than half of the 16 million Americans diagnosed with DM type 2 are aged above 65 years. Elderly patients with diabetes are at increased risk of developing vascular disease, including kidney disorders, complications with the retina of the eyes, myocardial ischemia (death in heart tissue), angina, myocardial infarction (heart attack), cerebrovascular accidents (strokes), and peripheral vascular disease, such as lower extremity ulcers.

Older patients do not always experience the classic symptoms of diabetes, which are polyuria (increased urination), polydipsia (increased thirst), and polyphagia (increased hunger). They may show a variety of problems, including unexplained weight loss, slow wound healing, recurrent bacterial or fungal infections, changes in mental state, cataracts, macular disease, muscle weakness and pain, angina (chest pain), and foot ulcers. The range of symptoms is caused by the gradual onset of diabetes in older people, who may have gradually developing high blood glucose for years before diagnosis.

Factors That Can Affect Diabetes Management in Older People

- Modifying lifestyle risk factors may be more difficult because of poor nutrition, inability to exercise, and long-standing habits such as smoking and a diet high in fat and calories.
- Previously diagnosed health conditions, such as hypertension and heart disease, in addition to an age-related decline in kidney and liver function, increase the challenge of treating diabetes.
- Older people are more likely to be prescribed multiple medications (polypharmacy), which increases the risk of adverse drug interactions.
- Elderly patients with diabetes are more prone to hypoglycemia and may not recognize and respond quickly to the signs of low blood glucose levels.
- Diabetic complications can develop quickly because of a long history of prediabetes before diagnosis.
- Older people may have decreased physical and/or mental abilities that make it difficult for them to understand and adhere to a complicated treatment regimen.
- Older patients may not be able to afford the medications and supplies needed to maintain health.

The treatment plan for aging patients with diabetes is the same as for other age groups; however, special consideration must be given to the patient's ability to understand and follow the plan. In addition, because the person may have other health problems that are being treated with medications, an aging patient newly diagnosed with diabetes may face a complicated treatment regimen that requires explicit instruction and continual follow-up (Box 31.2).

Gastrointestinal System

Age-related changes in the gastrointestinal system begin in the mouth with dental problems, a decrease in the number of taste buds and the production of saliva, and a diminishing sense of smell. Older people generally find eating less pleasurable, have a reduced appetite, and are unable to chew and lubricate their food well compared with younger people; this makes dysphagia (difficulty swallowing) a common age-related problem. Secretion of a protein that is needed for the absorption of vitamin B_{12} also declines, which affects the function of the nervous system and the formation of red blood cells, resulting in excessive fatigue. It is not unusual for aging patients to be seen in the physician's office regularly for vitamin B_{12} injections to hopefully increase their energy level.

Food passes more quickly through the small intestine, resulting in poorer absorption of vitamins and minerals. Peristalsis in the colon decreases, making aging patients more susceptible to constipation and disease of the intestine. Poor eating habits, a reduced fluid intake, and some medications (e.g., antidepressants, diuretics, and antacids containing aluminum or calcium) also contribute to constipation. The liver decreases in size and weight after age 70 years. It is still able to perform vital functions, but more time is required to metabolize drugs and alcohol. All of these factors combine to increase the potential for adverse drug reactions in older adults.

Aging individuals have a higher incidence of several gastrointestinal system diseases, such as gastroesophageal reflux disease (GERD), peptic ulcers, diverticulosis (related to lack of dietary fiber and constipation), cholelithiasis (gallstones), and colorectal cancer. Dietary counseling and annual screenings should be part of the routine care of aging patients.

Integumentary System

The skin is the body's first line of protection against infection, and it also is responsible for preventing the loss of body fluid and regulating body temperature. Changes in the appearance and function of the integumentary system usually are caused by a combination of ordinary age-related changes and environmental factors, especially the amount of sun exposure over time. Exposure to ultraviolet light from the sun frequently is the cause of wrinkles, age spots, blotches, and leathery, dry, loose skin, all of which are associated with aging. Changes caused by the ultraviolet light from the sun or by the normal aging process can affect all three layers of the skin: the epidermis (top layer of skin), dermis (main layer of skin), and subcutaneous tissue (layer just beneath skin).

The cells in the epidermis reproduce more slowly as people age, and this slower regrowth causes the skin to appear thinner. The skin becomes more prone to tearing and blistering. The risk of infections increases, the healing process takes longer, and older people are more susceptible to bruising. Because the skin can be easily torn, it is important to be very careful when performing phlebotomy or covering a wound on an older patient.

The dermis loses 20% of its mass during the aging process, resulting in the paper-thin or transparent skin seen in older adults. The number of collagen cells in the dermis also declines with age, causing the skin to sag and wrinkle. Because both sweat and sebaceous glands decrease in number, aging people have difficulty tolerating higher temperatures because they perspire less. At the same time, the blood supply to the dermis decreases; this makes it difficult to regulate the body temperature and leads to an increased susceptibility to both hypothermia and heat stroke in aging individuals. Any situation in which an older adult would be exposed to extremes of cold or heat should be avoided. Ensure that a blanket is available in the examining room if the air conditioning is on. Ask the person if he or she is too cold or too hot, and take the necessary steps to make the patient feel more comfortable.

Atrophy of the subcutaneous layer increases the skin's susceptibility to trauma, so patients bruise much more easily. The skin is denied natural lubrication, and dry skin is one of the most common complaints among older people. In addition, fat deposits increase in the abdomen in men and in the abdomen and thighs in women as they age.

Suggestions that might help older people prevent and treat dry skin include the following:

- Using a room humidifier to moisten the air
- Bathing less frequently and using warm rather than hot water
- Using a mild soap or cleansing cream (e.g., Aveeno®, or Dove®)
- Wearing protective clothing in cold weather
- Moisturizing dry skin
- Applying creams and moisturizers after getting out of the bathtub or shower to reduce the chance of falls

Pain receptors are distributed throughout the skin. Because of age-related changes in the receptors, older people have a higher pain threshold, or ability to handle pain longer than usual. They may not notice a cut or burn as quickly as a younger person would, so a more serious burn may occur before it is noticed. In addition, wound healing becomes a problem because of decreased blood flow to dermal tissues.

Other changes occur in the skin's attachments, such as hair and nails. Hair changes in color, growth, and distribution. Hair grays because of the decreased rate of melanin production and the replacement of pigmented (colored) hair with nonpigmented hair. Women lose hair on the trunk and have increased facial hair. Although alopecia (male balding) is caused by an inherited trait, aging also causes hair loss. Hair on the eyebrows, nose, and ears becomes coarser and longer in men. The nails of older people take longer to grow and are more brittle. Nails, particularly toenails, thicken as a result of trauma or nutritional deficiencies. It is not unusual for nails to split, making them more susceptible to fungal infections.

Seborrheic keratoses, usually referred to as "age spots," are one of the most common benign skin disorders found in the aging population. They appear as waxy, greasy papules that vary from tan to dark brown (Fig. 31.1) and typically are found in areas of sun exposure, such as the trunk, back, face, neck, extremities, and scalp. They are not dangerous but may be removed for cosmetic purposes.

Musculoskeletal System

As the body ages, changes occur in the muscles, bones, and joints that affect the individual's appearance, strength, and mobility (Box 31.3). The amount of change depends on diet, exercise, and heredity. Cartilage loss

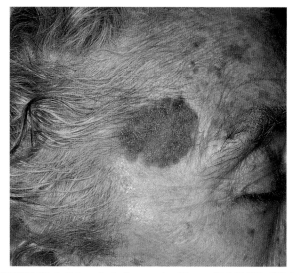

FIGURE 31.1 Seborrheic keratosis. (From Habif TP: *Clinical dermatology: a color guide to diagnosis and therapy,* ed 4, St. Louis, 2004, Mosby.)

and degeneration, producing osteoarthritis (degeneration, or breakdown of joint cartilage), commonly occur in the weight-bearing joints of older people. Joint range of motion is affected, and the disc spaces between the vertebrae of the back are decreased, causing loss of height as a person ages. A breakdown in joint structures may lead to inflammation, pain, stiffness, and deformity.

Aging brings a decrease in the strength and speed of muscle contractions in the extremities but only a slight decline in overall muscle endurance. Muscular changes in the aging patient are directly related to the individual's activity level. Research shows that musculoskeletal disease is not an inevitable result of the aging process; however, 40% to 50% of women aged above 50 years have a serious problem with bone demineralization. Men also experience bone loss but at a later age and a much slower rate than women.

Box 31.3	Suggestions for Helping the Older Adult With Mobility, Dexterity, and Balance

- Use assistive devices, such as adaptive silverware, tub seat or shower chair, electric razor, and reaching devices.
- Assist with gripping devices as needed (wait for the patient to place his or her hand around a cup or help him or her with it before letting go).
- Older adults may need more time to complete tasks but prefer to do so independently, so slow down.
- Stroke victims should be supported on the weak side when walking or transferring from a chair to the examination table.
- The physician may recommend physical therapy for range-of-motion exercises.
- Encourage activity; lack of activity causes a decline in the ability to function.

Osteoporosis

Osteoporosis, which is brittle and fragile bones, is the primary cause of hip fractures, which can lead to a loss of independence and complications that ultimately can end in death. The spinal vertebrae also can collapse, producing the stooped posture associated with "dowager's hump." Sometimes bones break because of the sheer weight of the body on them. Often people say that they fell and broke a bone, when in reality the bone fractured, causing them to fall. Multiple factors contribute to the development of osteoporosis, but it is most common in postmenopausal women. Risk factors for osteoporosis include the following:

- Female gender (women have a five times greater risk than men)
- Small-boned frame, thin
- Family history of osteoporosis
- Estrogen deficiency before age 45 years either from early menopause or removal of the female ovaries
- Estrogen deficiency resulting from an abnormal absence of menses (eating disorders, excessive aerobic exercise, fibrocystic ovaries)
- Racial background (Caucasian and Asian women have the highest risk)
- Aging
- Extended use of antiseizure drugs, steroids, and excessive thyroid hormone medications
- Sedentary lifestyle, smoking, excessive alcohol intake, and lack of calcium and vitamin D when growing up

Weight-bearing exercises, calcium and vitamin D supplements, and some medications are recommended to prevent demineralization of the bones.

Falls

The risk of injuries from falls increases with age; falls cause the greatest number of injuries in people aged above 70 years. Aging individuals are at greater risk of falling because of sensorimotor changes in vision and mobility, osteoporosis, and cerebrovascular accidents. Falls in older patients usually result in fractures, because a large percentage of them have osteoporosis. Serious fractures, such as those of the hip, require the patient to be immobile for extended periods, and this opens the door to a wide range of debilitating complications, such as pressure ulcers, pneumonia, placement in long-term care facilities, and even death. Falls are largely preventable. The patient care technician can play an active role in helping family members and patients become aware of risk factors and safety measures to avoid falls. Suggestions that can help patients prevent falls are as follows:

- Have regular hearing and vision tests.
- Understand the side effects of medications, especially those that cause vertigo.

- If you experience orthostatic hypotension, rise slowly and stand still for a moment with support before moving.
- Limit the use of alcohol.
- If needed, consistently use assistive devices, such as a cane or walker, for support.
- Wear low-heeled, rubber-soled shoes with good support.
- Avoid going outside in icy weather.
- Engage in regular weight-bearing exercise for muscle and bone strength.
- Keep hallways, stairs, and bathrooms well lit.
- Assess the home for possible danger areas; remove throw rugs; use handrails on steps and grab bars in bathrooms; keep emergency numbers handy.

Nervous System

Cognitive ability, the ability of a person to think, is influenced by many factors, including a person's general state of health, educational background, and genetic code. The normal process of aging may contribute to a change in the thinking process. The brain begins to get smaller at approximately age 50 years and continues to do so as we age because of a loss of fluid within the neurons (brain cells) and the shrinkage of nerve cells. Thinning of the dendrites makes transmitting messages from one neuron to the next more difficult. As a result of all of these factors, the aging brain weighs less, is smaller, and has started to pull away from the sheath or cortical mantle. Older neurons process information more slowly, so retrieving old information and learning new information takes longer. Reaction time also slows, and aging individuals are distracted more easily; however, recent research shows that the loss of brain cells is minimal and that the older brain is still capable of generating new neurons. Researchers believe that continued, moderate physical and mental activity can maintain the cognitive abilities of aging individuals.

Dementia, the severe loss of intellectual ability, is not a guaranteed part of aging but rather the result of a true disorder. Most men and women remain mentally competent until the end of their lives. Sudden loss of memory, disorientation (not knowing where you are, who you are, etc.), and trouble performing the daily tasks of life indicate a problem that should be investigated. Many conditions can cause signs and symptoms of dementia, including depression; reactions to prescription and over-the-counter drugs; alcoholism; malnutrition; thyroid, liver, heart, and vascular disorders; and Alzheimer's and Parkinson's disease. Multiple factors can interfere with mental judgment and motor skills, giving the impression of decreased mental status.

The best way to ensure mental functioning in later life is to remain mentally and physically stimulated. Exercise improves memory and thinking because of its positive effect on vascular health, increasing the amount of oxygen delivered to the aging brain. Other ways to maintain mental function are to keep socially active; practice stress-reduction activities; quit smoking; drink alcohol in moderation; use hearing aids and glasses if needed to stay in touch with the world; and receive treatment for depression, diabetes, hypertension, and high cholesterol levels. Risk factors for a decrease in cognitive function include the following:

- Hypertension, diabetes, and heart disease (these reduce blood flow to the brain)
- Environmental exposure to lead
- High stress levels
- Sedentary lifestyle and lack of social interaction
- Low education level
- Smoking and substance abuse

One of the most frequently used screening tools for dementia is the Mini-Mental State Examination, a 5-minute test designed to evaluate basic mental function in a number of different areas. The test assesses the patient's ability to recall facts, write, and calculate numbers. It gives the physician a quick way to determine whether more in-depth testing is needed. Each area of the examination is given a score, and these scores show whether the person is functioning within the expected range for his or her age (Fig. 31.2). The patient care technician may be asked to assist with his examination.

Alzheimer's Disease

Alzheimer's disease (AD) is a progressive deterioration of the brain caused by the destruction of central nervous system (CNS) neurons, leading to problems with memory, language, thinking, and behavior (Box 31.4). Cellular destruction is related to the buildup of plaque and tangled nerve fibers in the brain. Patients who show signs and symptoms of dementia are first evaluated for causes, such as disease or depression. AD has no definitive diagnostic test because it can be confirmed only through examination of the brain at autopsy. If the patient shows a gradual onset of progressive difficulty with memory, functional abilities, and behavior and has no evidence of other causes of these disturbances, the physician makes the diagnosis of AD. Imaging studies, including computed tomography (CT), magnetic resonance imaging (MRI), and positron emission tomography (PET), may help show the structural and functional changes in the brain that are associated with AD.

Researchers believe that as many as 5.4 million Americans suffer from AD. The disease typically begins after age 60 years, and the risk of developing the disorder increases with age, although younger people can be diagnosed with AD. An estimated 5% of people age 65 to 74 years have AD, and almost half of people age 85 years or older are diagnosed with the disease. Despite these statistics, AD is not considered a normal part of the aging process. AD is the seventh leading cause of death (across all ages) in the United States and the fifth leading cause of death for those age 65 years or older.

AD is a slowly progressive disease that begins with mild memory problems and ends with severe brain damage (Box 31.5). The course the disease takes and how fast changes occur varies among individuals, but on average, patients live for 8 to 10 years after they are diagnosed. Currently, no treatment can stop the progression of the disease. However, a great deal of research on the diagnosis and treatment of AD is underway.

The goal of treatment is to maintain normal activities as long as possible. There are some medications prescribed to improve the production of neurotransmitters in the brain. These drugs help prevent memory loss from becoming worse for a limited time. However, these drugs do not help everyone; as many as 50% of patients show no improvement in mental function. Individuals with AD frequently experience changes in behavior, so

| Box 31.4 | Signs and Symptoms of Alzheimer's Disease |

- Repeatedly asking the same questions
- Inability to remember common words or mixing up words when describing something
- Inability to complete simple tasks and misplacing items
- Becoming lost when driving familiar routes
- Sudden mood swings for no apparent reason
- Difficulty following simple directions

| Box 31.5 | Stages of Alzheimer's Disease |

- *First stage—Mild AD:* Occurs during the 2 to 4 years leading up to diagnosis; memory loss affects job performance; confusion and disorientation are common. Patient experiences mood or personality changes, difficulty making decisions, and paying bills; gets lost easily; withdraws from others; and loses things.
- *Second stage—Moderate AD:* Lasts 2 to 10 years after diagnosis; increased memory loss and confusion, shorter attention span, and restlessness are common. Patient makes constant repetitive statements; has problems with reading, writing, and numbers; may be irritable or suspicious; experiences motor problems; and has difficulty recognizing close friends and family members.
- *Terminal stage—Severe AD:* Lasts 1 to 3 years. Patient does not recognize family; experiences weight loss; is unable to care for self; is incontinent of bladder and bowel; and requires complete care.

medications may be prescribed to help control sleeplessness, agitation, wandering, anxiety, and depression. Treating these problems helps make the patient more comfortable while easing the burden on caregivers.

Supportive care for family members is absolutely essential, because they are faced with caring for a loved one who is suffering progressive memory loss. The patient care technician can be especially helpful in recommending educational workshops, support groups, and stress management skills for caregivers. Multiple resources are available, including online information and support groups, which family members may find helpful.

Pulmonary System

Maximum lung function decreases with age. The rate of airflow through the bronchi slowly declines after age 30 years, and the maximum force one is able to achieve on inspiration and expiration declines. The lungs lose their elasticity because of changes in elastin and collagen. They become smaller and flabbier. The alveoli enlarge, their walls become thinner, and the number of capillaries is reduced. As a result, the effective area for gas exchange in the lungs is reduced. The chest wall may stiffen from osteoporosis of the ribs and vertebrae and calcification of the rib cartilage. The respiratory muscles become weaker, making it harder to move air into and out of the lungs. To make up for this, older adults rely more on other muscles to help them breathe, such as the diaphragm. Weakening of the respiratory muscles and stiffening of the chest wall make it harder to cough deeply enough to clear mucus from the lungs. Pulmonary function tests reveal a decrease in vital capacity and an increase in residual volume. Sleep apnea and sleep disorders increase, causing a potential problem with decreased oxygen in the blood at night. All these factors combine to put the older adult at greater risk for respiratory infections and aspiration.

The larynx also changes with aging, causing a change in the pitch and quality of the voice. The voice sounds quieter and slightly hoarse. The individual's voice may sound weaker, but it should not interfere with the ability to communicate effectively.

Sensory Organs

Vision

By the time a person reaches age 50 years, structural and functional changes in the eye become noticeable (Table 31.2). The eyebrows and eyelashes start to gray. The skin around the eyelids wrinkles, and the loss of orbital fat allows the eye to sink deeper into the orbit. The cornea increases in thickness and has reduced refractive power. A yellow-gray ring (arcus senilis) may

	Age-Related	
Structure	**Change**	**Effects**
Lens	Thickens, becomes more opaque	Decreased refraction, causing blurred vision; decreased color acuity; cataracts
Anterior chamber	Decrease in size and volume	May develop increased intraocular pressure and glaucoma
Ciliary muscles	Affects pupil constriction and dilation	Limits light accommodation; night blindness
Cornea	Thickens, curve decreases	Problems with refraction
Retina	Decrease in number of rods and nerves	Decreased clarity; requires increase in minimum amount of light needed to see clearly

Table 31.2   Age-Related Changes in the Anatomic Structures of the Eye

develop on the outer edge of the cornea. The iris loses pigmentation, and as a result most older people appear to have gray eyes.

The lens of the eye continues to grow. As new lens fibers grow, old lens fibers are compressed and pushed to the center, causing the lens to become denser. The lens becomes flatter, thicker, less elastic, and more opaque, progressively yellowing with age. By age 70 years, the lens has tripled in mass. Clouding of the lens causes light rays to scatter, creating glare.

The pupil is designed to adjust to control the amount of light entering the eye. The ciliary muscle that causes the pupil to dilate weakens during the aging process. As a result, a reduction in the size of the pupil occurs, limiting the amount of light available to reach the retina. Tear production normally decreases. Tear glands do not make enough tears, or the tears are of poor quality and do not keep the eyes wet enough. Eye irritation and excessive tearing are a result of decreased lacrimation.

During the fourth decade of life, presbyopia develops, which makes it difficult to focus on detailed objects close at hand. This requires the use of corrective lenses to accommodate age-related farsightedness. The ability to refocus quickly from far to near or near to far decreases. Also, the ability to follow a moving object is decreased. The yellowing of the lens causes it to act like a filter, making it difficult to distinguish certain color intensities. Blues, greens, and violets are hard to differentiate, whereas yellows, reds, and oranges are easier to identify. The loss in the ability to discriminate closely related colors can affect the older person's ability to judge distances or his or her depth perception. This increases an aging person's susceptibility to falls and accidents. Stairs become a potential hazard because the edges of the steps cannot be seen clearly.

Older people need as much as six times more light to read; however, increasing the level of light does not completely compensate for visual decline, because the elderly also experience an increased sensitivity to glare. Glare is probably one of the most painful experiences for the aging eye. Exposed light bulbs, such as those used in chandeliers, and light from highly reflective surfaces, such as glass tables and floors, can produce excessive glare. The eye has a decreased ability to respond to abrupt changes from light to dark or dark to light. Going from a well-lit waiting room into a dim hallway or negotiating the way down dimly lit aisles in a movie theater could be treacherous for an older person.

Cataracts, Glaucoma, and Macular Degeneration

Eye diseases and disorders that occur frequently in older individuals are cataracts, glaucoma, and macular degeneration. Cataracts are cloudy or opaque areas in the lens that cause blurring of vision; rings or halos around lights and objects; and a blue or yellow tint to the visual field. Surgical lens extraction and implantation with an artificial lens improves vision in 95% of the cases. The procedure is performed in an outpatient facility using a small incision to remove the lens, laser therapy, or phacoemulsification (ultrasonic vibrations), which breaks up the lens and removes it without the need for an incision. Postoperatively patients must avoid bending or lifting heavy objects for 3 to 4 weeks; wearing an eye shield at night and glasses during the day helps protect the eye until it heals.

Glaucoma is a result of blockage of the outflow of aqueous humor, which causes an increase in intraocular pressure and damage to the optic nerve. If not treated, glaucoma can cause progressive loss of peripheral vision and ultimately lead to blindness; however, it can be treated with medication.

The macula is the part of the eye responsible for sharp vision and color. Damage to or breakdown of the macula is called *macular degeneration*, which causes progressive loss of the central field of vision. Macular degeneration is the leading cause of blindness in aging people, and at this time there is no effective treatment or cure.

Hearing

Hearing loss can have a huge psychologic effect on aging people, causing depression, social withdrawal, and feelings of loneliness. Hearing loss occurs gradually over a long period and may go undetected by the older person and healthcare providers. Lack of attention when addressed, inappropriate responses, asking to have statements repeated, and speaking too loudly or too softly often are signs of hearing loss. Changes in the ability to hear begin around age 30 years. By age 65 years, 25% of elderly adults have a hearing impairment,

---

Injury & Illness Prevention Box 31.1

- When escorting an older person, regardless of whether he or she is visually impaired, allow the patient to place his or her hand above your elbow. It is easier for the person to follow your movements. This method also provides a source of support and security.
- Use high levels of evenly distributed, glare-free light.
- Encourage the patient to ask the pharmacist to use large lettering when labeling medicine bottles.
- Use paper that has a nonglare finish and large print for forms and educational materials.
- Make distinct differences (e.g., size of containers or color coding with bright primary colors) for pills that are similar in size and color.
- Place all objects within the visual field and prevent clutter.

---

and the number increases to 65% of those over age 80 years. Age-related hearing loss usually is caused by a dysfunction or loss of hearing cells (sensory hair cells of the inner ear), resulting in an inability to hear high-frequency sounds and difficulty understanding speech. Hearing impairment is compounded by impacted ear wax, ear infections, Ménière's disease, long-term exposure to intense noise, and certain drugs that are toxic for the ear, such as aspirin.

Presbycusis is associated with normal aging and causes a decreased ability to hear high frequencies and to discriminate sounds. Parts of a conversation may be missed because the sound of the word goes above the 2000-cycle frequency. Often words that sound similar are difficult to differentiate. Consonants such as *g, f, s, sh, t,* and *z* produce high-pitched sounds that are more difficult to hear and differentiate. Low-frequency pitched sounds, such as the vowels *a, e, i, o,* and *u,* may be more easily heard by people with presbycusis. Inability to hear different frequencies, combined with low background noise from groups of people talking, noise from appliances, or busy public places, compromises an older person's ability to hear clearly. Hearing aids, which can be used to amplify speech, may increase background noises, resulting in sensory overload.

Another hearing disorder common among older people is tinnitus, a ringing or buzzing in the ear. It can be caused by impacted cerumen, an ear infection, use of antibiotics, a reaction to a medication, or a nerve disorder. Tinnitus can cause difficulty understanding conversational speech and can make sleeping difficult because of the continuous sensation of ringing in the ears.

Hearing loss, along with the isolation, is directly related to the development of depression in older adults. Treatable depression often is overlooked in elderly people because of coexisting physical illnesses that mask the symptoms of depression. The patient care

GERIATRIC DEPRESSION SCALE (SHORT FORM)

Choose the best answer for how you have felt over the past week:

1. Are you basically satisfied with your life? YES / **NO**
2. Have you dropped many of your activities and interests? **YES** / NO
3. Do you feel that your life is empty? **YES** / NO
4. Do you often get bored? **YES** / NO
5. Are you in good spirits most of the time? YES / **NO**
6. Are you afraid that something bad is going to happen to you? **YES** / NO
7. Do you feel happy most of the time? YES / **NO**
8. Do you often feel helpless? **YES** / NO
9. Do you prefer to stay at home, rather than going out and doing new things? **YES** / NO
10. Do you feel you have more problems with memory than most? **YES** / NO
11. Do you think it is wonderful to be alive now? YES / **NO**
12. Do you feel pretty worthless the way you are now? **YES** / NO
13. Do you feel full of energy? YES / **NO**
14. Do you feel that your situation is hopeless? **YES** / NO
15. Do you think that most people are better off than you are? **YES** / NO

Answers in **bold** indicate depression. Although differing sensitivities and specificities have been obtained across studies, for clinical purposes a score >5 points is suggestive of depression and should warrant a follow-up interview. Scores >10 are almost always depression.

FIGURE 31.3 Geriatric Depression Scale. (From Proctor D, Adams A: *Kinn's The Medical Assistant: an applied learning approach*, ed 12, St. Louis, 2014, Saunders.)

Injury & Illness Prevention Box 31.2

- Stand in the patient's direct line of vision and gently touch the person to get his or her attention.
- Use gestures, pictures, and large, bold print to communicate.
- Talk in short sentences into the ear with better hearing.
- Do not increase the volume of your speech; this also raises the frequency of the voice. Use expanded speech; lower the tone of your voice and talk in distinct syllables.
- Avoid background noise. Give instructions in a quiet room with the door closed. If the patient has a hearing aid, ensure that it is on.

technician may be able to contribute to information about depression in elderly patients through conversations with the individual and family members. The physician may use the Geriatric Depression Scale short form, which includes questions for the patient about daily activities, interests, and feelings to help diagnose depression in the ambulatory setting (Fig. 31.3).

Taste and Smell

During the aging process the abilities to taste and smell decline gradually. Deterioration and dying of the taste buds are part of the aging process. The ability to taste salt and sweet flavors is reduced, whereas the ability to detect bitter and sour flavors remains relatively the same. As a result, food frequently tastes bland and unappetizing. Patients receiving salt-restricted diets and patients with diabetes must be cautioned about the use of excessive amounts of salt and sugar. A decrease in the sense of smell accompanies the decrease in taste. Not only does this affect the individual's enjoyment of food, it also exposes the person to environmental dangers, such as gas leaks, smoke, and other dangerous odors that may go undetected. Checking for gas leaks around stoves and heaters and using smoke alarms reduce some of the danger. Also, dating food when it is put in the refrigerator is a good idea.

Nutritional Status

Because of the many environmental, social, economic, and physical changes of aging, older people are at greater risk for poor nutrition, which can negatively affect their health and energy level. It is estimated that 25% of the aging population suffers from malnutrition. Nutrition screening should be part of routine primary care to identify nutritional deficiencies and correct them before a disease process develops or to assist in the treatment of chronic disease. Patients with chronic conditions, such as cardiovascular disease, hypertension, and diabetes, can benefit from nutrition assessments and interventions. Malnourished older patients get more infections; their injuries take longer to heal; surgery is riskier for them; and their hospital stays are longer and more expensive.

The most effective method of assessing a patient's nutritional status is through a comprehensive patient interview that considers all potential stumbling blocks to adequate nutrition. The nurse will determine the nutritional status of older patients by considering many factors when conducting patient interviews.

Urinary System

As the body ages, structural changes in the kidneys cause the urinary system to become less efficient.

Between 40 and 80 years of age, the kidney loses about 20% of its mass. The number of functional nephron units decreases. Blood flow to the kidneys is reduced because of a decrease in cardiovascular efficiency. Because of the decrease in blood flow to the kidneys and the decreased number of kidney cells, the kidneys become less efficient at filtering waste from the blood. This results in a more diluted, less concentrated urine. The kidneys require more water to excrete the same amount of waste. Medication takes longer to be removed from the body. Older adults are at increased risk for toxic levels of medication in the bloodstream because of this reduced filtration rate.

Fibrous connective tissue replaces the smooth muscle and elastic tissue in the bladder. This thickening of the bladder wall reduces the bladder's ability to expand. The bladder's capacity to store fluid comfortably is reduced from 400 to 250 mL. These structural changes lead to increased frequency of urination and urinary retention. Older adults are at increased risk of urinary tract infections because of residual urine. Sleep is interrupted by the need to void during the night. The sensation of bladder fullness is not recognized as quickly by the older brain. Reduced time between awareness of the need to void and involuntary urination can cause anxiety. Often older adults reduce their fluid intake to prevent possible embarrassment. Unfortunately, this causes dehydration and an increased risk of urinary tract infections. Another change is loss of muscle tone in the urethra. In addition, the pelvic floor muscles in an aging woman relax as a result of decreased estrogen levels or previous pregnancy and childbirth.

Despite these changes, the kidneys are able to continue functioning normally. Urinary incontinence, the involuntary loss of urine, is a significant problem for aging patients but is not a normal part of the aging process. Changes in the urinary system make older people more vulnerable to incontinence, but factors such as infection, confusion, difficulty with mobility, and side effects of medications contribute to the development of the problem. Incontinence is both an emotional and a physical problem. To avoid the risk of an embarrassing accident, people with this problem may avoid social occasions or activities they enjoy. Often people are too embarrassed to admit that they have this condition, or they believe that it is just part of aging. Once the condition has been diagnosed by a urologist, pelvic floor muscle exercises, medication, or surgery may be recommended.

Reproductive System

Aging brings a decrease in circulating levels of the female hormones estrogen and progesterone, whereas androgen (male hormones) levels increase. The results of this decrease are changes in the genital tract. The vagina diminishes in width and length and becomes less elastic. The cervix, uterus, and ovaries decrease in size. Vaginal secretions decline; therefore lubrication diminishes, resulting in vaginal dryness. Bacterial or yeast infections may occur because vaginal secretions are less acidic. Estrogen cream applied to vaginal tissue may be prescribed by the physician for help with dryness and thinning of the vaginal tissue. The patient should discuss the benefits and risks of estrogen replacement therapy with the physician to determine whether it should be used.

Even though sperm production may decline in men aged above 50 years, men remain virile well into old age. However, they experience a change in hormonal levels of testosterone, and these changes can affect the prostate gland. The prostate enlarges over time and presses down on the urethra, causing difficulty with urination. Surgery may be required to remove excess portions of the gland. Unfortunately, the operation may cause impotence, which can be treated medically with erectile dysfunction medications.

Men experience some changes in sexual functioning as they age. It takes longer for the penis to become erect, longer for an orgasm to occur, and longer to recover. Direct stimulation may be required before an erection occurs, and when it does, it may be less firm than that in younger years.

Some drugs and illnesses can interfere with sexual function. Drugs used to control high blood pressure, antihistamines, antidepressants, and some stomach acid blockers, in addition to the diseases diabetes, arthritis, and arteriosclerosis, can have a negative effect on sexual function. Often people who have had heart surgery or a heart attack are concerned about sexual activity. Patients need to feel comfortable and should not be embarrassed to discuss their concerns openly with their physician. It is important for healthcare providers to dismiss the myth that older patients have lost the desire for and interest in sexual intercourse.

Sleep Disorders

Complaints of sleeping difficulties increase with age. The amount of time spent sleeping may be slightly longer than that in a younger person, but the quality of sleep declines. Older people often are light sleepers and have periods of wakefulness in bed. Rapid eye movement (REM) sleep is the stage of sleep when people experience dreaming. Non-REM sleep is the period of deepest sleep. The amount of time spent in the deepest stages of sleep decreases with age. Sleep that is disturbed or that leaves the person feeling tired is not part of the aging process and may indicate some underlying emotional or physical problem. Lack of sleep can result in restlessness, disorientation, "thick" speech, and mispronounced words. Often these symptoms are mistaken as signs of dementia. Other factors that might influence sleep patterns are medications, caffeine, alcohol, depression, and environmental or physical changes.

Common sleep problems in older adults include periodic limb movement disorder (PLMD), in which periodic jerking of the legs occurs during sleep, and sleep apnea, which is common among overweight individuals and can occur frequently during the night, interrupting sleep. Numerous medical conditions can interfere with sleep, including joint and bone pain; Parkinson's disease (because of difficulty changing positions); congestive heart failure; chronic obstructive pulmonary disease; diabetes mellitus, which increases nocturia; depression; and certain medications (e.g., beta blockers can cause nightmares, antidepressants increase PLMD, and barbiturates may result in nightmares or hallucinations).

It is important to be aware of the effect of sleep problems because often these can be confused with dementia. Patients who are experiencing difficulty with sleeping should be encouraged to document their sleeping patterns, napping patterns, medications, diet, exercise routines, and any events that have resulted in a change of lifestyle. They should discuss this problem with their physician. Simple modification of behavioral patterns may resolve the problem. Taking fewer naps, completing exercise several hours before bedtime, changing eating times, reducing the amount of alcohol and caffeine ingested, drinking a glass of milk before bedtime, or changing medications or the time they are taken all are suggestions that might alter the factors responsible for sleep disturbances.

If behavioral approaches are not effective, medications may be considered for short-term use only, because they have a high incidence of physical and psychologic dependence. Elderly people are especially susceptible to side effects from these drugs, such as next-day drowsiness and temporary memory loss.

Living Arrangements

At any given time, only 5% of the elderly population lives in long-term care facilities. According to information published by the National Institute on Aging, most older people live close to their children and are in frequent contact with them. People prefer to age in place; that is, they want to live in their own home environment as long as possible. Individuals are admitted to nursing homes because they are no longer able to perform activities of daily living, such as bathing, dressing, eating, walking, and maintaining bladder and bowel continence. They also have difficulty with grocery shopping, housekeeping, and money management. Chronic health conditions and accidents interfere with the older person's ability to perform these tasks.

Many resources are available to help seniors to maintain their independence. Outreach programs, such as

Meals on Wheels, deliver nutritious meals to the homes of older adults. Senior centers serve as a focal point for many activities and as a source of information. Transportation services provide rides to doctors' appointments, day care centers, shopping centers, and community events. Home health agencies provide several types of services, including personal care, shopping, transportation, and meal preparation. Some home health agencies provide a range of activities, from patient education to IV therapy; medical-social services; physical, speech, and occupational therapies; and nutrition and dietary counseling. Advanced technology allows people to receive services at home that formerly were provided only at a hospital or a physician's office.

Adult day care centers provide socialization, recreation, meals, and, in some centers, physical therapy, occupational therapy, and transportation. These centers offer supervision for older adults who may be taken care of by family members in the evening but need care during the day. They also serve as respite for a caregiver.

Assisted-living facilities can be retirement homes or board and care homes. These facilities are appropriate for older adults who need assistance with some activities of daily living, such as bathing, dressing, and walking. Skilled nursing facilities provide 24-hour medical care and supervision. In addition to medical care, residents receive care that may include physical, occupational, and speech therapies. The objective of treatment is to improve or maintain the person's abilities.

THE PATIENT CARE TECHNICIAN'S ROLE IN CARING FOR THE OLDER PATIENT

Elderly patients in the healthcare setting often need extra help by the healthcare team. For example, aging patients typically require more time to perform tasks and have questions answered. The patient care technician may be tempted to hurry along to perform tasks so that they can move on to the next patient. Keeping the best interests of the patient in mind, the PCT should treat the eldery patient with respect, providing time to prepare for the examination, ask questions and receive answers, and have procedures explained. A healthcare system that is sensitive to the needs of older patients schedules longer periods for appointments; has adequate lighting in the patient's room; provides forms in large print; and has an examination room equipped with furniture, magazines, and treatment folders especially designed for older adults.

The primary issue in elder care is effective use of communication. How you communicate with people is often influenced by what you know or do not know about them. Older people are subject to many changes that affect how they are able to interact with their environment. It is important to recognize these changes and to investigate one's personal perception of older people to break down the barriers that prohibit effective communication.

As people age, they often experience a loss of control over their lives because of physical disabilities, financial constraints, and institutional living. Part of our job is to help aging people maintain their dignity and independence while in the healthcare setting. Remember, each patient, regardless of his or her education, socioeconomic status, or age, deserves to be treated with compassion and respect. Ask the patient directly what is wrong rather than discussing the patient with family members. It also is important to listen carefully and to be specific and sincere when responding. When a patient is talking, take time to allow him or her to complete the sentence; do not finish it for the person. Give the patient your full attention rather than continuing with other tasks while he or she is speaking. Older people may take a little longer to process information, but they are capable of understanding. Do not hurry through explanations or questions; rather, take time to review a form or give instructions as needed.

Patient Education

The patient care technician must keep the sensorimotor changes that accompany aging and respectful patient communication in mind when conducting patient education with older patients (Box 31.6). Remember, the aging process does not affect a person's ability to learn; it just may take longer to process the information, and the material may need to be repeated for understanding. Showing sensitivity to the needs of aging learners ensures successful patient education and improves compliance with prescribed treatment plans. The aging population generally is respectful toward authority; therefore if the patient care technician cannot gain the patient's cooperation, the physician may be able to provide authoritative reinforcement of material. General guidelines for effective patient education with older adults include the following:

- The patient may have short-term memory loss, so you may need to repeat the information using different words.

Box 31.6   **Suggestions for Effective Communication With Aging Patients**

- Address the patient by Mr., Mrs., or Miss unless the patient has given you permission to use his or her first name.
- Introduce yourself and explain the purpose of a procedure before performing the procedure.
- Face the aging person and softly touch the individual to get his or her attention before beginning to speak.
- Use expanded speech, gestures, demonstrations, or written instructions in block print.
- If the message must be repeated, paraphrase or find other words to say the same thing.
- Observe the patient's nonverbal behavior for cues indicating whether he or she understands.
- Provide adequate lighting without glare.
- Allow patients time to process information and take care of themselves unless they ask for assistance.
- Conduct communication in a quiet room without distractions.
- Involve family members as needed for continuity of care.
- When leaving a telephone message, remember to speak slowly and clearly and repeat the message in the same manner. It is difficult to interpret a message, and even more difficult to write it down, if the message was delivered in a hurried manner.
- Use referrals and community resources for support, such as the following:
  - Alzheimer's Association (1-800-272-3900)
  - American Council of the Blind (1-800-424-8666)—provides referrals to state and other organizations that provide services and equipment for the blind

- American Speech-Language-Hearing Association (1-800-638-8255)—offers information on hearing aids, hearing loss, and communication problems in older people and provides a list of certified audiologist and speech pathologists
- Arthritis Foundation Information Line (1-800-283-7800)—makes referrals to local chapters and provides information
- Eldercare Locator (1-800-677-1116)—run by the National Association of Area Agencies on Aging; help line provides information on contacting local chapters that oversee services to older adults
- National Institute on Aging Information Center (1-800-222-2225)—provides information on geriatric health issues
- National Meals-on-Wheels Foundation (1-800-999-6262)
- Hospice Helpline (1-800-658-8898)—provides information about hospice care and makes referrals to local hospices

- The patient may be distracted more easily, so learning in a group may be difficult.
- The patient may take longer to process information, so teach at a pace that matches the patient's needs.
- Provide the patient with handouts that have large print and block letters for reviewing information at home.
- Involve family members as needed for continuity of care.

Legal and Ethical Issues

All patients have the right to know about the medications, treatments, and alternatives available to them. The Patients' Bill of Rights informs the patient of those rights in a healthcare setting. They include the right to privacy about personal and medical information and the right to informed consent, which holds the physician accountable for explaining clearly the advantages and risks of any procedures, tests, or treatments. The patient must give permission for medical care and has the right to refuse treatment. The patient has the right to be informed about his or her condition and treatment and the chances of recovery. The patient also has the right to have advance directives explained to him or her.

Consent must be given by the individual undergoing the procedure as long as he or she is judged to be competent, that is, as long as the patient is able to understand the consequences of the procedure. In an emergency situation or if a court has ruled that the patient is incompetent, someone else must give consent. This may be a person who already was designated to hold the durable power of attorney, a close family member (spouse, adult child, parent, sibling), or a court-appointed guardian.

Most states have legal documents available that provide written instructions specifying the type of medical care a person wants in the event she or he becomes incapacitated; these are called *advance directives*. The document designates a person who has a durable power of attorney; this is an authorization for making medical decisions on an individual's behalf if he or she is unable to make treatment decisions. The document provides a list of specific instructions for the proxy to follow.

Various issues may be covered in these documents. A "do not resuscitate" (DNR) order allows a patient to refuse attempts to restore a heartbeat. The patient also may decide to withdraw life-sustaining treatment, such as respirators or feeding tubes. A copy of the directive should be kept on file as part of the patient's medical record. It is important to check the laws of the state in which you practice with regard to advance directives, because they vary from state to state (Fig. 31.4).

Another legal issue in the care of aging patients is the possibility of elder abuse. Mistreatment of aging people occurs at all social, racial, and economic levels. The abuse may be physical, mental, sexual, material, or financial; it may involve neglect or failure to provide adequate care, or it may involve self-neglect when aging people are unable or refuse to care for themselves. Abuse of elders by their caregivers may be difficult to identify. The aging victim could feel embarrassed, guilty, or afraid to report the abuse. Indications that a patient may be a victim of elder abuse are as follows:

- Poor general appearance and poor hygiene
- Pattern of changing doctors and frequent emergency department visits
- Skin lesions, signs of dehydration, bruises (signs of new and old bruising together), abrasions, welts, burns, or pressure sores
- Recurrent injuries caused by accidents
- Signs of malnutrition and weight loss without related illness
- Any injury that does not fit the given history

Delegation and Documentation Box 31.1

- If a patient tells you that someone is abusing him or her, report it to the nurse at once.
- Document exactly what was stated by the patient, being as descriptive as possible, under the guidance of the nurse.
- Report the abuse to the appropriate authorities, under the direction of the nurse, and according to hospital policy and state laws.

Directive made this _____ th day of _____ in the year _____ .
(day)   (month)   (year)

I, _____ , being of sound mind, willfully and voluntarily make known my desire that my life shall not be artificially prolonged under the circumstances set forth in this directive.

If at any time I should have

— an incurable or irreversible condition caused by injury,
— disease,
— or illness certified to be a terminal condition by two physicians

and if the application of life-sustaining procedures would serve only to artificially postpone the moment of my death, and if my attending physician determines that my death is imminent or will result within a relatively short time without the application of life-sustaining procedures. I direct that those procedures be withheld or withdrawn, and that I be permitted to die naturally.

In the absence of my ability to give directions regarding the use of those life-sustaining procedures, it is my intention that this directive be honored by my family and physicians as the final expression of my legal right to refuse medical or surgical treatment and accept the consequences from that refusal.

If I have been diagnosed as pregnant and that diagnosis is known to my physician, this directive has no effect during my pregnancy. This directive is in effect until it is revoked.

I understand the full import of this directive and I am emotionally and mentally competent to make this directive. I understand that I may revoke this directive at any time.

I request that only comfort care be provided to me, no antibiotics, no artificial nutrition, no mechanical ventilation, and no hydration. It is my strong preference to be allowed to die outside of a care facility if possible, even if that preference is determined by my physician to shorten my period of dying. The only condition under which I desire these preferences for end of life care to be altered is in the case of possible organ and tissue donation. I request that any and all organs and tissue that may be salvaged be provided for transplant. My remains may then be cremated.

Signed _____ in the City of _____ etc.

I am not a person designated by the declarant to make a treatment decision. I am not related to the declarant by blood or marriage. I would not be entitled to any portion of the declarant's estate on the declarant's death. I am not the attending physician of the declarant or an employee of the attending physician.

I have no claim in against any portion of the declarant's estate on the declarant's death. Furthermore, if I am an employee of the health care facility in which the declarant is a patient, I am not involved in providing direct patient care to the declarant and am not an officer, director, partner, or business office employee of the heath care facility or of any parent organization of the health care facility.

Witness _____

Witness _____

FIGURE 31.4 Sample advance directive. (From Proctor D, Adams A: *Kinn's The Medical Assistant: an applied learning approach*, ed 12, St. Louis, 2014, Saunders.)

CHAPTER SUMMARY

More than 40 million Americans are 65 years of age or older. The most rapidly growing age group is the "oldest old," those older than 85 years. By the middle of the 21st century, more than 72 million people will be older than 65 years. Most older people have at least one chronic medical condition, and many have multiple conditions. The aging population will affect all aspects of society.

Normal age-related changes are expected, and the individual can compensate for them. However, these changes intensify with poor health habits and chronic disease. Age-related changes can be managed through regular exercise, a healthy diet, prevention of sun damage, and annual physical examinations with health screening.

Major health issues of older people are related to an increase in atherosclerosis and potential cardiovascular disease; hypertension; diabetes mellitus type 2; integumentary system changes; arthritis; osteoporosis; an increased risk of injury from falls; dementia attributable to metabolic or cardiovascular disease or AD; pneumonia, aspiration, and reactivation of tuberculosis; cataracts, glaucoma, and macular degeneration; depression; malnutrition; urinary tract abnormalities; menopausal changes; and sleep disorders.

A commonly used screening tool for dementia is the Folstein Mini-Mental State Examination, a 5-minute screening test that is designed to evaluate basic mental function. The physician may use the Geriatric Depression Scale short form, which questions the patient about daily activities, interests, and feelings. Nutritional status can be assessed through a comprehensive patient interview that considers all potential problems preventing adequate nutrition.

Complaints of sleeping difficulties increase with age. The amount of time spent in the deepest stages of sleep declines with age. Factors that might influence sleep patterns are medications, caffeine, alcohol, depression, and environmental or physical changes. Common sleep problems in older adults include PLMD and sleep apnea.

Aging people prefer to remain in their home environment for as long as possible. Adult day care centers can provide supervision for older adults who may be taken care of by family members in the evening but need care during the day. Assisted-living facilities are appropriate for older adults who need assistance with some activities of daily living. Skilled nursing facilities provide 24-hour medical care and supervision.

The patient care technician's role in caring for the older patient is to develop effective communication skills that accommodate age-related sensorimotor changes; to allow time for longer appointments; to provide adequate lighting and forms in large print; and to develop appropriate in-service training as requested by the physician. Examination rooms should have furniture and treatment folders especially designed for the elderly patient. Referrals and community resources should be used for patient and family support.

Effective communication with aging patients includes addressing the patient with an appropriate title; introducing yourself and explaining the purpose of a procedure before touching the patient; establishing eye contact and getting the patient's attention before beginning to speak; using expanded speech, gestures, demonstrations, or written instructions in block print; repeating the message as needed for understanding; observing the patient's nonverbal behaviors for cues that indicate whether he or she understands; allowing time to process information; preventing distractions; and involving family members as needed. Legal and ethical issues associated with aging patients include adequate informed consent, the use of advance directives, and staying alert for signs of possible elder abuse.

Case Scenario

The family of Rita Schaeffer, a 73-year-old patient, is concerned about the risk of falls. Mrs. Schaeffer recently was diagnosed with osteoporosis, and she lives alone. What information should the patient care technician give the family to help them prevent accidents in their mother's home? Also, Mrs. Schaeffer's 43-year-old daughter is concerned about developing osteoporosis. Can she prevent the disease?

REVIEW QUESTIONS

1. As people get older, they require how much sleep at night?
   a. They require as increased amount of sleep.
   b. They require as decreased amount of sleep.
   c. The amount of sleep required does not change as one gets older.
   d. The amount of sleep required is the same as an infant.

2. A ringing in the ears of an older adult is known as what?
   a. Presbycusis
   b. Presbyopia
   c. Tinnitus
   d. Impacted earwax

3. The fastest growing older group of adults is in what age range?
   a. 40 to 50 years old
   b. 50 to 60 years old
   c. 60 to 70 years old
   d. 85 years and older

4. As adults get older, how is their vision affected?
   a. They require additional lighting to see well.
   b. Their vision is unchanged as long as they do not have diabetes.
   c. They require less lighting to see well.
   d. They see better at night than during the day.

5. Alzheimer's disease is known as what type of disease with regard to how it appears?
   a. Sudden and mild loss of function
   b. Sudden and fast loss of function
   c. Progressive and mild loss of function
   d. Progressive and fast loss of function

Caring for Patients With Mental Health Needs

LEARNING OBJECTIVES

1. Describe the mental health continuum.
2. Identify defining characteristics of people who are mentally healthy and those who are mentally ill.
3. Identify sources of stress.
4. List five warning signs of suicide.
5. Discuss the history of alcoholism.
6. Describe the purpose of Alcoholics Anonymous.

KEY TERMS

abuse To misuse something that has a bad effect

addiction Being addicted to a particular substance, thing, or activity

Alcoholics Anonymous (AA) An international nonprofit organization that began in 1935 as a way for abstinent alcoholic people to help other alcoholic people become and stay sober through group support, shared experiences, and faith in a power greater than themselves

alcoholism The addiction to alcohol

anxiety A vague feeling of apprehension that results from a perceived threat to the self, although the source is often unknown

behavior The manner in which a person performs any or all of the activities of daily life

club drugs Substances that people frequently take for euphoric effect at parties, concerts, dance clubs, or all-night raves

depression A mood disturbance characterized by exaggerated feelings of sadness, despair, lowered self-esteem, loss of interest in former activities, and hopeless, negative thoughts

detoxification Medical treatment of an alcoholic or drug addict involving keeping alcohol or drugs from entering the body until the bloodstream is free of toxins

displacement The unconscious transfer of an intense emotion from its original object to another one

group therapy A form of psychotherapy in which a group of patients meet to describe and discuss their problems together under the supervision of a therapist.

hallucination Is a sensory experience without a stimulus trigger (involves the senses; may be auditory, visual, olfactory [smell], and tactile [touch])

illusions False interpretation of extreme sensory stimuli, usually visual or auditory, such as a mirage in the desert or the sound of voices in the wind

mental health A person's ability to cope with and adjust to the recurrent stresses of everyday living

mental health continuum A range of wellness to illness with regard to mental health; moving from being constructive with mental health, to destructive with mental illness

mental illness An inability to cope with a situation that an individual finds overwhelming

raves Dance parties with extremely loud music

street drugs Substances that users buy from illegal drug dealers

stress The nonspecific response of the body to any demand made on it

stressor A situation, activity, or event that produces stress

A patient care technician (PCT) is likely to use mental health nursing principles in a variety of healthcare settings. Basic mental health concepts are useful for understanding a patient's behavioral responses to disease and dysfunction. Behavior can be defined as the manner in which a person performs any or all of the activities of daily life. Individuals respond differently to changes in daily activities, such as the changes created by illness and hospitalization. All individuals have unique personalities and resources that affect their behavior in dealing with changing situations and the changing environment. An individual's mental health sometimes varies depending on the situation and the available support systems. Someone who has a strong support system in place is more likely to cope with illness better.

Mental health can be defined as a person's ability to cope with and adjust to the recurrent stresses of everyday living. Mental health is ever-changing and moves along a continuum. Mentally healthy individuals are individuals who are able to enjoy life's activities, adapt successfully to changes, set realistic goals, solve problems, have satisfying working relationships, and maintain interpersonal relationships with family and friends (Fig. 32.1).

Factors affecting mental health include inherited characteristics, how much someone was nurtured during the childhood, and life's circumstances. The influence of these factors on the individual's response to daily stressors in life is sometimes positive and sometimes negative. Possible positive influences include an adequate coping ability, mother–child bonding at birth, success in school, good physical health, and how financially secure someone may be at any point in his or her life. Possible negative influences include mental illness, extreme sibling rivalry, rejection from parents such as not receiving adequate love from one's mother, poor physical health, poverty, and dysfunctional relationships.

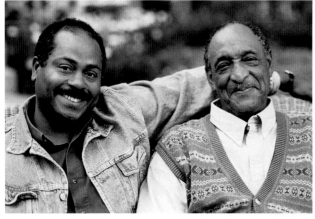

FIGURE 32.1 Maintaining interpersonal relationships with family members provides a positive influence that affects mental health. (From Lewis SL, Heitkemper MM, Dirksen SR, et al.: *Medical-surgical nursing: assessment and management of clinical problems,* ed 5, St. Louis, 2000, Mosby.)

Evidence of mental illness often consists of a pattern of behaviors that are obvious, threatening, and disruptive of relationships or that are very different from behaviors that are considered socially and culturally acceptable.

Changes in society and in the economy have altered the status and situation of many individuals. According to the National Institute of Mental Health (n.d.), 13.4% of adults in the United State received treatment for a mental health problem in 2008. This population includes all adults who received inpatient or outpatient care or used prescription medication for mental or emotional problems. Twice as many people actually have a mental health disorder. An astounding 50% of people in the United States will develop a mental health disorder in their lifetime (www.nimh.nih.gov). The difference between individuals seeking treatment and those not treated for mental illness should serve as an alert to the healthcare team who in their practice encounter patients and families who have mental health concerns (Centers for Disease Control and Prevention [CDC], 2011). Members of the healthcare team may have daily contact with battered spouses, abused children, people who are homeless as a result of mental illness, substance abusers, or patients experiencing depression, anxiety, or other mental health alterations. Regardless of the practice setting, all members of the healthcare team often encounter patients who are in need of emotional support.

MENTAL HEALTH CONTINUUM

Mental health and mental illness are the opposite ends of a mental health continuum (Fig. 32.2). Functioning is normal on the healthy end of the mental health continuum. Mental health is characterized by an assertive communication style, acceptance of strengths and weaknesses, and available energy to deal with life's situations. The influences of daily stressors, although affecting the mentally healthy individual, do not normally disrupt mental health functioning. Continued stressor exposure results in a deterioration of mental health and alterations in behaviors. The longer and the more intense the stressors are, the more likely behaviors are to become dysfunctional. Loss of contact with reality can result when an individual is at the illness end of the continuum. The middle point on the continuum represents normal mental health. Although a person at this point probably

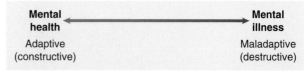

FIGURE 32.2 Mental health continuum. (From Cooper K, Gosnell K: *Foundations of nursing,* ed 7, St. Louis, 2015, Mosby.)

Box 32.1	Characteristics Identified in Mental Illness

- Poor self-concept
- Feelings of inadequacy
- Dependent behavior resulting from feelings of inadequacy
- Pessimism that is constant
- Poor judgment
- Inability to cope with daily events
- Irresponsibility
- Inability to accept responsibility for actions
- Avoidance of problems (no attempt to handle them)
- Inability to recognize own talents
- Inability to recognize limitations
- Inability to perceive reality
- Maladaptive behavior
- Demanding or seeking immediate gratification
- Inability to establish a meaningful relationship

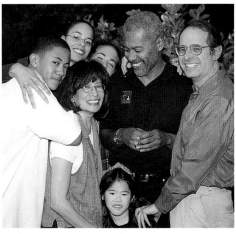

FIGURE 32.3 Recognition and use of a support system of family and friends is one of the mental health components that determine placement on the mental health continuum. (From Varcarolis EM: *Foundations of psychiatric mental health nursing*, ed 5, Philadelphia, 2006, Saunders.)

displays some lack of insight, this middle point level is characterized by adequate coping skills, problem-solving ability, and satisfactory responses or adjustments to life changes with some growth or possibly some mild regression. Although many individuals function in a relatively healthy manner, periods of crisis or biochemical imbalance have potential to decrease functional capacity, moving one toward the illness end of the continuum (Box 32.1).

To determine a patient's placement on the continuum, it is necessary to look at several components of mental health. These components include a positive self-concept, awareness of responsibility for one's own behavior and its consequences, taking care of satisfying interpersonal relationships, being willing to adapt to change, communicating effectively, having awareness and acceptance of emotions and their expression, effective problem-solving, and recognition and use of supportive systems (Fig. 32.3).

A person may be deemed to be mentally ill by the behavior the person displays, as well as the context or setting in which the behavior occurs. Mental illness results from an inability to cope with a situation that an individual finds overwhelming. The maladaptive behavior is often part of a response to acute anxiety (see Box 32.1).

Stress

People are continually exposed to a variety of situations that produce stress, and their mental health fluctuates along with their ability to adapt to and deal with life situations or events. Any event that requires change leads to a degree of stress. It is possible for the event to be either pleasant or unpleasant. Stress is the nonspecific response of the body to any demand made on it. An individual's response to a stressful situation or event is often a learned or conditioned behavior and is experienced differently by each individual.

A stressor is a situation, activity, or event that produces stress. Stressors are physical, social, economic, chemical, spiritual, or developmental, or some combination of all of these. The meaning of the stress to an individual determines whether that individual feels distress. Stress is highly subjective, meaning that it depends on what the patient says it is. Stress is uniquely perceived by the person experiencing it and is not usually the same for each person. Stress in itself is neither good nor bad; however, it has both positive and negative effects. Stress that results in individual growth and development and promotes change and adaptation brings positive results. Some stressors have potential to be overwhelming, which then causes negative results and characteristic of ineffective coping.

Mental health nursing concerns itself with behavior, particularly a person's response to stressors. Health factors affect this response. The stress of being ill greatly influences a person's emotional well-being and coping ability. How a person perceives stress determines whether the stress produces anxiety. A person's response to a stressful situation or event is often a result of learned behavior and thus is, at least in theory, able to change.

Anxiety

Anxiety can be defined as a vague feeling of apprehension that results from a perceived threat to the self, although the source is often unknown. Anxiety is said to be a universal emotion and is a response to a stressful event. Anxiety is something felt from within that a person experiences when there is a real or a believed threat to the physical body or self-concept. Anxiety is a major part of all mental health disturbances. In mild forms, anxiety prepares the body for action and reaction to danger. Mild levels of anxiety enable the body to meet stressful demands by promoting problem-solving and effective action. Higher levels of anxiety can paralyze coping skills and result in emotional chaos. In severe forms, anxiety interferes with daily activities.

Anxiety is usually described in terms of levels, and each level is associated with certain behaviors (Box 32.2). Signs of higher levels of anxiety include vocal changes; rapid speech; increased pulse, respirations, and blood pressure; tremors; restlessness; increased perspiration; nausea; decreased appetite; diarrhea; frequent urination; and, occasionally, vomiting.

Anxiety arises as the result of inner conflict, and thus the behavior stems from the anxiety. Negative behavior is often a defense against anxiety. Individuals learn a variety of ways to respond to anxiety as they move through the various stages of growth and development.

Box 32.2   Levels of Anxiety

An individual's response in a given situation depends on the level of anxiety.

Mild
- Slight increase in vital signs measurements and an awareness of danger
- Ability to think and make connections; heightened awareness
- Readiness for action
- Increased motivation

Moderate
- Feeling of tension
- Decreased perception
- Continuing alertness, but only to specific information
- May display a proneness to arguing, teasing, or complaining
- Appearance (often) of physical signs and symptoms: headache, diarrhea, nausea, vomiting, low back pain, and stronger vital signs

Severe
- Feeling of impending danger
- Significant narrowing and distortion of perceptual field
- Possible distortion of communication and difficulty in making self understood
- Feeling of fatigue
- Changes in vital signs, potentially evident on assessment

Panic
- Extreme terror
- Possible immobilization
- Distortion of reality
- Potential further disintegration of personality
- Potential to cause harm to self and others

Behavior shown in response to stress and anxiety results from many factors. The degree of anxiety experienced is influenced by the following:

- How the person views the stressor
- The number of stressors the individual is handling at one time
- Previous experience with similar situations
- The amount of change that the event represents for the individual
- The degree of physical and emotional health being experienced at the time of the stress

Events that have the potential to bring about feelings of anxiety include the following:

- *Threats to physical integrity:* Decreased ability to perform activities of daily living; impending physiologic disability (surgery, diagnosis of a life-threatening disorder, pain, infection, trauma)
- *Threats to self-esteem and negative hits to the identity:* Loss of significant relationships, loss of spouse, difficulty at work, loss of job, change in jobs, relocation to a new home

Anxiety is relieved through various coping and mental mechanisms. These mechanisms are partly conscious and partly unconscious; they serve to protect individuals from situations perceived as dangerous. Anxiety is an inevitable part of life. Part of the emotional growth process is to learn to deal with stress and anxiety in an adaptive or corrective manner.

Depression

Depression is a mood disturbance characterized by exaggerated feelings of sadness, despair, lowered self-esteem, loss of interest in former activities, and hopeless, negative thoughts. Depression is more than a state of mind; it is an illness that affects about 1 in 20 people every year (CDC, 2014). Depression is found in all races, ethnic groups, age groups, and socioeconomic levels. Women are affected twice as often as men.

Depression can be so severe at times that an affected person will think about, or actually succeed at, committing suicide. Suicide falls in the top 10 leading causes of death in the United States, where the statistic falls in the top 10 depends on the age group (CDC, 2014). Many deaths supposedly caused by accidental overdoses, automobile accidents, and refusal of medical care might be viewed as hidden suicides even though they are not reported as such. Suicide attempts also are not included in the statistics. Although the highest rate of suicide is among the older population, suicide among teenagers is on the rise in this country. It is essential that children be taught effective coping skills.

To help prevent suicide, the PCT needs to recognize warning signs and learn the kinds of actions that can

Box 32.3   Suicide Warnings and Precautions

Warning Signs of Suicide

- Withdrawing from family or friends
- Talking about death, the hereafter, or suicide
- Giving away prized possessions
- Drug or alcohol abuse
- Personality changes, such as unusual anger, boredom, or apathy
- Unusual neglect of appearance; difficulty concentrating on work or school; complaints of physical problems that have no organic cause; disturbed sleeping or eating patterns; loss of self-esteem; feelings of helplessness, hopelessness, extreme anxiety, or panic
- Previously failed attempts with verbalized regrets of failure

Suicide Precautions in the Hospital Environment

- Remove articles that can be used for suicide: belts, straps, shoelaces, sheets, breakable items for sharp edges, razor blades, curtain cords, bed coils, and personal care items.
- Remove any furniture that can be used for self-injury, as well as doors to closets. Ensure that windows are shatterproof.
- Designate a room close to the front desk of the unit or a room with a closed TV monitor.
- Check the patient approximately every 15 minutes on an irregular schedule around the clock.
- Instruct visitors not to leave gifts in the room until the staff examines them for anything that can be used for self-injury.
- Ensure that the patient swallows all medications administered. Administer liquid forms when available. Administer injectables if the patient refuses oral forms as ordered.
- Attend the patient during meals, and keep track of eating utensils and dinnerware. Ensure that used trays are not sitting where the patient has the opportunity to walk by and remove tableware.
- Make frequent therapeutic verbal contact.

often prevent suicide attempts (Box 32.3). Consider verbal statements such as "I wish I were dead" or "You won't see me coming back here again" and questions about specific methods of suicide to be warning signals. Actions such as giving away possessions, refusing medications, or neglecting hygiene are also possible warning signals. Many people have anxiety because of a moral conflict within themselves. Many suicidal individuals manage to leave that anxiety behind by making the decision to commit suicide.

The Role of the Sitter

As a PCT, you may be asked to serve as a sitter for a patient who may be experiencing thoughts of hurting oneself. This is a very important role and one that can be very serious if not followed. If you are asked to spend your shift as a sitter for a particular patient, this typically means that you will spend the entire shift in the patient's room, ensuring that the patient does not hurt himself or herself. This can be a difficult shift, especially if it is during the night-time hours, because you are sitting still and it is important that you do not fall asleep, or lose your focus on the patient.

Delegation and Documentation Box 32.1

- As a sitter, you are responsible for monitoring the patient's activity while remaining in the room with him or her.
- Most facilities will have you document the patient's activity every hour on a flow sheet.
- Always record accurate results; never make assumptions. If vital signs are required every hour, take the vital signs every hour. Never guess.

It is often appropriate for you to watch television with the patient or engage in conversation. Their rights should be respected and they should not be pressured to talk to you about how they feel. They may just want to be silent. Another staff member may come to relieve you for a dinner break or bathroom break. It is imperative that you do not leave until that person arrives. You can be held liable for the patient's safety if you leave the patient alone and he or she hurt himself or herself. If you need assistance while in the patient's room, activate the call light and ask for help. If the person is in the process of hurting himself or herself, it is appropriate to activate the emergency call system.

Injury & Illness Prevention Box 32.1

- Anytime a patient makes statements such as "I wish I were dead" or "I won't want to live anymore," report it directly to the nurse at once.
- Never leave a patient alone if you are responsible for sitting with the patient who is on suicide precautions, also known as suicide watch.

Post-traumatic Stress Disorder

Post-traumatic stress disorder (PTSD) describes a response to an intensely traumatic experience beyond the usual range of human experiences. These experiences—such as war, rape, a major motor vehicle accident, being tortured or observing someone being tortured, or witnessing a violent death—tend to bring about feelings of terror and helplessness. One such experience was witnessing the attack on New York City's World Trade Center on September 11, 2001. The people who escaped the World Trade Center towers before the collapse and emergency personnel who responded to the attack were the most likely to suffer from PTSD. Also at high risk are veterans returning from Iraq, Afghanistan, and other war-torn areas of the world. The experience is often repeatedly relived in dreams or flashbacks. Flashbacks often arise in response to a trigger, a stimulus that resembles the experience or perhaps the anniversary of the event. Flashbacks sometimes include illusions (false interpretation of extreme sensory stimuli, usually visual or auditory, such as a mirage in the desert or the sound of voices in the wind) and hallucinations. Avoidance behavior associated with this disorder sometimes includes emotional detachment, guilt about being a survivor, amnesia (forgetting) of the event, insomnia (inability to sleep), irritability, difficulty concentrating, and extreme caution. Physical response to severe anxiety occurs with each relived episode. Depression and substance abuse often occur in association with PTSD.

There are three types of PTSD: acute, chronic, and delayed. In acute PTSD, symptoms occur within 6 months of the event and last about 6 months. Chronic PTSD is characterized by symptoms that last 6 months or longer. Delayed PTSD involves symptoms that start 6 months or more after the event.

Treatment for PTSD includes antidepressant or anti-seizure medications; cognitive therapy, which focuses on breaking negative thought patterns; and behavioral therapy, which aims to break off a conditioned response that has become automatic.

Limits of Confidentiality

Confidentiality is sometimes a problem when effectiveness of care depends on the patient's willingness to talk about feelings and thoughts. It is important that the patient knows that each member of the healthcare team will share any information he or she receives with the others. No one member of the team keeps any secrets from the others. This practice also keeps patients from manipulating the staff or pitting one staff member or patient against another.

Just as the healthcare team has a duty to report child abuse, they also have a duty to warn. Sometimes a patient will express intent to kill someone when he or she is released, and the PCT is obligated to notify the appropriate authorities. Families of victims have filed—and won—lawsuits against healthcare workers for not warning the victim.

ADDICTION

Problems associated with the abuse or misuse of alcohol, tobacco, caffeine, nicotine, and other drugs consume a major proportion of current healthcare dollars. Many patients seeking care from acute care facilities and a variety of outpatient settings also suffer from some type of addictive behavior. It is not uncommon for patients to deny or hide their substance abuse problem. Substance abuse may not be addressed until withdrawal symptoms become apparent. Patients suffering with chronic pain have a high risk of developing tolerance of and addiction to the pain medicines they take. Patients suffering from anxiety and depression sometimes self-medicate with alcohol, marijuana, or other substances. It is important for the nurse to investigate what the patient does to relieve stress or pain when the nurse collects data about the patient. These data often help identify addictive behavior patterns that can slow down the patient's recovery from acute illness. As the PCT, it is beneficial for you to understand what addiction is so that you can recognize it and report certain behaviors to the nurse. You may also work on a unit that specializes in helping patients become free from addiction.

Addiction consists of four elements: (1) excessive use or abuse of a substance, (2) display of psychologic disturbance, (3) decline of social and economic function, and (4) uncontrollable consumption of the substance, indicating dependence (not able to live without the substance). Alcoholism is the addiction to alcohol. It is possible to suffer from more than one addiction at the same time. For example, an alcoholic person may also be a smoker and a compulsive gambler.

In the adult population (age 18 years and older), 56% report having consumed alcohol in the past month. About 24% of these current drinkers admit to binge drinking in the past month, and an additional 6.9% admit to heavy drinking within the past month (www.niaaa.nih.gov, 2014). The age when one begins to drink is strongly predictive of the development of alcohol dependence in the life span: Of people who start drinking at the age of 14 years or younger, 44% will develop alcoholism. Alcohol and drug abuse are increasing in the older population. Older adults sometimes turn to alcohol, prescription and nonprescription drugs, caffeine, and nicotine to help cope with physiologic and sociologic changes associated with aging. Aging causes changes in how the body absorbs, metabolizes, and eliminates drugs; thus the risk of misuse and abuse increases with age.

Alcohol is involved in 31% of all deaths caused by motor vehicle accidents and fatal intentional injuries such as suicides and homicides. About 88,000 deaths each year are related to alcohol consumption (www.niaaa.nih.gov, 2014).

The use of alcohol and drugs has been around practically forever. In different cultures from around the world, alcohol and drugs have been used as medicine, in celebrations, and as a part of worship services. In the history of the United States, legal positions on the use of alcohol have varied. The temperance movement in the 1800s stressed moderation in or total avoidance of the use of alcohol. The Eighteenth Amendment to the

U.S. Constitution, known as *Prohibition,* which forbade the production, transport, and sale of alcoholic beverages, was passed in 1919 and later repealed in 1933. There has been a decrease in alcohol use over the years that experts attribute to education of the public and laws set forth to limit availability of alcohol to minors.

Although there has been a long-term decline in overall alcohol use, many people still use illicit drugs. In 2013 in the United States, 9.4% of the population acknowledged that they had used illicit drugs in the previous month. In 2013, there were approximately 19.8 million who admitted to using marijuana, the most commonly used illicit drug (https://www.drugabuse .gov/publications/drugfacts/nationwide-trends). This is increased from 14.5 million in 2007. The goal of the Comprehensive Drug Abuse and Controlled Substance Act of 1970 (commonly referred to as the *Controlled Substance Act*) was to provide legal control over drugs that previous federal drug-related laws did not cover. The Bureau of Drug Abuse Control moved from the U.S. Food and Drug Administration to the Department of Justice and later merged into the Drug Enforcement Agency, which today is the leading agency responsible for enforcing the 1970 act. All prescribing physicians and dispensing pharmacies register with the Drug Enforcement Agency. Smuggling and other illegal activities provide the public with illicit drugs.

Alcohol Abuse and Alcoholism

Alcoholism is a national health problem that is right behind heart disease and cancer in terms of the number of lives it affects. No one theory explains the cause of alcoholism. Several factors probably contribute to the development of alcoholism. Some believe that people are more likely to develop alcoholism because of some biologic reason, such as an inner urge controlled by the nervous system or a dysfunction of the endocrine system. Alcoholism is, in part, genetically determined. The incidence of alcoholism in members of certain families is high: The sons of alcoholic men are four times more likely to develop alcoholism over their lifetime (National Council on Alcoholism and Drug Dependence, https://www.ncadd.org). Deficiencies in some liver enzymes necessary to metabolize alcohol contribute to the development of alcoholism in some people. Many Asians and Native Americans do not have enough of these enzymes; alcoholism rates are higher in these ethnic groups than in the general public. Jews, Mormons, and Muslims have very low rates of alcoholism, whereas people of French descent and those of Irish descent have high rates.

Wide cultural differences concerning drug and alcohol use have been found in U.S. society. Most young people in the United States have their first drink at an early age. The average age that a girl has her first drink

is 13 years, and for boys the age is 11 years (http:// www.helpguide.org/harvard/the-dangers-of-teenage -drinking.htm). Alcohol sometimes serves as a rite of passage into adulthood. Drinking beer or other alcoholic beverages is the way many Americans celebrate certain holidays (e.g., St. Patrick's Day). Experts consider drinking to be the leading health problem in the African American community. Hispanic populations and many other ethnic groups celebrate life while drinking alcohol. Alcohol often serves as a gateway drug. Many multi-drug users began by abusing alcohol and progressed to abusing other substances.

Etiology and Pathophysiology

Alcohol is a central nervous system (CNS) depressant. Judgment is impaired; however, memory of pleasure is retained. As a person continues to drink alcohol, it affects the most primitive part of the brain that regulates hunger, thirst, and sexual desire. Repeated alcohol consumption affects the part of the brain, where compulsion controls are located, leading to obsessive-compulsive behavior. Rapid, large-quantity consumption of alcohol can lead to unconsciousness, during which respiration is sometimes affected. Death from acute alcohol poisoning is possible.

The active ingredient of alcoholic beverages is ethyl alcohol, or ethanol. There are similar amounts of alcohol in 12 ounces of beer, 4 ounces of wine, and $1\frac{1}{2}$ ounces of hard liquor. Alcohol does not require digestion, and the body absorbs it readily in the stomach and the intestines. An empty stomach increases the rate of absorption. After ingestion, the body loses small amounts through breathing and in the urine, but 90% is metabolized by the liver.

Alcohol has a diuretic effect, causing frequent urination. The urine of a heavy drinker sometimes contains increased amounts of electrolytes, especially potassium, magnesium, and zinc. Prolonged use of alcohol has a toxic effect on the intestinal mucosa that results in decreased absorption of vitamin B_1 (thiamine), vitamin B_9 (folic acid), and vitamin B_{12} (cobalamin).

Alcohol does provide the body with calories but no minerals or vitamins. One ounce of alcohol provides 200 kcal but no other nutritional value. Blood alcohol levels depend on the amount of alcohol ingested and the size of the individual. Most states designate blood alcohol serum levels of 80 mg/dL (0.08%) as the legal limit for driving a motor vehicle. Increasing blood alcohol serum levels have increasingly serious side effects.

Alcohol Withdrawal Syndrome

Alcohol withdrawal syndrome occurs in a person who has developed physiologic dependence and quits drinking abruptly. The risk for having alcohol withdrawal syndrome is highest in older adults, malnourished people, and people who have another acute illness. The range of possible signs and symptoms varies from mild tremor and flulike signs and symptoms to severe agitation and hallucinations. Signs and symptoms associated with the cessation of alcohol consumption include diaphoresis; tachycardia; hypertension; tremors; nausea or vomiting, or both; anorexia; restlessness; disorientation; hallucinations; and seizures.

The tremors from alcohol cessation occur 6 to 48 hours after the last drink and sometimes last for 3 to 5 days. Tremors usually occur in the hands but may also be present in the tongue, the chin, the trunk, and the feet. Seizures can occur 12 to 24 hours after alcohol cessation.

Care for the addicted patient starts with detoxification, the removal of the poisonous effects of a substance. A controlled setting in which the patient can be observed closely and treated for any complications is important during this acute phase of recovery.

Safety of the patient is a primary concern. If the patient is intoxicated, an open airway must be maintained. The side-lying position and oral suctioning should be considered if oral secretions can be aspirated or if vomiting could occur. If swallowing is intact, the head of the bed should be elevated at least 30 degrees to encourage better air exchange. Intravenous (IV) fluids may be administered by the nurse to correct the patient's fluid and electrolyte imbalance. The IV site must be monitored often, especially if the patient is restless. The facility's seizure precautions—such as padded side rails, floor pads, and moving patient to a room close to the nurse's station—should be instituted. You may be asked, as the patient care technician, to assist with making sure seizure precautions are in place.

Practitioners usually treat tremors, nervousness, and restlessness with medications. Environmental stimuli, such as lights and sounds, should be reduced. The patient should be allowed to ambulate or perform other activities that will help ease nervousness, but the patient must refrain from doing too much, known as overexertion. The patient should be accompanied by the patient care technician or other staff member while ambulating if he or she is unsteady from coordination disturbance or lack of conditioning. As weakness decreases, a regular exercise program will typically be included in the care plan.

Explanations to the patient should be kept simple, and the PCT should speak in a calm voice, planning time for the patient's verbalizations. Therapeutic conversation techniques are used to assist the patient in understanding himself or herself. Denial is confronted in a nonjudgmental manner. The family is encouraged to participate in planning for sobriety. Counselors sometimes initiate individual therapy to assist the patient into the rehabilitation phase of recovery.

Disorientation is possible, especially at night. Nightlights in the room and frequent visits by PCTs tend to help. If a patient is not able to sleep at night, he or she should sit up and have a snack; then the PCT may give the patient a back rub and encourage him or her to rest. If the patient appears fearful or panicky and unable to reacquire orientation to reality, the supervising nurse should be notified. Vital signs (including temperature) should be checked before the healthcare provider is notified. Physical restraints have the potential to make aggressive behavior worse, but are sometimes necessary if the patient poses a risk for harm to self or others. Restraints can be applied only after a physician's order is given and appropriate precautions for surveillance of the patient are implemented, per the facility's policy and procedure. The nurse will notify you if the patient is going to have restraints applied.

Many addicted patients are malnourished and suffer from loss of appetite. Incorporating nutritious foods and inquiring about food preferences will help meet nutritional deficits. Providing between-meal snacks is also helpful.

Rehabilitation

After detoxification, the acute phase of recovery, it is time to start rehabilitation. The object of rehabilitation is to help the patient abstain from substance abuse. Because there is no cure for addiction, abstinence is the practical equivalent to the control of the disease. Treatment programs often include family members in part of the treatment plan. Some of these programs are inpatient, and some are outpatient or day-treatment programs.

Group Therapy

Group therapy is an effective treatment modality. Group therapy provides a caring, emotionally supportive atmosphere in which the patient is able to acknowledge the relationship of substance abuse with negative consequences in his or her life. The group tends to point out negative defense mechanisms such as denial or displacement and to offer possible solutions to its members. Families should be encouraged to attend support groups to help the patient and family to grow together, not apart. Group therapy sometimes continues after completion of an inpatient program. Group therapy is an important part of all recovery programs.

Alcoholics Anonymous

Alcoholics Anonymous (AA) is an international nonprofit organization that began in 1935 as a way for abstinent alcoholic people to help other alcoholic people become and stay sober through group support, shared experiences, and faith in a power greater than themselves. There are regular meetings in most communities.

Listings for local AA chapters may be found in the telephone book, in the newspaper, or on the Internet. The foundation of AA is a 12-step program that assists the dependent person in admitting powerlessness over alcohol (Box 32.4). Other groups have followed up on the success of AA, usually using similar models for rehabilitation; these groups include Overeaters Anonymous, Al-Anon (for friends and family of alcoholic people), and Narcotics Anonymous.

Treatment Centers

Residential treatment centers provide the opportunity for detoxification. There is no direct medical intervention; instead, trained nurses provide close physical monitoring with the assistance of counselors and recovered peers. After detoxification, the patient enters a drug- and alcohol-free residence. A primary goal of this type of treatment is the rebuilding of social skills that do not involve drug use as the primary method of interaction. The length of the stay in a treatment center ranges from 1 to 6 months; most centers operate on an ability-to-pay basis, with some governmental funding.

Drug Abuse

Although alcohol abuse is present most frequently in patients fighting addiction or in patients who are being treated for other health problems, drug abuse is also a growing problem in the nation. Many people think only of illegal drugs when drug abuse is mentioned, but abuse of prescription and over-the-counter drugs is common. Prescription drugs are sometimes traded or shared. Drug abusers may seek excessive prescriptions from their healthcare providers, purchase them on the streets, or divert them from the supplies of friends or family members. Rationalizations such as "If it worked for me, it will work for my friend" and "If one pill works, two pills will work better" often serve to deny or justify misuse or abuse of many prescription and over-the-counter drugs.

When a person takes drugs for reasons other than medical issues or in a dose higher than recommended, the term *misuse* or *abuse* applies. Club drugs refer to substances that people frequently take for euphoric effect at parties, concerts, dance clubs, or all-night raves (also called trance parties: dance parties with extremely loud music). Club drugs are often street drugs. Street drugs are substances that users buy from illegal drug dealers. These drugs come from illegal manufacturers without strict controls, are illegally obtained prescription drugs, or are not approved for use in the United States. Chronic abuse has the potential to lead to psychologic or physical dependence, or both. Commonly abused drugs include depressants, opioids, stimulants, hallucinogens, cannabis, and inhalants (Box 32.5).

Homelessness

One major stressor to the person is homelessness. Homelessness is a public health issue and affects many. On any given night, approximately, 564,708 people are experiencing homelessness—meaning that they were sleeping outside or in an emergency shelter or transitional housing program. From 2013 to 2014, a period of ongoing recovery from the Great Recession, overall homelessness decreased by 2.3% and homelessness decreased among every major subpopulation: unsheltered persons (10%), families (2.7%), chronically homeless individuals (2.5%), and veterans (10.5%). The Great Recession is over, the economy is bouncing back, and

---

Box 32.4 Twelve Steps of Alcoholics Anonymous

1. We admitted we were powerless over alcohol—that our lives had become unmanageable.
2. Came to believe that a Power greater than ourselves could restore us to sanity.
3. Made a decision to turn our will and our lives over to the care of God *as we understood Him*.
4. Made a searching and fearless moral inventory of ourselves.
5. Admitted to God, to ourselves, and to another human being the exact nature of our wrongs.
6. Were entirely ready to have God remove all these defects of character.
7. Humbly asked Him to remove our shortcomings.
8. Made a list of all people we had harmed, and became willing to make amends to them all.
9. Made direct amends to such people wherever possible, except when to do so would injure them or others.
10. Continued to take personal inventory and when we were wrong promptly admitted it.
11. Sought through prayer and meditation to improve our conscious contact with God *as we understood Him*, praying only for knowledge of His will for us and the power to carry that out.
12. Having had a spiritual awakening as a result of these Steps, we tried to carry this message to alcoholics, and to practice these principles in all our affairs.

The Twelve Steps are reprinted with permission of Alcoholics Anonymous World Services, Inc. ("A.A.W.S"). Permission to reprint the Twelve Steps does not mean that A.A.W.S has reviewed or approved the contents of this publication, or that A.A necessarily agrees with the views expressed herein. A.A is a program of recovery from alcoholism only—use of the Twelve Steps in connection with programs and activities which are patterned after A.A, but which address other problems, or in any other non-A.A context, does not imply otherwise.
(From Alcoholics Anonymous: Alcoholics Anonymous, ed 4, New York, 2001, Alcoholics World Services, Inc.)

Box 32.5	Commonly Abused Drugs and Their Street Names*

Amphetamines: Speed, truck drivers, copilots, black beauties, crank, go

Barbiturates: Reds, blues, yellow jackets, rainbows, bluies

Benzodiazepines: Downers, chill pill, vitamin V

Chloral hydrate: Mickey Finn, mickey

Cocaine: Snow, crack, blow, coke, nose candy, toot, white dust, toot sweet

Gamma-hydroxybutyrate (GHB): Soap, easy lay, Georgia homeboy, liquid ecstasy

Heroin: H, smack, scag, junk, caca

Ketamine: Special K, vitamin K

Lysergic acid diethylamide (LSD): Acid, windowpane, gelcap, microdots, blotter, purple haze

Marijuana: Pot, reefer, grass, dope, weed, green, cannabis, Jamaican, Acapulco gold

Methamphetamine: Speed, crystal, ice

3,4-Methylenedioxymethamphetamine (MDMA): Ecstasy, E, XTC, hug, love bug, beans, Adam, Molly

Nitrous oxide: Nitrous, whippets

Phencyclidine (PCP): Angel dust, rocket fuel, wack, ozone

Psilocybin: Shroom, magic mushroom

Rohypnol: Roofies, rough, rope, roach

there are fewer people homeless in America. There are, however, too many people who are at risk of homelessness (www.endhomelessness.org).

The fastest growing section of the homeless population is the family with children. This includes families who have two parents and children, as well as single-parent families. Poverty, mental illness, physical illness, and lack of affordable housing are primary reasons for homelessness (National Coalition for the Homeless, 2010). Homelessness severely affects the functioning, health, and well-being of the family and its members. Children of homeless families are often in fair or poor health and have higher rates of illness. They often enter the healthcare system for treatment through the emergency department, because they have no funds or insurance for physician offices, and they know that they cannot be turned away from the emergency department without at least being seen. Children of homeless families are less likely to attend school, more likely to drop out of school, and less likely to become employable. It can be a cycle that continues if not broken. Homeless families and their children are at serious risk for developing long-term health, psychologic, and socioeconomic problems.

Some patients become homeless because of their choice to use substances, such as alcohol. Any money that is earned may be spent on purchasing alcohol rather than paying necessary bills to maintain housing. Over time, this may result in losing the housing because of the inability to pay.

As the PCT, you may be able to assist the patient in seeking housing upon discharge from the hospital. Consult with the nurse to see if there are any opportunities for the patients with regard to housing. Demonstrate a caring attitude that is nonjudgmental.

CHAPTER SUMMARY

All behavior has meaning. An individual's behavior is the best that person is capable of, based on his or her exposure to his or her current environment. Anxiety is a universal response to a real or imagined threat to self.

Stress is the nonspecific response of the body to demands. Stressors are factors causing stress. High or chronic stress has the potential to hamper the immune response to illness. It is possible to view mental health and illness as existing on a continuum.

Physical illness affects the mental health of an individual. Behavior incorporating the sick role and dependency until recovery occurs allows the individual to cope with body image changes and keep the self-intact. The use of therapeutic communication is a dynamic method of interaction with patients for problem-solving and growth.

Many patients who enter acute care facilities with other diagnoses also have problems of drug and alcohol abuse. *Substance abuse* and *drug dependency* are terms often used interchangeably in reference to addiction. Alcoholism is a chronic, incurable, progressive disease. Maintaining a professional, nonjudgmental attitude when communicating about use sometimes allows the user to be honest about use.

The goal of detoxification is to keep the patient free from complications while ridding the body of the substance. Safety is of primary concern during detoxification. Malnourishment occurs in many people who chronically abuse alcohol or drugs.

Like illegal drugs, over-the-counter drugs and prescription drugs are abused. Street drugs pose a risk of severe side effects and sometimes permanent damage because there are no controls in the manufacturing of these drugs.

Case Scenario

Ms. K, a patient on the psychiatric unit who has been pacing the halls, is now staring out the window. She has a diagnosis of anxiety. She is toying with a ring on her finger. You notice that Ms. K is vigorously tapping one foot on the floor. Complete the dialog between you and the patient using effective communication.

REVIEW QUESTIONS

1. Besides feelings of sadness or despair, which is also a sign or symptom of depression?
   a. Extreme fatigue
   b. Restlessness
   c. Flight of ideas
   d. Hallucinations

2. An early age at the onset of drinking alcohol is a strong risk factor for developing which disorder?
   a. Alzheimer's disease
   b. Alcohol or substance abuse
   c. Resistance to chemical dependency
   d. Immunity to alcohol

3. In all deaths related to motor vehicles and fatal intentional injuries, alcohol is involved in what percentage of them?
   a. 7%
   b. 10%
   c. 17%
   d. 38%

4. A patient has begun attending AA meetings. Which statement reflects the patient's understanding of the purpose of this organization?
   a. "They claim they will help me stay sober."
   b. "I'll dry out in AA, and then I can have a social drink once in a while."
   c. "AA is only for people who have reached the bottom."
   d. "If I lose my job, AA will help me find another."

5. A patient admitted to the emergency department is complaining of an anxiety attack. What signs are consistent with an anxiety attack?
   a. Hypotension
   b. Lethargy
   c. Hyperventilation
   d. Hallucinations

Caring for Patients With Chronic Conditions

1. Describe the pathology of cerebrovascular diseases.
2. Describe the chronic diseases of the respiratory system.
3. Summarize the risk factors for the development of heart disease.
4. Compare and contrast prediabetes, diabetes type I, and diabetes type II.
5. Discuss the different types of hepatitis.
6. Summarize the characteristics of HIV infection.
7. Discuss the risk factors for breast cancer.

angina Chest pain

ataxia Failure or irregularity of muscle actions and coordination

bronchiectasis Dilation of the bronchi and bronchioles associated with secondary infection or ciliary dysfunction

bronchospasm A sudden narrowing of the airways reducing the amount of air that can pass

chronic bronchitis Recurrent inflammation of the membranes lining the bronchial tubes

diplopia Double vision

endemic Term describing a disease or microorganism that is specific to a particular geographic area

gluconeogenesis The formation of glucose in the liver from proteins and fats

glycogen The sugar (starch) formed from glucose; it is stored mainly in the liver

glycosuria The abnormal presence of glucose in the urine

Kaposi sarcoma Kaposi sarcoma is a cancer of the blood vessels or lymph system and is known for producing reddish or purple plaques on the skin. The most common form of Kaposi sarcoma is associated with infection by the human immunodeficiency virus (HIV), the virus that causes AIDS

lymphedema A condition of localized fluid retention and tissue swelling caused by a compromised lymphatic system

paresthesia An abnormal sensation of burning, prickling, or stinging

polyphagia Increased appetite

tracheostomy A surgical opening made through the neck into the trachea to allow breathing

tubercle A nodule produced by the tuberculosis bacillus

virulent Exceedingly pathogenic, noxious, or deadly

wasting syndrome Physical deterioration resulting in profound weight loss, fatigue, anorexia, and mental confusion

Chronic conditions account for a significant portion of hospital and outpatient clinic visits. According to the Centers for Disease Control and Prevention (CDC), about half of adults have at least one chronic condition. A chronic condition is one that lasts longer than 6 months. Heart disease and cancer accounted for 48% of all deaths in 2010. Obesity is a serious concern that also leads to the development of chronic diseases, such as diabetes or hypertension. During 2009 to 2010, one third of all adults, or more than 78 million, were obese (defined as body mass index [BMI] ≥30 kg/m²). Lack of exercise and increased use of technology has led to the increase in the number of those who are overweight or obese.

This chapter will provide an overview of the most prevalent or often occurring chronic conditions in America today. The patient care technician should be knowledgeable of these, as it is highly likely that some of the patients cared for in the healthcare facility will have one or more of these conditions.

CEREBROVASCULAR ACCIDENT

A cerebrovascular accident (CVA), commonly referred to as a *stroke,* occurs when a vessel in the brain either ruptures or becomes blocked and the tissue on the other side of the damaged vessel becomes oxygen deprived. Cerebral artery ruptures are caused by uncontrolled hypertension or hemorrhaging of a weakened section of an artery in the brain. As a result of the rupture, the surrounding brain tissue fills with blood, damaging and possibly destroying the affected tissue. A blockage occurs when an embolus or thrombus (clot) becomes wedged in an artery and obstructs the flow of blood to an area of the brain (Fig. 33.1).

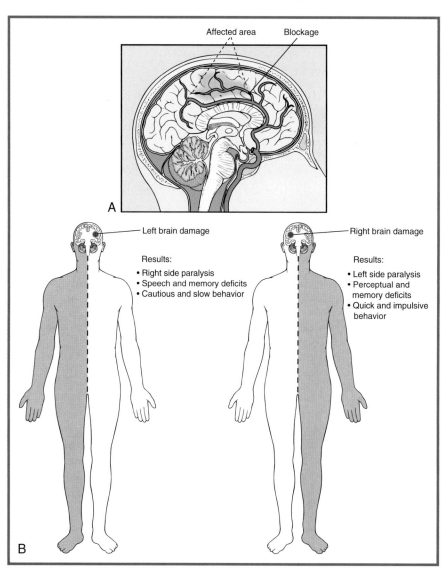

FIGURE 33.1 Cerebral artery occlusion (A) and hemiplegia (B). (Modified from Frazier MS, Drzymkowski JW: *Essentials of human diseases and conditions,* ed 6, St. Louis, 2016, Saunders.)

Thrombotic stroke: A blood clot (thrombus) forms in a cerebral artery and blocks distal blood flow.
Embolic stroke: A blood clot from somewhere else in the body (e.g., the lower leg) or a piece of plaque (typically from the carotid arteries) breaks away and flows through the bloodstream to the brain; the embolus eventually blocks a cerebral artery, causing distal ischemia.
Cerebral hemorrhage: An artery in the brain ruptures, possibly because of untreated or uncontrolled hypertension or a congenital aneurysm.

The patient's subsequent symptoms depend on the location of the arterial occlusion or rupture (Box 33.1). Some of the more common symptoms include slurred speech; unexplained confusion; sudden, severe headache; difficulty swallowing; vertigo; diplopia; loss of consciousness; personality change; loss of bowel or bladder control; and paralysis on one side of the body.

Treatment of a stroke requires immediate emergency transport to the hospital. The initial emphasis is on minimizing the long-term disabilities often seen with strokes by providing immediate treatment to save as much brain tissue as possible. Drugs that dissolve the clot may be given if the cause of the stroke was a thrombus or an embolus. However, timing is important, as these medications may be effective only if given within the first 3 to 6 hours after it began. If cerebral edema is present, the patient is treated with medicines to decrease inflammation and edema, which may reverse the swelling. An important part of the recovery to follow is extensive treatment in a stroke rehabilitation program that includes physical, occupational, and speech therapies. Identification early on is the best treatment so that medications can be given as soon as possible. The patient care technician may be asked to assist with transporting the patient who presents to the emergency department with complaints of a stroke to radiology for scans of the brain. Timing is of the essence so that treatment can begin as soon as possible.

Any of the following factors can increase the risk of a stroke:

- Hypertension
- Diabetes (increases the risk by two to three times)
- Hypercholesterolemia
- Cigarette smoking (increases the risk by 50%)
- Obesity
- Family history of stroke and chronic diseases such as diabetes
- Endocarditis (infection and inflammation within the heart)
- Arteriosclerosis and atherosclerosis
- Heart disease (e.g., atrial fibrillation, which increases the risk by five times)
- Sleep apnea
- Sickle cell anemia
- Cocaine abuse

Individuals with three or more of the following five health conditions are twice as likely to have a cerebrovascular accident: obesity, low high-density lipoprotein (HDL) cholesterol levels, high triglyceride levels, blood pressure of 130/85 mm Hg or higher, and diabetes and/or prediabetes (fasting blood glucose between 100 and 125 mg/dL).

Multiple Sclerosis

Multiple sclerosis is an autoimmune reaction that causes progressive inflammation and deterioration (demyelination) of the myelin sheath, leaving nerve fibers uncovered and resulting in a scattering of the nervous message as it passes down within the nerve cell. Early symptoms may include numbness, paresthesia, diplopia, ataxia, and bladder control problems. As the disease progresses, patients experience increased spasticity, vertigo, depression, gait problems, joint pain, fatigue, and varying degrees of paralysis. It most often begins in women between 15 and 60 years of age. The cause remains unknown; however, it is more common in northern climates, and it may be associated with a viral infection (www.mayoclinic.org). Multiple sclerosis frequently is diagnosed by the exacerbation (flare-up) and remission (temporary recovery) of neurologic symptoms characteristic of the condition. Patients cycle through remission and relapse, and an ever-increasing degree of dysfunction occurs after each episode. An MRI study may show plaques on nerve fibers where the myelin sheaths have been destroyed and areas of sclerosis from scar tissue at the inflammation sites.

Multiple sclerosis has no cure; therefore treatment focuses on alleviating symptoms and delaying the progression of the disease. Medications used to treat the disease include corticosteroids during periods of exacerbation, interferon (Betaseron, Avonex) to reduce the frequency and severity of relapses, and additional medications to treat fatigue, pain, spasticity, and bladder control problems. Some patients live an essentially normal life with only occasional attacks, whereas others experience rapidly progressive disability.

Chronic Conditions of the Respiratory Tract

According to the CDC, approximately one third of the world's population is infected with tuberculosis (TB) (http://www.cdc.gov/tb/statistics/, 2015). TB causes more deaths than any other infectious agent in the world. For more than 50 years, the incidence of TB in the United States steadily declined; however, from the late 1980s through the 1990s, a resurgence in reported cases occurred. This increase was believed to be the result of increased travel and immigration; an increase in the number of individuals with AIDS (discussed later in this chapter), who have little resistance to disease; an increase in the number of homeless and malnourished people; and the overwhelming proliferation of drug-resistant TB bacilli. An international TB vaccine, bacille Calmette-Guérin (BCG), is available, but it is rarely used in the United States. The vaccine does not always provide protection from the disease and those who are vaccinated may have a positive Mantoux test result.

TB is caused by the bacterium *Mycobacterium tuberculosis*. This organism is covered with a waxy substance that enables it to survive outside a living host for a long time. It is transmitted by droplets of sputum expectorated (coughed) into the environment by an infected host that are inhaled by another person. In the warm, moist respiratory tract, these organisms again can become active if the individual is susceptible to the disease. TB also can be spread when an infected person coughs or sneezes, releasing airborne infected droplets, which are inhaled and cause an infection if the person is susceptible.

TB develops in two stages. The primary infection occurs when the person is first infected with the bacteria and the lungs become inflamed. Cell-mediated immunity ensues, isolating the bacteria and forming a tubercle. At this point a healthy individual sometimes can stop the spread of the infection, causing the TB bacillus in the tubercle to become inactive. In this situation, the person was exposed to the pathogen but never developed active disease and so is said to have a *latent* TB infection. Individuals with latent TB are asymptomatic and are not infectious (Box 33.2). However, because an exposed person develops antibodies to the disease, he or she consistently tests positive on TB skin screening tests. Therefore rather than the purified protein derivative (PPD), or Mantoux test, these patients should have chest x-ray studies to diagnose active TB.

At any time the bacilli in the tubercles can be reactivated, and secondary, or active, TB can develop. The patient now is actively infected with the disease, which can spread to the bones, brain, and kidneys (see Box 33.2). Some people develop active TB soon after becoming infected, before the immune systems can fight the TB bacteria; others develop it later in life, when the immune systems are weakened for other reasons.

TB is diagnosed most frequently in people living in crowded conditions with poor hygiene, those who are malnourished, and those who have other chronic conditions. It spreads most rapidly in large cities, and among the elderly, alcoholics, and the homeless. Symptoms of

---

Box 33.2   Signs and Symptoms of Latent and Active Tuberculosis

Latent Tuberculosis Infection
- Does not feel sick
- Not infectious
- Positive purified protein derivative (PPD) test result
- Positive QuantiFERON-TB Gold blood test result
- Chest x-ray studies with normal findings
- Negative sputum culture

Active Tuberculosis Disease
- Symptoms include cough, fatigue, weight loss, anorexia, fever with chills, and night sweats
- Infectious (highest risk of infection is with close family members or associates)
- Positive PPD and QuantiFERON-TB Gold blood tests
- Chest x-ray studies with abnormal findings and/or positive sputum culture

(From the Centers for Disease Control and Prevention. Accessed September 30, 2016. Available at www.cdc.gov/tb/publications/factsheets/general/LTBIandActiveTB.htm.)

---

an active infection include an intermittent fever that peaks in the afternoon, night sweats, weight loss, and general malaise. As the infection becomes virulent in the host, a productive cough develops, and thick, dark, frequently blood-tinged mucus is expectorated.

The primary diagnosis of TB is established through the patient's signs and symptoms. The infection is suspected with a positive chest x-ray film but is confirmed with a sputum culture. Traditional culture methods originally took 4 to 6 weeks, and this extended period allowed a potentially infectious individual to continue to spread the disease. New culture techniques identify the bacterium in as little as 36 to 48 hours. A physician also may order a blood test, the QuantiFERON-TB Gold test (QFT), to diagnose TB infection. The QFT measures the response to TB proteins when they are mixed with a small amount of blood. A two-step Mantoux test is recommended for individuals who are aged above 45 years and have never had a Mantoux test; those who have been vaccinated with BCG; and employees of hospitals and long-term-care facilities. When this test is ordered by a healthcare provider, an initial intradermal skin test is administered and read in 48 to 72 hours. If the result is negative, a second Mantoux is performed on the opposite arm 1 to 3 weeks after the first test and again read in 48 to 72 hours.

Once a diagnosis of TB has been confirmed, the patient is prescribed long-term treatment with a combination of drugs to eradicate the bacilli. If the patient has tested positive for TB but does not have an active infection, the physician prescribes isoniazid (INH) and rifampin (RIF) for 6 months to treat any possible tubercle formations. If the patient has active pulmonary TB, the CDC recommends a four-drug regimen—INH, RIF, pyrazinamide, and ethambutol—daily for 2 months; this is then reduced to two drugs for an additional 4 to 7 months, depending on sputum culture outcomes. It is crucial that patients being treated with TB medications strictly comply with medication orders to prevent the creation of multidrug-resistant TB (MDR-TB). Resistant strains of TB develop because of skipped doses or failure to take the medication as long as prescribed. MDR-TB requires at least 2 years of drug therapy with medications that can cause serious side effects, especially liver damage. All tuberculin-negative healthcare workers should have a PPD annually; workers who show a positive reaction but are not actively infected with TB should have an annual chest x-ray evaluation to screen for the disease.

Chronic Obstructive Pulmonary Disease

Chronic obstructive pulmonary disease (COPD) is a group of diseases with the common characteristic of chronic airway obstruction. COPD is the fourth leading cause of death in America, and most of those deaths are related to smoking. Among the diseases in this group are chronic bronchitis, bronchiectasis, asthma, and emphysema. Although the way the obstruction occurs may vary, a patient with COPD is unable to ventilate the lungs freely, which results in an ineffective exchange of respiratory gases, dyspnea, and productive cough. Over time, eliminating carbon dioxide from the lungs during expiration becomes increasingly difficult. Many patients who have COPD will have a dependence on oxygen in order for the brain to remain oxygenated.

Asthma

Asthma attacks occur in response to a number of triggers that cause inflammation and a spasm of the bronchus within the lung that results in airflow obstruction. Asthma can develop into a chronic disease characterized by increased activity or sensitivity of the bronchial tubes to external factors, such as environmental irritants, poor air quality, and allergies, or to internal factors, such as stress, exercise, infection, and allergen inhalation. Asthma also has a strong hereditary factor.

Asthma attacks can be mild to severe and can last minutes to days. Bronchospasms trap air in the lungs while the inflammatory response creates edema and causes secretion of mucus into the constricted bronchioles. A patient with asthma complains of a nonproductive cough, dyspnea (difficulty breathing), expiratory wheezing, and chest tightness. Because the individual has difficulty breathing, tachycardia, pallor, and diaphoresis also may occur. The patient can speak only a few words at a time, stopping intermittently to breathe in.

When the chest is auscultated, the physician hears diminished breath sounds with wheezes and rhonchi in the lungs. Chest x-ray studies may show changes in the lungs from mucous obstructions. Blood tests include a complete blood cell count with a differential count to determine whether the attack is allergy related. The patient care technician may be asked to obtain a blood sample for the patient experiencing an asthma attack who presents to the emergency department.

Regardless of their age, patients with asthma should be actively involved in the day-to-day management of their disease. Peak flow meters assess the individual's ability to move air into and out of the lungs. The physician may want the patient to keep a log of daily peak flow results or to use the instrument as an at-home monitoring device when chest tightness and wheezing occur. The meter measures the peak expiratory flow rate, which is the fastest speed at which the patient can blow air out of the lungs after taking in as big a breath as possible. Peak flow readings provide an evaluation of bronchiole function that the patient can perform at home with limited assistance. Readings can help predict an asthma attack if levels are falling; can measure the degree of bronchospasm; and provide the physician with feedback regarding the effectiveness of asthma treatment.

The physician uses three zones of measurement to interpret peak flow rates. This type of system is referred to as a stop-light system of measurement. A stop light has three lights; green, which indicates go; yellow, which indicates caution; red, which indicates one must stop. This makes it easier for the adult and child to manage their respiratory status with use of a flow meter. The green zone is considered normal: the reading is 80% to 100% of normal peak flow rates, indicating that the patient's asthma is under control. The yellow zone signals caution: The patient's highest reading is 50% to 80% of normal. The physician makes treatment decisions and recommendations at this point, or the patient may already be instructed on how to manage medications if readings are within these levels. The red zone includes readings below 50% of the normal level, and immediate action must be taken to prevent severe bronchospasms.

If the patient is having an asthma attack, the bronchioles are constricting, becoming edematous, and filling up with mucus, so the patient is unable to exhale strongly enough to raise the peak flow indicator to a normal level. If readings are below normal, the physician prescribes a treatment plan that may include contacting the physician when peak flow levels are below a certain point or starting nebulizer treatments. The physician may recommend an increase in antiinflammatory medication if more than a 20% variation from normal is seen in the readings. The medication therapy chosen depends on the severity and frequency of acute attacks, but management is necessary to prevent

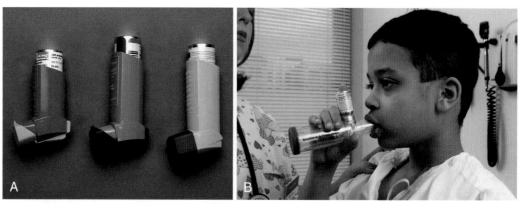

FIGURE 33.2 A, Inhalers. B, An inhaler with a spacer. (From Proctor D, Adams A: *Kinn's The Medical Assistant: an applied learning approach,* ed 12, St. Louis, 2014, Saunders.)

permanent lung damage and emphysema-like changes in the lungs.

The treatment of asthma consists of a regimen of medications, including "rescue" inhalers (e.g., ipratropium bromide [Atrovent] or albuterol [Ventolin]), which are used to relieve bronchospasms or for exercise-induced asthma (Fig. 33.2). Tissue inflammation can be treated with steroid inhalers (e.g., flunisolide [Aerobid], triamcinolone acetonide [Azmacort], or fluticasone [Flovent Diskus]) and/or an oral leukotriene-receptor antagonists such as zafirlukast (Accolate) or montelukast sodium (Singulair) taken daily. Another option is a combination inhaler, such as fluticasone and salmeterol (Advair Diskus), that contains both types of medications to prevent and treat bronchiole inflammation. A severe attack may require injections of epinephrine, oral corticosteroids (prednisone), and/or nebulizer treatments with a bronchodilator. A nebulizer forces compressed air through a medication chamber that converts liquid medication (albuterol or budesonide [Pulmicort]) into an aerosol or mist form that can be inhaled though a mask or mouthpiece.

The physician prescribes an inhaler dose according to the number of "puffs" of a metered-dose inhaler (MDI) the patient should administer (Box 33.3). MDIs consist of a pressurized canister containing medication and a mouthpiece. Most MDIs hold about 200 doses of medication combined with a pressurized gas propellant, which forces the drug out of the canister. When the canister is inverted and depressed, a metered dose (premeasured) is delivered through the mouthpiece in aerosol form. Patient teaching is very important to ensure that the patient operates the device correctly so that the medication can be administered as ordered. If both a steroid and a bronchodilator have been prescribed, the bronchodilator should be taken first, because this opens the airways so that the steroid is better distributed throughout the lungs. The nurse or respiratory therapist will typically administer all asthma medications to include inhalers and nebulizers; however, depending on facility policy, this may be delegated to

Box 33.3 Patient Education for a Metered-Dose Inhaler

Instruct the patient in the use of a metered-dose inhaler as follows:

1. Shake the canister vigorously and place it into the mouthpiece device.
2. Open your mouth and hold the inhaler approximately 1 inch away. (If the patient places the mouthpiece in the mouth, the gas propellant causes the drug to bounce off the back of the throat, and much of it will be lost around the mouth.)
3. Exhale normally. Then, while beginning to inhale slowly, depress the canister, releasing a metered dose of medication.
4. Continue to breathe in until your lungs are full; hold the breath to a count of 10, if possible, and then breathe out normally.
5. If a second dose has been prescribed, wait at least 1 minute between puffs.

Some inhalers come attached to spacers or can be adapted to meet the needs of children or older patients who have difficulty managing the technique. When the canister is depressed, the medication stays in the spacer, and the patient can take more time to inhale the particles (see Fig. 33.2B).

the patient care technician. See Procedure 33.1 for administering a nebulizer treatment.

Emphysema

Emphysema is a progressive obstructive disease of the pulmonary system that is irreversible. Emphysema causes loss of elasticity in the walls of the alveoli, and eventually these walls stretch and break, creating air spaces that cannot conduct the oxygen–carbon dioxide exchange. The remaining alveoli become overinflated, and as time progresses, exhaling completely becomes very difficult. Cigarette smoking is the primary contributing factor, although patients who develop emphysema

PROCEDURE 33.1

Administer a Nebulizer Treatment

1. Plug the nebulizer into a properly grounded electrical outlet.
2. Introduce yourself and confirm the patient's identity.
3. Explain the purpose of the treatment.
4. Sanitize your hands.
5. Measure the prescribed dose of drug into the nebulizer medication cup.

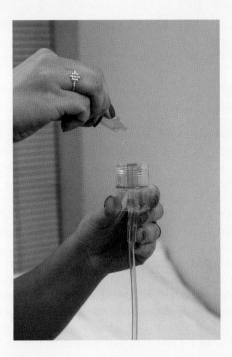

6. Replace the top of the medication cup and connect it to the mouthpiece or face mask.
7. Connect the disposable tubing to the nebulizer and the medication cup.
8. The patient should be sitting upright to allow for total lung expansion.
10. Turn on the nebulizer. If using a mask, position it comfortably but securely over the patient's mouth and nose.

11. If using a mouthpiece, instruct the patient to hold it between the teeth with the lips pursed around the mouthpiece.

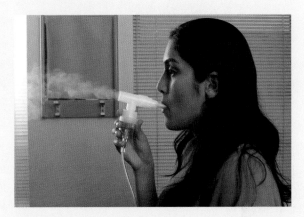

12. Encourage the patient to take slow, deep breaths through the mouth and to hold each breath 2 to 3 seconds to allow the medication to disperse through the lungs.
13. Continue the treatment until aerosol is no longer produced (approximately 10 minutes).
14. **CAUTION:** If the patient is receiving a bronchodilator (albuterol), he or she may experience dizziness, tremors, or tachycardia. Continue the treatment unless otherwise notified by the nurse.
14. Turn off the nebulizer.
15. Encourage the patient to take several deep breaths and to cough loosened secretions into disposable tissues.
16. Dispose of the mouthpiece or mask and tubing in a biohazard container and instruct the patient also to dispose of the contaminated tissues in the biohazard container.
17. Sanitize your hands.
18. Record the nebulizer treatment; the patient's response, including the amount of coughing and whether coughing was productive or nonproductive; and any side effects of the medication.

---

at an early age may have a genetic predisposition to the disease. Other contributors include exposure to pollutants or chronic respiratory disorders (chronic bronchitis or asthma).

Symptoms may not be seen until irreversible damage has occurred. When signs and symptoms occur, they include dyspnea, shortness of breath (SOB), wheezing, production of thick mucus, restlessness, fatigue, anorexia, persistent cough (productive or nonproductive), and peripheral cyanosis with clubbing (Fig. 33.3). The condition typically is diagnosed from presenting signs and symptoms and a chest x-ray examination, as

well as a pulmonary function test (PFT) that shows increased residual volume and decreased forced expiratory volume.

Patients with emphysema are encouraged to avoid respiratory irritants, and individuals with respiratory infections to stop smoking. Many of these patients require oxygen therapy and benefit from postural drainage and chest percussion to enable the patients to expectorate trapped mucus. Nebulizer treatments also may be prescribed.

Patients with emphysema expend a great deal of energy just to expel air from the lungs, so they should

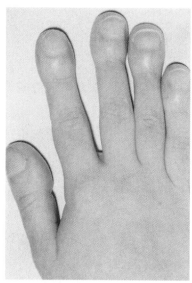

FIGURE 33.3 Clubbing. (From Zitelli B, Davis H: *Atlas of pediatric physical diagnosis*, ed 6, Philadelphia, 2012, Mosby.)

Box 33.4	Common Signs and Symptoms of Obstructive Sleep Apnea

- Excessive daytime sleepiness (hypersomnia)
- Persistently loud, disruptive snoring
- Snoring, choking, or gasping sounds while asleep
- Episodes of breathing cessation during sleep
- Dry mouth or sore throat on awakening
- Morning headache

consume a high-calorie, high-fluid diet and perform certain exercises, such as pursed-lip breathing, to help them conserve energy. A patient with emphysema requires continuous care and support; therefore encouraging family involvement in the treatment plan is important. Referral to a pulmonary rehabilitation program or support group can benefit both patient and family members.

Obstructive Sleep Apnea

Obstructive sleep apnea occurs when the muscles in the posterior pharynx that support the soft palate, uvula, tonsils, and tongue relax during sleep. This relaxation causes the trachea to narrow or close with inhalation, momentarily stopping breathing. Blood oxygen levels are lowered, and the brain senses hypoxemia, so it stimulates the patient from sleep to reopen the trachea. The patient is awake so briefly that he or she is not aware of the arousal, but this occurs repeatedly throughout the night, preventing the person from achieving a deeper, more restful level of sleep. Because of this interrupted sleep, the individual frequently complains of sleepiness during the day (Box 33.4).

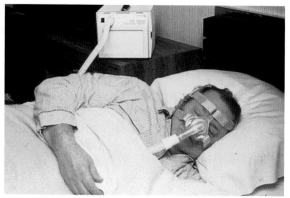

FIGURE 33.4 Patient with a continuous positive airway pressure (CPAP) machine. (Courtesy Philips Respironics, Murrysville, Pennsylvania.)

Individuals are at greater risk of developing obstructive sleep apnea if they are overweight, because a fat or thick neck may narrow the trachea; if they have enlarged adenoids or tonsils; if they are male, because men develop sleep apnea twice as frequently as women; if they have a family history of sleep apnea; and if they drink alcohol or take sedatives, because these chemicals relax throat muscles.

Patients with suspected sleep apnea report chronic fatigue (from the constant startling out of a restful sleep) and pronounced snoring. Sleep apnea is diagnosed after the patient has been monitored during a sleep study, a process called *nocturnal polysomnography*. The patient is connected to equipment that monitors the pulse rate, brain activity, breathing patterns, blood oxygen levels, and limb movements during sleep.

Multiple complications in addition to chronic daytime fatigue can occur because of sleep apnea. Patients are more susceptible to hypertension and resultant heart disease because hypoxic episodes during sleep raise blood pressure and put a strain on the heart. Individuals with sleep apnea also tend to complain of memory problems, morning headaches, depression, and nocturia.

Sleep apnea typically is treated with a continuous positive airway pressure (CPAP) machine (Fig. 33.4), which delivers air pressure through a mask placed over the mouth or through a cannula in the nose. The air pressure created by the machine is greater than that of the surrounding air, and it forces the upper airway passages open and prevents tracheal collapse. Although CPAP is the preferred method of treatment, it can be awkward and uncomfortable, making it difficult to sleep. Patients may have to experiment with different types of masks and need to be encouraged to follow through with the recommended treatment. Individuals with mild obstructive sleep apnea can try alternative treatment with a dental device that opens the throat by bringing the jaw forward. Surgery may also be an option to remove the uvula, tonsils, and adenoids, as well as excess tissue from the nose and back of the throat that vibrates during sleep, resulting in snoring.

Cancer of the Respiratory System

The most prevalent cancers of the respiratory system are lung cancer and carcinoma of the larynx. Although there continues to be no cure for cancer, there are many advanced treatment options that have led to better outcomes for those with cancer and perhaps longer lives.

Lung Cancer

Lung cancer is the leading cause of cancer-related deaths for both men and women in the United States. It is estimated that 90% of lung tumors are linked to cigarette smoking; other risk factors include chronic exposure to second-hand smoke, carcinogens (e.g., radon gas and asbestos), and a genetic predisposition. The risk of developing cancer is higher for patients who started to smoke at a young age and who have smoked more than a pack a day for a long period. Individuals who quit smoking can significantly lower their risk of lung cancer; after 10 years, the risk is reduced by one third. Female smokers are at greater risk of lung cancer than male smokers.

The lung is a common site of secondary tumors from metastasis in addition to primary carcinomas. Several different cellular types of tumors can develop in the lungs, but the one seen most frequently is bronchogenic carcinoma, which originates in the epithelial lining of the bronchioles. The early symptoms of lung cancer (i.e., a chronic, productive cough; SOB; and chest tightness) are masked by symptoms regularly displayed by habitual smokers. A tumor may be discovered accidentally during a routine chest x-ray evaluation or may not be discovered until metastatic symptoms, such as anemia, weight loss, and fatigue, lead to the diagnosis of a primary lung tumor. Patients who show symptoms usually display local effects of a tumor in the chest, such as bronchial obstruction, atelectasis, hemoptysis, chest pain, and pleural membrane involvement. Unless the tumor is diagnosed very early, lung cancer has a poor prognosis. Treatment consists of surgery, radiation therapy, and chemotherapy.

Carcinoma of the Larynx

Carcinoma of the larynx is pathologically linked to smoking and chronic alcohol consumption. Ninety percent of cases of laryngeal cancer occur in men; most of those affected are 60 to 70 years of age. Patients show early signs of hoarseness, loss of voice, and dysphagia (difficulty swallowing), and occasionally, respiration becomes impaired. Because of these early symptoms, most laryngeal tumors are discovered in the early stages and can be removed, resulting in a very good prognosis. Surgical treatment consists of a partial or total laryngectomy. With a total laryngectomy, the voice is permanently lost, and a tracheostomy is performed. Patients undergoing such procedures need comprehensive preparation and benefit from meeting a laryngectomy survivor, in addition to participating in a support group to deal with postsurgical adjustments.

Diseases and Disorders of the Heart

Many diseases and disorders affect the heart and its blood vessels. Cardiac disease has multiple risk factors; some of these cannot be changed, and others people can change or seek to have treated. The more risk factors a person has, the greater his or her risk of developing cardiovascular disease.

CHRONIC CONDITIONS OF THE CARDIAC SYSTEM

Coronary artery disease (CAD) causes more than 1 million deaths in the United States every year. When CAD occurs, the formation of atherosclerotic plaques narrows the arteries supplying the myocardium, or the muscle layer of the heart. Atherosclerotic plaque buildup is primarily related to cholesterol blood levels. Anginal chest pain is pain behind the sternum that is precipitated by activity but that can be relieved either by rest or by sublingual nitroglycerin.

Patients may be asymptomatic until the disease becomes fully developed. The first symptom may be angina, followed by pressure or fullness in the chest, syncope, shortness of breath, edema, unexplained coughing spells, and fatigue. A patient reporting any

Box 33.5   Risk Factors for Heart Disease

Risk Factors That Cannot Be Changed

- *Advancing age:* Most people who die of heart disease are aged 65 years or older; older women are more likely to die of myocardial infarctions (MIs) than are older men.
- *Gender:* Men are at greater risk of MIs and experience heart attacks earlier in life; women are at greater risk after menopause.
- *Family history and race:* The children of parents with heart disease are more likely to develop it; African Americans are at greater risk of developing hypertension and heart disease associated with it; Mexican Americans, Native Americans, native Hawaiians, and some Asian Americans also are at greater risk.

Lifestyle Risk Factors That Can Be Modified or Treated

- *Smoking:* Male smokers develop heart disease three times more often than women; female smokers develop heart disease six times more often than those who have never smoked. Smoking is associated with sudden cardiac death. Exposure to secondhand smoke also increases the risk.
- *High blood cholesterol:* The risk of heart disease rises with rising blood cholesterol levels.
- *Hypertension:* Hypertension increases the amount of work the heart must do to circulate blood throughout the body.
- *Sedentary lifestyle:* Regular exercise helps prevent cardiovascular disease.
- *Obesity and overweight:* Excess weight, especially increased body fat at the waist, is associated with an increased risk of heart disease and stroke; losing as little as 10 pounds can lower the risk.
- *Diabetes mellitus:* The risk of heart disease is even greater if blood glucose levels are not controlled; at least 68% of people with diabetes die of some form of heart disease; 16% die of stroke.

(Adapted from the American Heart Association. Accessed 9/30/2016. Available at www.heart.org/HEARTORG/Conditions/HeartAttack/UnderstandYourRiskofHeartAttack/Understand-Your-Risk-of-Heart-Attack_UCM_002040_Article.jsp.)

Box 33.6   Signs and Symptoms of Myocardial Infarction in Women

In addition to angina, the signs and symptoms of a heart attack in women may start weeks before the actual cardiac injury and could include the following:

- Abdominal, neck, shoulder, or upper back pain
- Jaw pain
- Shortness of breath
- Vertigo (dizziness)
- Sweating
- Indigestion or nausea and vomiting
- Extreme fatigue
- Aching in both arms

associated with the method of plaque buildup in women; the plaque tends to develop as an evenly spread layer along the entire lumen of the blood vessels rather than as a localized plaque buildup, as is seen in men. Women with heart disease typically experience this diffuse atheroma buildup in smaller vessels, which causes more subtle symptoms than the crushing chest pain associated with classic myocardial infarctions (Box 33.6).

The major concern in heart disease is the lack of blood to the myocardium, which occurs when a vessel becomes totally blocked. Ischemia, or lack of oxygen-rich blood, over a prolonged period leads to necrosis (death) of a portion of the myocardium, resulting in an MI, or heart attack. Symptoms of an MI are similar to those of angina; however, an MI is identified by pain that lasts longer than 30 minutes and is not relieved by rest or nitroglycerin tablets. An MI is a life-threatening event; intervention must begin within the first hour, or death may occur.

Diagnostic and Therapeutic Procedures

An MI is diagnosed by ECG changes and elevated cardiac enzymes. The blood test most often ordered to confirm myocardial damage is the creatine kinase (CK) level. The patient care technician may be asked to perform blood tests at the bedside of the patient in the emergency room who is experiencing angina. This may include drawing blood for CK levels, as well as troponin levels. Creatine kinase levels begin to increase approximately 6 hours after the start of a heart attack and reach their peak in about 18 hours; they return to normal in 24 to 36 hours. The more severe the cardiac damage, the longer it takes for CK levels to peak and then return to normal. Determination of the troponin levels is a more sensitive blood test that can detect minor myocardial damage not evident with CK levels. Troponins increase in the bloodstream within 4 to 6 hours after the initial myocardial damage and peak in 10 to 24 hours. In the case of minor myocardial damage, troponin levels remain elevated up to 10 to 14 days, allowing for later

of these symptoms should be seen by the physician immediately.

In recent years the rate of heart disease has declined in men but not in women. Traditional risk factors negatively affect both genders; however, women are at greater risk if they have metabolic syndrome (a combination of hypertension, elevated insulin levels, excess body fat around the waist, and high blood cholesterol levels); if they have increased levels of stress and/or depression; if they smoke (female smokers are at much greater risk than male smokers); and if they have reduced estrogen production before menopause (Box 33.5). The difference in female risks and symptoms is

diagnosis of the event. Patients found to have an MI typically are hospitalized immediately, started on oxygen, and continuously monitored by ECG.

Medical treatment includes the use of thrombolytic medications, such as alteplase (Activase) and reteplase (Retavase), to dissolve coronary artery blockage and prevent permanent myocardial damage. To be most effective, this treatment must be started within 3 hours of the episode; however, it is still helpful if administered within 12 hours of initial symptoms. This timetable makes it extremely important that patients be diagnosed and treated as soon as possible. As the patient care technician, your role is valuable in obtaining the blood samples and ECG necessary for the physician to plan treatment for the patient. The patient who is experiencing angina should be prioritized to the top of your list with reference to which patient you see first. Thrombolytic medications are administered intravenously (IV) along with heparin to prevent clots that are being dissolved from reforming. Aspirin also is used to prevent the formation of blood clots in affected blood vessels. Additional pharmaceutical treatment includes the use of nitroglycerin to dilate the coronary arteries so that more blood can be delivered to the myocardium; beta blockers (atenolol [Tenormin], metoprolol [Lopressor], or propranolol [Inderal]) to slow the heart rate and lower blood pressure; anticoagulants (warfarin [Coumadin]) for 3 to 6 months to prevent thrombus formation; and anticholesterol agents to lower blood cholesterol levels and prevent subsequent formation of atherosclerotic plaques.

When the coronary arteries that supply blood to the myocardium are blocked, or occluded, either percutaneous transluminal coronary angioplasty (PTCA) or coronary artery bypass grafting (CABG) may be indicated. (These surgical procedures are discussed later in this chapter.)

After discharge from the hospital, patients with CAD that has resulted in an MI face multiple lifestyle changes to prevent another episode. Recommendations include no smoking; regular light exercise, such as walking 30 minutes a day, 5 days a week; a diet low in salt, fat, and cholesterol; maintaining a healthy weight; controlling hypertension; reducing stress; and limiting alcohol intake to one or two drinks a day. The patient care technician should be prepared to provide encouragement and to reinforce the importance of lifestyle changes to prevent future heart problems. If ordered by the physician, professional referrals to a cardiac rehabilitation program and dietitian can also be helpful.

Endocrine Dysfunction of the Pancreas: Diabetes Mellitus

Diabetes mellitus is a common hormonal imbalance that has reached epidemic proportions in the United States.

In 2012, approximately 21.9 million Americans, or 9.3% of the population, have DM, and the number is growing (http://www.diabetes.org/diabetes-basics/statistics/). Diabetes occurs in people of all ages and races but is more common in older adults (25.9% of individuals aged above 65 years) and in African Americans, Latinos, Native Americans, and Asian Americans/Pacific Islanders. Diabetes mellitus is characterized by chronic hyperglycemia and problems with carbohydrate metabolism. This problem with glucose management is caused by a lack of insulin production and/or resistance to insulin at the target cell level. The pancreas contains islets of Langerhans, which produce and secrete the hormones insulin and glucagon. When the blood glucose level is too high, beta islet cells secrete insulin, which is sent through the bloodstream to the target tissue site to conduct glucose into the cell. When blood glucose levels are low, glucagon is secreted by the alpha islet cells to stimulate the liver to convert glycogen (stored glucose) into circulating glucose.

If there is resistance to insulin at the target cell membrane or if not enough insulin is available to help transport glucose from the blood into the cells, the person experiences a variety of symptoms, including glycosuria, polyuria, polydipsia, polyphagia, rapid weight loss, drowsiness, fatigue, itching of the skin, visual disturbances, and skin infections. The American Diabetes Association has identified four major types of diabetes: prediabetes, DM type I, DM type II, and gestational diabetes. If left untreated or managed poorly, DM can have serious, life-threatening consequences, such as cardiovascular disease, stroke, hypertension, blindness, kidney disease, nervous system disorders, amputations, pregnancy complications, and diabetic coma. Patient education is crucial for compliance with treatment and prevention of life-threatening complications.

Prediabetes

Prediabetes is a condition in which a person's blood glucose level is higher than normal but not high enough for a diagnosis of diabetes type II. It is estimated that 54 million adults in the United States have prediabetes. Some of the long-term damage to vascular and cardiac systems may be occurring during prediabetes. Studies indicate that most individuals with prediabetes develop diabetes type II within 10 years. However, if patients lower their blood glucose levels, they can delay or prevent its onset. Experts recommend that patients with prediabetes lose 5% to 10% of their weight and perform moderate physical activity for 30 to 60 minutes daily. A loss of just 10 to 20 pounds can make a huge difference in blood glucose levels.

Two tests are used to diagnose prediabetes: the fasting plasma glucose (FPG) test and the oral glucose tolerance test (OGTT) (Box 33.7). A person with prediabetes has a

- Plasma glucose level ≥200 mg/dL (norm is 80 to 120 mg/dL) with the classic symptoms of polyuria, polydipsia, and unexplained weight loss
- Fasting plasma glucose level ≥126 mg/dL (norm is 70 to 110 mg/dL) on more than one occasion
- Two-hour oral glucose tolerance test (OGTT) result ≥200 mg/dL
- Urinalysis positive for glucose and possibly ketones
- Glycosylated hemoglobin (HbA$_{1c}$) >7% (normal is 4% to 6%)

fasting blood glucose level between 100 and 125 mg/dL; individuals with an FPG level of 126 mg/dL or higher are diagnosed as diabetic. A person with prediabetes has a 2-hour OGTT result of 140 to 199 mg/dL; diabetes is diagnosed if the OGTT is 200 mg/dL or higher.

Type I Diabetes

Diabetes type I most often develops in children and young adults. This disease previously was known as either *juvenile-onset diabetes* or *insulin-dependent diabetes*. In DM type I the pancreas is unable to produce insulin because of the destruction of the beta islet cells from autoimmune, genetic, or environmental factors. Type I affects 5% to 10% of patients with diabetes, and it typically has an acute onset. Treatment of diabetes type I requires insulin administration. The goal for insulin therapy is to maintain blood glucose levels as close to normal as possible without causing hypoglycemia. Many types and brands of insulin are available, but to prevent allergic reactions, only genetically engineered human insulin should be used. At this time, the only method of insulin administration is injection, because gastrointestinal processes destroy insulin if it is given by mouth. However, multiple studies are underway on buccal (by cheek), inhaled, and patch forms of the hormone. An inhaled form of insulin had been released but is no longer available because of concerns that the drug is associated with decreased pulmonary function.

- *Insulin pump:* An insulin pump is a computerized device that administers a constant dose of insulin using a small portable pump. The pump is programmed to deliver a measured dose of insulin by continuous subcutaneous infusion through a catheter, which is placed in the abdomen or buttocks areas. This method more closely resembles the body's normal surge of insulin and is designed to maintain blood glucose levels consistently within normal limits.
- *Injector pen:* Injector pens are preloaded with insulin cartridges for easy use (Fig. 33.5). Insulin pens are disposable or refillable and easily portable and therefore can be used by patients with diabetes when they are away from home.

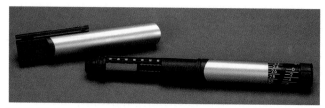

FIGURE 33.5 NovoPen. (From Proctor D, Adams A: *Kinn's The Medical Assistant: an applied learning approach,* ed 12, St. Louis, 2014, Saunders.)

Successful treatment of DM type I involves a complicated treatment plan in which various types of insulin are given in multiple injections (typically four) throughout the day. The insulin type and dosage are balanced by the patient's typical exercise regimen and diet (Box 33.8). The patient must monitor blood glucose levels with a glucometer periodically throughout the day to determine whether the levels are within the normal range. The physician typically prescribes glucometer testing in the morning before breakfast, before dinner, and possibly before lunch and at bedtime if the patient is having difficulty keeping blood plasma levels stabilized. The nurse may ask you to observe the patient performing glucometer screening. If any errors are noted when the patient assesses his or her own blood glucose you would need to notify the nurse so that he or she may perform additional teaching.

Glucometers are palm sized and use very small amounts of capillary blood from a site in the finger, forearm, upper arm, or abdomen (see Chapter 24). Many different types of glucometers are available, but all display test results within seconds, and the results are stored in the memory function of the machine for future reference. Some patients will prefer to bring their glucometers with them to the hospital because that is the equipment they are used to. Depending on facility policy, this may or may not be allowed. Some healthcare facilities use glucometers that sync with the electronic health record, which would prevent the patient from using his or her own.

Patients with diabetes also need to find the best method of disposing of their syringes and lancets. Local pharmacies or hospitals may offer assistance with disposal of used sharps. If the patient does not have access to a sharps return program, a puncture-resistant container with an opening that can be easily and tightly sealed before disposal is a good choice.

Regardless of the type of diabetes, for treatment to be successful, patients must play an active role in the management of their disease. The ideal is to maintain blood plasma levels as close to the norm as possible to prevent complications. The American Diabetes Association recommends blood levels between 90 and 130 mg/dL before meals and below 180 mg/dL 2 hours after starting a meal, with a glycated (glycosylated) hemoglobin level (HbA$_{1c}$) below 7%.

Type II Diabetes

Diabetes mellitus type II, once called *adult-onset* or *non-insulin-dependent diabetes,* usually develops in adults but may be seen at any age. Factors that increase the risk of developing DM type II include a family history, a history of gestational diabetes, impaired glucose tolerance, physical inactivity, and obesity. In this type of DM, the pancreas produces insulin, but not enough, and/or the target cells are resistant to insulin action. Diabetes type II is responsible for 95% of cases of diabetes mellitus.

This form of diabetes frequently goes undetected for many years because of the gradual onset of hyperglycemia and the absence of classic diabetic symptoms. However, because of this insidious onset over time, patients with diabetes type II are at even greater risk of developing vascular complications. Insulin resistance at the target cell level may improve with weight reduction and/or pharmacologic treatment.

Treatment for diabetes type II includes weight loss, exercise, dietary restrictions, and oral hypoglycemic medications that act to stimulate insulin production and/or improve tissue response to insulin. Medications for diabetes type II have multiple functions, including stimulating insulin secretion from pancreatic islet cells in patients with some pancreatic function; reducing insulin resistance at the cellular level; improving sensitivity to insulin in muscle and adipose tissue; and inhibiting hepatic gluconeogenesis.

As with diabetes type I, the goal of treatment is to maintain blood glucose levels within the normal range. For some patients, exercise, diet, and weight loss are sufficient to control blood glucose levels. Sometimes just the loss of 10 to 20 pounds is enough to bring blood glucose levels under control. Other patients may need medication to maintain normal blood glucose levels; however, levels must be monitored daily with a glucometer to determine the success of treatment. Over time,

the individual with diabetes type II may require insulin to control hyperglycemia.

Chronic Gastrointestinal Disorders

Inflammation of the liver, called *hepatitis,* may be caused by a localized infection (viral hepatitis), a systemic infection, chemical exposure, or a complication of drug metabolism. Mild inflammation temporarily impairs function, but severe inflammation may lead to necrosis and serious complications.

Viral Hepatitis

Acute viral hepatitis is an infection of the liver that causes a sudden onset of hepatocyte inflammation. Several forms of the hepatitis virus are categorized as hepatitides A, B, C, D, E, and G (Table 33.1). Hepatic cells can regenerate; therefore, depending on the degree of liver involvement, the patient may recover completely or could develop widespread necrosis, cirrhosis, and liver failure. Chronic inflammation, defined as the presence of the disease for longer than 6 months, can occur with hepatitis B, C, or D. This usually results in permanent liver damage and an associated increased risk of liver cancer. Individuals infected with hepatitis B, C, or D may become lifelong carriers of the disease. Hepatitis carriers are asymptomatic but can transmit the virus to others (Box 33.9).

The hepatitis A virus (HAV) is transmitted through contaminated water or shellfish. Some parts of the world are endemic for the disease, and a vaccine is available. The hepatitis B virus (HBV) has a relatively long incubation period, which makes tracking the source of the infection difficult. Because the virus is found in all blood and body fluids, it can be transmitted in many ways, including needlesticks, human bites from individuals infected with the virus, sexual contact, and maternal-fetal transmission. Immunization of individuals at increased risk is highly recommended. All healthcare personnel are included in this group, because they are

Box 33.9	Groups at Risk for Hepatitis A, B, and C

- **Hepatitis A:** day care workers and clients, institutionalized residents, individuals traveling to infected areas
- **Hepatitis B:** IV drug users, homosexual men, hemodialysis patients, hemophiliac individuals, healthcare workers, individuals with a history of frequent sexual partners
- **Hepatitis C:** patients receiving frequent blood transfusions, homosexual men, IV drug users, healthcare workers

Table 33.1	Characteristics of the Types of Viral Hepatitis		
Hepatitis Type	**Mode of Transmission**	**Incubation Period**	**Symptoms**
A	Fecal-oral (food or water contaminated by feces from infected person); contaminated raw shellfish; infected household members or sexual partners	2 to 7 weeks	Fatigue, weakness, anorexia; some patients have joint pain, hepatomegaly, lymphadenopathy, jaundice
B (serum hepatitis)	Blood and body fluids; placental transfer	1 to 6 months	General malaise, joint swelling, pruritic rash, hepatomegaly, anorexia, nausea, vomiting, dark yellowish-brown urine, jaundice; may become chronic
C (non-A non-B)	Blood and body fluids; most frequent type of posttransfusion hepatitis	2 weeks to 6 months	Acute onset of fever, chills malaise, nausea, vomiting; frequently becomes chronic
D (delta virus)	Blood and body fluids	Seen only in patients with hepatitis B	Similar to those of hepatitis B; increases the severity of hepatitis B
E	Fecal-oral	2 to 9 weeks	Similar to those in hepatitis A; seen in India, Asia, Africa, and Central America; mild form but can cause death in pregnant women
G	Blood and blood products	Not known	Similar to those of hepatitis C; may become chronic but does not appear to be an important cause of clinical liver disease

at increased risk for infection through exposure to blood or blood products and body fluids. Hepatitis B virus immunization is included as part of the pediatric immunizations.

As a healthcare professional, the patient care technician cares for sick people on a daily basis who may be carriers of the hepatitis virus. Changing dressings, collecting specimens, holding a patient's hand that was just used to cover the mouth, and discarding a wet baby diaper all are possible ways that exposure can occur. The first line of defense, regardless of whether the patient care technician has been immunized, is frequent washing and sanitization of the hands and wearing gloves when exposure to blood or body fluids is possible.

Diagnosis and Treatment

Hepatitides A, B, and C are diagnosed through identification of the virus or antibodies to the virus in the blood. Another useful diagnostic test is a liver biopsy. Once the infection has been diagnosed, liver function tests are done periodically throughout the course of the disease to determine the degree of liver damage. Patients with hepatitis B, C, or D must be monitored for possible chronic hepatitis and the development of a carrier state. Prescription medications include interferon, which stimulates the immune response, and antiviral drugs (e.g., telbivudine [Tyzeka], entecavir [Baraclude]) to prevent viral cell replication. Otherwise, the treatment for all forms of hepatitis generally consists of bed rest and a high-protein diet.

The best form of treatment for hepatitis B is prevention through vaccination against the disease. The vaccine is given intramuscularly in three doses. The first two are given 30 days apart, and the third is given 6 months after the first. The Occupational Safety and Health Administration (OSHA) requires healthcare employers to make the vaccine available to employees free of charge. Patient care technician programs encourage students to be vaccinated, because they also are at risk for acquiring the disease.

CHRONIC IMMUNOLOGIC & ONCOLOGIC DISORDERS

Acquired Immunodeficiency Syndrome

Acquired immunodeficiency syndrome (AIDS) is the deadly sexually transmitted disease. It is caused by the human immunodeficiency virus (HIV; www.std-gov.org). The virus invades CD4 T lymphocytes, destroying their ability to fight infection on the cellular level. Individuals may be without symptoms when first exposed to HIV. Those who do develop symptoms may complain of a fever, arthralgia (joint pain), myalgia (muscle pain), lymphadenopathy, rash, night sweats, and malaise approximately 2 to 6 weeks after exposure to the virus.

The goal of treatment of HIV infection is to reduce the amount of virus in the body with antiretroviral drugs, thereby slowing the destruction of the immune system. Individuals with an early diagnosis and consistent, appropriate medical treatment with advanced drug therapy can remain HIV positive without developing AIDS, and can live near-normal life expectancies. Acquired immunodeficiency syndrome is diagnosed when evidence appears of a wide range of opportunistic infections that develop because of depressed T-cell counts. These include *Pneumocystis carinii* pneumonia

(PCP), candidiasis (yeast infection), Kaposi sarcoma, dementia, and wasting syndrome. A patient is considered to be HIV positive when antibodies to the virus are detected; however, the diagnosis of AIDS is not made until the CD4 T-cell count drops below 200 mm^3 (the normal count is 600 to 1000 mm^3) and/or opportunistic infections have been diagnosed. Current HIV management includes monitoring of CD4 T-cell counts at diagnosis and every 3 to 6 months thereafter.

HIV is transmitted when infected blood or blood products, semen, or vaginal secretions come in contact with the mucous membranes or the broken skin of an uninfected person. It also can be passed in utero from an infected mother to her fetus, during delivery, or by breast-feeding. Intravenous drug users who share needles and anyone who has unprotected sex of any kind are at increased risk for contracting HIV. Healthcare workers are also at risk for accidental exposure in the workplace and should consistently follow standard precautions to protect themselves and their patients from this deadly disease. HIV is a fragile virus; it cannot survive outside the body, and it is easily destroyed by chemical disinfectants such as household bleach.

All HIV tests screen for antibodies to the virus, and any positive result, regardless of the type of test used, is followed up with the more definitive Western blot test before a positive diagnosis is made. The most widely used screening test for HIV infection is the enzyme immunoassay (EIA; also called the *enzyme-linked immunosorbent assay* [ELISA]), which typically is performed on a venous blood sample. ELISA tests also can be done on other body fluids, including oral fluid and urine, although urine screening is not as accurate or as sensitive to antibody levels. The physician may also order a viral load test that reflects the amount of HIV in the blood. Generally, the higher the viral load, the more aggressive the HIV infection.

Newer developments in rapid HIV screening use either blood or oral fluid (not the same as saliva) and can produce results within 20 to 60 minutes with accuracy rates similar to those of traditional EIA screening tests. Many emergency departments have the patient care technician perform this screening on patients who may meet the criteria for HIV. This rapid test has improved the response time to patients in the emergency care setting.

The U.S. Food and Drug Administration (FDA) has approved the OraQuick Advance HIV1/2 Antibody Test for use on both oral fluid and plasma specimens. To perform the oral test, a single gentle swab is done around both upper and lower outer gums, the swabbing device is inserted into a vial containing a developer solution, and the result is positive if two reddish purple lines appear in a small window after 20 minutes. This test is not designed for home screening, because it is restricted to use by trained individuals, such as patient care technicians. However, an FDA-approved home test

called the *Home Access HIV-1 Test System* is available at most drug stores. The kit provides the materials for collection of a specimen at home rather than in a healthcare facility. To perform the test, the individual pricks a finger, places a blood drop on a specially treated card, and then mails the card to a licensed laboratory for testing. The individual uses an identification number provided with the kit to call the laboratory for results. As with all other HIV screening tools, a positive result must be followed by a Western blot test to confirm the diagnosis.

HIV infection can be treated with medications, but it cannot be cured. However, recent research indicates that HIV-positive individuals taking antiretroviral medications are less contagious than those not being treated. Once patients begin antiretroviral treatment, they must continue to take these drugs for the rest of their lives. The medications must be taken at the time and frequency prescribed to be effective in controlling the spread of the virus and to prevent drug-resistant strains from developing. The FDA currently has approved more than 30 medications for the treatment of HIV infection in adults and adolescents. Unfortunately, HIV medications can cause multiple side effects, including fever, nausea, fatigue, liver abnormalities, diabetes mellitus, hypercholesterolemia, decreased bone density, skin rash, pancreatitis, and neurologic disorders.

The psychosocial needs of a patient found to have HIV infection are demanding. Treatment is designed to control duplication of the virus in the body, but the patient will always be infectious. Transmission of the disease is prevented by sexual abstinence or consistent use of condoms and precautions with blood spills; these options must be discussed and consistently reinforced by the nurse with the patient. Community organizations can serve as a source of counseling and support for patients who test HIV positive and for their families. As mandated by federal law, the patient care technician must remember that all information regarding a patient's HIV status must be kept in strict confidence, and no documentation in the medical record can indicate the patient's HIV or AIDS status.

HIV cannot reproduce outside a living host, and no record exists of infection from environmental contact. Also, no evidence indicates that the virus can be transmitted by insects. Latex or polyurethane condoms used consistently and correctly provide a highly effective mechanical barrier to HIV. According to 2014 data, HIV is most prevalent in gay and bisexual men (70% of existing cases); African Americans represent approximately 14% of the U.S. population but accounted for 49.4% of new HIV infections; Hispanic/Latinos remained stable between 2010 and 2014 of all new infections, and 24% of new cases were reported in heterosexuals. Individuals with a sexually transmitted infection (STI) are at two to five times greater risk of contracting HIV if exposed; if an HIV-infected individual has another STI, HIV transmission is more likely. Treating STIs in HIV-infected individuals decreases the amount of HIV in genital secretions.

HIPAA Applications

Staying up-to-date on confidentiality restrictions regarding a patient's HIV status is a major challenge. The Health Insurance Portability and Accountability Act (HIPAA) provides minimum requirements for protecting personal health information, but state laws can override HIPAA regulations if the state law is considered more stringent. In addition, individual healthcare institutions (hospitals, universities, physicians' practices) may have their own policies and procedures for managing confidential information about HIV and AIDS. For example, if a physician believes that a person who tests HIV positive will not disclose his or her HIV status to significant others, most states permit the physician to act. First, the physician must attempt to notify the patient that the information is going to be disclosed. Then the physician can inform the patient's spouse, sexual partner or partners, child, or needle-sharing partner or partners at risk of being infected with HIV about their risk of exposure. However, the state may limit this disclosure by not permitting the physician to identify the name of the individual who is HIV positive.

- Confidential HIV information includes any records that could reasonably identify the individual as a person who has had an HIV test, is HIV positive, has opportunistic diseases related to HIV, or has AIDS.
- The HIPAA protects the patient's confidential *information*, not just the paper or electronic records of that information. This means that verbal disclosure of the individual's HIV and AIDS status is limited to only the personnel who have the right to that information according to individual state laws. For example, if you learn about your neighbor's HIV status at work and you go home and discuss it with your family, your employer is responsible for your disclosure of this information, and both you and your employer may be fined by the state or sued by the patient.
- Disclosure of HIV and AIDS status for treatment, payment, or healthcare operations can be made only with the specific written consent of the patient.
- Depending on state laws, written consent may not be needed to release HIV information if a court order for the information is issued; if the case is being reported to state or local vital statistics or public health agencies; or if the information is to be provided to certain employees of correctional institutions or residential treatment facilities, funeral directors, or emergency personnel.

BREAST CANCER

Breast cancer is the second leading cause of cancer deaths in women. According to the American Cancer Society, 1 in 8 women has a lifetime risk of developing breast cancer and a 1 in 36 risk of dying from the disease (www.cancer.org). Predisposing factors include a family history of breast cancer (especially in the mother or a sister), early onset of monthly menstrual cycles and late menopause, first pregnancy after age 30 years or no pregnancy, prolonged use of estrogen replacement therapy, excess alcohol intake, smoking, and obesity.

Because recent research has failed to link reduced death rates from breast cancer with monthly breast self-examinations (BSE), the American Cancer Society now recommends that women have their physician perform a clinical breast examination (CBE) rather than rely on monthly BSEs for early detection. However, although a monthly BSE is now considered optional, women still should be aware of the normal appearance and texture of the breasts and should immediately report to the physician any changes or new breast symptoms. Clinical breast examination should be done every 3 years from age 20 to 39 years and annually from 40 years of age. A mammogram should be done annually starting at age 40 years and each year after that. If a woman has an increased risk of breast cancer (e.g., family history), the physician may recommend annual mammography screening before age 40 years or other diagnostic procedures, such as ultrasonography or magnetic resonance imaging (MRI). An MRI scan can reveal tumors too small to detect with a breast examination that may not show up clearly on a mammogram. The American Cancer Society recommends MRI screening for women at high risk for developing breast cancer.

Indications of breast cancer include a palpable breast mass that is firm and immovable, breast pain, tissue thickening, nipple retraction or dimpling, nipple discharge, and axillary lymphadenopathy. If a breast mass is palpated, a mammogram or ultrasonography of the area is ordered and, if indicated, a biopsy is performed. The physician may perform a needle biopsy to remove cells and/or tissue from a palpated mass for evaluation by the pathologist. If a nonpalpable mass is found on a mammogram, a guided needle aspiration is done, and surgical biopsy is a possible follow-up. During this procedure, the physician uses a mammogram to guide the needle toward the suspicious mass, from which a biopsy sample can be taken. If a tissue sample cannot be obtained through a needle, wire localization may be done to pinpoint the areas of concern from the mammogram. During this diagnostic procedure, a thin wire is passed through the breast to the point of concern (based on mammogram visualization). This wire marking is used during a surgical procedure to pinpoint tissue that was suspicious on the mammogram. If a biopsy shows malignant cells, the physician orders

Box 33.10 Inflammatory Breast Cancer

- Inflammatory breast cancer is a rare, aggressive cancer that causes the sudden onset of discoloration and warmth in the affected breast, along with edema, dimpling of the skin, enlarged axillary lymph nodes, and pain.
- The condition is easily confused with a breast infection, so patients should contact their physician as soon as symptoms appear.
- Cancer cells spread rapidly and block lymph vessels in the skin, which results in the classic symptoms.
- The condition is diagnosed by an excisional biopsy to confirm the presence of clumped cancer cells in the area lymph vessels.
- Inflammatory breast cancer typically is diagnosed as stage II, which means that the cancer has spread to local lymph nodes. However, one third of patients are found to have stage IV carcinoma, in which metastasis already has occurred.

an estrogen and progesterone receptor test to determine whether hormones affect the way the cancer grows. If the cancer cells increase growth patterns when exposed to hormone levels, the physician may recommend treatment with a drug such as tamoxifen, which prevents estrogen from binding to these sites.

Treatment of breast cancer depends on the type of carcinoma and its staging (Box 33.10). Treatment almost always begins with surgery, but the type of surgery and the extent of the tissue removed depend on several factors. Breast-saving surgeries include lumpectomy, in which only the suspicious mass plus a surrounding area of normal tissue is removed, and radiation therapy is used as a follow-up to destroy any remaining cancerous cells. A partial mastectomy may be done for more advanced cases; this procedure involves removal of the tumor and tissue surrounding it, part of the chest muscle beneath the mass, and some of the lymph nodes in the

axillary region. A complete mastectomy, which involves removal of the entire breast, chest muscle, and axillary lymph nodes, may still be indicated if the mass has spread. However, removal of multiple axillary lymph nodes greatly increases the risk that subsequent lymphedema and recurrent infections will develop in the arm on the affected side. New techniques recommend the removal of the sentinel lymph node, the first lymph node to which the cancer is likely to spread from the tumor. The sentinel node is found by injecting a blue dye near the tumor; the lymph vessels absorb the dye and carry it toward the lymph nodes, and the first node to receive the dye and turn blue is the one that is removed for pathologic testing. If the sentinel node is cancer-free, there is very little chance that the breast tumor has metastasized, and no other nodes need to be removed. If cancer cells are evident, further diagnostic procedures are indicated to determine possible locations of metastatic tumors.

Many patients now opt for breast reconstruction after a partial or complete mastectomy. This procedure typically is performed by a plastic surgeon and can be done using a variety of methods, including implantation of a silicone or gel material or the use of fat and other tissue from another part of the body, such as the abdomen, to reconstruct breast tissue. After the breast has been re-formed, the physician uses tattoo techniques to create the areola and nipple. The patient must discuss these options with her surgeon before the mastectomy is performed; therefore the PCT may be involved in the referral process.

When caring for a patient in the postoperative phase of a mastectomy, it is important that the patient care technician is aware of precautions to take to avoid causing complications to the operative site, or increasing the patient's chance of lymphedema. Because of the involvement of the lymph nodes, the affected side is typically avoided when taking blood pressure or performing needle sticks. This is usually posted as a sign above the patient's bed as a precautionary measure.

CHAPTER SUMMARY

As individuals age they can experience a variety of chronic illnesses depending on their current level of health. Ways to decrease incidence of these chronic illnesses may include weight management, a healthy diet, health screenings, avoidance of alcohol and tobacco, and reducing stress as much as possible. When patients have a chronic incidence, how they care for themselves and whether they follow their treatment plan can determine the effect the illness has on their body. The patient care technician can play a supportive role in caring for those with chronic illnesses.

Case Scenario

Dr. Samuelson is the primary care physician for a nursing home in the area. He is concerned because one of the employees you work with has had a positive result on a Mantoux test. What other tests will Dr. Samuelson order to confirm the diagnosis? If those tests come back positive, how will the employee be treated? What about the other employees and residents of the nursing home? Should you worry that you are going to get TB?

REVIEW QUESTIONS

1. A blood clot (thrombus) forms in a cerebral artery and blocks distal blood flow. This is known as what type of stroke?
   a. Thrombotic
   b. Embolitic
   c. Cerebral hemorrhage
   d. Transient ischemic attack

2. When the pancreas is unable to produce insulin because of the destruction of the beta islet cells, this is known as what type of diabetes?
   a. Gestational diabetes
   b. Prediabetes
   c. Type I diabetes
   d. Type II diabetes

3. The peak flow meter is used in what type of disease to determine respiratory status?
   a. Asthma
   b. Tuberculosis
   c. Chronic obstructive pulmonary disease
   d. Emphysema

4. How can HIV be cured?
   a. Medications
   b. Vaccination
   c. Safe sexual practices
   d. There is no cure.

5. What is a predisposing risk factor for breast cancer in women?
   a. Taking multivitamins
   b. Drinking soft drinks
   c. Obesity
   d. X-ray use

End-of-Life Care

1. Discuss the philosophy of hospice care.
2. Differentiate between palliative care and curative care.
3. Discuss four criteria for admission to hospice care.
4. Name the members of the interdisciplinary team, and explain their roles.
5. Describe the stages of dying.
6. Describe the interventions required in providing postmortem care.
7. Discuss the role of hospice in families' bereavement period.
8. Discuss two ethics issues in hospice care.

autopsy Examination performed after a person's death to confirm or determine the cause of death.

bereavement A period of mourning or an expression of grief in reaction to the death of someone close.

curative treatment Aggressive care in which the goal and intent is curing the disease and prolonging life at all cost.

holistic Pertaining to the total patient care in which the physical, emotional, social, economic, and spiritual needs of the patient are considered.

hospice A facility or program designed to provide a caring environment for meeting the physical and emotional needs of the terminally ill.

interdisciplinary team A multiprofessional health team whose members work together in caring for a terminally ill patient.

mortician Person trained in the care of the dead.

palliative care The active, complete care of a patient whose disease has not responded to curative therapy.

postmortem care Care for the patient's body after death.

primary caregiver A member of the immediate family, such as the spouse or adult child, who assist in the decision making for someone who is nearing the end of life.

psychosocial A combination of psychologic and social factors.

respite care A period of relief from responsibilities of caring for a patient.

terminal illness A disease in an advanced stage with no known cure and poor prognosis.

Box 34.1   A Hospice Nurse's Perspective

Frequently I am asked whether it is depressing to work with terminally ill patients and death every day. Frankly, I cannot think of doing anything else. Death is as much a part of life as is birth, and through hospice, I am challenged to find very individualized and innovative ways to give back the control that dying patients have lost while being treated for various kinds of terminal illnesses.

As a hospice nurse, I am guided by a dedicated interdisciplinary team to achieve symptom control so that quality of life can again be realized. Many hopes and dreams can become reality once a patient is comfortable. Frequently comfort enables our patients to take one more family trip, attend a great family reunion, and go to a special wedding, graduation, or anniversary. What could be more rewarding than playing a part in that and seeing the joy it brings? Together we rejoice in the celebration of life, see families reunited, see peace made with God, review each triumph, and weep over each disappointment and loss. Families are enabled to say all the things they could not find words for before: "Thank you"; "I'm sorry"; "Forgive me"; "I love you"; and finally the good-byes.

Of course there is sadness, but there are also reconciliation, peace, and beauty, for this is a part of life and these are the important things in life. Daily, I feel so personally grateful for every person I have known and loved and lost, for I know that I have learned far more about living from them than I could ever teach them about dying. Through it all, I have become closer to God, more compassionate, more open to people, and more sensitive to the needs of others. Hospice nursing has given me direction and hope.

Kathleen Carsten, CRNH
Hospice Nurse

The philosophy of hospice is to provide care and support to patients with a terminal illness (a disease in an advanced stage with no known cure and poor prognosis) and their families. An interdisciplinary team promotes comfort, care, and support through compassion, interest, and genuine concern (Box 34.1) in order to promote quality of life as the end approaches (Hospice Association of America, n.d.). With hospice support, the patient and the family recognize that dying is a natural part of life. The goals are to maximize the quality of life and keep the patient as comfortable as possible in the home or setting that he or she chooses.

HISTORICAL OVERVIEW

"Hospice" is from the Latin word *hospitium,* meaning "hospitality" and "lodging." The concept originated in Europe, where hospices were resting places for travelers. Monks and nuns believed that service to one's neighbor was a sign of love and dedication to God. Typical medieval hospices run by monks and nuns were a combination guesthouse and infirmary for the sick. They were places of refuge for the poor, the sick, and travelers on religious journeys. They provided food, shelter, and care to ill guests until the guests were strong enough to continue their journey or died. As centuries passed and hospices developed into hospitals, the emphasis on physical care increased, and spiritual care became less important.

The idea of hospice was renewed in the 1960s in London, when Dame Cicely Saunders, a nurse and physician, realized that terminally ill patients needed a different kind of care. She had a patient who was dying of a terminal illness, and she found that quality of life was not the main emphasis of his care. She then devoted her life to improving pain management and symptom control for people who were dying. She believed that it is important for each patient to know his or her own contribution to life and that his or her life had meaning. She began her work at St. Joseph's Hospice, operated by the Irish Sisters of Charity. In 1968, St. Christopher's Hospice of London was opened, and this hospice continues to serve as a national and international education, training, and research center for professionals involved in the hospice approach to care of terminally ill patients.

The philosophy of hospice migrated to the United States in the early 1970s; the first hospice program opened in Connecticut in 1971. Since then, more than 2 million healthcare providers, nurses, clergy, social workers, and many nonprofessional volunteers have worked together to provide home and hospice care to more than 12 million patients throughout the United States (http://www.nahc.org/).

Hospices serve patients with various primary disease processes, the most common being dementia, which accounts for 14.8% of the patient population. Heart disease processes account for 14.7% of the client population, and lung diseases account for almost 9.3% of the primary diagnoses of the patients served by hospice (National Hospice and Palliative Care Organization, 2015).

Hospices vary in structure and organization. Some hospices are based in a hospital. On occasion, a hospice patient goes into the hospital and receives hospice services for control of acute pain or for 5-day respite care for the family or care provider occasionally. Patients sometimes receive hospice care intermittently and sometimes continuously (Smeltzer et al., 2010). There are also freestanding hospices, in which the atmosphere is more like that of a friendly dormitory than that of a hospital. The patients usually wear their own clothes, move about the hospice as they choose, and socialize with each other and with the staff. The kitchen is always open for individually prepared food, as well as for conversation.

- The Hospice Medicare Benefit covers all expenses for palliative care related to the terminal illness, including professional staff visits, medication, equipment, occasional short periods of respite for caregivers, and acute care when needed for the control of symptoms.
- Hospice often provides dying older adults with a higher level of control and dignity than do other types of healthcare.
- The primary caregiver is often a member of the immediate family, such as the spouse or adult child.
- The Hospice Medicare Benefit provides for bereavement follow-up care for up to 1 year after the patient's death.

(Centers for Medicare & Medicaid Services: Coverage of hospice services under hospital insurance. Medicare benefit policy manual (Publication No. 100-02). Retrieved from www.cms.gov/Regulations -and-Guidance/Guidance/Manuals/downloads/bp102c09.pdf 2012, p. 238.)

Some hospices are operated by a home health agency or community-based organization in which care is usually provided in the patient's home, wherever that home may be. Hospice care may also be given in a long-term care setting. Skilled team members, including healthcare providers, nurses, hospice aides, social workers, spiritual leaders, bereavement coordinators, and volunteers, make visits to the home or wherever the patient most often resides. The team provides comfort measures, as well as medications and therapy. The team members also educate the patient and the caregiver with regard to disease processes, medication administration, and how to provide daily care. Expert help and support is available to the patient and the caregiver 24 hours a day, either by phone or in person.

The Medicare Hospice Benefit came into effect in 1983, and today hospice services are reimbursable through Medicare, Medicaid, and most private insurance companies. Medicare certification or state licensure ensures quality hospice services (Box 34.2).

PALLIATIVE VERSUS CURATIVE CARE

Palliative care, as defined by the World Health Organization, is the active, complete care of a patient whose disease has not responded to curative therapy (Fig. 34.1). Palliative care emphasizes the control of pain, relief of symptoms, and provision of psychologic, social, and spiritual assistance (World Health Organization, n.d.). It is possible to begin palliative care earlier in the dying process, whereas hospice is usually available only in the last 6 months of life. This type of pain and symptom control is viewed by the World Health Organization (2011) as an urgent humanitarian need. The palliative care process maintains the patient as the center of this interdisciplinary approach to patient care (Center to Advance Palliative Care, 2011; Ellison, 2012). Palliative care can serve as a bridge between curative care and hospice (Smeltzer et al., 2010).

When a patient with a life-threatening illness has undergone all reasonable treatment and the disease has not been arrested or cured, it is necessary for the patient to decide whether continued active therapy is feasible or beneficial. By this time, the patient may already have experienced many physical and emotional symptoms that keep them from being able to do much on their own, as a result of the treatments or the progression of the disease.

This situation leads the patient and family to decide whether to continue with these treatments or to transition to palliative measures. Curative treatment is aggressive care in which the goal and intent is curing the disease and prolonging life at all cost. Palliative care is not curative in nature but aims to relieve pain and distress and to control symptoms of the disease. It is important to give the patient and caregiver honest and accurate information so that they are able to make appropriate decisions.

CRITERIA FOR ADMISSION TO HOSPICE

The patient is required to meet certain criteria to be admitted into hospice:

- The healthcare provider must certify that the patient's illness is terminal and that the patient has a prognosis of 6 months or less to live. The healthcare provider must have a degree in medicine or osteopathy to make the prognosis determination.
- For the patient to qualify for Medicare or Medicaid assistance, two healthcare providers are required to verify that the patient is dying and has less than 6 months to live. This must be documented by the medical provider in a narrative that supports the reason for the limited life expectancy. The hospice patient who continues to live beyond the estimated period still qualifies for Medicare if hospice criteria are still met (Centers for Medicare & Medicaid Services, 2012).
- It is mandatory that the patient desires and agrees that the services are needed and requested; this respects their right to deny care. The patient and caregiver must understand that all treatment will be palliative and that no further curative treatment will be rendered.
- The patient and caregiver are required to understand and agree that hospice staff will plan the care according to comfort and that they will not necessarily perform life-support measures.

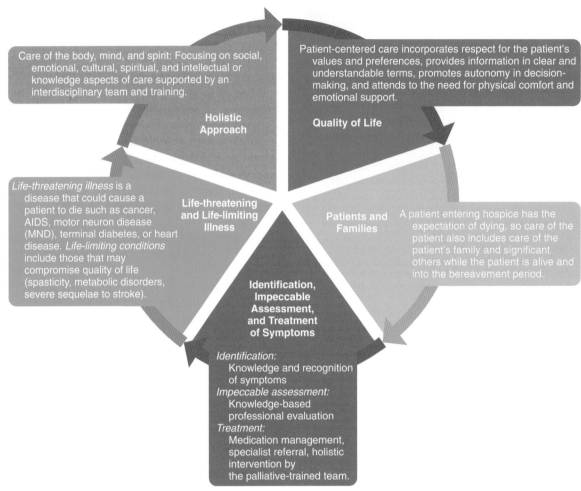

Care of the body, mind, and spirit: Focusing on social, emotional, cultural, spiritual, and intellectual or knowledge aspects of care supported by an interdisciplinary team and training.

Holistic Approach

Patient-centered care incorporates respect for the patient's values and preferences, provides information in clear and understandable terms, promotes autonomy in decision-making, and attends to the need for physical comfort and emotional support.

Quality of Life

Life-threatening illness is a disease that could cause a patient to die such as cancer, AIDS, motor neuron disease (MND), terminal diabetes, or heart disease. *Life-limiting conditions* include those that may compromise quality of life (spasticity, metabolic disorders, severe sequelae to stroke).

Life-threatening and Life-limiting Illness

Patients and Families

A patient entering hospice has the expectation of dying, so care of the patient also includes care of the patient's family and significant others while the patient is alive and into the bereavement period.

Identification, Impeccable Assessment, and Treatment of Symptoms

Identification: Knowledge and recognition of symptoms
Impeccable assessment: Knowledge-based professional evaluation
Treatment: Medication management, specialist referral, holistic intervention by the palliative-trained team.

FIGURE 34.1 Components of palliative care. (Abernethy AP, Wheeler JL, Bull J: Development of a health information technology–based data system in community-based hospice and palliative care, *American Journal of Preventive Medicine* 40(5 Suppl 2):S217-S224, 2011.)

• The patient and caregiver—or, if the patient is unable to participate, the caregiver—are required to understand the outlook for the patient and be willing to participate in the planning of care.

Many hospices in the United States request that the patient have a primary caregiver (a person who assumes ongoing responsibility for health maintenance and therapy for the illness). The caregiver is sometimes an immediate family member and sometimes a significant other, a friend, or a hired caregiver. Caregiver services become required when patients are no longer able to care for themselves safely. If a patient resides in a freestanding hospice residence, a long-term care facility, or a residential home, the nursing staff is designated as the primary caregiver.

Once the criteria are met and a patient is admitted to hospice, the staff performs complete physical, psychosocial, and spiritual assessments, and those involved discuss the care openly. The patient and caregiver receive a complete explanation of the hospice program and the philosophy of hospice, along with the interdisciplinary team concept.

GOALS OF HOSPICE

To provide effective hospice care, an understanding of the philosophy and its relationship with the patient's responses and points of view is beneficial. The basic goals of hospice address the following:

• Controlling or relieving the patient's symptoms
• Allowing the patient and caregiver to be involved in the decisions regarding the plan of care
• Encouraging the patient and caregiver to live life to the fullest
• Providing continuous support to maintain patient and family confidence
• Educating and supporting the primary caregiver in the home setting that the patient chooses

INTERDISCIPLINARY TEAM

In the hospice approach, holistic (pertaining to the total patient care in which the physical, emotional, social, economic, and spiritual needs of the patient are considered) care is performed by an interdisciplinary team that manages the problems encountered during the patient's admission into hospice (Fig. 34.2). The interdisciplinary team (a multiprofessional health team whose members work together in caring for a terminally ill patient) develops and supervises the plan of care in conjunction with all those involved with the care. The core interdisciplinary team members are the medical director, the nurse coordinator, the social worker, and the spiritual coordinator. To provide support to the dying patient and the caregiver, the interdisciplinary team considers all aspects of the family unit. The team includes the family in all decisions and care planning because families also experience the stresses related to the terminal illness and death of the patient (Fig. 34.3). These stresses also extend into the bereavement period after the patient dies.

Each hospice patient is assigned a primary team that consists of the patient's own healthcare provider, the primary hospice nurse, the social worker, a primary hospice aide, a primary volunteer, and a spiritual leader. This group of professionals, along with the interdisciplinary team, develops and is responsible for carrying out the plan of care. Regular and frequent team meetings are held to discuss the patient's physical, mental, and spiritual conditions; the plan of care is revised as needed. The effectiveness of the plan of care is also discussed. The team meeting is the forum for bringing together all members' observations and thoughts respectfully, and the team strives to function as a cohesive unit to use all expertise and resources in the interest of providing quality patient care (Tables 34.1 and 34.2).

Medical Director

The medical director has a doctoral degree in medicine (MD) or osteopathy (DO) and assumes overall responsibility for the medical component of the hospice

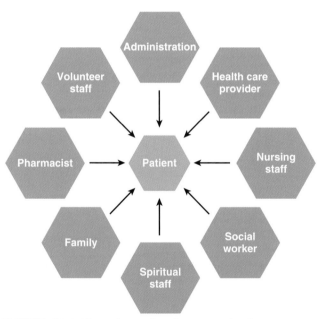

FIGURE 34.2 The relationship between the hospice team members and the patient. (From Cooper K, Gosnell K: *Foundations of nursing*, ed 7, St. Louis, 2015, Mosby.)

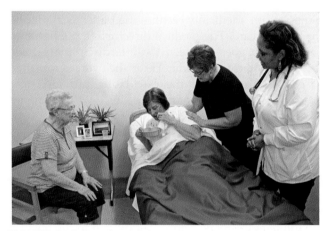

FIGURE 34.3 Family member participation with the hospice care team. (From Cooper K, Gosnell K: *Foundations of nursing*, ed 7, St. Louis, 2015, Mosby.)

Table 34.1	Core Interdisciplinary Hospice Team	
Team Member	**Background**	**Function or Responsibility**
Medical director	Licensed physician	Mediates between the hospice team and attending medical provider Provides consultation relative to the medical aspect of care
Nurse coordinator	Licensed registered nurse	Manages the patient's care Explains the service, admits the patients, assigns the primary team
Social worker	Bachelor's degree in social work	Evaluates the patient's psychosocial needs Serves as resource for potential community services Assists with counseling in grief issues
Spiritual coordinator	Seminary degree	Serves as liaison between the patient and the spiritual community Coordinates spiritual support

Table 34.2	Primary Hospice Team	
Team Member	**Background**	**Function or Responsibility**
Volunteer coordinator	Experience in volunteer work	Recruits and trains the volunteers
		Coordinates assignments of volunteers
Bereavement coordinator	Professional with grief experience	Assesses and supports the bereaved survivor
		Facilitates support groups
Hospice pharmacist	Licensed registered pharmacist	Provides drug consultation
Primary healthcare provider	Licensed physician	Responsible for the medical aspect of symptom control for patient
Primary nurse	Licensed registered nurse	Serves as liaison between (1) patient and (2) caregiver, healthcare provider, and interdisciplinary team
		Evaluates patient's response to treatment
		Educates the patient and family in disease process and care
		Assesses symptom management
		Provides emotional support to patient and caregiver
Primary spiritual leader	As required by religious group	Supports patient and caregiver in coping with fears and uncertainty about spiritual issues
Hospice volunteer	Completion of volunteer training	Provides companionship for patient and caregiver
		Available for short periods of respite care
Hospice aide	Certified as a home health aide	Administers personal care and assistance with bathing

patient's care program. The medical director does not take the place of the patient's healthcare provider but acts as a consultant for the healthcare provider. The medical director, with consultation from the interdisciplinary team, medically certifies the patient's eligibility for hospice care. The medical director is a mediator, or liaison, who goes between the interdisciplinary team and the healthcare provider. He or she oversees the plan of care, ensuring that the care being provided and ordered is palliative in nature.

Nurse Coordinator and Hospice Nurses

The nurse coordinator is a registered nurse (RN) who coordinates the implementation of the plan of care for each patient. The nurse coordinator often performs the initial assessment, admits the patient to the hospice program, and develops the plan of care along with the interdisciplinary team. The nurse coordinator also ensures that the plan of care is being followed, coordinates assignments of the hospice nurses and aides, facilitates meetings, and determines methods of payment.

Hospice nurses coordinate services of the hospice team, which includes hospice healthcare providers, pharmacists, dietitians, physical therapists, social workers, clergy, certified nursing assistants, and hospice volunteers. Hospice nurses must possess compassion, excellent teaching skills, and the ability to adapt therapeutically to the hospice patients' many needs. It is also necessary for a hospice nurse to be especially adept in pain and symptom control (Hospice and Palliative Nurses Association, n.d.).

Social Worker

The social worker evaluates and assesses the psychosocial (a combination of psychologic and social factors) needs of the patient. The social worker assists with accessing community resources and filing of insurance papers, supports the patient and caregiver with emotional and grief issues, and, in some cases when communication difficulties are present, also assists with counseling. The social worker provides these services under the direction of the healthcare provider and in accordance with the plan of care.

Spiritual Coordinator

The spiritual coordinator, who may be affiliated with any religious preference of the patient and family, is the spiritual liaison between the interdisciplinary team and the hospice patient. The spiritual coordinator assists with the spiritual assessment of the patient and, in keeping with patients' and families' beliefs, develops the plan of care with regard to spiritual matters. If the patient desires spiritual assistance and does not have a spiritual home, the spiritual coordinator assists in finding the spiritual support desired. The spiritual coordinator is vital with assisting the patient and caregiver cope with fears and uncertainty. Possible support includes dealing with unfinished business and regrets and providing opportunities for reconciliation, prayer, and spiritual healing. Funeral planning and performing funeral services are also included in this role, as is continued support for the family throughout the bereavement period. In addition, the spiritual

Box 34.3   Cultural Considerations: Death and Dying

- The United States is becoming increasingly multicultural, and hospice care is challenged to meet the needs of people from other cultures.
- Compassionate and empathic care is often a universal language regardless of the culture, but it is necessary to learn as much as possible about a patient's culture so as to provide appropriate assistance. Each person has a different reaction and tradition regarding death and dying, but all people experience grief.
- A cultural assessment of the patient and the family must include factors such as the following (Center to Advance Palliative Care, 2011):
  - Religious beliefs
  - Primary decision-making person and process
  - Dietary preferences
- Preferred language and the need for translation services as needed, as well as written information provided in the language of preference for the patient and the family
- Support measure preferences such as alternative medicine, as well as who is allowed to support the patient
- The patient's perspective of death, dying, and burial
- The family's grief processes, burial practices, and perspective of death
- The team may need to be prepared for a change in expectations regarding the death of the patient because of differences in belief systems between the patient and the surviving family members.
- Changes regarding the plan of care must not be made without discussing them with all family members.

coordinator is one resource to assist with cultural differences (Box 34.3). The following sections describe additional members of the team whose services are needed to provide adequate care for the patient.

Volunteer Coordinator

The volunteer coordinator must have experience in volunteer work. The volunteer coordinator assesses the patient and caregiver for services that might be offered through volunteers and volunteer agencies. When families are responsible for the total care of the patient in the home, caregiver "burnout" becomes a concern. This is when the services of volunteers become vital. They provide companionship, caregiver relief through respite care (a period of relief from responsibilities of caring for a patient), and emotional support. Appropriate services for the volunteer to provide are what are considered typical of a good neighbor: perhaps grocery shopping, yard work, reading to the patient, or keeping the patient company while the caregiver leaves the home for short periods. The volunteer coordinator ensures that the volunteer is adequately trained and prepared for working with the dying patient. Responsibilities also include assigning the proper volunteer to the appropriate patient. Each year, more than 400,000 hospice volunteers donate time to hospice patients (Hospice Foundation of America, n.d.).

Bereavement Coordinator

Bereavement is a period of mourning or an expression of grief in reaction to the death of someone close. The bereavement coordinator is a professional who has

experience in dealing with grief issues. The bereavement coordinator assesses the patient and the caregiver at the time of admission to the hospice program and identifies potential risk factors that may arise after the death of the patient. The bereavement coordinator follows the plan of care for the bereaved caregiver for at least a year after the death. The bereavement coordinator facilitates support groups and assigns bereavement volunteers to visit the caregiver.

The bereavement coordinator sometimes also provides counseling but has the option to refer the family to other counseling if the issues are too extensive. The goals of bereavement counseling for loved ones during the patient's illness and after the death are (1) to provide support and (2) to assist survivors in the transition to a life without the deceased person. It is appropriate to incorporate grief support into the plan of care.

Hospice Pharmacist

The hospice pharmacist must be a licensed pharmacist and available for consultation about the drugs the hospice patient may be taking. The pharmacist evaluates for drug-drug or drug-food interactions, appropriate drug doses, and correct administration times and routes. The pharmacist typically gives information and advice about common drugs used, administration time, and doses.

Nutrition Consultant

Licensed medical nutritional therapists (LMNTs) or licensed dietitians are available for hospice consultations and for diet counseling. The hospice nurse performs the nutritional assessment at the patient's admission. If the nurse notes nutritional problems, a referral may be made to the LMNT or dietitian for assistance with diet counseling and meal planning. The LMNT or dietitian also assists with educating the caregiver about nutritional issues in end-stage diseases. Most patients' dietary preferences change when they are approaching the end of their life.

Hospice Aide

The hospice aide is a certified nurse's aide (CNA) or patient care technician (PCT) who works under the supervision of the hospice nurse. The hospice aide follows the plan of care that the interdisciplinary team develops and assists the patient with bathing and hygiene, including hair, nail, oral, and skin care. The hospice aide sometimes also assists the patient or the caregiver with light homemaker services. The patient and the hospice aide often develop a close relationship, and in some cases, the patient shares feelings with the aide more easily than with any other member of the team.

Other Services

Other services, if needed, are available from a physical therapist, a speech-language pathologist, and an occupational therapist. These services are available not for rehabilitative purposes but to assist with improving the quality of life and care for the patient and the caregiver. The physical therapist assists with teaching the caregiver transferring skills, exercises that are sometimes useful to relieve muscle cramps, and wheelchair fittings. The speech-language pathologist helps with difficulties in communication or swallowing. The occupational therapist helps with positioning for comfort, providing adaptive equipment for the patient, or other assistance for comfort and for activities of daily living.

PALLIATIVE CARE/HOSPICE

The goal and emphasis of hospice is symptom management and palliative care. The team of caregivers routinely assesses, reassesses, and documents the severity, the treatment, and the control of symptoms of the illness.

When the patient is admitted and with each subsequent visit, the nurse and the team must assess the comfort level of the patient. One assessment tool that is often used is the Edmonton Symptom Assessment System. This tool addresses the areas of pain, tiredness (lack of energy), drowsiness, nausea, appetite, shortness of breath, depression (feeling sad), anxiety or nervousness, and overall feeling of well-being. The patient is

asked to rate each of these areas on a scale of 0 to 10. Having the patient participate in this way allows the patient to say where he or she has the most discomfort or area of greatest concern (Alberta Health Services and Covenant Health, 2010).

Pain

Of all the symptoms that a dying patient experiences, pain is the most dreaded and feared; therefore pain management is a priority in hospice. Pain is considered the fifth vital sign. It disrupts activities as well as the quality and enjoyment of life. To a healthy person, pain is usually temporary and tolerable, but to a terminally ill patient, it can be excruciating, constant, and terrifying. Pain takes many forms, such as physical, psychosocial, and spiritual, and addressing and alleviating it is correct and proper. It is all too easy for the caregiver caring for people experiencing pain to become frustrated and feel helpless as he or she tries to control the discomfort, which leads to feelings of guilt and inadequacy. There are a variety of medications the hospice nurse will administer to patients in order for them to be as comfortable as possible. The pain medicine may be delivered in the form of a pill, oral solution, or perhaps through an IV. Intramuscular injections are typically avoided when the patient is nearing the end of life. Sometimes patches are used, which are placed on the patient's skin.

An individualized approach is needed to successfully manage pain. Various alternative pharmacologic and nonpharmacologic options are available. Radiation therapy, nerve blocks, and psychologic or physical methods all can be tried in appropriate circumstances. Hot or cold packs at the site of discomfort, repositioning the patient, music therapy, relaxation techniques, acupuncture, and even transcutaneous electric nerve stimulation (TENS) are sometimes good alternatives.

Nausea and Vomiting

Nausea and vomiting tend to be very upsetting to both the patient and the caregiver. Many patients consider nausea to be worse than vomiting because at times it is noticeable only to the patient and therefore is overlooked by caregivers and healthcare professionals. It is important to assess for the cause of nausea and vomiting, and to remove the cause if at all possible. Nausea is a possible side effect of chemotherapy and can result from an obstruction, a tumor, uncontrolled pain, constipation, and even food smells. At times, the treatment of the nausea is as simple as bringing in food already prepared so that the cooking smells do not bother the patient. Sometimes the drugs used for pain control cause nausea; medications known as antiemetics, which relieve nausea, may be administered with the pain medicine. Nausea is a common side effect with the initiation of some pain medications. This side effect usually subsides after a time, and the best response is to use an antiemetic rather than discontinue the pain medicine. Anxiety has also been known to cause nausea, which then leads to vomiting. Patients who vomit are typically anxious about why they are vomiting, which often worsens the symptoms.

Eating slowly and in a pleasant atmosphere, with relaxation and rest periods after eating, is a good way to control the nausea. If vomiting occurs, the PCT should discourage eating for a short time until it stabilizes. When the nausea and vomiting have subsided, the patient may begin drinking liquids to avoid dehydration or start eating soft, bland foods. Small, light, bland meals should be served, and sweet, greasy, spicy, or strong-smelling foods should be avoided. If anxiety and fear are causing nausea and vomiting, verbalizing the fears is often helpful. Under no circumstances is it ever acceptable to force the patient to eat food or drink fluids if he or she has no desire to eat because this also has potential to compromise dignity and be detrimental to the patient's well-being.

Constipation

One of the most common problems of terminally ill patients is constipation. Constipation has many possible causes. Sometimes this problem causes more anxiety and discomfort than pain itself. Because constipation has the ability to cause other symptoms, such as abdominal pain, nausea, or vomiting, prevention of the problem is important. Factors that contribute to constipation are poor dietary intake, poor fluid intake, tumor compression of the bowel, use of pain medications, and a decrease in physical activity.

Psychosocial and Spiritual Issues

Spiritual unrest and issues are often combined with psychosocial problems and have the potential to surface, especially when symptoms are uncontrolled. It is always necessary to respect any religious or spiritual concerns and meet the patient's wishes if at all possible. Spiritual assessments conducted by the nurse are meant to gather information regarding the patient's feelings and needs. When confronted with a terminal illness, some patients question their faiths and beliefs, and some search for the spiritual support that they have never had. Many symptoms, such as depression, the need to suffer, bitterness, anger, hallucinations, or dreams of fire, are, in some cases, indicative of unmet spiritual needs.

Spiritual issues should be referred to the spiritual coordinator and not used as an opening to share personal feelings and beliefs unless the patient specifically asks for that perspective. The hospice organization determines whether the nurse or the spiritual coordinator performs the spiritual assessment. It is essential for the assessor to be nonjudgmental and accepting of the patient's and the caregiver's spiritual beliefs. The social worker may also assist with the relationship between the patient and the caregiver and provide counseling to resolve conflict. The social worker does not "fix" the conflicts but assists in problem-solving. The development of trust between the patient and the interdisciplinary team is critical and is invaluable in dealing with these issues.

Other Common Signs and Symptoms

Weight loss and dehydration sometimes lead to a decrease in soft tissue, especially on the bony areas of knees, hips, elbows, and buttocks, which can lead to skin impairment.

Increased weakness is also significant in the last stages of a terminal illness; it often leads to activity intolerance and causes the patient to spend most of the time reclining. This leads to a risk for skin impairment and the formation of pressure ulcers. Poor nutrition, decreased circulation, and decreased mobility all contribute to an increased risk for skin impairment. Education provided frequently to the family and the patient is necessary to promote integrity of the skin. The caregiver should observe the patient's skin and report any erythema or impairment. The nurse instructs the caregiver to reposition the patient for comfort, use alternating air or egg-crate mattresses, and to perform good hygiene to prevent skin impairment. As the PCT, you can encourage the patient to change positions regularly, and can assist with placement of additional pillows, cushions, and so on.

Weakness is accompanied by instability and falling and often leads to safety issues. Patients often exhibit signs of depression and may make comments regarding suicide. Comments regarding suicide do not always come from the actual desire to kill oneself but are, in some cases, rather a statement of a desire for independence. Sleeplessness, also known as insomnia, sometimes occurs as a result of an accumulation of signs and symptoms, and exhaustion has the potential to cause an exacerbation of all other signs and symptoms.

It is important at this time to ensure that the patient has good skin care. Cleanliness promoted by bathing is often refreshing, as well as helpful in promoting comfort and the feeling of self-worth. The skin should be inspected frequently and kept as dry and clean as possible. An egg-crate mattress, sheepskin, or an air-flotation mattress, as well as heel and elbow protectors, help cushion the bony areas. The hospice aide, or PCT, is often very helpful to the patient in assisting with personal care, hygiene, and bathing. Caregivers must be able to prevent falls and injuries, and the nurse should provide information regarding home safety. Listening and providing emotional support are important nursing interventions for the patient with depression and suicidal thoughts. The social worker is influential in these situations.

The hospice interdisciplinary team realizes that a terminal illness is potentially the most difficult time in a person's life. The team takes as honest and straightforward an approach as possible in all matters affecting the patient and caregiver. It is thought that the fear of the unknown is always greater than the fear of the known. Because of this, education is an important part of the care that the team provides to the patient. Educating the caregiver about symptom management, hands-on care of the patient, caring for body functions, and the signs and symptoms of approaching death are important to help relieve fears (Table 34.3).

THE DYING PATIENT

Communicating With the Dying Patient

When dealing with a dying patient in hospice, the PCT shows respect for the patient and offers appropriate reassurance and support when using therapeutic communication. Supportive words without a supportive attitude are empty in meaning and fail to provide comfort. Verbal and nonverbal communication should match. Reassurance that is unrealistic or given merely to calm a patient does not work. Stating that "everything will be just fine" when this is untrue or uncertain only increases the patient's anxiety and violates trust in the nurse. The PCT should not offer false reassurance.

Therapeutic communication also requires the PCT to pay careful attention to what the patient expresses verbally and nonverbally. Always verify with the patient any interpretations or summaries of the patient's thoughts and feelings to ensure that they are both accurate and effective.

If patients prefer not to communicate at a particular time, PCTs should accept and respect their wishes. Indicate a willingness to return at another time when the patient is feeling more comfortable. Be available to listen actively, without judgment, and with acceptance. Allow the patient to express emotions and feelings without fear.

Behavior that indicates listening to the patient is called "attending behavior." It includes appropriate eye contact, attentive body language, and verbal following. Nurses should show attentiveness in nonverbal as well as verbal ways. For instance, sit in a chair close to the patient's bed to reduce the physical distance and the emotional distance it implies. When appropriately used, touching is a highly effective means of communication. Later in the illness, when strength for or interest in verbal communication has dwindled, a patient derives particular benefit from being touched. Holding a hand, patting an arm, gently wiping away a tear—all indicate attending behavior, and concern and care.

It is important to remember that the PCT cannot "solve" the problem of dying. The PCT can have a positive impact on the dying patient's feelings and fears.

Table 34.3	Signs and Symptoms of Approaching Death

Signs and Symptoms	Interventions
The arms and legs of the body sometimes become cool to the touch, and the underside of the body sometimes becomes darker.	Keep warm blankets on the patient to prevent feeling of coldness.
The patient may spend more and more time sleeping during the day and at times is difficult to arouse.	Assist caregiver in planning time to be with the patient when the patient is most alert.
The patient may become increasingly confused about time, place, and identity of close and familiar people.	Reorient the patient as appropriate to the time of day and who is present. Do not upset the patient.
Incontinence of urine and bowel movements often happens when death is imminent. Sometimes there is a significant decrease in urine output.	Educate the caregiver in keeping the patient clean and dry. Provide pads or adult diapers as needed.
Oral secretions sometimes become more profuse and collect in the back of the throat. This produces the sound often referred to as the "death rattle."	Provide a cool-mist humidifier to increase the humidity in the room when oral secretions build up. Elevate the head of the bed with pillows or obtain a hospital bed to make breathing easier.
Clarity of hearing and vision decrease slightly.	Keep lights on in the room when vision decreases, and never assume that the patient is not able to hear you.
Restlessness, pulling at the bed linen, and having visions of people or things that do not exist sometimes occur.	Talk calmly and assuredly with the confused patient so as not to startle or frighten him or her further.
The patient's need for food and drink decreases.	Inform the caregiver that the patient will not starve to death or die of dehydration. Much reassurance is needed in this area.
Breathing patterns change to an irregular pace; there are sometimes 10- to 30-second periods of no breathing (apnea).	Elevating the head of the bed often relieves the patient who has irregular breathing patterns.
Changes in vital signs occur, with decreased blood pressure and elevated pulse.	Inform the family that these changes are normal and expected and are not uncomfortable for the patient.

Communicate openly and sensitively with the patient. By doing so, the PCT not only facilitates the expression of emotion but also affirms that the patient is a living human who has the PCT's support and compassion.

One of the most important tasks is to empower patients and families to participate in the final act of living. Communicate reassurance, confidence, and support for the vulnerable patient and family by sustaining nursing assessment practices, continuing to communicate, and providing skilled physical care.

Assisting the Patient in Saying Good-Bye

One of the most difficult tasks a terminally ill patient faces is leaving loved ones behind. The patient who is aware of dying needs to say good-bye, whether in a verbal, nonverbal, concrete, or symbolic way. For their part, family members must also work through the process of acknowledging the impending parting. Good-byes help them move toward the completion of unfinished business with the patient that could otherwise complicate their transition through the grieving process. The PCT's assistance in this area is important to both the dying person and the family.

First, provide a private, comfortable environment. Sometimes, emotional expression becomes overwhelming for the patient, the family, or both; offer to remain present or nearby to help support the family member or loved one and the patient. Various ways are available to assist patients in saying their good-byes, such as role-playing, letter writing, or making audio or video recordings. Help patients focus on what they want to say. One way to facilitate this is to ask them to talk to their loved ones as if they were going to be separated for a long time. Encourage them to express those feelings and thoughts they most want their loved ones to know in their absence. Help the dying person to formulate appropriate letters or tape recordings by asking, "What would you want to say to your 6-year-old when the child is 12?" Often dying patients become depressed because they do not have a purpose in life. Working on tasks such as poems, letters, and recordings affords patients feelings of control and productivity in their last days.

Adjusting the environment to increase comfort and safety is paramount. Use side rails for safety and, when possible, to assist weak patients to adjust their own positions.

Assessments and Interventions Related to Impending Death

Of all the needs of the dying patient, the three most important needs are the need for love and affection, for the control of pain, and for the preservation of dignity and self-worth.

Delegation and Documentation Box 34.1

The task of supporting patients and families in grief should not be delegated to the PCT. A professional nurse has the responsibility for recognizing a patient's grief and knowing the appropriate communication and counseling strategies to use. The PCT should do the following:

- Inform the nurse when the patient expresses behaviors of grief (e.g., crying, anger, loss of appetite).
- Conduct conversations with patients but to inform the nurse when patients express needs or concerns.
- Inform the nurse when family members arrive so that the nurse can meet with them and assess how they are coping.

A professional nurse is responsible for assessment of patient symptoms and a determination of what symptoms can be independently managed and what symptoms need medical intervention. Certain symptom therapies can be delegated to the PCT, such as positioning and environmental controls, hygiene approaches, and hydration. Therapies such as administration of medications require a nurse's intervention. The nurse provides PCTs with instruction and assistance regarding the following:

- When to notify the nurse if the patient's symptoms worsen or change in nature
- Potential adverse effects of medications and what to report to the nurse
- The need to maintain communication with dying patients who still retain the sense of hearing

Certain aspects of care of the body after death are delegated to the PCT. Also, care after death can, in fact, begin before the actual death so that patients and families can preserve cultural practices. Check agency policy regarding which staff members are permitted to remove invasive tubes or lines. At the time of death, it may be best for the nurse and PCT to work together in preparing the body (Procedure 34.1).

- Inform other care providers of any preference the family might have because of cultural, religious, or ethnic beliefs that influence the routine procedures of caring for the patient's body.
- Reinforce the importance of handling the body with respect.

(Modified from Perry A, Potter P, Ostendorf W: Clinical nursing skills and techniques, ed 8, St. Louis, 2014, Elsevier.)

The patient near death continues to need careful nursing interventions. Because of the increased weakness and deterioration of the body, the patient's physical needs are important. Ideally, the nurse also helps patients recognize and accept death as a reality of life so that they can undertake their last task in life with self-esteem and dignity. Ensuring support by others can help prevent a patient from being left to die alone.

The nurse will assess the patient for impending death. Although patients may appear comatose, unconscious, or unresponsive, this appearance is often a result

PROCEDURE 34.1

Care of the Body After Death

1. Gather equipment.
2. Wash hands.
3. Don clean gloves.
4. Close patient's eyes and mouth if needed.
5. Remove all tubing and other devices from patient's body.*
6. Place patient in supine position. Elevate the head. Do not place one hand on top of the other.
7. Replace soiled dressings with clean ones.
8. Bathe patient as necessary.
9. Brush or comb hair. Apply clean gown.
10. Care for valuables and personal belongings. If wedding band is to remain on the deceased, secure ring to finger with a small strip of tape over ring.
11. Allow family to view body and remain in room. A sheet or light blanket placed over the body with only the head and upper shoulders exposed maintains dignity and respect for the deceased. Remove unneeded equipment from the room. Provide soft lighting and offer chairs.
12. After the family has left the room, attach special label if patient had a contagious disease. Close door to room.
13. Await arrival of ambulance or transfer to morgue. (Some agencies use a shroud to enclose the body before transfer to the morgue [Fig. 34.4].)
14. Document procedure and disposition of patient's body and of belongings and valuables.

*Some situations require that all tubing remain in the body (e.g., when an autopsy is scheduled). Know agency policy.

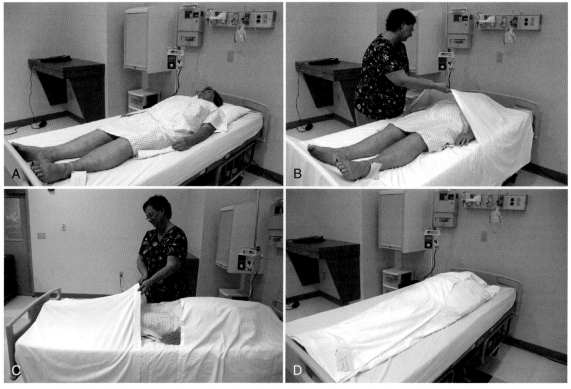

FIGURE 34.4 Care of the body after death. (From Cooper K, Gosnell K: *Foundations of nursing,* ed 7, St. Louis, 2015, Mosby.)

of extreme fatigue, and the nurse may find that patients are aware of activities that occur around them. Sometimes the patient may become restless and pick or pull at the bed linens. Remember that this is among the signs and symptoms of decreased oxygenation. Discoloration of arms and legs is a result of impaired circulation.

Changes in vital signs are observed, including (1) slow, weak, and thready pulse; (2) lowered blood pressure; and (3) rapid, shallow, irregular, or abnormally slow respirations. Mouth breathing occurs, which leads to dry oral mucous membranes. The patient often has a detached look in the eyes. Diminished sensory and motor function is seen in the lower extremities, which progresses to the upper extremities. Touch sensation diminishes while pressure and pain sensations may remain intact. As death becomes imminent, the pupils become dilated and fixed, Cheyne-Stokes respirations occur, the pulse becomes increasingly weaker and more rapid, and the blood pressure continues to fall. Peripheral circulation diminishes. The skin is cool and clammy; profuse diaphoresis may occur. If mucus collects in the patient's throat, noisy respirations are heard. This sound is referred to as the *death rattle*. A period of peace may immediately precede the moment of death. The clinical signs of death are given in the following list:

1. Unreceptivity and unresponsiveness
2. No movement or breathing
3. No reflexes
4. Flat line encephalogram (brain activity)
5. Absence of apical pulse
6. Cessation of respirations

Postmortem Care

In most states, the healthcare provider is responsible for certifying a death in the medical record. The healthcare provider notes time of death and records a description of therapies or actions taken in the medical record. The healthcare provider may request permission from the family for the autopsy (examination performed after a person's death to confirm or determine the cause of death). Autopsies are required in circumstances of unusual death (e.g., violent trauma or unexpected death in the home).

Because of the therapeutic nurse–patient relationship, the nurse and the PCT may be the best persons to provide postmortem care (care for the patient's body after death). Keep in mind the need to care for the patient's body with dignity and sensitivity. Provide postmortem care as soon as possible after death to prevent tissue damage or disfigurement. If the family has requested organ donation, take immediate measures as appropriate. Know the state laws and the policies and procedures of the employing institution.

Prepare the body and the room to keep the stress of the experience to a minimum, after the patient has been pronounced dead by a healthcare provider or professional nurse and before the family views the body. Remove supplies and equipment from sight. Remove, clamp, or cut tubes that remain in the body to within 1 inch (2.5 cm) of the skin, and tape them in place. Care of tubes and specimens depends on agency policy and whether an autopsy will be performed. Never, however, remove tubes, dressings, drains, and other equipment that is in place on or in the patient when an autopsy is to be performed. Clear away soiled linen and other clutter. Use spray deodorizer to help eliminate unpleasant odors.

Prepare the body by making it look as natural and comfortable as possible. Place the body in the supine position with arms at the sides, palms down or across the abdomen (but not one hand over the other); this helps the mortician (person trained in the care of the dead) better prepare it for interment. Discoloration of the face can result if blood is allowed to pool; to prevent this, place a small pillow or folded towel under the head. The eyelids usually remain closed if gently held down for a few seconds. If not, a moistened cotton ball can hold them in place. Insert the patient's dentures to maintain normal facial features. A rolled-up towel under the chin keeps the mouth closed (see Procedure 34.1). The cultural considerations box on care of the body after death presents culturally related attitudes toward preparation of the body (Box 34.4).

At the time of death, make a notation of any valuables, such as watch, rings, or money, and secure these articles so that they may be delivered to the family according to agency policy. Documentation of all valuables and their disposition in the patient's medical record is required (Box 34.5).

Offer the family the opportunity to view the body. An often helpful suggestion is that this is an opportunity to say good-bye to their loved one, especially if they were not present at the time of death. If the family hesitates to view the body, let them think about it. If they decide not to view the body, accept their decision without judgment. If the family decides to view the body, assure them that they will not be alone if they prefer the nurse be present. Offer to accompany them, or ask to call on someone else to be present if they would like. Spend as much time as possible assisting the grieving family, and offer to contact other support services, such as social services and the spiritual adviser. (Many healthcare facilities employ a full-time chaplain who may be summoned in the event of death.) The family now becomes the patient.

Documentation

Document the care given to the dying patient objectively, completely, legibly, and accurately. As death approaches, make frequent documentation, and include the signs of impending death as they occur. Recording who was present at the time of the patient's death is important. Continue documentation until the last entry, which states where and to whom the body was transferred (see Box 34.5).

Bereavement Period

Hospice care does not end once the patient dies but usually continues for up to 1 year with bereavement support (Center to Advance Palliative Care, 2011). The family, especially the primary caregiver, continues to need support after the patient dies. Even though the family feels they have prepared for the death, facing the

---

Box 34.4   Cultural Considerations: Care of the Body After Death

1. *African Americans:* Most families prefer to have members of the healthcare team clean and prepare the loved one's body. Some may have misgivings about organ donation but may agree to an autopsy. Cremation is usually not done.
2. *Chinese Americans:* Some families may prefer to bathe the deceased themselves. Often they feel the body should remain intact; organ donation and autopsy are uncommon.
3. *Filipino Americans:* Some families may prefer to wash the body themselves and are likely to want time for all family members to say good-bye. The family may not permit organ donation or autopsy.
4. *Hispanics or Latino Americans:* Family members may want to help with care of the body and are likely to want to say good-bye. Organ donation and autopsy are uncommon.
5. *Jews:* The dying person may want to make a deathbed confession or desire prayers. Observant Jews usually oppose autopsies but may consider organ donation. The body must not be left unattended until burial; a family member may remain present while the body is prepared by nursing staff, during transport

to and while in the morgue, and then to the funeral home.
6. *Roman Catholics:* The dying person may desire to receive the sacraments of Reconciliation and Anointing of the Sick within 30 days before death. The Roman Catholic faith does not oppose autopsies or organ donation.
7. *Muslims:* When close to death, a devout Muslim may wish to recite the Islamic Creed with help from others. After death, the person's eyes and mouth should be closed and the limbs should be straightened.
8. *Hindus:* The dying person should be in a peaceful room if not at home. The patient or someone else should recite the Gita. Family members may prefer to wash the body and may feel that organ donation is an individual choice.
9. *Buddhists:* An ordained monk or nun should care for the dying person. After death, the body should be covered with a cotton sheet. The body should not be touched or manipulated. The eyes and the mouth should not be closed. No noise, talking, or crying is allowed. Buddhists consider organ donation to be an individual choice.

(Data from Mazanec P, Tyler MK: Cultural considerations in end-of-life care, *American Journal of Nursing 103(3):50, 2003; Giger JN, Davidhizar RE:* Transcultural nursing: assessment and interventions, *ed 5, St. Louis, 2008, Mosby; and Gift of Hope Organization:* Religious viewpoints, *2003. Retrieved from www.giftofhope.org/about_donation/religious_viewpoints_list.htm#c.)*

Box 34.5   Documentation of End-of-Life Care

Documentation includes the following:
- Time of death and actions taken to prevent the death if applicable
- Who pronounced the death of the patient
- Any special preparation and type of donation, including time, staff, and company
- Who was called and who came to the hospital: donor organization, morgue, funeral home, chaplain, or individual family members making any decisions
- Personal articles left on the body and taped to skin or tubes left in
- Personal items given to the family and specific names and description of items
- Time of discharge and destination of the body
- Location of name tags on the body
- Special requests by the family
- Any other personal statements that might be needed to clarify the situation

future without the person who died is difficult. Many people believe that four full seasons must pass before bereaved persons are able to think of the deceased without feeling intense emotional pain, but this period is different for everyone. The death of a loved one is a

devastating agony that takes time to heal and subside. Depending on the size of the program, special bereavement teams with counselors may be available for the caregiver and family. Some teams facilitate a bereavement support group that meets regularly, providing these families the opportunities to communicate and share their feelings. Volunteers and pastors keep in touch by visits, phone calls, cards, and remembering the bereaved person on holidays and anniversaries.

The hospice staff also goes through a grieving period for each patient who dies. It is a good idea to attend funeral services, attend memorials, or visit the caregivers as appropriate after the death to help ease their grief. Each hospice provides support to its staff with support meetings and time to vent their feelings and to heal.

ETHICS ISSUES IN HOSPICE CARE

Ethics issues that sometimes arise when dealing with hospice patients include withholding or withdrawing nutritional support, the right to refuse treatment, and do-not-resuscitate (DNR) orders. Families find it difficult to discontinue food and water, even when death is clearly approaching. If the patient is unconscious, decision making regarding these issues sometimes falls on one family member, which has potential to create guilt feelings if other family members disagree. There are no simple answers to any of these concerns. It is helpful when the patient makes his or her wishes known in advance, as in a living will or an advance directive, or assigns a durable power of attorney.

An advance directive is a document prepared while an individual is alive and competent. It provides guidance to the family and the healthcare team in the event that the individual is no longer capable of making decisions. The directive states the individual's preferences concerning life-support measures and organ donations and sometimes gives authority to another person to make decisions for the individual, who at that point may be in a coma.

A hospice patient may have suffered many losses throughout the illness: health, job, independence, self-esteem, family, and financial security. Hospice attempts to assist the patient in maintaining dignity and control. Hospice places the emphasis on living and not dying. It is important for the hospice team to be sensitive to the patient's and the caregiver's needs and to maintain honesty at all times. The team must make sure to include the patient and the caregiver in all aspects of care and decision making. The nurse should provide opportunities for expressing concerns and fears because this will make the process less fearful and threatening. Allowing the patient and the caregiver to live fully, comfortably, and with dignity until death occurs naturally is the main goal of hospice care.

THE FUTURE OF HOSPICE CARE

Trends indicate that as more patients and families are educated about its many benefits, hospice is increasingly attractive as an alternative to facing death in a clinical setting. Nevertheless, a small amount of people who have the option of hospice care choose to participate in it. Healthcare providers, patients, and family members are often unwilling to begin hospice care for several reasons. The patient or family sometimes believe that availing themselves of the services of hospice denotes giving up hope, and some healthcare providers are hesitant to prescribe hospice care if they perceive the patient's worsening condition a personal failure on their part (Lewis et al., 2007). It is necessary for healthcare providers and nurses caring for patients with terminal illnesses in clinical facilities to open the dialog with families about the option of hospice and its possible benefits to patients and their caregivers.

CHAPTER SUMMARY

Hospice is a philosophy of care about providing support to patients with a terminal illness and to their families. "Hospice" is derived from the Latin word *hospitium,* meaning "hospitality" and "lodging." Hospice care is appropriate when active treatment is no longer effective and supportive measures are necessary to assist a terminally ill patient through the dying process.

The Hospice Medicare Benefit covers all expenses for palliative care related to the terminal illness, including professional staff visits, medication, equipment, respite care, and acute care.

Hospice care emphasizes quality, not quantity, of life. Palliative care is appropriate when a cure is not possible but care is still necessary. The goal of palliative care is to control pain and other symptoms for the prevention of distress. Palliative care is the treatment used to relieve or reduce discomfort of disease processes and may be used at any point during treatment, but is most often used when curative therapy has failed.

Entering a hospice program is the decision of a patient and family. An important criterion for the patient to be admitted into hospice is certification by the attending healthcare provider and a second healthcare provider that the patient has a prognosis of 6 months or less to live.

Hospice care consists of a blending of professionals and nonprofessionals to meet the total needs of the patient and family. Hospice care is delivered by an interdisciplinary team because no individual or individual profession is able to meet all the needs of terminally ill patients and families all the time. Hospice care accounts for all aspects of the lives of patients and their families. Stresses and concerns have the potential to arise in many ways when families are faced with a terminal illness.

In a hospice care program, the patient and family are considered together as the unit of care because families experience much stress and pain during the terminal illness of one of their members. Family participation in caregiving is an important part of palliative care. Hospice care is available 24 hours a day, 7 days a week, because needs may arise at any time.

Hospice care entails respect for all patient and family belief systems, wherein resources to meet the physical, psychosocial, and spiritual needs of the family unit are sought. Hospice care for the family continues into the bereavement period. Needs of the family continue after the patient dies.

Continuing to speak to and include patients in their care is essential because as death approaches, the dying patient becomes weaker. Patients may appear comatose yet be aware of activities around them.

Signs of impending death are (1) slow, thready, and weaker pulse; (2) lowered blood pressure; (3) rapid, shallow, irregular, or abnormally slow respirations; and (4) mottling of lower extremities. Postmortem care is the care administered to the body after death. Follow procedures, including cleansing, positioning, and labeling the body.

REVIEW QUESTIONS

1. The _____ is the mediator between the hospice team and the attending healthcare provider.
   a. family member
   b. patient care technician
   c. nurse
   d. medical director

2. _____ is considered the fifth vital sign and must be assessed at every hospice visit.
   a. Pain
   b. Temperature
   c. Heart rate
   d. Respiratory rate

3. The patient has never attended church and on hospice admission requested no spiritual support. Now he is within days of death and voiced some spiritual concerns to the PCT. What should the PCT do at this time?
   a. Share personal spiritual beliefs with him.
   b. Advise him that it is too late and no church would accept him.
   c. Contact the hospice nurse to voice the patient's concerns.
   d. Communicate this information to the social worker.

4. The patient died peacefully and with dignity, but his wife is still having problems dealing with the death. What services by the hospice team can be anticipated?
   a. Continue bereavement support for her for the next year.
   b. Dismiss the wife from all hospice services.
   c. Encourage her to begin to explore activities outside of the home.
   d. Have the hospice aide continue with her visits to the home.

5. The nurse is caring for a dying patient. What are clinical signs of death? (Select all that apply.)
   a. Slow thready pulse
   b. Absence of apical pulse
   c. Cessation of respirations
   d. Cessation of bowel sounds
   e. Flat encephalogram

Appendix: Medical Terminology

COMBINING FORMS: PREFIXES AND SUFFIXES

Medical terminology is similar to a foreign language. Like a foreign language, it can be analyzed and studied until it becomes a comfortable part of the vocabulary. The main purpose of medical terms is to communicate ideas in such a way that everyone understands exactly what is meant. Many medical terms are derived from Latin and Greek sources. They often consist of two or more simple words or word elements. A word root or **combining form** may be put together with a **prefix** and a **suffix.**

Root: The basis of a word
Example: *nephr*/o/tic (degenerative changes in the kidney)
Root: nephr- (kidney)
Linking vowel: A vowel that joins the combining form to the suffix or another combining form
Example: nephr/*o*/sis (disease of the kidneys)
Linking vowel: o
Prefix: The beginning of a word
Example: *hyper*/active (excessively active)
Prefix: hyper- (excessive)
Suffix: The ending of a word
Example: nephr/*itis* (inflammation of the kidney)
Suffix: -itis (inflammation)
Combining form: The union of a word root with a linking vowel
Example: *hepato*/megaly (enlargement of the liver)
Combining form: hepato- (liver)

COMMON PREFIXES

Prefix	Definition
a-	without
ab-	away from
ad-	toward
ambi-	both
an-	not
ana-	up
ante-	before, in front of

Prefix	Definition
anti-	against
auto-	self
bi-	two
brady-	slow
cata-	down
circum-	around
co-	with, together
con-	with, together
contra-	against
de-	from, lack of
dia-	through, across
diplo-	double, twofold
dis-	to free or undo
dys-	bad, painful, difficult, abnormal
ec-	out, out from
ecto-	outside
em-	in
endo-	in, within
enter-	intestine
epi-	above, upon
eu-	good, normal
ex-	out, away from
exo-	outside
extra-	outside
gastr-	stomach
hemi-	one half
hetero-	different
homo-	same
hyper-	excessive, above normal
hypo-	under, below normal
im-	not
in-	in, not
infra-	under, below
inter-	between
intra-	in, within
macro-	large
mal-	bad
medi-	middle
mesa-	middle
meta-	beyond, change
micro-	small
mono-	one
multi-	many, much
neo-	new
osteo-	bone
pan-	all
para-	near, beside, beyond
per-	through, by
peri-	around
poly-	many, much
post-	after, behind
pre-	before, in front of

Prefix	Definition
primi-	first
pro-	before, in front of
pseudo-	false
quadri-	four
re-	back
retro-	backward, behind
scler-	hardening
semi-	one half
sub-	under, below
super-	above, excessive
supra-	above, excessive
sym-	together
syn-	union, together, joined
tachy-	rapid
therm-	heat
trans-	through, across
tri-	three
ultra-	beyond, excess
uni-	one

COMMON SUFFIXES

Suffix	Definition
-ac	pertaining to
-al	pertaining to
-algia	painful condition, pain
-ar	pertaining to
-ary	pertaining to
-blast	embryonic
-cele	hernia, swelling, sac
-centesis	puncture of a cavity
-clasis	break, fracture
-clysis	irrigation, washing
-coccus	berry shaped
-crit	to separate
-cyte	cell
-desis	fusion, binding, fixation
-drome	to run
-dynia	pain
-ectasis	expansion, dilation
-ectomy	excision, removal of a body part
-emesis	vomiting
-emia	blood
-er	one who
-gen	forming, producing, origin
-genesis	forming, producing, origin
-genic	origin, formation
-grade	to go
-gram	the record made, mark
-graph	instrument for recording, machine
-graphy	the process, process of recording
-ia	condition
-iasis	morbid condition
-iatry	treatment, medicine
-ic	pertaining to
-icle	small, minute
-ism	condition
-ist	one who specializes in, specialist
-itis	inflammation
-lith	stone, calculus
-logist	specialist in the study of
-logy	process of study
-lysis	dissolution, setting free
-malacia	softening, soft
-megaly	enlargement

Suffix	Definition
-meter	instrument for measuring
-metry	act of measuring
-odynia	pain
-oid	form, shape
-ole	small, minute
-ology	study or science of
-oma	tumor
-opsy	viewing
-or	one who
-orrhea	flow, discharge
-osis	condition, disease
-ous	pertaining to
-para	to bear (offspring)
-paresis	partial paralysis
-pathy	disease, suffering
-penia	deficiency, lack of, decrease
-pexy	fixation
-phagia	eating, swallowing
-phasia	speech
-philia	attraction for
-phobia	fear
-physis	to grow
-plasia	formation, growth
-plasm	growth, formation
-plasty	mold, shape, repair
-plegia	paralysis
-poiesis	formation, production
-ptosis	downward displacement, falling
-ptysis	spitting
-rrhage	bursting forth
-rrhagia	bursting forth
-rrhaphy	suture
-rrhea	flow, discharge
-rrhexis	rupture
-scope	instrument to visually examine
-scopy	process of examining, visual examination
-sis	state of, condition
-spasm	involuntary spasm
-stalsis	constriction
-stasis	control, constant level, stop
-stenosis	narrowing, stricture
-stomy	creation of an opening
-therapy	treatment
-tic	pertaining to
-tome	instrument for cutting
-tomy	process of cutting, incision
-toxic	poison
-tresia	opening
-tripsy	surgical crushing
-trophy	nourishment
-ula	small, minute
-ule	small, minute
-y	process

ABBREVIATIONS AND ACRONYMS

Health care workers use a vast array of abbreviations and acronyms. It is wise to learn those that are used in the facility and on the units where you work. The first list presents the most common general abbreviations and acronyms encountered in the health care field. These are used in patient charts and during the course of conversation and shift report. The following lists organize the abbreviations related to time, to measurements, and to medications.

Abbreviation/ Acronym	Definition
a	before
aa	of each
AB	abortion
ABD	abdomen
ABGs	arterial blood gases
ACTH	adrenocorticotropic hormone
ADFC	aid to families with dependent children
ADH	antidiuretic hormone
ad lib	as desired, at liberty
ADLs	activities of daily living
AFP	alpha-fetoprotein
A/G ratio	albumin-globulin ratio
AHRQ	Agency for Healthcare Research and Quality
AIDS	acquired immunodeficiency syndrome
AKA	above-the-knee amputation
ALL	acute lymphocytic leukemia
ALS	amyotrophic lateral sclerosis
AMA	American Medical Association
AMB	ambulate, ambulatory
AML	acute myelocytic leukemia
ANA	American Nurses' Association; antinuclear antibody
ANCC	American Nurses Credentialing Center
AP	anteroposterior
APTT	activated partial thromboplastin time
ARC	American Red Cross
ARDS	acute (or adult) respiratory distress syndrome
ARF	acute renal failure
ASHD	arteriosclerotic heart disease
AST	aspartate aminotransferase
ATN	acute tubular necrosis
AV	atrioventricular
AVM	arteriovenous malformation
AVR	aortic valve replacement
BE	barium enema (x-ray film)
BKA	below-the-knee amputation
BM	bowel movement
BMR	basal metabolic rate
BP, B/P	blood pressure
BPH	benign prostatic hypertrophy
BRP	bathroom privileges
BS	bowel sounds
BUN	blood urea nitrogen
Bx	biopsy
C	Celsius
c̄	with
Ca	cancer; calcium
CABG	coronary artery bypass graft
CAD	coronary artery disease
CAPD	continuous ambulatory peritoneal dialysis
CAL	chronic airflow limitation
cal	calories
CAT	computed axial tomography
CBC	complete blood count
CC	chief complaint
CCPD	continuous-cycle peritoneal dialysis
CCRN	certified critical care registered nurse
CCU	coronary care unit
CDC	Centers for Disease Control and Prevention
CEA	carcinoembryonic antigen
CHF	congestive heart failure
Cl	chloride
CLL	chronic lymphocytic leukemia
CML	chronic myelocytic leukemia

Abbreviation/ Acronym	Definition
CMV	cytomegalovirus
CNA	certified nursing assistant
CNS	central nervous system
C/O	complains of
CO	cardiac output
COLD	chronic obstructive lung disease
COPD	chronic obstructive pulmonary disease
CP	cerebral palsy
CPK	creatine phosphokinase
CPR	cardiopulmonary resuscitation
CRF	chronic renal failure
crit	hematocrit
CRNA	certified registered nurse anesthetist
CS	central service; central supply
CSF	cerebrospinal fluid
CVP	central venous pressure
D & C	dilation and curettage
DEA#	Drug Enforcement Administration number
DIC	disseminated intravascular coagulation
Diff	differential white blood cell count
DOB	date of birth
DON	Director of Nurses
DJD	degenerative joint disease
DM	diabetes mellitus
DOA	dead on arrival
DOE	dyspnea on exertion
DPT	diphtheria, pertussis, tetanus toxoid (also DTP)
DRGs	diagnosis-related groups
DVT	deep vein thrombosis
Dx	diagnosis
EBV	Epstein-Barr virus
ECG, EKG	electrocardiogram
ECT	electroconvulsive therapy
ED	emergency department
EDC	expected date of confinement
EEG	electroencephalogram
EENT	eye, ear, nose, and throat
EMG	electromyogram
ENT	ear, nose, and throat
EOM	extraocular movement
ER	emergency room
ERCP	endoscopic retrograde cholangiopancreatography
ERT	estrogen replacement therapy
ESL	extracorporeal shock-wave lithotripsy
ESR	erythrocyte sedimentation rate
ESRD	end-stage renal disease
EST	electroshock therapy
F	Fahrenheit
FBS	fasting blood sugar
FDA	Food and Drug Administration
FH	family history
FHR	fetal heart rate
FHT	fetal heart tone
FS	frozen section
FSBS	finger stick blood sugar
FUO	fever of unknown origin
Fx	fracture
GB	gallbladder
GBS	Group Beta Streptococcus
GC	gonorrhea
GI	gastrointestinal
GTT	glucose tolerance test
GU	genitourinary
gyn	gynecology
hct	hematocrit

Abbreviation/ Acronym	Definition
HAI	health care–associated infection
HDL	high-density lipoprotein
Hgb, HG	hemoglobin
HIV	human immunodeficiency virus
HMO	health maintenance organization
HNP	herniated nucleus pulposus
H2O	water
HPV	human papillomavirus
HRC	human rights committee
HSV	herpes simplex virus
Ht	height
HTN	hypertension
HVA	hepatitis A virus
HVB	hepatitis B virus
hx	history
IABP	intra-aortic balloon pump
ICU	intensive care unit
ICP	intracranial pressure
ICS	intercostal space
I & D	incision and drainage
INR	international normalized ratio
I & O	intake and output
IOP	intraocular pressure
IUD	intrauterine device
IVP	intravenous pyelogram
JVD	jugular venous distention
K	potassium
KUB	kidney, ureters, bladder (x-ray)
lab	laboratory
LDL	low-density lipoprotein
LLL	left lower lobe
LLQ	left lower quadrant
LMP	last menstrual period
LOC	level of consciousness
LP	lumbar puncture
LPN	licensed practical nurse
LRQ	lower right quadrant
LUQ	left upper quadrant
LVN	licensed vocational nurse
lytes	electrolytes
MD	medical doctor
MI	myocardial infarction
MRI	magnetic resonance imaging
MS	multiple sclerosis
MVA	motor vehicle accident
MVP	mitral valve prolapse
MVR	mitral valve replacement
Na	sodium
NANDA-I	North American Nursing Diagnosis Association–International
NAPNES	National Association for Practical Nurse Education and Service
NCI	National Cancer Institute
NFLPN	National Federation of Licensed Practical Nurses
NIH	National Institutes of Health
NLN	National League for Nursing
noc	night
NPH	neutral protamine Hagedorn (insulin)
NPO	nothing by mouth (per os)
NSAID	nonsteroidal anti-inflammatory drug
O	oxygen
OA	osteoarthritis
OB	obstetrics
OB-GYN	obstetrics-gynecology
OBS	organic brain syndrome
OOB	out of bed
OR	operating room

Abbreviation/ Acronym	Definition
ORIF	open reduction–internal fixation
ORT	orthopedics
os	mouth
OSHA	Occupational Safety and Health Administration
OT	occupational therapy
OV	office visit
P	pulse
PA	posteroanterior
PAC	premature atrial contraction
PACU	postanesthesia care unit
Pap	Papanicolaou smear
PAR	postanesthesia recovery (unit)
path	pathology
PCA	patient-controlled analgesia
PE	physical examination
PEEP	positive end-expiratory pressure
per	through, by
PERRLA	pupils equal, round, reactive to light and accommodation
PFT	pulmonary function test
PH	past history
PID	pelvic inflammatory disease
PMH	past medical history
PMI	point of maximal impulse
PMS	premenstrual syndrome
PND	paroxysmal nocturnal dyspnea
PO	orally
postop	postoperative
PP	postprandial (after meals)
preop	preoperative
PRN	as needed
pro time	prothrombin time
PSA	prostate-specific antigen
pt	patient
PT	prothrombin time; physical therapy
PTCA	percutaneous transluminal coronary angioplasty
PTT	partial thromboplastin time
PVC	premature ventricular contraction
PVD	peripheral vascular disease
R	respirations
RBC	red blood cells, red blood (count)
RBS	random blood sugar
RDA	recommended dietary allowance
REM	rapid eye movement
RLL	right lower lobe
RLQ	right lower quadrant
R/O	rule out
ROM	range of motion
rom	rupture of membranes
ROS	review of systems, review of symptoms
RN	registered nurse
RR	recovery room
Rx	prescription
S̄	without
SA	sinoatrial
SAH	subarachnoid hemorrhage
SBE	subacute bacterial endocarditis
sed rate	sedimentation rate
SIADH	syndrome of inappropriate secretion of antidiuretic hormone
SLE	systemic lupus erythematosus
SNF	skilled nursing facility
SOB	short of breath
sol	solution
sono	sonogram, sonography
S/P	status post

Abbreviation/ Acronym	Definition
sp gr	specific gravity
SSE	soapsuds enema
SSRI	selective serotonin reuptake inhibitor
staph	staphylococcus
stat	immediately
STD	sexually transmitted disease
strep	streptococcus
subcut	subcutaneous
T	temperature
T & A	tonsillectomy and adenoidectomy
TAH	transabdominal hysterectomy
TB	tuberculosis
TENS	transcutaneous electrical nerve stimulation
THA	total hip arthroplasty
THR	total hip replacement
TIA	transient ischemic attack
TJC	The Joint Commission (formerly JCAHO)
TKA	total knee arthroplasty
TKR	total knee replacement
TPN	total parenteral nutrition
TPR	temperature, pulse, respiration
TURP	transurethral resection of the prostate
TWE	tap water enema
Tx	treatment, traction
UA	urinalysis
UAP	unlicensed assistive personnel
UGI	upper gastrointestinal
ULQ	upper left quadrant
ung	ointment
URI	upper respiratory infection
US	ultrasound
UTI	urinary tract infection
VA	Veterans Affairs
VD	venereal disease
VDRL	Venereal Disease Research Laboratories test
VLDL	very-low-density lipoprotein
VNA	Visiting Nurse Association
VS	vital signs
WBC	white blood cell (count)
WNL	within normal limits
Wt	weight

ABBREVIATIONS RELATED TO TIME

Abbreviation	Definition
ac, AC	before meals
A.M.	before noon
bid	twice a day
h, H	hour

Abbreviation	Definition
MN	midnight
pc, PC	after meals
P.M.	after noon, evening
q 1 hr (or q1h, etc.)	every hour
q 2 hr	every 2 hours
q 3 hr	every 3 hours
q 4 hr	every 4 hours
q 6 hr	every 6 hours
q 8 hr	every 8 hours
qid	four times a day
tid	three times a day

ABBREVIATIONS RELATED TO MEDICATIONS

Abbreviation	Definition
ac, AC	before meals
amp	ampule
cap	capsule
comp	compound
dil	dilute
elix	elixir
ext	extract
H	hypodermic, hypodermic injection
ID	intradermal
IM	intramuscular
IV	intravenous
pc, PC	after meals
PP	postprandial
tab	tablet

ABBREVIATIONS RELATED TO MEASUREMENTS

Abbreviation	Definition
cm	centimeter
g, gm	gram
gr	grain
kg	kilogram
L	liter
mcg	microgram
mEq	milliequivalent
mg	milligram
mL	milliliter
oz	ounce
Tbsp	tablespoon
tsp	teaspoon

REVIEW QUESTION ANSWERS

CHAPTER 1: TODAY'S HEALTH CARE

1. A
2. B
3. B
4. A
5. A
6. C
7. D
8. A
9. A
10. A

CHAPTER 2: THE ROLE OF THE PATIENT CARE TECHNICIAN

1. B
2. A
3. C
4. B
5. B

CHAPTER 3: PROFESSIONALISM AND WORK ETHICS

1. B
2. B
3. A
4. A
5. A

CHAPTER 4: COMMUNICATING WITH THE HEALTH CARE TEAM

1. B
2. A
3. B
4. B
5. C

CHAPTER 5: UNDERSTANDING THE PATIENT AS A PERSON

1. B
2. C
3. B
4. D
5. B

CHAPTER 6: PATIENT RIGHTS, ETHICS AND LAWS

1. C
2. A
3. A
4. B
5. D
6. B
7. D
8. D

CHAPTER 7: BODY STRUCTURE AND FUNCTION/ GROWTH AND DEVELOPMENT

1. C
2. A
3. D
4. D
5. A
6. C
7. B
8. C
9. B
10. B
11. D
12. B
13. C
14. B
15. C
16. C

CHAPTER 8: PAIN MANAGEMENT, COMFORT, REST, AND SLEEP

1. B
2. A
3. C
4. D
5. C

CHAPTER 9: ASEPSIS AND INFECTION CONTROL

1. A
2. C
3. D
4. A
5. C
6. A

CHAPTER 10: WORKPLACE SAFETY AND BODY MECHANICS

1. D
2. D
3. A
4. A
5. C
6. B

CHAPTER 11: PATIENT SAFETY

1. A, D
2. D
3. C
4. D
5. B

CHAPTER 12: MOVING, POSITIONING, AND PREVENTING FALLS

1. A
2. A
3. D
4. A
5. C
6. D

CHAPTER 13: BASIC EMERGENCY CARE

1. A
2. C
3. B
4. A
5. B

CHAPTER 14: ASSISTING WITH THE PHYSICAL EXAMINATION

1. A
2. D
3. B
4. B
5. D

CHAPTER 15: MEASURING AND RECORDING VITAL SIGNS

1. 37.2; 100.4; 38.9; 103.1
2. B
3. B
4. B
5. B
6. A

CHAPTER 16: OBTAINING AND MONITORING AN ELECTROCARDIOGRAM

1. A
2. A
3. A
4. B
5. D

CHAPTER 17: ASSISTING WITH ADMISSIONS AND DISCHARGE

1. D
2. D
3. D
4. C
5. A

CHAPTER 18: BED MAKING AND HYGIENE

1. D
2. D
3. B
4. D
5. A
6. C

CHAPTER 19: ASSISTING WITH GROOMING

1. C
2. A
3. A
4. B
5. A

CHAPTER 20: ASSISTING WITH NUTRITION AND FLUIDS

1. A
2. A
3. D
4. A
5. B

CHAPTER 21: ASSISTING WITH URINARY ELIMINATION

1. B
2. D
3. C
4. C
5. B

CHAPTER 22: ASSISTING WITH BOWEL ELIMINATION

1. C
2. D
3. C
4. B
5. B

CHAPTER 23: ASSISTING WITH OXYGEN NEEDS

1. A, B, D
2. A
3. C
4. D
5. A

CHAPTER 24: BLOOD COLLECTING AND PROCESSING

1. C
2. A
3. C
4. A
5. A
6. C
7. C
8. B
9. C
10. C

CHAPTER 25: SPECIMEN COLLECTING AND TESTING

1. A
2. B
3. C
4. D
5. C

CHAPTER 26: CARE OF THE SURGICAL PATIENT

1. D
2. D
3. B
4. C
5. B

CHAPTER 27: HEAT AND COLD APPLICATIONS

1. B
2. D
3. A
4. C
5. B

CHAPTER 28: CARE OF WOUNDS AND PRESSURE ULCERS

1. D
2. C
3. C
4. D
5. C

CHAPTER 29: REHABILITATIVE AND RESTORATIVE CARE

1. C
2. A
3. A
4. D
5. C

CHAPTER 30: CARE OF WOMEN AND CHILDREN

1. D
2. C
3. A
4. C
5. A
6. B
7. C
8. D

CHAPTER 31: CARING FOR THE OLDER ADULT

1. B
2. C
3. D
4. A
5. C

CHAPTER 32: CARING FOR PATIENTS WITH MENTAL HEALTH NEEDS

1. A
2. B
3. D
4. A
5. C

CHAPTER 33: CARING FOR THE PATIENT WITH CHRONIC CONDITIONS

1. A
2. C
3. A
4. D
5. C

CHAPTER 34: END-OF-LIFE CARE

1. D
2. A
3. A
4. A
5. B, C, E

GLOSSARY

abduction The movement of a limb or other part away from the midline of the body, or from another part

accountability Being responsible for one's own actions

acrocyanosis When the hands and feet of a newborn may appear slightly blue because of poor peripheral circulation

active transport Chemical activity that allows the cell to admit larger molecules than would otherwise be possible

acuity The measurement of the intensity of nursing care required by a patient

acute pain Pain that is intense and of short duration, usually lasting less than 6 months

adduction Movement toward the midline of the body; also applies to movements inward and across the body

admission Entry of a patient into the healthcare facility

adoptive family A family unit with adopted children

Affordable Care Act The landmark health reform legislation passed by the 111th Congress and generally referred to as Obamacare

ageism A form of discrimination and prejudice against the older adult

aggressive communication Occurs when an individual interacts with another in an overpowering and forceful manner to meet one's own personal needs at the expense of the other

alba Vaginal drainage that is slightly yellow to white

Alcoholics Anonymous (AA) An international nonprofit organization that began in 1935 as a way for abstinent alcoholic people to help other alcoholic people become and stay sober through group support, shared experiences, and faith in a power greater than themselves

alcoholism The addiction to alcohol

alignment The process of adjusting body parts so that they are in proper relative position

alopecia An area of the scalp where there is hair loss or no hair; also known as baldness

anatomy The study, classification, and description of structures and organs of the body

angina Chest pain

anorexia Lack of appetite

anticoagulant therapy Medications that increase the tendency to bleed

antiseptic A substance that tends to inhibit the growth and reproduction of microorganisms and may be used on humans

anxiety A vague feeling of apprehension that results from a perceived threat to the self, although the source is often unknown

apical heart rate Measure of heart function that is completed by placing a stethoscope at the apex, or bottom left, of the heart

apnea Absence or cessation of breathing

arrhythmia An abnormality or irregularity in the heart rhythm

arteriosclerosis Thickening, decreased elasticity, and calcification of arterial walls

asepsis The condition of being free from infection

assertive communication Interaction that takes into account the feelings and needs of the patient, yet honors the technician's rights as an individual

assertiveness One's ability to confidently and comfortably express thoughts and feelings while still respecting the legitimate rights of the patient

ataxia Failure or irregularity of muscle actions and coordination

atria The two upper chambers of the heart

atrioventricular (AV) node The part of the cardiac conduction system between the atria and the ventricles

auditors People appointed to examine patient charts and health records to assess quality of care

auscultation The act of listening to body sounds, typically with a stethoscope, to assess various organs throughout the body

autopsy Examination performed after a person's death to confirm or determine the cause of death

axilla The underarm area or armpit

bandage A strip or roll of cloth or other material that can be wound around a part of the body in a variety of ways for multiple purposes

basal metabolic rate (BMR) The body's use of energy to maintain bodily functions

base of support A stance with feet shoulder-width apart

bedpan A shallow container used for urination or defection while in the bed

behavior The manner in which a person performs any or all of the activities of daily life

beneficence The duty to protect life

benefits A payment or gift made by the healthcare institution, such as healthcare insurance and paid time off

bereavement A period of mourning or an expression of grief in reaction to the death of someone close

bilirubinuria The presence of bilirubin in the urine

binder A bandage that is made of large pieces of material to fit a specific body part

bioterrorism The use of biologic agents to create fear and threat; healthcare facilities must be prepared to treat mass casualties from such an attack

blended (reconstituted) family When adults remarry and bring together children from previous marriages

blood pressure The pressure of blood in the circulatory system

bounding Term used to describe a pulse that feels full because of increased power of cardiac contraction or as a result of increased blood volume

bradycardia A slow heartbeat; a pulse below 60 beats per minute

bradypnea Respirations that are regular in rhythm but slower than normal in rate

bronchiectasis Dilation of the bronchi and bronchioles associated with secondary infection or ciliary dysfunction

bronchospasm A sudden narrowing of the airways reduces the amount of air that can pass

bruit An abnormal sound or murmur heard on auscultation of an organ, vessel (such as a carotid artery), or gland

bundle of His Specialized muscle fibers that conduct electrical impulses from the AV node to the ventricular myocardium

canthus Corner of the eye

career ladder A stepwise progression from entry level to a more advanced role, and may include more pay, more authority, and more responsibility

cathartics Drugs that stimulate bowel evacuation (see laxatives)

cell The smallest living unit of structure and function in our body

Centers for Disease Control and Prevention (CDC) A federal agency that provides facilities and services for the investigation, identification, prevention, and control of disease

cephalocaudal Growth and development that proceeds from the head toward the feet

certification Confirmation that one has the knowledge and/or skill pertaining to a particular area or subject usually through the successful completion of a certification examination

certified nursing assistant Someone who helps patients with healthcare needs under the direction of a nurse

cerumen A waxy secretion in the ear canal; commonly called *ear wax*

characteristics Distinguishing traits, qualities, or properties

chart (healthcare record) A legal record that is used to meet the many demands of the health, accreditation, medical insurance, and legal systems

charting The process of adding information to the chart

chromosomes Spindle-shaped rods in a cell that carry genetic information in the form of genes

chronic bronchitis Recurrent inflammation of the membranes lining the bronchial tubes

chronic illness An irreversible lifelong disease state or impairment for which disease management programs may offer supportive care, function, and prevention of further disability

chronic obstructive pulmonary disease (COPD) A progressive, irreversible lung condition that results in diminished lung capacity

chronic pain Pain lasting longer than 6 months

circumorbital Circular area around the eye

clitoris A small, elongated erectile body above the urinary meatus at the superior point of the labia minora

closed posture A more formal, distant stance, generally with the arms, and possibly the legs, tightly crossed

clubbing Abnormal enlargement of the distal phalanges (fingers and toes) associated with cyanotic heart disease or advanced chronic pulmonary disease

codes A system of notification to be transmitted rapidly

cohabitation Living together without being married

coitus Sexual union between male and female; also called *intercourse*

collagen The protein that forms the inelastic fibers of tendons, ligaments, and fascia

colonoscopy Procedure in which a fiberoptic scope is used to examine the large intestine

colony-forming units (CFUs) A term used when reporting bacteriuria; one CFU represents one bacterium present in the urine sample

colostomy Surgical creation of a stoma on the abdominal wall to where the colon is surgically attached

colostrum A thin, yellow, milky fluid secreted by the mammary glands a few days before and after delivery

commensurate Corresponding in size, amount, extent, or degree; equal in measure; proportionate

Commission on Accreditation of Rehabilitation Facilities A nonprofit, private, international standard-setting and accreditation body whose mission is to promote and advocate the delivery of quality rehabilitation

communication A reciprocal process in which messages are sent and received between people

competent Having adequate or requisite capabilities

computer on wheels Point-of-care computer devices sometimes housed on wheeled carts

conception (fertilization) The union of a sperm with an ovum (egg)

connotation An implication; something suggested by a word or thing

connotative meaning When one sometimes receives a message differently from how the sender meant it to be received

contamination The entry of infectious materials into a previously clean or sterile environment

continuing education units (CEUs) Credits earned for attending sessions that have some educational information relating to a particular topic

continuity of care Continuing of established patient care from one setting to another

contracture When muscles, ligaments, and tendons are not shortened and lengthened with movement, a permanent shortening of these structures may occur

costal Pertaining to the ribs

credibility The quality or power of inspiring belief

cross-training Where one individual is trained to do a variety of skills in a variety of areas

cultural competence The awareness of one's own cultural beliefs and practices and their relation to those of others, which may be different

culturally competent care Providing care to patients that is individual and specific to their cultural beliefs and practices

culture A set of learned values, beliefs, customs, and practices that are shared by a group and are passed from one generation to another

culture and sensitivity (C&S) A procedure performed in the microbiology laboratory in which a specimen is cultured on artificial media to detect bacterial or fungal growth, followed by appropriate screening for antibiotic sensitivity

curative treatment Aggressive care in which the goal and intent is curing the disease and prolonging life at all cost

cyanosis A blue coloration of the mucous membranes and body extremities caused by lack of oxygen

cytoplasm A sticky, gel-like substance that contains 70% water, as well as nutrients, minerals, enzymes, and other specialized materials

dandruff An excessive amount of flaking skin that appears white in color

decubitus ulcers Sores or ulcers that develop over a bony prominence as the result of ischemia from prolonged pressure; also called *bed sores*

defecation The act of eliminating feces

dehiscence Rupture of the wound at the incisional line

dehydration When the body loses more water than it takes in

demeanor Behavior toward others; outward manner

denotative meaning The commonly accepted definition of a particular word

dentures A set of artificial teeth not permanently implanted

deposition When witnesses are required to undergo questioning by the attorneys

depression A mood disturbance characterized by exaggerated feelings of sadness, despair, lowered self-esteem, loss of interest in former activities, and hopeless, negative thoughts

detoxification Medical treatment of an alcoholic or drug addict involving keeping alcohol or drugs from entering the body until the bloodstream is free of toxins

detrimental Obviously harmful or damaging

development A lifelong process that begins at conception, the beginning of pregnancy, and ends with death

diastole The relaxation of the chambers of the heart during which blood enters the heart from the vascular system and the lungs

diffusion A process in which solid particles in a fluid move from an area of higher concentration to an area of lower concentration, resulting in an even distribution of the particles in the fluid

dilation The opening of the cervix through the process of labor, measured as 0 to 10 cm dilated

diplopia Double vision

disability Any restriction in or lack of ability to perform an activity in the manner or within the range considered normal as the result of impairment

disaster manual Sometimes called the emergency response plan or emergency management plan

disaster situation An uncontrollable, unexpected, psychologically shocking event that is unique and likely to have a significant impact on a variety of healthcare facilities

discharge The exiting of a patient from a healthcare facility; when a patient leaves the hospital to go home or to another facility

discharge planning The systematic process of planning for patient care after discharge from a hospital or healthcare facility

discretion The quality of being discreet; having or showing good judgment or conduct, especially in speech

disinfection The use of a chemical that can be applied to objects to destroy microorganisms

disorientation Mental confusion characterized by inadequate or incorrect perception of place, time, and identity

displacement The unconscious transfer of an intense emotion from its original object to another one

disseminated To disburse; to spread around

diurnal rhythm Pattern of activity or behavior that follows a day-night cycle

doctrine of informed consent Full disclosure of the facts the patient needs to make an intelligent (informed) decision before any invasive treatment or procedure is performed

documenting Recording the interventions carried out to meet the patient's needs

dorsal Toward the back (see posterior)

dorsal (supine) Lying flat on the back

dorsal recumbent Supine position with patient lying on back, head, and shoulder with extremities moderately flexed; legs are sometimes extended

dorsiflexion To bend or flex backward

drainage The removal of fluids from a body cavity, wound, or other source of discharge by one or more methods

drug of choice The drug an abuser uses most frequently to satisfy the craving for a certain feeling; the user's preferred drug

drug tolerance The need to use more and more of a substance to get the same feeling as the body learns to tolerate the drug

dysphagia Difficulty swallowing

dyspnea Difficult or painful breathing

ectopic Originating outside the normal tissue

effacement The thinning of the cervix during labor, measured in percentages from 0% to 100% effaced

elastin An essential part of elastic connective tissue; when moist, it is flexible and elastic

electrocardiogram A graphic record of electrical conduction through the heart

electronic health record (EHR) The electronic version of a patient's chart; also known as the electronic medical record (EMR)

empathy Ability to recognize and to some extent share the emotions and state of mind of another and to understand the meaning and significance of that person's behavior

emphysema Pathologic accumulation of air in the alveoli, which results in alveolar destruction and overall oxygen deprivation; in the lungs, the bronchioles become plugged with mucus and lose elasticity

endemic Term describing a disease or microorganism that is specific to a particular geographic area

endogenous Growing within the body

enema Instillation of a solution into the colon via the anus

epithelialization The formation of new cells during wound healing

ergonomics The science of matching workplace conditions and job demands to the capabilities of workers, especially in regard to musculoskeletal disorders and their prevention

eschar A piece of dead tissue that is cast off from the surface of the skin, particularly after a burn injury, but also seen in an ulcer

essential hypertension Elevated blood pressure of unknown cause that develops for no apparent reason; sometimes called *primary hypertension*

ethics Refers to values that influence a person's behavior and the individual's feelings and beliefs about what is right or wrong

ethics dilemmas Situations that do not have a clear right or wrong answer

ethnicity A group of people who share a common social and cultural heritage based on shared traditions, national origin, and physical and biologic characteristics

ethnocentrism A belief that the beliefs and practices of one's particular culture are best

euthanasia The practice of intentionally ending a life in order to relieve pain and suffering

exogenous Growing outside the body

extended family Consists of the nuclear or traditional family and additional family such as grandparents, grandchildren, aunts, and uncles who live in the same household

extension Movement of certain joints that decreases angle between two adjoining bones

exudate Fluid, cells, or other substances that have been slowly exuded, or discharged, from cells or blood through small pores or breaks in cell membranes

family-centered care A philosophy that recognizes the important role of the family in the lives of children with disabilities or other chronic conditions

fear of retribution Having a fear of being punished

febrile Condition characterized by an elevated body temperature

fecal impaction A collection of feces in the rectum in the form of a mass that becomes so large or hard that the patient is unable to pass it voluntarily

fibrillation Rapid, random, ineffective contractions of the heart

filtrate The fluid that remains after a liquid is passed through a membranous filter

filtration The movement of water and particles through a membrane by force from either pressure or gravity

flatulence The presence of air or gas (flatus) in the intestinal tract

flexion The action of bending or the condition of being bent, especially the bending of a limb or join

folk health belief system A system that believes that health and illness are controlled by supernatural forces; they may be secular or sacred, or a combination of both

fomite A nonliving object that can harbor microorganisms, such as computers or chairs

foster family A family formed when the biologic parents are unable or unwilling to provide adequate, safe care for their children

Fowler's Posture assumed by patient when head of bed is raised 45 to 60 degrees

functional limitation Any loss of ability to perform tasks or activities of daily living

fundus The curved, top portion of the uterus; the fundal height can be used as a measurement of fetal growth and estimated gestation

gait Manner or style of walking

genupectoral Also known as knee-chest; patient kneels so that weight of body is supported by knees and chest, with abdomen raised, head turned to one side, and arms flexed

gerontologic rehabilitation nursing A specialty practice that focuses on the unique requirements of older adult rehabilitation patients

gestures Movements people use to emphasize the idea they are attempting to communicate

glomerular filtration rate (GFR) Is a test used to check how well the kidneys are working; specifically, it estimates how much blood passes through the glomeruli in each minute

gluconeogenesis The formation of glucose in the liver from proteins and fats

glycogen The sugar (starch) formed from glucose; it is stored mainly in the liver

glycosuria The abnormal presence of glucose in the urine

gold standard The paragon of excellence; the diagnostic test against which all others are compared

grandfamilies Families with children under the age of 18 years who live with or in the custody of grandparents

granulation A sign of healing; soft, pink, fleshy projections that consist of capillaries surrounded by fibrous collagen

grooming Taking care of one's personal needs

growth An increase in size and may involve the entire being or parts within

hallucination Is a sensory experience without a stimulus trigger (involves the senses; may be auditory, visual, olfactory [smell], and tactile [touch])

handicap A physical, mental, or emotional impairment or disability that interferes with a person's normal functioning

health To be without illness or to be free from disease

health disparity A greater difference that has been discovered between one group compared with another group, meaning that one group is suffering more than another group

Health Insurance Portability and Accountability Act (HIPAA) Enacted in 1996 as a way to protect everyone's privacy

health literacy The degree to which people can understand basic health information in order to make their own decisions about treatment options

health promotion Strategies that aim at keeping a person healthy from the beginning

healthcare facility Any agency that provides healthcare

healthcare system A network of agencies, facilities, and providers involved with healthcare in a specified geographic area

hemoconcentration A condition in which the concentration of blood cells is increased in proportion to the plasma

hemolysis The destruction or dissolution of red blood cells, with subsequent release of hemoglobin

holistic Pertaining to the total patient care in which the physical, emotional, social, economic, and spiritual needs of the patient are considered

holistic healthcare A system of comprehensive or total patient care that considers the physical, emotional, social, economic, and spiritual needs of a person

homeostasis The process of keeping body fluids in balance

homosexual family A family comprised of a same-sex couple

hospitalist A physician, nurse practitioner, or physician's assistant who provides care to patients who are hospitalized

host An organism in which another organism is nourished and harbored

human chorionic gonadotropin (HCG) A hormone secreted by the placenta that is found in the urine of pregnant females

hydration Maintenance of a balance of fluid

hygiene The activities to maintain personal cleanliness

hyperextension Extreme or abnormal extension

hyperpnea An increase in the depth of breathing

hypertension High blood pressure

hyperventilation Abnormally prolonged and deep breathing, usually associated with acute anxiety or emotional tension

hypotension Blood pressure that is below normal (systolic pressure below 90 mm Hg and diastolic pressure below 50 mm Hg)

hypoxia Reduced oxygen content in tissue and cells

ice collar A bag or pack that is filled with ice that can be wrapped around a part of the body

idiopathic Pertaining to a condition or a disease that has no known cause

ileostomy Opening in the ileum, the distal part of the small intestine

illness A disease or sickness that affects the body and/or mind

illusions False interpretation of extreme sensory stimuli, usually visual or auditory, such as a mirage in the desert or the sound of voices in the wind

immobility The inability to move around freely

impairment Any loss or abnormality of psychologic, physical, or anatomic structure or function

incision A cut produced surgically by a sharp instrument that creates an opening into an organ or space in the body

infarction An area of tissue that has died from lack of blood supply

infection Invasion of body tissues by microorganisms, which then proliferate and damage tissues

infiltration Leaking of intravenous fluid into the tissue surrounding the vein

informatics The study of information processing

initiative Energy or aptitude to cause or facilitate the start of something or to cause something to happen

injury prevention Strategies that focus on prevention of injuries

insubordination Disobedience to authority

interdisciplinary rehabilitation team A team that collaborates to identify individuals' goals and features a combination of expanded problem-solving beyond the boundaries of the individual disciplines, together with discipline-specific work toward goal attainment

interdisciplinary team A multiprofessional health team whose members work together in caring for a terminally ill patient

intermittent pulse A pulse in which beats occasionally are skipped

intravenous (IV) Taking place in, or being administered into, a vein

ischemia Decreased blood flow to a body part or organ, caused by constriction or blockage of the supplying artery

jargon Commonplace "language" or terminology unique to people in a particular work setting, such as a hospital, or to a specific type of work, such as nursing

Kaposi's sarcoma Kaposi's sarcoma is a cancer of the blood vessels or lymph system and is known for producing reddish or purple plaques on the skin; the most common form of Kaposi sarcoma is associated with infection by the human immunodeficiency virus (HIV), the virus that causes AIDS

Kardex (or Rand) A system used by some facilities to consolidate patient orders and care needs in a centralized concise way

labia majora Larger fold or lip of tissue connecting to the vagina

labia minora Smaller fold or lip of tissue connecting to the vagina

lacrimation The secretion or discharge of tears

lactation Function of secreting milk or period during which milk is secreted

lanugo Downy, fine hair characteristic of the fetus between 20 weeks of gestation and birth

laws Prescribe proper behavior in society; they sanction acceptable behavior and prohibit unacceptable behavior

laxatives A drug that stimulates the evacuation of the bowels (see cathartics)

liability Legal responsibility

liable See liability

life expectancy The number of years an individual will probably live, based on the average for others with similar characteristics

lithotomy Patient lies supine with hips and knees flexed and thighs abducted and rotated externally

lochia Bloody vaginal discharge after a delivery that consists of blood, tissue, and mucus

macerated The softening and breaking down of skin resulting from prolonged exposure to moisture

malpractice Professional negligence, or not taking care of someone in the manner he or she should be cared for based upon established standards and medical practices

manipulation Movement or exercising of a body part by means of an externally applied force

meconium The newborn's initial stools that are odorless, black-green, and sticky

medical asepsis The principles of using clean technique

medication administration record (MAR) The report that serves as the legal record of the drugs administered to a patient at a facility by a healthcare professional

mental health A person's ability to cope with and adjust to the recurrent stresses of everyday living

metabolite The product of the metabolism of a substance, such as a drug

microorganisms Tiny, usually microscopic, entities capable of carrying on living processes

mitosis A type of cell division

mobility A person's ability to move around freely in his or her environment

mononuclear white blood cells Leukocytes with an unsegmented nucleus; monocytes and lymphocytes in particular

mons pubis The fat pad that covers the symphysis pubis

morale The mental and emotional condition, enthusiasm, loyalty, or confidence of an individual or group with regard to the function or tasks at hand

mortician Person trained in the care of the dead

multidisciplinary rehabilitation team A rehabilitation team that develops discipline-specific goals, clear boundaries between disciplines, and outcomes that are the sum of each discipline's efforts

multiparous Pertaining to women who have had two or more pregnancies

murmur Abnormal sound heard during auscultation of the heart that may or may not have a pathologic origin; it is associated with valve disease or a congenital heart defect

myocardial Pertaining to the heart muscle

myocardium The muscular lining of the heart

narrative charting Recording of patient care in descriptive form

nasal cannula A simple, two-pronged plastic device that is used to deliver low concentrations of oxygen

nodules Small lumps, lesions, or swellings that are felt when the skin is palpated

nomenclature Classification system of technical or scientific names and terminology

nonmaleficence To do no harm

non–rapid eye movement Phase of sleep necessary for body tissue restoration and healthy cardiac function

nonverbal communication Transmitted without the use of words (either oral or written)

noxious Injurious to physical health

nuclear family A family unit that consists of parents and their biologic offspring, or children

nucleus The largest organelle within the cell responsible for cell reproduction and control of the other organelles

nurse A licensed person trained to care for the sick

nursing care plan Plan that outlines the proposed nursing care based on the nursing assessment and nursing diagnoses to provide continuity of care

Occupational Safety and Health Administration (OSHA) A federal organization that provides guidelines to help reduce safety hazards in the workplace

ombudsman Someone who is appointed to represent a person to ensure that the rights of the patient are being maintained

Omnibus Budget Reconciliation Act (OBRA) Standards for long-term care facilities and nursing homes or assisted living facilities to ensure that residents would be able to achieve and maintain their highest level of well-being possible

one-way communication Communication in which the sender is in control and expects and gets very little response from the receiver

open posture When one takes a relaxed stance with uncrossed arms and legs while facing the other individual

optimistic Inclined to put the most favorable construction on actions and events or to anticipate the best possible outcome

oral hygiene Care of the oral cavity

orthopnea Condition in which an individual must sit or stand to breathe comfortably

orthopneic A posture assumed by the patient sitting up in bed at 90-degree angle, or sometimes resting in forward tilt while supported by pillow on overbed table

orthostatic (postural) hypotension A temporary fall in blood pressure when a person rapidly changes from a recumbent position to a standing position

osmosis The passage of water across a selectively permeable membrane, with the water molecules going from the less concentrated solution to the more concentrated solution

ostomy An artificial opening

otitis externa Inflammation or infection of the external auditory canal (swimmer's ear)

palliative care The active, complete care of a patient whose disease has not responded to curative therapy

palpation The use of touch during the physical examination to assess the size, consistency, and location of certain body parts

palpitations A pounding or racing of the heart; may or may not indicate a serious heart disorder

paresthesia An abnormal sensation of burning, prickling, or stinging

parturition The act or process of giving birth to a child

PASS The mnemonic (Pull the pin, Aim low, Squeeze handle, Sweep the unit) that will help the patient care technician remember how to operate the fire extinguisher

passive transport The movement of small molecules across the membrane of a cell by diffusion

pathogenic Disease-producing

patient A person receiving medical treatment

patient care technician A health technician working under the supervision of a registered nurse, physician, or other health professional to provide basic patient care

patient-controlled analgesia A portable, computerized pump with a chamber for a syringe that allows patients to self-administer medication when they feel that they need it

pediculosis capitis Head lice

perineal care Care of the genitalia

peripheral Term that refers to an area outside of or away from an organ or structure

perks Those things that are more attractive or interesting, such as having weekends off

persona An individual's social facade or front that reflects the role in life the individual is playing; the personality a person projects in public

personal health record An extension of the electronic health record (EHR) that allows patients to input their own information into an electronic database

personal hygiene The self-care measures people use to maintain health and prevent disease

phagocytosis The process that permits a cell to engulf (or surround) any foreign material and to digest it

phenylalanine An essential amino acid found in milk, eggs, and other foods

phlebitis Inflammation, or swelling, of the walls of a vein

phlebotomy The practice of drawing blood

physiatrist Physicians specializing in physical medicine or rehabilitation

physical disuse syndrome Inactivity that can lead to deterioration of many body functions

physician A person who provides and practices medicine

physiology The processes and functions of the various structures and how they interrelate

pinocytosis The process by which extracellular fluid is taken into the cell

plasma The liquid portion of whole blood that contains active clotting agents

podiatrist A doctor who specializes in the care of the feet

point of care Taking place at the patient rather than away from the patient; typically at the bedside

point-of-care testing Tests that can be completed quickly with results able to be obtained quickly so that treatment can begin as soon as possible; typically performed at the bedside

poison Any substance that is harmful to your body when ingested (eaten), inhaled, injected, or absorbed through the skin

polymorphonuclear white blood cells Leukocytes with a segmented nucleus; also known as *polymorphonuclear neutrophils* (PMNs) or *segmented neutrophils*

polyphagia Increased appetite

postmortem care Care for the patient's body after death

posttraumatic stress disorder (PTSD) A psychologic reaction to the experience of trauma outside the normal range of human experience

posture The way that an individual sits, stands, and moves

presbycusis A decreased ability to hear high frequencies and to discriminate sounds

presbyopia A difficulty in being able to focus on detailed objects close at hand

primary care physician A physician who treats patients, typically in an outpatient setting, for a broad range of diseases, across all age ranges

primary caregiver A member of the immediate family, such as the spouse or adult child, who assists in the decision making for someone who is nearing the end of life

primary intention Wound healing that occurs when wound edges are close together and little tissue is lost, such as those made surgically

professionalism The conduct or qualities characterized by or conforming to the technical or ethics standards of a profession; exhibiting a courteous, conscientious, and generally businesslike manner in the workplace

prolactin A hormone secreted by the anterior pituitary gland that is responsible for stimulating milk production in the mammary alveolar cells

pronation Rotation of the hand or forearm so that the surface of the palm is facing downward or toward the back

prone Lying face down in horizontal position

proximodistal Growth and development that originates in the center of the body and moves toward the outside

psychosocial A combination of psychologic and social factors

pulse deficit Condition in which the radial pulse is less than the apical pulse; may indicate a peripheral vascular abnormality

pulse pressure The difference between systolic and diastolic blood pressures (30 to 50 mm Hg is considered normal)

puncture A stab wound for a drainage system

purulent Producing or containing pus

pyrexia Febrile condition or fever

quality assurance, assessment, and improvement An audit in healthcare that evaluates services provided and the results achieved compared with accepted standards

quarks The building blocks of protons and neutrons that comprise the atom

race A group of people who share biologic physical characteristics

RACE Rescue patients, sound the Alarm, Confine the fire, and Extinguish or Evacuate

rales Abnormal or crackling breath sounds during inspiration

range of motion (ROM) Normal movement that any given joint is capable of making

rapid eye movement Phase of sleep that is believed to be functionally important, more vivid, and elaborate, allowing a person to clarify emotions and prepare the mind for events of the next day

Rapid Response Team A team of medical personnel who respond to a patient whose condition may be rapidly getting worse

rapport Development of a relationship with a person who feels that you understand the feelings of that person

receiver The person or people to whom the message is conveyed

recording Recording the interventions carried out to meet the patient's needs

referred pain Pain that is felt at a site other than the injured or diseased organ or part of the body

renal thresholds Levels above which substances cannot be reabsorbed by the renal tubules and therefore are excreted in the urine

reproach An expression of rebuke or disapproval; a cause or occasion of blame, discredit, or disgrace

reservoir Any natural habitat of a microorganism that promotes growth and reproduction

residual urine Amount of urine left in the bladder after they void

respiratory Relating to respiration, or the act of breathing

respite care A period of relief from responsibilities of caring for a patient

rhonchi Abnormal rumbling sounds on expiration that indicate airway obstruction by thick secretions or spasms

safety reminder device (SRD) Formerly referred to as restraints

sanguineous Composed of or pertaining to blood

SBAR/traditional (block) chart Situation, background, assessment, and recommendation is a method of communication among healthcare workers and is considered to be a part of documentation

sclera The white part of the eye that forms the orbit

secondary hypertension Elevated blood pressure resulting from another condition, typically kidney disease

secondary intention Wound healing that occurs when a wound must granulate during healing, occurs when skin edges are not close together (approximated) or when pus has formed

sediment Insoluble material that settles to the bottom of a urine specimen

semi-Fowler's Posture assumed by patient when head of bed is raised approximately 30 degrees

sender One who conveys the message in communication

sentinel event Any unexpected occurrence involving death or serious physical or psychologic injury, or the risk thereof

separation anxiety Fears and apprehension caused by separation from familiar surroundings and significant people

serosa Vaginal discharge that is pink to brown in color

serosanguineous Thin and red, composed of serum and blood

serous Thin and watery, composed of the serum portion of blood

serum The liquid portion of whole blood that remains after the blood has clotted

Sims' Position in which patient lies on side with knee and thigh drawn upward toward chest

simulation The acting out of a scenario or situation on a manikin in an effort to gain confidence and improve skill before participating with a real person

sinoatrial (SA) node The pacemaker of the heart; it is located in the right atrium

sinus arrhythmia Irregular heartbeat that originates in the sinoatrial node (pacemaker)

skin turgor The degree of elasticity of skin

social Contract family (see cohabitation)

society A nation, community, or broad group of people who establish particular aims, beliefs, or standards of living and conduct

spinal cord injury (SCI) Any injury in which the spinal cord undergoes compression by fracture or displacement of vertebrae, by bleeding, or by edema

spirometer Instrument that measures the volume of air inhaled and exhaled

spore The reproductive cell of some microorganisms, such as fungi or protozoa

standard precautions A set of guidelines designed to reduce the risk of transmission of microorganisms from both recognized and unrecognized sources of infections

standards of care Acts whose performance is required, permitted, or prohibited

stat The medical abbreviation for immediately; at this moment

stereotype A generalized expectation about forms of behavior, an individual, or a group

sterilization Complete destruction of all forms of microbial life

stertorous Term that describes a strenuous respiratory effort marked by a snoring sound

street drugs Substances that users buy from illegal drug dealers

stress The nonspecific response of the body to any demand made on it

stressor A situation, activity, or event that produces stress

subculture Shares many characteristics with the primary culture but has characteristic patterns of behavior and ideals that distinguish it from the rest of a cultural group

supination The kind of rotation that allows the hand to turn up

supine Lying face-up

surgical asepsis The complete destruction of organisms on instruments or equipment that will enter the patient's body

syncope Fainting; a brief lapse in consciousness

synergistic A relationship in which the actions of two or more substances or organs achieve an effect that cannot be achieved by an individual substance or organ

system An organization of varying numbers and kinds of organs arranged to perform complex functions of the body

systole The contraction of the heart; blood is pumped from the heart to the lungs and the rest of the body

tachycardia A rapid but regular heart rate; one that exceeds 100 beats per minute

tachypnea Condition marked by rapid, shallow respirations

teratogen A substance, agent, or process that interferes with normal prenatal development, causing the formation of one or more developmental abnormalities in the fetus

terminal illness A disease in an advanced stage with no known cure and poor prognosis

terrorism A violent or dangerous act used to intimidate or coerce a person or government to further a political or social agenda

tertiary intention A type of wound healing where the practitioner leaves a contaminated wound open and closes it later, after the infection is controlled, by suturing two layers of granulation tissue together in the wound

therapeutic diet A diet used as a medical treatment

third-party payers Entities (people or elements) other than the giver or receiver of service responsible for payment; e.g., Medicare or insurance company

thixotropic gel A material that appears to be a solid until subjected to a disturbance, such as centrifugation, whereupon it becomes a liquid

thready Term that describes a pulse that is scarcely perceptible

tinea capitis Also known as ringworm, a fungal infection of the skin

tinnitus A ringing or buzzing in the ears

tissue An organization of many similar cells that act together to perform a common function

tracheostomy A surgical opening made through the neck into the trachea to allow breathing

transcutaneous electric nerve stimulation A pocket-sized, battery-operated device that provides a continuous, mild electric current to the skin via electrodes that are attached to a stimulator by flexible wires

transdisciplinary rehabilitation team A rehabilitation team that participates in cross-training of their staff to minimize any duplication of effort toward individual goal attainment

transfer Moving a patient from one unit to another (interagency transfer) or moving a patient from one healthcare facility to another (interagency transfer)

transillumination Inspection of a cavity or organ by passing light through its walls

trauma Physical injury or a wound caused by an external force or violence

traumatic brain injury (TBI) A type of injury to the brain that can result in temporary or permanent damage

Trendelenburg's Patient's head is low and the body and legs are on inclined plane

T-tube A drainage tube into the duct to maintain a free flow of bile

tubercle A nodule produced by the tuberculosis bacillus

two-way communication Communication that requires that both the sender and the receiver participate in the interaction

umbilical cord The lifeline connecting the mother to the baby; it is whitish blue-gray with three vessels (one vein and two arteries) and contains a gelatinous tissue called Wharton jelly

umbilicus The depressed point in the middle of the abdomen

urinal A device for collecting urine from male patients; urinals for female patients are also available

urination The act of emptying the bladder

vasoconstriction Narrowing of the blood vessels

vasodilation Dilation of the blood vessels

vector A person or animal that does not become ill but harbors and spreads an organism, causing disease in others

vehicle The means by which microorganisms are carried about and transported to the next host, once they have left the reservoir

ventral To face forward; the front of the body

ventricles The two lower chambers of the heart

verbal communication Involves the use of spoken or written words or symbols

verdict A decision made in a lawsuit or medical malpractice case

vernix A yellowish white, cream cheese–like substance that covers a newborn

versatile The person can perform multiple tasks in one setting, or in multiple settings

vertigo Dizziness

virulent Exceedingly pathogenic, noxious, or deadly

visual analog scale A pain scale used when the patient marks a spot on a horizontal line to indicate pain intensity (intensity increases as the line moves from left to right)

vulva The external female genitalia, which begins at the mons pubis and terminates at the anus

wasting syndrome Physical deterioration resulting in profound weight loss, fatigue, anorexia, and mental confusion

wellness The state of being in good physical and mental health

wheezing A high-pitched sound heard on expiration; indicates obstruction or narrowing of respiratory passages

work ethics A set of values based on the moral virtues of hard work and diligence

wound Any injury to the body's tissues that involves a break in the skin

zygote The developing ovum from the time it is fertilized until, as a blastocyst, it is implanted in the uterus

REFERENCES

Chapter 1
American Association of Colleges of Nursing: Nursing shortage, 2012.
American Hospital Association: *The patient care partnership: understanding expecatations, rights and responsibilities* (website). http://www.aha.org/content/00-10/pcp_english_030730.pdf. Accessed August 3, 2016.
Centers for Medicare & Medicaid Services: *Centers for Medicare & Medicaid Services* (website). https://www.cms.gov/. Accessed August 3, 2016.

Chapter 2
Egan DJ, Nakao JH, VanLeer PM, et al: Increased rates of rapid point-of-care HIV testing using patient care technicians to perform tests in the ED, *Am J Emerg Med* 32:651–654, 2014.
Small A, Okungu LA, Joseph T: Continuing education for patient care technicians: a unit-based RN-led initiative, *Am J Nurs* 112:51–55, 2012.
Vachharajani TJ: Hemodialysis vascular access care in the United States: closing gaps in education of patient care technicians, *Semin Dial* 24:92–96, 2011.

Chapter 4
Adams JM, Osborne-McKenzie T: Advancing the evidence base for a standardized provider handover structure: using staff nurse descriptions of information needed to deliver competent care, *J Contin Educ Nurs* 43(6):261–266, 2012. doi: 10.3928/00220124-20120215-88.
American Hospital Association: *Communicating with patients*, n.d. Retrieved from: www.aha.org/advocacy-issues/communicatingpts/index.shtml.
Balzer Riley J: *Communication in nursing*, ed 7, St. Louis, 2012, Mosby.
Kaiser Permanente: *Shifting perspectives: Kaiser Permanente's nurse knowledge exchange ensures smooth, consistent and postitive patient hand-offs* (website). https://share.kaiserpermanente.org/article/shifting-perspectives/. Accessed August 3, 2016.
Maier-Lorentz MM: Transcultural nursing: its importance in nursing practice, *J Cult Divers* 15(1):37–43, 2008.
Menon AS, Greenwald S, Ma TJ, et al: Patient and physician willingness to use personal health records in the emergency department, *West J Emerg Med* 13(2):172–175, 2012.
National Alliance for Health Information Technology: *Defining key health information technology terms*, 2008. Retrieved from: http://cdm16064.contentdm.oclc.org/cdm/singleitem/collection/p266901coll4/id/2086/rec/10.
The Office of the National Coordinator for Health Information Technology (ONC) Office of the Secretary, United States Department of Health and Human Services: *Report to congress* (website). https://www.healthit.gov/sites/default/files/rtc_adoption_and_exchange9302014.pdf. Accessed August 3, 2016.

Chapter 6
Benak LD, Applegate S: Informed consent and issues surrounding lack of capacity, *J Forensic Nurs* 2(1):48, 2006. http://www.ncbi.nlm.nih.gov/pubmed/17073401.
Motacki K, Burke K: *Nursing delegation and management of patient care*, ed 1, St. Louis, 2011, Mosby.
Reising DL, Allen PN: Protecting yourself from malpractice claims, *American Nurse Today* 2(2):39–44, 2007. https://americannursetoday.com/protecting-yourself-from-malpractice-claims/.

Chapter 7
American Academy of Child & Adolescent Psychiatry (AACAP): *The adopted child*, 2011. Retrieved from: www.aacap.org/page.ww?name=The+Adopted+Child&section=Facts+for+Families.
American Academy of Pediatrics (AAP): *AAP reaffirms breastfeeding guidelines*, 2012. Retrieved from: www.aap.org/en-us/about-the-aap/aap-press-room/pages/AAP-Reaffirms-Breastfeeding-Guidelines.aspx.
American Dental Association: *Healthy habits*, 2013. Retrieved from: www.mouthhealthy.org/en/babies-and-kids/healthy-habits.aspx.
Centers for Disease Control and Prevention (CDC): *Basics about childhood obesity*, 2012. Retrieved from: www.cdc.gov/obesity/childhood/basics.html.
Centers for Disease Control and Prevention (CDC): *Genomics and health*, 2011. Retrieved from: www.cdc.gov/genomics/public/faq.htm#couple.
Central Intelligence Agency: *CIA world factbook*, 2012. Retrieved from: https://www.cia.gov/library/publications/the-world-factbook/rankorder/2102rank.html?countryName=Tuvalu&countryCode=tv&regionCode=aus&rank=168.
Hoyert DL, Xu JQ: Deaths: preliminary data for 2011, *Natl Vital Stat Rep* 61(6), 2012. Retrieved from: www.cdc.gov/nchs/data/nvsr/nvsr61/nvsr61_06.pdf.

Moskowitz C: What is the smallest thing in the universe? *LiveScience* 2012. Retrieved from: www.livescience.com/23232-smallest-ingredients-universe-physics.html.
Nix S: *Williams' basic nutrition and diet therapy*, St. Louis, 2013, Mosby.
Patton KT, Thibodeau GA: *Anatomy & physiology and anatomy & physiology online package*, ed 8, St. Louis, 2013, Mosby.
Torbati YJ: Census: fewer than 10 percent of all city households are nuclear families, *The Baltimore Sun* 2010. Retrieved from: http://articles.baltimoresun.com/2010-12-18/news/bs-md-census-households-20101217_1_nuclear-families-census-data-young-professionals.
U.S. Census Bureau: *Expectation of life at birth, and projections*, 2012. Retrieved from: www.census.gov/compendia/statab/cats/births_deaths_marriages_divorces/life_expectancy.html.
U.S. Department of Health and Human Services (US DHHS): *About healthy people*, 2012. Retrieved from: www.healthypeople.gov/2020/about/default.aspx.

Chapter 8
Acello B: Meeting JCAHO standards for pain control, *Nursing* 30(3):52, 2000.
American Pain Society (APS): *Principles of analgesic use in the treatment of acute and chronic pain: a concise guide to medical practice*, ed 2, Glenview, Ill, 1995, Author.
Lowery F: Chronic, noncancer pain boosts suicide risk, *Medscape* 2013. Retrieved from: http://www.medscape.com/viewarticle/804832.
Mayer DM, Torma L, Byock I, et al: Speaking the language of pain, *Am J Nurs* 101(2):44, 2001.
McCaffery M, Pasero C: *Pain: clinical management*, ed 3, St. Louis, 2003, Mosby.
McCance KL, Huether SE: *Pathophysiology: the biological basis for disease in adults and children*, ed 6, St. Louis, 2009, Mosby.
Potter PA, Perry AG: *Fundamentals of nursing*, ed 7, St. Louis, 2009, Mosby.
The Joint Commission (TJC): *Facts about pain management*, 2013. Retrieved from: www.jointcommission.org/assets/1/18/Pain_Management1.PDF.

Chapter 9
Centers for Disease Control and Prevention (CDC): *Updated U.S. Public Health Service guidelines for the management of occupational exposure to HIV and recommendations for postexposure prophylaxis*, Washington, D.C., 2005, Author.
Jensen PA, Lambert LA, Iademarco MF, et al: Guidelines for preventing the transmission of Mycobacterium tuberculosis in health-care settings, *MMWR Morb Mortal Wkly Rep* 54:RR–17, 2005.
U.S. Department of Labor, Occupational Safety and Health Administration (OSHA): *Respiratory precautions*, 2009. Retrieved from: www.osha.gov/pls/oshaweb/owadisp.show_document?p_table=STANDARDS&p_id=12716.

Chapter 10
Ahrens M: *Fires in health care facilities*. National Fire Protection Association Fire Analysis and Research Division, 2012. Retrieved from: www.nfpa.org/assets/files//MbrSecurePDF/OS.HealthCareFacilities.pdf.
Centers for Disease Control and Prevention: *Recommended vaccines for healthcare workers* (website). http://www.cdc.gov/vaccines/adults/rec-vac/hcw.html. Accessed.

Chapter 11
Environmental Protection Agency (EPA): Managing radioactive materials and waste, 2012. Retrieved from: www.epa.gov/radiation/manage.html.

Chapter 12
Howard NL: Patient handling: fact vs. fiction, *American Nurse Today* 5(7):2010. Retrieved from: www.americannursetoday.com/article.aspx?id=6908.

Chapter 15
Cicek HS, et al: Effect of nail polish and henna on oxygen saturation determined by pulse oximetry in healthy young adult females, *Emerg Med J* 28(9):783, 2010.
Nesseler N, et al: Pulse oximetry and high-dose vasopressors; a comparison between forehead reflectance and finger transmission sensors, *Intensive Care Med* 38(1718):2012.
WHO: World Health Organization Pulse Oximetry Training Manual. (2011) Obtained from: http://www.who.int/patientsafety/safesurgery/pulse_oximetry/who_ps_pulse_oxymetry_training_manual_en.pdf.
Yont, et al: Comparison of oxygen saturation values and measurement times by pulse oximetry in various parts of the body, *Appl Nurs Res* 24(4):2011.

Chapter 17
Maslow A: *Motivation and personality*, ed 2, New York, 1970, Harper & Row.
The Joint Commission (2008) https://www.acep.org/clinical---practice
-management/the-joint-commission-(tjc)/.

Chapter 18
AHRQ (2016). http://www.ahrq.gov/professionals/systems/hospital/
pressureulcertoolkit/putool1.html.

Chapter 24
CLSI: *Procedures for the collection of diagnostic blood specimens by venipuncture:
approved standard*, 6th ed, CLSI document GP41-A6. Wayne, PA, 2007,
Clinical and Laboratory Standards Institute.
CLSI: *Tubes and additives for venous and capillary blood specimen collection;
approved standard*, 6th ed, CLSI document GP39-A6. Wayne, PA, 2010,
Clinical and Laboratory Standards Institute.

Chapter 28
Agency for Healthcare Research and Quality(AHRQ): *Preventing pressure ulcers
in hospitals: A toolkit for improving quality of care*, 2011. Retrieved from:
www.ahrq.gov/professionals/systems/long-term-care/resources/
pressure-ulcers/pressureulcertoolkit/putool1.html.
Jones V, Grey JE, Harding KE: Wound dressings, *BMJ* 332(7544):777–780, 2006.
Medscape: *A closer look at pressure ulcers: "Reasonably preventable,"* 2008.
Retrieved from: www.medscape.org/viewarticle/574206_2.

Chapter 29
American Association of Physiatrists: About the AAP, 2013. Retrieved from:
www.physiatry.org.
American Physical Therapy Association (APTA): Early rehab in ICU generates
net financial savings in hospitals, PT in Motion, 2014. Retrieved from:
www.apta.org/PTinmotion/newsnow/2014/1/15/earlyrehabstudy.
American Psychiatric Association (APA): *Diagnostic and statistical manual of
mental disorders*, ed 3, Washington, D.C., 1980, American Psychiatric Press.
Association of Rehabilitation Nurses: Definitions and scope of practice, 2014.
Retrieved at: www.rehabnurse.org/certification/content/Definition-and-
Scope.html.
Clark CC: Posttraumatic stress disorder: how to support healing, *Am J Nurs*
97(8):27–33, 1997.
Cultural Competency Advisory Group: *Establishing a culturally competent
master's and doctorally prepared nursing workforce*, Washington, D.C., 2009,
American Association of Colleges of Nursing.
Glass AJ: Introduction. In Bourne PG, editor: *The psychology and physiology of
stress*, New York, 1969, Academic Press.
Handicap [definition], n.d. Retrieved from: www.yourdictionary.com/
handicap#medical.
Lipshutz AKM, Engel H, Thornton K, et al: Early mobilization in the intensive
care unit, 2012. Retrieved from: www.icu.sagepub.com.
Mayo Clinic: Post-traumatic stress disorder, 2011. Retrieved from: www.
mayoclinic.org/diseases-conditions/post-traumatic-stress-disorder/
basics/definition/CON-20022540.
National Center for PTSD: Treatment of PTSD, 2013. Retrieved from:
www.ptsd.va.gov.
National Heart, Lung, and Blood Institute: What is cardiac rehabilitation?
2013. Retrieved from: www.nhlbi.nih.gov.
National Heart, Lung, and Blood Institute: What is pulmonary rehabilitation?
2010. Retrieved from: www.nhlbi.nih.gov/health/health-topics/topics/
pulreh.
National Institute of Mental Health: What is post-traumatic stress disorder? n.d.
Retrieved from: www.nimh.nih.gov/health/topics/post-traumatic-stress-
disorder-ptsd/index.shtml.
Nelson AL: Polytrauma: a new frontier in rehabilitation nursing, *Rehabil Nurs*
33(5):191–192, 2008.
Pennardt A: Blast injuries. Medscape, 2011. Retrieved from: http://emedicine.
medscape.com.
PubMed Health: Fact sheet: Disease management programs—
Structured treatment programs for people with chronic diseases
[summary of scientific report published by Institute for Quality and
Efficiency in Health Care (IQWiG), Cologne, Germany], 2007; updated
December 2012. Retrieved from: www.ncbi.nlm.nih.gov/pubmedhealth/
PMH0005155.
Rehabilitation Institute of Chicago: The role of nurses in rehabilitation
care, 2013. Retrieved from: www.ric.org/about/people/
nurses.
Rosdahl CB, Kowalski MT: *Texbook of basic nursing*, Philadelphia, 2012, Wolters
Kluwer Health/Lippincollt, Williams, and Wilkins.
Rosenfeld JV, Ford NL: Bomb blast, mild traumatic brain injury and
psychiatric morbidity: A review, 2013. Retrieved from: www.
noninvasiveicp.

Smeltzer SC, Bare BG, Hinkle JL, et al: *Textbook of medical-surgical nursing*, ed
12, Philadelphia, 2010, Wolters Kluwer Health/Lippincott, Williams, &
Wilkins.
United States Department of Health and Human Services: 2020 Topics and
objectives, 2013. Retrieved from: http://healthypeople.gov/2020/topics
objectives2020/default.aspx.
Zheng X, Chen G, Song X, et al: Twenty-year trends in the prevalence of
disability in China.

Chapter 30
American Academy of Pediatrics: Circumcision Policy Statement,
PEDIATRICS Volume 130, Number 3, September 2012.
Goodman J: Jewish Circumcision: an alternative perspective, *BJU Int* 83:22–27,
1999.

Chapter 32
Centers for Disease Control and Prevention (CDC): CDC report: Mental illness
surveillance among U.S. adults, 2011. Retrieved from: www.cdc.gov/
mentalhealthsurveillance.
Centers for Disease Control and Prevention (CDC): 10 Leading causes of
death by age group, United States—2014. Retrieved from: http://www.
cdc.gov/injury/images/lc-charts/leading_causes_of_death_age_group
_2014_1050w760h.gif.
Centers for Disease Control and Prevention (CDC): An estimated 1 in 20 U.S.
adults report depression, 2014. Retrieved from: http://www.cdc.gov/
mentalhealth/basics/mental-illness/depression.htm.
National Coalition for the Homeless: *Homeless families with children: NCH fact
sheet*, Washington, DC, 2010, The Coalition. Retrieved from: http://www
.nationalhomeless.org/publications/facts. Accessed August 19, 2010.
National Institute on Alcohol Abuse and Alcoholism, 2014 https://www
.niaaa.nih.gov/alcohol-health/overview-alcohol-consumption/alcohol
-facts-and-statistics.
National Institute of Mental Health: Use of mental health services and
treatment among adults, n.d. Retrieved from: www.nimh.nih.gov/
statistics/3use_mt_adult.shtml.

Chapter 33
Gaddam S, Gunukula SK, Mador MJ: Post-operative outcomes in adult
obstructive sleep apnea patients undergoing non-upper airway surgery: a
systematic review and meta-analysis, *Sleep Breath* 2013.

Chapter 34
Alberta Health Services and Covenant Health: Guidelines for using the
revised Edmonton Symptom Assessment System (ESAS-r), 2010. Retrieved
from: www.palliative.org/newpc/_pdfs/tools/ESAS-r%20guidelines.pdf.
Center to Advance Palliative Care: A guide to help palliative care programs
successfully complete The Joint Commission (TJC) certification process,
2011. Retrieved from: www.capc.org/palliative-care-professional
-development/Licensing/joint-commission/tjc-guide-2011.pdf.
Center to Advance Palliative Care: Policies and tools for hospital palliative
care programs: A crosswalk of National Quality Forum preferred practices,
2011. Retrieved from: www.capc.org/capc-resources/capc_publications/
nqf-crosswalk.pdf.
Centers for Medicare & Medicaid Services: Chapter 9—Coverage of
hospice services under hospital insurance. Medicare Benefit Policy
Manual (Publication No. 100-02), 2012. Retrieved from: www.cms
.gov/Regulations-and-Guidance/Guidance/Manuals/downloads/
bp102c09.pdf.
Ellison D: Report from the CAPC conference 2012, 2012. Retrieved from:
www.theonc.org/author.asp?section_id=2004&doc_id=255012.
Hospice and Palliative Nurses Association: Hospice/palliative care nurses,
n.d. Retrieved from: www.nursesource.org/hospice.html.
Hospice Association of America: Hospice fact sheet, n.d. Retrieved from:
www.nahc.org/haa/facts.
Hospice Foundation of America: Volunteering and hospice, n.d. Retrieved
from: www.hospicefoundation.org/pages/page.asp?page_id=171081.
Lewis SL, Heitkemper MM, Dirksen SR: *Medical-surgical nursing: assessment
and management of clinical problems*, ed 6, St. Louis, 2007, Mosby.
National Hospice and Palliative Care Organization: Hospice care in America,
2013. Retrieved from: www.nhpco.org/sites/default/files/public/
Statistics_Research/2013_Facts_Figures.pdf.
Smeltzer SC, Bare BG, Hinkle JL, et al: *Textbook of medical-surgical nursing*,
ed 12, Philadelphia, 2010, Wolters Kluwer Health/Lippincott, Williams, &
Wilkins.
World Health Organization (WHO): World Hospice and Palliative Care Day,
2011. Retrieved from: www.who.int/cancer/events/palliative_care_day/
en.
World Health Organization (WHO): Palliative care is an essential part of
cancer control, n.d. Retrieved from: www.who.int/cancer/palliative/en.

INDEX

Page numbers followed by "*f*" indicate figures, "*t*" indicate tables, and "*b*" indicate boxes.